MW01047990

Professional Nursing Practice

Concepts and Perspectives

THIRD EDITION

Barbara Kozier
Glenora Erb
Kathleen Blais

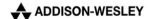

ADDISON-WESLEY

An Imprint of Addison Wesley Longman, Inc.

Menlo Park, California • Reading, Massachusetts • New York • Harlow, England
Don Mills, Ontario • Sydney • Mexico City • Madrid • Amsterdam

Senior editor: Erin Mulligan
Editorial assistant: Kim Crowder
Managing editor: Wendy Earl
Production editor: David W. Rich/Edit San Jose
Text and cover designer: Brad Greene/Greene Design
Composition supervisor: Vivian McDougal
Senior manufacturing supervisor: Merry Free Osborn

Copyright © 1997 by Addison Wesley Longman, Inc.

All rights reserved. No part of this publication may be reproduced, stored in a
retrieval system, or transmitted, in any form or by any means, electronic, mechanical,
photocopying, recording, or any other media or embodiments now known or
hereafter to become known, without the prior written permission of the publisher.
Manufactured in the United States of America. Published simultaneously in Canada.

Care has been taken to confirm the accuracy of the information presented in this
book. The authors, editors, and publisher, however, cannot accept any responsibility
for errors or omissions or for consequences from application of the information in
this book and make no warranty, express or implied, with respect to its contents.

The authors and publisher have exerted every effort to ensure that drug selection
and dosages set forth in this text are in accord with current recommendation and
practice at time of publication. However, in view of ongoing research, changes in
government regulations, and the constant flow of information relating to drug therapy and drug reactions, the reader is urged to check the package inserts of all drugs
for any change in indications of dosage and for added warnings and precautions.
This is particularly important when the recommended agent is a new and/or
infrequently employed drug.

Library of Congress Cataloging-in-Publication Data

Kozier, Barbara.
     Professional Nursing Practice : concepts and perspectives /
Barbara Kozier, Glenora Erb, Kathleen Blais. — 3rd ed.
       p.   cm.
     Includes bibliographical references and index.
     ISBN 0-8053-3523-4
     1. Nursing—Philosophy. I. Erb, Glenora Lea, 1937– .
II. Blais, Kathleen.
    RT84.5.K69 1997
    610.73—dc20   96-17922
                                          CIP

ISBN 0-8053-3523-4
1 2 3 4 5 6 7 8 9 10–RMV–00 99 98 97 96

♦♦ Addison Wesley Longman, Inc.
2725 Sand Hill Road
Menlo Park, California 94025

CONTRIBUTORS

Suzanne C. Beyea, RN, CS, PhD
Associate Professor
Saint Anselm College
Manchester, NH

Fay L. Bower, DNSc, FAAN
President
Clarkson College
Omaha, NE

Jean Niland Candela, RN, BSN (C), CC
Staff Nurse II (Specialty)
Memorial Regional Hospital
Hollywood, FL

Divina Grossman, RN, PhD, ARNP, CS
Associate Professor and Department Chairperson
Adult/Gerontological and Psychiatric Nursing
Florida International University
Miami, FL

Carol R. Kneisl, RN, MS, CS
President and Educational Director
Nursing Transitions, Inc.
Williamsville, NY

Sandra L. Lobar, PhD, ARNP
Associate Professor and Chairperson
School of Nursing
Florida International University
Miami, FL

Ruth A. Pease, RN, MSN, EdD
Professor of Nursing and Assistant Department Chair
Division of Nursing, School of Health
California State University - Dominguez Hills
Carson, CA

Suzanne Phillips, EdD, ARNP
Associate Professor
School of Nursing
Florida International University
Miami, FL

Elizabeth A. Riley, RN, MS, CS
Assistant Clinical Director, Adult Services
Four Winds - Saratoga
Saratoga Springs, NY

Diane Whitehead, RN, BSN, MSN, EdDc
Department Head Nursing
Broward Community College
Davie, FL

REVIEWERS

Martha S. Buhler, RN, EdD
Chair, Department of Baccalaureate Degree Nursing
School of Nursing
Georgia Southwestern College
Americus, GA

Patricia A. Burks, RN, BSN
Instructor
Department of Nursing
Western Oklahoma State College
Altus, OK

Kristen S. Cameron, RN, MS
Assistant Professor
Nursing Department
Paco Hernando Community College
Brooksville, FL

Margaret A. Droste, MSN, PhD
Assistant Professor
Department of Nursing
Webster University
St. Louis, MO

Margaret Kettman-Thomas, RN, MSN, MEd
Director of Nursing Education
Department of Nursing
Western Oklahoma State College
Altus, OK

Mary M. Lambert, RN, BSN, MSEd
Instructor
Department of Nursing
Western Oklahoma State College
Altus, OK

Sherry L. Merrow, EdD, RN, CS
Associate Dean of Health Sciences
Endicott College
Beverly, MA

Patricia C. Serenko, RN, MSN
Assistant Professor of Nursing
Department of Nursing
Mt. Aloysius College
Cresson, PA

Preface

To meet the demands of a dramatically changing health care system, nurses must change and grow. They need skills in communication and interpersonal relations to become effective members of a collaborative health care team. They need to think critically and be creative in implementing nursing strategies with clients of diverse cultural backgrounds in increasingly diverse settings. They need skills in teaching, leading, managing, politics, and using power. They need to be prepared to provide home- and community-based nursing care. They need to continue their unique role that demands a blend of nurturance, sensitivity, caring, empathy, commitment, and skill based on broad knowledge. In addition, they need to understand holistic healing modalities and complementary therapies. In this book we address concepts on which students can build their repertoire of prefessional nursing knowledge. These concepts include, but are not limited to, wellness, health promotion, and disease prevention; holistic care; multiculturalism; nursing theories and conceptual frameworks; nursing research; and professional empowerment and politics.

Professional Nursing Practice: Concepts and Perspectives, 3rd edition is intended as a text for registered nurses who are in transition or bridge programs to pursue a baccalaureate degree in nursing. It may also be used in generic nursing programs. This text has been revised extensively, and the change in title is intended to reflect the content changes. A new organization in the text emphasizes the nature of professional nursing, professional nursing roles, the processes guiding professional nursing practice, elements of professional practice, and visions for the future of nursing.

NEW TO THIS EDITION

- **Thirteen New Chapters** New chapters focus on important topics and concepts for today's student. They include: Chapter 4 "Collaboration in Health Care;" Chapter 10 "Leader and Manager;" Chapter 11 "Research Consumer;" Chapter 12 "Critical Thinking and Decision Making;" Chapter 16 "Promoting Health of Individuals and Family;" Chapter 17 "Providing Care in the Home and Community;" Chapter 19 "Enhancing Healing;" Chapter 20 "Intervening in Crises;" Chapter 21 "Managing Family Violence;" Chapter 22 "Professional Empowerment and Politics;" Chapter 23 "Advanced Nursing Education and Practice;" and Chapter 24 "Looking Into the Future."

- **Increased Emphasis on Wellness and Health Promotion** Many chapters in the new edition focus on the importance of health and wellness in nursing care. See Chapter 3 "Health and Wellness;" Chapter 8 "Health Promoter;" Chapter 16 "Promoting the Health of Individuals and Families;" and Chapter 19 "Enhancing Healing."

- **New Information on Home and Community Care** Chapter 17 "Providing Care in the Home and Community" provides a comprehensive overview of current realities in home and community settings.

- **Coverage of Managed Care and Critical Pathways** Chapter 4 includes information about managed care and critical pathways as well as a sample critical pathway.

- **New Critical Thinking Chapter** A new chapter, Chapter 12, defines and discusses critical thinking and includes cognitive critical thinking skills, attitudes that foster critical thinking, elements and standards of critical thinking, applications of critical thinking in problem solving and decision making, and ways to develop critical thinking attitudes and skills.

- **Two-Color Design** For the first time, the 3rd edition of this text uses two colors throughout the book, making the text more appealing and easier to use.

- **Practicing Nurse Profiles** Practicing nurse profiles occur in two chapters, Chapter 17 "Providing Care in the Home and Community" and Chapter 23 "Advanced Nursing Education and Practice." The profiles include information about why these practitioners chose their specific practice areas, what qualities they think are necessary to be a nurse in this setting, what their job entails, and what encouragement they would offer a nurse considering practice in this setting. The profiles provide a useful first-person perspective for students.

- **"Consider…" Sections** In each chapter, "Consider…" sections present questions or ideas for students to consider and discuss. Items are related to the content presented and are intended to stimulate critical thinking. These sections can be used as a basis for group discussions in a classroom setting or for independent learning.

- **Readings for Enrichment Boxes** Boxes in each chapter provide annotated readings to supplement the learner's knowledge. The readings come from a variety of professional sources and were chosen to pique student interest in exploring new resources.

HALLMARK FEATURES

The 3rd edition of *Professional Nursing Practice: Concepts and Perspectives* retains several of the features that have been well-received by the readers of previous editions.

- Updated nursing research notes in each chapter describe relevant studies and relate them to clinical practice.

- Historical perspectives of nursing are now included in Chapter 1 "Perspectives of Professional Practice."

- Hallmark chapters have been completely updated including Chapter 2 "Nursing Theories and Conceptual Frameworks;" Chapter 3 "Health and Wellness;" Chapter 5 "Values, Ethics, and Advocacy;" Chapter 6 "Legal Rights and Responsibilities;" Chapter 7 "Socialization to Professional Nursing Roles;" Chapter 9 "Learner and Teacher;" Chapter 13 "Change Process;" Chapter 14 "Nursing Process;" Chapter 15 "Group Process;" and Chapter 18 "Supporting Cultural Needs."

ORGANIZATION

This edition is organized into five units. Units and chapters can be used independently or in any sequence. The steps of the nursing process are a major organizational element in many chapters and particularly in Unit 2 and Unit 4.

- Unit 1 "Nature of Professional Nursing" focuses on the concepts of profession and professionalism, historical and societal influences on nursing, ethical and legal issues, selected nursing issues, nursing theories and conceptual frameworks for nursing, concepts of health and wellness, and the collaborative process in health care.

- Unit 2 "Professional Nursing Roles" includes the socialization process related to the professional nurse as caregiver, teacher, counselor, client advocate, change agent, manager, researcher, consultant, case manager, and quality care evaluator. Separate chapters focus on selected professional roles: health promoter, learner and teacher, leader and manager, and research consumer.

- Unit 3 "Processes Guiding Professional Practice" includes chapters about critical thinking and decision making, the change process, the nursing process, and the group process.

- Unit 4 "Elements of Professional Practice" includes chapters devoted to promoting the health of individuals and families in the community, supporting cultural needs, enhancing healing through holistic care, intervening in a crisis, and managing family violence. The latter three chapters were added to this revision in response to users' requests.

- Unit 5 "Visions for the Future of Nursing" includes three chapters on professional empowerment and politics, advanced nursing education and practice, and the final chapter, "Looking Into the Future," written by Fay Bower. This chapter discusses past events that have affected nursing, future events that will affect nursing, what we have learned about health care that can help us in the future, and visions of tomorrow.

We hope this book helps learners from diverse backgrounds to appreciate nursing's proud heritage, to understand what is meant by "professional," to view nursing as a profession, and to develop knowledge and abilities that will contribute to the advancement of the profession. In addition, we hope the knowledge gained will help nurses provide quality care in a constantly changing health care arena.

ACKNOWLEDGEMENTS

We extend sincere thanks to the talented and committed team of people who worked on this book.

- The contributions, whose expertise has broadened both the scope and depth of the text: **Suzanne Beyea** for Chapter 4 "Collaboration in Health Care," **Diane Whitehead** for Chapter 10 "Leader and Manager;" **Divina Grossman** for Chapter 11 "Research Consumer;" **Ruth Pease** for Chapter 12 "Critical Thinking and Decision Making;" **Suzanne Phillips** and **Sandra Lobar** for Chapter 16 "Promoting Health for Individuals and Families" and Chapter 17 "Providing Care in the Home and Community;" **Carol Kneisl** and **Elizabeth Riley** for Chapter 20 "Intervening in Crises;" **Jean Candela** for Chapter 23 "Advanced Nursing Education and Practice;" and **Fay Bower** for Chapter 24 "Looking Into the Future."

- All the reviewers, who provided many discerning comments and suggestions that expanded our thinking and writing. Please see page iii for a list of the reviewers.

- **Erin Mulligan,** senior editor, whose commitment to the manuscript, understanding of writing demands, and flexibility in rearranging schedules contributed positively to this revision. Her attention to detail and developmental suggestions for every chapter were also greatly appreciated.

- **Kim Crowder,** editorial assistant, for her gracious, capable assistance whenever it was needed. Her prompt replies rescued us on many occasions.

- **Mary Tobin,** typist, for her continuing help in meeting the demands of manuscript deadlines. Her competency and efficiency are greatly valued.

- **Wendy Earl,** managing editor, for the indispensable behind-the-scenes coordination of all the production activities.

- **David Rich,** production editor, for his organizational and communication skills, conscientious attention to detail, and high standards. It was a pleasure to work with him again.

- **Sally Peyrefitte,** copyeditor, for the excellent contributions to the writing style and syntax, and the many inquiries for clarity. The copyedit was exceptional and we feel fortunate to have had her work on another of our books.

- **Brad Greene,** cover and text designer, for his visual interpretation and talents that have made this third edition very appealing.

- **Joan Andrews, Carole MacFarlane,** and **Linda Edge,** library personnel, for their continuing assistance in obtaining the many reference materials for the manuscript.

Barbara Kozier
Glenora Erb
Kathleen Blais

Contents

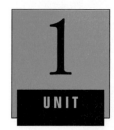

UNIT

Nature of
Professional Nursing

Perspectives of Professional Nursing

"Nursing encompasses an art, a humanistic orientation, a feeling for the value of the individual, and an intuitive sense of ethics and of the appropriateness of action taken."

— Myrtle Aydelotte, 1992

For the past century, nursing has undergone dramatic change and has ardently pursued legitimization and recognition as a full profession. This chapter presents criteria that have been developed by experts in the social sciences to help assess whether nursing has become a full profession.

- Many factors have influenced the development of nursing practice, education, and research. These factors include the status and roles of women, religious values, societal attitudes, and technology.
- Nursing practice roles have always encompassed care and nurturing, but they now encompass much more.
- Nursing education programs have evolved from apprenticeship programs in hospitals to formal education in higher institutions of learning.
- Nursing research has gained considerable momentum in the latter part of this century to generate new knowledge and improve client care.

PROFESSIONALISM

Three terms related to profession need to be differentiated: professionalism, professionalization, and profession. **Professionalism** refers to professional character, spirit, or methods. It is a set of attributes, a way of life that implies responsibility and commitment. Nursing professionalism owes much to the influence of Florence Nightingale (1820–1910). **Professionalization** is a process of becoming professional—that is, of acquiring characteristics considered to be professional. **Profession** has been defined in dictionaries as an occupation that requires extensive education or a calling that requires special knowledge, skill, and preparation. A profession is generally distinguished from other kinds of occupations by (a) its requirement of prolonged, specialized training to acquire a body of knowledge pertinent to the role to be performed and (b) an orientation of the individual toward service, either to a community or to an organization. The standards of education and practice for the profession are determined by the members of the profession, rather than by outsiders. The education

---

Criteria of a Profession

Flexner (1915)

Professional activity is basically intellectual.

Activities are practical, not theoretical.

Work can be learned because it is based on a body of knowledge.

Techniques can be taught.

A strong organization is in place.

Work is motivated by altruism.

Bixler and Bixler (1945)

Body of knowledge is specialized.

Body of knowledge is increasing.

New knowledge is developed to improve education and practice.

Practice is autonomous.

Education takes place in higher institutions.

Service is considered to be more important than personal gain.

Compensation comes through freedom to act, continuing professional growth, and economic security.

Barber (1965)

A vast amount of systematic general knowledge.

Oriented primarily to community interest rather than self-interest.

Strong behavioral self-control supported by codes of ethics and internalized through work socialization and through organizing and conducting voluntary associations operated by work specialists.

A system of rewards: monetary and honorary.

Pavalko (1971)

Work is based on a systematic body of theory and abstract knowledge.

Work has social value.

Work is a service to the public.

Education is required for specialization.

Autonomy.

Commitment to the profession.

Group identity and subculture.

A code of ethics.

TABLE 1–1   Position of Nursing on the Occupation-Profession Model

Category	Occupation	Profession	Nursing
1. *Theory*	Absent	Present	Beginning stages
2. *Relevance to social values*	Not relevant	Relevant	Relevant
3. *Training period*	Short, not specialized	Long and specialized	Varied in length; some specialization
4. *Motivation*	Self-interest	Service	Service, but varies
5. *Autonomy*	Absent	Complete	Incomplete
6. *Commitment*	Short-term	Long-term	Varies; relatively short
7. *Sense of community*	Low	High	Developing
8. *Code of ethics*	Undeveloped	Highly developed	Highly developed

SOURCE: Adapted from *Sociology of Occupations and Professions* by R. M. Pavalko, 1971, Itasca, IL: F. E. Peacock, p. 26. Reprinted by permission of the publisher; *Professionalization of nursing current issues and trends* by M. M. Moloney, 1986, Philadelphia: Lippincott, p. 27. Reprinted with permission.

of the professional involves a complete socialization process, more far-reaching in its social and attitudinal aspects and its technical features than is usually required in other kinds of occupations.

Is Nursing a Profession?

The debate about whether nursing already is a profession or has yet to reach that status continues. Traditionally, only medicine, law, and theology have been considered professions, but nursing has been called a profession for many years. In fact, Strauss (1966, p. 60) refers to a magazine article about nursing reform published in 1882 titled, "A New Profession for Women." Experts in the social sciences have developed criteria against which an occupation can be judged to ascertain its professional status. See the box on page 3.

Using Pavalko's eight criteria of a profession, nursing's position in the occupation-profession model is described in Table 1–1. As the table shows, some professional characteristics are not as highly developed in nursing as they are in other professions.

Pavalko's Occupation-Profession Continuum Model

In his occupation-profession model, Pavalko (1971) identifies eight categories that serve as criteria to determine whether an occupation is a profession (see Table 1–1).

1. *Theory*. The work group is judged on the extent to which its work is based on a systematic body of knowledge. This knowledge is developed through research.

   As a profession, nursing is establishing a well-defined body of knowledge and expertise. A number of nursing conceptual frameworks (discussed in Chapter 2) contribute to the knowledge base of nursing and give direction to nursing practice, education, and ongoing research.

   Increasing research in nursing is contributing to this body of knowledge. In the 1940s, nursing research was at a very early stage of development. In the 1950s, increased federal funding and professional support helped establish centers for nursing research. Most early research was directed to the study of nursing education. In the 1960s, studies focused chiefly on the nature of the knowledge base underlying nursing practice. Since the 1970s, nursing research has focused largely on practice-related issues. Nursing research as a dimension of the nurse's role is discussed further in Chapter 11.

2. *Relevance to social values*. This category suggests that a profession justifies its existence by close association with values that society as a whole

embraces, such as life and happiness. Since its inception, nursing has been truly altruistic in that it has existed to serve others. In the early history of nursing, in fact, nurses were expected to devote most of their lives to nursing. Contemporary nursing still emphasizes service to others, but today's nurses expect just compensation and a life separate from nursing.

Nursing embodies the characteristics of relevance to social values because it values health, well-being, and caring, which are values held by society at large. People recognize that nurses *care* and therefore most hold nurses in high esteem; however, society often more readily values the physician's role in *cure* and may overlook the role nurses play in helping clients to attain health and prevent illness. Nursing is thought generally to meet this characteristic even though not all members of society may consider it a profession.

3. *Training (education) period.* Training or education is the third characteristic in Pavalko's occupation-profession model. This category has four subdivisions: the educational content, length of education, the use of symbolic and ideational processes, and degree of specialization that is related to practice.

According to Florence Nightingale, nursing education should involve theory and practice. Over the years, nursing has evolved to include both these dimensions. However, the length of study required for entry to practice is still an issue of controversy.

Historically, nurses were educated in hospitals. In modern times, the trend has shifted toward providing nursing education programs in colleges and universities. Many nursing educators believe that the undergraduate nursing curriculum should include liberal arts education in addition to the biologic and social sciences and the nursing discipline. The *Standards for Professional Nursing Education* developed by the American Nurses Association (ANA, 1984, p. 1) states that the "education for those preparing to become nurses as well as those already licensed to practice nursing should take place in institutions of higher education." In 1983, the National League for Nursing (NLN) voted at its convention to retain the baccalaureate degree as the minimal academic preparation for the professional nurse (Lewis, 1983, pp. 246–247).

In the United States today, there are five levels of entry into registered nursing: hospital diploma, associate degree, baccalaureate degree, generic master's degree, and generic doctoral degree. At this time it appears that there is no consensus among nurses about the appropriate length for nursing education programs. At present, education programs vary from 2 years for an associate degree to 4 or 5 years for a baccalaureate degree. There is also controversy surrounding specialization issues, for example, whether a master of science degree should be the entry level for specialization or whether a doctorate in nursing should be required.

4. *Motivation.* Motivation to work is Pavalko's fourth category. In this instance, Pavalko refers not to the motivation of the individual but to the group as a whole. Motivation means the extent to which the nursing group emphasizes service to others rather than service to self as its primary goal. There is a point of view that today's young people are more centered on self than young people of 50 years ago. Butter (1989, p. 40) has pointed out that college freshmen tend to value more highly careers in fields that are associated with status, power, and money, rather than service. Traditionally, these characteristics have not been associated with nursing. However, many nurses do have a service orientation toward their clients as well.

5. *Autonomy.* Pavalko's fifth category is autonomy: the freedom of the group to regulate and control its own work behavior. Styles wrote in 1982 that many sociologists view *autonomy* as the sole differentiating characteristic of a profession (Styles, 1982, p. 27).

A profession is autonomous if it regulates itself and sets standards for its members. Providing autonomy is one of the purposes of a professional association. If nursing is to have professional status, it must function autonomously in the formation of policy and in the control of its activity. To be autonomous, a professional group must be granted legal authority to define the scope of its practice, describe its particular functions and roles, and determine its goals and responsibilities in delivery of its services. The amount of autonomy a professional group possesses depends on its effectiveness at governance. **Governance** is the establishment and maintenance of social, political, and economic arrangements by which practitioners control their practice, their self-discipline, their working conditions, and their professional affairs.

To practitioners of nursing, autonomy means independence at work, responsibility, and accountability for one's actions. Usually, nurses are not strictly autonomous: although they have self-regulation through the professional state boards of nursing in the United States or provincial associations in Canada (in Ontario, Canada, the College of Nursing performs this function), most nurses are employed by institutions that allow them only limited control over their practice. Some nurses, however, recognize autonomy involving their identity, authority and independence as related to their clinical judgments, in practice. These nurses do believe they function autonomously in hospitals and home care.

In addition, there are nurses who function independently, such as nurse midwives and nurse anesthetists (see Chapter 23). Other nurses, such as those working in intensive care units and emergency departments, function collaboratively with physicians and other health professionals. Their knowledge and expertise is recognized by others (see Chapter 4 for a discussion of collaborative care).

6. *Commitment.* Pavalko's sixth category is commitment toward work. In this context, people who are committed to their work view it as more than a stepping stone to another type of work or as intermittent work. For people who engage in an occupation, commitment tends to be absent; professionals, in contrast, tend to commit to their work for a lifetime or long period of time.

Commitment in nursing has tended to be low. Nurses, most of whom are women, often have conflicting obligations, such as family. However, in recent years, nurses have tended to remain in

RESEARCH NOTE

Is Professional Autonomy Related to Any Nurse Characteristics?

In one study, researchers explored the relationship between demographic characteristics and professional nursing autonomy. The study's sample included 2000 RNs, with subsamples of 500 nurses from Idaho, Missouri, Florida, and Maryland. Surveys included demographic data and items from the Nursing Activity Scale (NAS) (Schutzenhofer, 1987) and the Personal Attributes Questionnaire (PAQ) (Spence, Helmreich & Stapp, 1974).

Demographic characteristics considered were sex, basic level of nursing education, highest level of education, marital status, years in practice as an RN, years since graduation from a basic (generic) nursing program, employment status, employment setting, staffing models in the clinical setting, clinical specialty, position/job title, and nursing organization membership. The NAS is a 30-item scale that describes clinical nursing situations applicable to a variety of clinical specialties in which a nurse must exercise some degree of professional nursing autonomy. The PAQ is a 24-item questionnaire of gender-stereotyped expressive and instrumental personality qualities. The scale is composed of three subscales of eight items each. The "M" scale consists of things judged to be more characteristic of men than women and socially desirable for both men and women to some degree. The "F" scale consists of items more characteristic of women than men, but socially desirable to some degree for both. The third scale,

the "M-F" scale, reflects characteristics that stereotypically differentiate men and women and have different social desirability ratings.

Findings revealed significant relationships between autonomy and nursing education, practice setting, clinical specialty, functional role, membership in professional organizations, and gender-stereotyped personality traits. Those who had the greatest sense of autonomy were those with graduate education; those who worked in a public health setting rather than a hospital setting; those whose major clinical specialty was psychiatric/mental health; those who had the title CNS or NP; those who were members of professional organizations; and those who had personality traits typically associated with men. Age and years of nursing experience were not shown to have any relationship to autonomy.

Implications: Nurses can look to higher education and specific clinical settings as factors that can enable them to achieve professional autonomy in the workplace. In addition, nurse administrators, educators, managers, and advanced clinical practitioners can serve as role models for autonomous practice.

SOURCE: "Nurse Characteristics and Professional Autonomy" by K. K. Schutzenhofer and D. B. Musser, Fall 1994, *Image: Journal of Nursing Scholarship*, 26, 201–204.

the workforce, taking part-time employment instead of leaving to raise families, as many did in the past. Career-oriented nurses value commitment to people and continued education to broaden their own and nursing's power base; job-oriented nurses, in contrast, chiefly value the income they earn from the job. Increasingly, more nurses are becoming committed to nursing, thus moving nursing toward professional status.

7. *Sense of community.* A sense of community means that members of a group share a common identity and destiny and possess a distinctive subculture. In the past, nurses have sported many symbols of their profession, such as a cap, white uniform, and pin. Although many of these symbols have disappeared, nurses do have a strong sense of professional identity.

One way nurses can develop a sense of community is to join associations and groups.

There are two types of organizations: professional and nonprofessional. "A professional organization is an organization of practitioners who judge one another as professionally competent and who have banded together to perform social functions which they cannot perform in their separate capacities as individuals" (Merton, 1958, p. 50).

Styles (1983) writes that nursing organizations must perform the following five functions for the preservation and development of the profession:

a. *Defining and regulating the profession through setting and enforcing standards of education and practice for the generalist and the specialist.* In the United States and Canada, regulation is achieved largely through the licensure of individual nurses, certification, and accreditation. (See the section on credentialing of nurses in Chapter 6.) Regulation is also achieved through the adoption of codes of ethics and norms of conduct (Styles, 1983, p. 570).

b. *Developing the knowledge base for practice in its broadest and narrowest components.* One significant contribution to nursing knowledge is the work of the North American Nursing Diagnosis Association (NANDA). This group is generating and expanding a taxonomy of nursing diagnoses. Research is required to determine the validity and reliability of these diagnoses.

c. *Transmitting values, norms, knowledge, and skill to nursing students, new graduates, and members of the profession for application in practice.* This func-

tion is largely performed through the education of nurses and the socialization process.

d. *Communicating and advocating the values and contributions of the field to several publics and constituencies.* This function requires that nursing organizations speak for nurses from a position of broad agreement. It is essential for nurses to participate actively in formulating health legislation and policy.

e. *Attending to the social and general welfare of their members.* Professional associations give their members social and moral support to perform their roles as professionals and to cope with professional problems. Association journals disseminate updated knowledge, new ideas, and professional concerns. By participating in the collective bargaining process, nurses can improve their economic and working conditions.

Nursing organizations are established at local, national, and international levels. The functions of the ANA are shown in the box on page 8.

8. *Code of ethics.* The existence of a code of ethics is the final category in Pavalko's model. Occupations are not likely to have a written code of ethics that sets forth standards of behavior and relationships between its members and the public they serve. Established professions, in contrast, do have formal codes of ethics. Nurses have traditionally placed a high value on the worth and dignity of others. The nursing profession requires integrity of its members; that is, a member is expected to do what is considered right regardless of the personal cost. Nurses must respect the professional judgment of others and must develop nursing standards and establish mechanisms for identifying and dealing with unethical behavior. The International Council of Nurses (ICN), the ANA, the Canadian Nurses Association (CNA), and other national nursing associations have codes of ethics.

An examination of nursing in relation to Pavalko's eight criteria shows that the most likely evaluation is that nursing is an emerging profession. In the categories of social values (2) and ethics (8), nursing appears to have met the professional criteria. In other categories, nursing appears to be at various stages of development toward professional status. Gains are being made, but nursing must continue to work to become completely professional.

SOURCE: American Nurses Association, *American Nurses Association Bylaws*, as revised June 30, 1991, Washington, DC: ANA. Used by permission.

Functions of the American Nurses Association (ANA)

- Establish standards of nursing practice, nursing education, and nursing services

- Establish a code of ethical conduct for nurses

- Ensure a system of credentialing in nursing

- Initiate and influence legislation, governmental programs, national health policy, and international health policy

- Support systematic study, evaluation, and research in nursing

- Serve as the central agency for the collection, analysis, and dissemination of information relevant to nursing

- Promote and protect the economic and general welfare of nurses

- Provide leadership in national and international nursing

- Provide for the professional development of nurses

- Conduct an affirmative action program

- Ensure a collective bargaining program for nurses

- Provide services to constituent members

- Maintain communication with members through official publications

- Assume an active role as consumer advocate

- Represent and speak for the nursing profession with allied health groups, national and international organizations, governmental bodies, and the public

- Protect and promote the advancement of human rights related to health care and nursing

CONSIDER...

- ways of increasing your autonomy in your practice setting.
- comparing nursing with other professions, such as law or medicine. How are they similar in education and practice? How do they differ? What changes would you recommend for the nursing profession as a result of these comparisons?
- Flexner's criterion that in a profession, "work is motivated by altruism." What are your thoughts about this criterion?
- Barber's criterion that a profession is "oriented primarily to community interest rather than self-interest." What do you think of this criterion?

Standards of Clinical Nursing Practice

Establishing and implementing standards of practice are major functions of a professional organization. The purpose of **standards of clinical nursing practice** is to describe the responsibilities for which nurses are accountable. The standards (a) reflect the values and priorities of the nursing profession, (b) provide direction for professional nursing practice, (c) provide a framework for the evaluation of nursing practice, and (d) define the profession's accountability to the public and the client outcomes for which nurses are responsible (ANA 1991b, p. 3). In 1991, the ANA developed standards of clinical nursing practice that are generic in nature and provide for the practice of nursing regardless of area of specialization. Various specialty nursing organizations have further developed specific standards of nursing practice related to the practice of nursing in a specialty area.

The profession's responsibilities inherent in establishing and implementing standards of practice include (a) to establish, maintain, and improve standards, (b) to hold members accountable for using standards, (c) to educate the public to appreciate the standards, (d) to protect the public from individuals who have not attained the standards or willfully do not follow them, and (e) to protect individual members of the profession from each other (Phaneuf & Lang 1985, p. 2).

Nursing standards clearly reflect the specific functions and activities that nurses provide, as opposed to the functions of other health workers. The ANA's standards of clinical nursing practice consist of both standards of care and standards of professional performance. *Standards of care* describe the competence of nursing care demonstrated by the components of the nursing process. These six standards with related measurement criteria are provided throughout Chapter 14. *Standards of professional performance* describe the competence level of professional role behaviors. These standards are shown in the accompanying box.

When standards of professional practice are implemented, they serve as yardsticks for the measurements used in licensure, certification, accreditation, quality assurance, peer review, and public policy.

ANA Standards of Professional Performance

I. Quality of Care
The Nurse systematically evaluates the quality and effectiveness of nursing practice.

II. Performance Appraisal
The Nurse evaluates his/her own nursing practice in relation to professional practice standards and relevant statutes and regulations.

III. Education
The Nurse acquires and maintains current knowledge in nursing practice.

IV. Collegiality
The Nurse contributes to the professional development of peers, colleagues, and others.

V. Ethics
The Nurse's decisions and actions on behalf of clients are determined in an ethical manner.

VI. Collaboration
The Nurse collaborates with the client, significant others, and health care providers in providing client care.

VII. Research
The Nurse uses research findings in practice.

VIII. Resource Utilization
The Nurse considers factors related to safety, effectiveness, and cost in planning and delivering client care.

SOURCE: American Nurses Association, *Standards of Clinical Nursing Practice* (Washington, DC: ANA, 1991). Used with permission.

HISTORICAL PERSPECTIVES

Nursing has undergone dramatic change in response to societal needs and influences. A look at nursing's beginnings can reveal its continuing struggle for autonomy and professionalization. In the words of Fahy (1995, p. 5), "If you don't know where you've been, how do you know where you are going?" In recent decades, a renewed interest in nursing history has produced a growing amount of related literature.

This section highlights only selected aspects of events that have influenced nursing practice, nursing education, and nursing research.

Nursing Practice

Recurring themes of women's roles and status, religious (Christian) values, war, science and technology, societal attitudes, and visionary nursing leadership have influenced nursing practice in the past. Many of these factors still exert their influence today.

Women's Roles

Traditional female roles of wife, mother, daughter, and sister have always included the care and nurturing of other family members. From the beginning of time, women have cared for infants and children; thus, nursing could be said to have its roots in "the home." Additionally, women, who in general occupied a subservient and dependent role, were called upon to care for others in the community who were ill. Generally, the care provided was related to physical maintenance and comfort. Thus, the traditional nursing role has always entailed humanistic caring, nurturing, comforting, and supporting.

In ancient civilizations midwives provided care for the mother and infant during birthing, and wet nurses often suckled and cared for infant children of wealthy families. Often these roles were filled by female slaves. The slave-nurse was dependent on the master, healer, or priest for instruction or direction in the care of her charge.

Religion

Religion has also played a significant role in the development of nursing. Although many of the world's religions encourage benevolence, it was the Christian value of "love thy neighbor as thyself" and Christ's parable of the Good Samaritan that had significant impact on the development of Western nursing. During the third and fourth centuries, several wealthy matrons of the Roman Empire, including Marcella, Fabiola, and Paula, converted to Christianity and used their wealth to provide houses of care and healing (the forerunner of hospitals) for the poor, the sick, and the homeless. Women were not, however, the sold providers of nursing services. In the third century, in Rome an organization of men called the Parabolani Brotherhood provided care to the sick and dying during the great plague in Alexandria.

The Crusades saw the formation of several orders of knights, including the Knights of Saint John of Jerusalem (also known as the Knights Hospitalers), the Teutonic Knights, and the Knights of Lazarus. These brothers in arms provided nursing care to their sick and injured comrades. These orders also built hospitals, the organization and management of which set a standard for the administration of hospitals throughout Europe at that time.

During the Middle Ages (A.D. 500–1500), male and female religious, military, and secular orders formed with the primary purpose of caring for the sick. Conspicuous among them were the Augustinian sisters, who comprised the first purely nursing order; the aforementioned Knights of Saint John (Knights Hospitalers); and the Alexian Brotherhood.

In 1633, the Sisters of Charity were founded by Saint Vincent de Paul in France. The Order of the Sisters of Charity sent nursing sisters to provide care in the New World, establishing hospitals in Canada, the United States, and Australia.

The deaconess groups, which had their origins in the Roman Empire of the third and fourth centuries, were suppressed during the Middle Ages by the Western churches. However, these groups of nursing providers resurfaced occasionally throughout the centuries, most notably in 1836, when Theodor Fliedner reinstituted the Order of Deaconesses and opened a small hospital and training school in Kaiserswerth, Germany. Florence Nightingale received her "training" in nursing at the Kaiserswerth School.

Early religious values, such as self-denial, spiritual calling, and devotion to duty and hard work, have dominated nursing throughout its history. Nurses' commitment to these values often has resulted in exploitation and few monetary rewards. For some time, nurses themselves believed it was inappropriate to expect economic gain from their "calling."

War

Throughout history wars have accentuated the need for nurses. During the Crimean War (1854–1856), the inadequacy of care given to soldiers led to public outcry in Great Britain. The role Florence Nightingale played in addressing this problem is well known. She was asked by Sir Sidney Herbert of the British War Department to recruit a contingent of female nurses to provide care to the sick and injured in the Crimea. Nightingale and her nurses transformed the military hospitals by setting up kitchens, a laundry, recreation centers, and reading rooms and by organizing classes for orderlies. Nightingale, called the "Lady with the Lamp" is credited with performing miracles in Crimea; the mortality rate in the Barrack Hospital in Turkey, for example, was reduced to 1%.

During the American Civil War (1861–1865), several nurses emerged who were notable for their contributions to a country torn by internal strife. Harriet Tubman and Sojourner Truth provided care and safety to slaves fleeing to the North on the "Underground Railroad." Mother Biekerdyke and Clara Barton (who is credited with founding the American Red Cross) searched the battlefields and gave care to injured and dying soldiers. Noted authors Walt Whitman and Louisa May Alcott volunteered as nurses to give care to injured soldiers in military hospitals. They chronicled their experiences in their writings as a permanent record of nursing's contribution during this time.

World War II casualties created an acute shortage of care. It was at this time that auxiliary health care workers became prominent. "Practical" nurses, aides, and technicians provided much of the actual nursing care under the instruction and supervision of better-prepared nurses. At the same time, medical specialties arose to meet the needs of hospitalized clients. Health care focused on the problem of "the disability, the disease, the diagnosis, not on the person, his family, his needs, his wholeness or his humanity" (Bevis, 1989, p. 39). A focus on the client's wholeness and individuality gained prominence in nursing in the mid 20th century. This view has expanded to include empowerment of clients and helping them become participative decision makers in their care (see Chapter 4).

Science and Technology

Technologic advances have affected many areas of nursing practice. For example, in 1860 Louis Pasteur confirmed the presence of airborne bacteria. In 1865, Joseph Lister applied Pasteur's discoveries to the field of surgery and used carbolic acid (phenol) successfully in treating a compound fracture (Dolan, Fitzpatrick & Herrmann, 1983, p. 230). His contributions led to widespread use of chemicals in controlling bacterial invasion. Other discoveries led to the growing, or culturing, of microorganisms and the production of antitoxins to prevent disease. The discovery of ether as an anesthetic in the late 1800s also affected nursing practice. Nurses were recruited to give anesthesia. This development was the origin of the role of nurse anesthetist (Dolan et al., 1983, p. 238).

The knowledge explosion of the 20th century brought forth many other changes that today have become standard practice. For example, intravenous infusion pumps, cardiac and fetal monitoring devices, and computerized equipment all enhance the nurse's ability to make expert clinical judgments and manage care.

Technologic change also creates challenges for nurses. For example, dangerous equipment or harmful chemical residues that are prevalent in some industries present hazardous conditions for employees. Trauma (injury) and disease can be a direct result of advanced technology; the classic example is automobile accidents, which are among the top five causes of death in North America. In addition, the modern life-style frequently creates high levels of stress, which has been associated with major physical illnesses (e.g., heart disease, cancer, and gastrointestinal disturbances), as well as psychologic problems (e.g., depression).

Although technologic advances are often greeted with approval, they are also often considered counterproductive to human interaction and holistic care. To preserve these important aspects of care, nurses are placing greater emphasis on the "high touch" aspect of a "high tech" environment, recognizing that clients require human interactions, such as warmth, care, acknowledgment of self worth, and collaborative decision making.

Technology has affected nursing practice in many other ways. The ability to prolong life—and, in a sense, also to prolong death—has created ethical dilemmas. Increases in life expectancies have led to an increase in the complexity of care for older adults, who are living longer with multiple health problems. More people of all ages are living longer with chronic illness because medical advances have forestalled the progression of many diseases that formerly resulted in speedy death. In addition, the educational requirements of nurses (both continuing education and basic preparation) have changed to ensure the provision of effective, safe nursing practice, and nursing practice is becoming more specialized.

Societal Attitudes

Society's attitudes about nurses and nursing have significantly influenced professional nursing. In *The Changing Image of the Nurse*, Kalisch and Kalisch indicate that the public's attitudes toward nurses and nursing are closely related to the images of nurses reflected in literature and the mass media (1987, p. x). Awareness of these portrayals, which are often both persuasive and unrealistic, can help nurses correct the public's inaccurate beliefs, ideas, and impressions of nurses and nursing.

Before the mid 1800s, nursing was without organization, education, or social status; the prevailing attitude was that a woman's place was in the home and that no respectable woman should have a career. The role for the Victorian middle-class woman was that of wife and mother, and any education she obtained was for the purpose of making her a pleasant companion to her husband and a responsible mother to her children. Nurses in hospitals during this period were women of the lower classes, who often were poorly educated or even incarcerated criminals. Society's attitudes about nursing during this period are reflected in the writings of Charles Dickens. In his book *Martin Chuzzlewit* (1896), Dickens refers to the nursing care given by criminals and women of low moral standards. Sairy Gamp, the central character in this book, epitomizes the nurses of the day, who lived and worked in appalling environments. Their work was considered a repugnant form of domestic service, for which little or no special training was required. This portrayal greatly influenced attitudes toward nurses and training.

Kalisch and Kalisch (1987) identify five dominant images of mass media portrayals of nurses since the 1920s: the Angel of Mercy, Girl Friday, Heroine, Wife and Mother, and Sex Object. To counter these portrayals, they propose a new image of the nurse as Careerist.

The *Angel of Mercy* image arose in the latter part of the 19th century, largely because of the work of Florence Nightingale during the Crimean War. After Nightingale brought respectability to the nursing profession, nurses were viewed as noble, moral, religious, dedicated, and self-sacrificing. Novelists characterized this new breed of nurses as refined young ladies who were "angels of mercy" rather than educated, skilled professionals. Nursing was raised to the level of a divine calling.

In the 1920s, after women gained the right to vote, women, including wives and mothers, demonstrated their capacity to hold jobs outside their homes above the level of domestic servant or file clerk. They began to compete with men as skilled bookkeepers, typists, and machine operators, and employers made the most of women as inexpensive laborers in factories and offices. In terms of nursing, the public's conception of the nurse as Angel of Mercy continued, but it was joined by a different antiprofessional image—the *Girl Friday*. The media portrayed nurses as subordinate to physicians and more interested in romance and love than in their work.

The public image of the nurse in the 1930s and 1940s was elevated considerably in the embodiment of the *Heroine* representation. During this decade, women were rarely portrayed as only wives and mothers; they were promoted to higher-status employment as journalists and business executives. Nurses appeared as courageous, committed, competent, calm and poised in the face of crisis, skilled, and professional. This Heroine portrayal was magnified by nurses' acts of bravery in World War II and their contributions in fighting poliomyelitis—in particular, the work of the Australian nurse Elizabeth Kenny.

After World War II, many women who had shared the camaraderie of the fighting services resumed their roles of wives and mothers. The deprivation associated with the war years made family life attractive, and returning veterans replaced millions of women in the workforce. A sexual division of labor became evident: Most women in the workforce were stenographers, secretaries, teachers, or nurses. Even in teaching there was a division of labor: In the primary grades, most teachers were women; in high school, most teachers were men. Women were notably underrepresented in the professions of medicine, law, engineering, and scientific research. In the media, the nurse's role was largely underplayed; nursing tasks were seen as involving minimal skill and no judgment—the nurse's job was primarily to support the physician in a servant or a "wife-like" role.

After the mid 1960s, the dominant media image of nurses was the *Sex Object*. Nurses were characterized as sensual, romantic, frivolous, irresponsible, hedonistic, and even promiscuous. For example, in the "MASH" series, the nurse Margaret Houlihan was referred to as "Hot Lips." The "Carry On" series emphasized bedpan humor, jokes about enemas, and doctors and male patients who lusted after nurses. On the rare occasions when nurses were shown engaging in actual nursing work, the portrayal often cast the nurse in a demeaning and subordinate role.

Kalisch and Kalisch (1982) perceive the *Careerist* as the new ideal image for the 1980s onward. They describe the careerist as an "intelligent, rational, progressive, sophisticated, empathetic, sincere, kind, and assertive person who is committed to attaining higher and higher standards of health care for the public" (p. 189). They contend that the principal goal of career nurses may not be so much to support and advance their families as it is to achieve self-actualization. Although transition to the Careerist image may not be easy, it is important for nurses to strive to communicate this new image, rather than passively accepting the definitions and descriptions of others. Kalisch and Kalisch suggest that perhaps on an unconscious level, nurses have contributed to the maintenance of "dysfunctional stereotypes" and that nurses themselves need to focus on a status that truly reflects their education, role, and professional commitment.

Unfavorable unprofessional media portrayals of nurses have had and continue to have serious consequences for the nursing profession. Kalisch and Kalisch (1987, p. 187) point out four implications of these consequences:

1. The public are unaware of the changed role of the nurse and the many services that nurses provide.

2. The quality and quantity of individuals who choose nursing as a career is affected. A demeaning image of nursing casts nursing as an undesirable profession.

3. The decisions of policy making relative to nursing are influenced. Legislation that gives nurses more autonomy in their practice or allocates scarce resources to advance the role of the nurse is hindered by legislators who may view the nurse as an unintelligent hand-maiden to the physician.

4. Nurses' self-image can be damaged by unfavorable media portrayals.

During the past few decades, the nursing profession has taken steps to improve the image of the nurse. Many media watch groups have evolved at local and national levels to monitor the media, to voice opinions, and to supplant outdated images with accurate accounts of today's nurse.

In the early 1990s, the Tri-Council for Nursing (the American Association of Colleges of Nursing, the American Nurses Association, the American Organization of Nurse Executives, and the National League for Nursing) initiated a national effort (titled "Nurses of America") to improve the image of nursing. Through a quarterly newsletter, *Media Watch: A Publication of Nurses of America*, nurses are asked to complete Television Program Surveillance Forms. The organization has also implemented a Media Training Project. These trained representatives of nursing will assist in presenting programs on nursing to consumers.

Young (1992, p. 50) states that nursing's image can be changed through professionalism. In addition, individual nurses need to develop a professional self-image (see Chapter 7).

Nursing Leaders

Florence Nightingale, Clara Barton, Lillian Wald, Lavinia Dock, Margaret Sanger, and Mary Breckenridge are among the leaders who have made notable contributions in influencing both nursing's history and women's history. These women were all politically astute pioneers. Their skills at influencing others and bringing about change remain models for political nurse activists today. Contemporary nursing leaders, such as Virginia Henderson, who created a modern worldwide definition of nursing, and Martha Rogers, a catalyst for theory development, are discussed in Chapter 2.

Nightingale (1820–1910) Florence Nightingale's contributions to nursing are well documented. Her achievements in improving the standards for the care of war casualties in the Crimea earned her the title "Lady with the Lamp." Her efforts in reforming hospitals and in producing and implementing public health policies also made her an accomplished political nurse. She was the first nurse to exert political pressure on government. Through her contributions to nursing education—perhaps her greatest achievement—she is also recognized as nursing's first scientist/theorist for her work *Notes on Nursing: What It Is, and What It Is Not*.

Nightingale was born to a wealthy and intellectual family. Her education included the mastery of several ancient and modern languages, literature, philosophy, history, science, mathematics, religion, art, and music. It was expected that she would follow the usual path of a wealthy and intelligent woman of the day: marry, bear children, and maintain a gracious and elegant home. Nightingale, however, believed she was "called by God to help others … [and] to improve the well-being of mankind" (Schuyler, 1992, p. 4). She was determined to become a nurse, in spite of opposition from her family and the restrictive societal code for affluent young English women. As a well-traveled young woman of the day, she visited Kaiserswerth in 1847, where she received 3 months' training in nursing. In 1853, she studied in Paris with the Sisters of Charity, after which she returned to England to assume the position of superintendent of a charity hospital for ill governesses.

When she returned to England, Nightingale was given an honorarium of £4500 by a grateful English public. She later used this money to develop the Nightingale Training School for Nurses, which opened in 1860. The school served as a model for other training schools. Its graduates traveled to other countries to manage hospitals and institute nurse training programs.

Barton (1812–1912) Clara Barton was a schoolteacher who volunteered as a nurse during the American Civil War. Her responsibilities were to organize the nursing services. Barton is noted for her role in establishing the American Red Cross, which linked with the International Red Cross when the United States Congress ratified the Treaty of Geneva (Geneva Convention). It was Barton who persuaded Congress in 1882 to ratify this treaty so that the Red Cross could perform humanitarian efforts in time of peace.

Wald (1867–1940) Lillian Wald is considered the founder of public health nursing. Wald and Mary Brewster were the first to offer trained nursing services to the poor in the New York slums. Their home among the poor on the upper floor of a tenement, called the Henry Street Settlement and Visiting Nurse Service, provided nursing services, social services, and organized educational and cultural activities. Soon after the founding of the Henry Street Settlement, school nursing was established as an adjunct to visiting nursing. Again, Wald was involved, along with Lina E. Rogers. Another of Wald's notable contributions was the creation of the United States Children's Bureau in 1912 to monitor fair child labor laws (Hall-Long, 1995, p. 25).

Dock (1858–1956) Lavinia Dock was a feminist, prolific writer, political activist, suffragette, and friend of Wald. She actively participated in protest movements for women's rights that resulted in the 1920 passage of the Nineteenth Amendment to the U.S. Constitution, which granted women the right to vote. In addition, Dock campaigned for legislation to allow nurses rather than physicians to control their profession. In 1893, Dock, with the assistance of Mary Adelaide Nutting and Isabel Hampton Robb, founded the American Society of Superintendents of Training Schools for Nurses of the United States and Canada, a precursor for the current National League for Nursing.

Sanger (1879–1966) Margaret Higgins Sanger, a public health nurse in New York, has had a lasting impact on women's health care. Imprisoned for opening the first birth control information clinic in America, she is considered the founder of Planned Parenthood. Her experience with the large number of unwanted pregnancies among the working poor was instrumental in addressing this problem.

Breckinridge (1881–1965) After World War I, the Frontier Nursing Service (FNS) was established by a notable pioneer nurse, Mary Breckinridge. In 1918, she worked with the American Committee for Devastated France, distributing food, clothing, and supplies to rural villages in France and taking care of sick children. In 1921, Breckinridge returned to the United States with plans to provide health care to the people of rural America. She had initially prepared herself by taking courses at Teachers' College in New York and midwifery training in London and by developing prominent social contacts for fundraising. In 1925, Breckinridge and two other nurses began the FNS in Leslie County, Kentucky. Within this organization, Breckinridge started one of the first midwifery training schools in the United States.

CONSIDER...

- how nursing might have developed differently if the majority of nurses were male and/or baccalaureate prepared.
- what societal and personal values influence your individual nursing practice.
- what perceptions your clients or family members and friends have of your nursing role. Is the perception professional or unfavorable? What can you do to convey an accurate image?

Nursing Education

Diploma Programs

After Florence Nightingale established the first school of nursing (the Nightingale Training School for Nurses) at St. Thomas's Hospital in England in 1860, the concept traveled quickly to North America. Hospital administrators welcomed the idea of training schools as a source of free or inexpensive staffing for the hospital. Nursing education in the early years largely took the form of apprenticeships. With little formal classroom instruction, students learned by doing, that is, by providing care to clients in hospitals. There was no standardization of curriculum and no accreditation. Programs were designed to meet the service needs of the hospital, not the educational needs of the students.

The first training programs for nurses at hospital schools were opened in the 1860s at the New England Hospital for Women and Children in Boston, at Women's Hospital in Philadelphia, at Bellevue Hospital in New York, and at Johns Hopkins in Baltimore. The number of diploma programs rose quickly after these initial programs, from 15 in 1890 to 432 in 1900 (Bullough, Bullough, & Soukup, 1983). By 1920 there were almost 2300 diploma programs (Fitzpatrick, 1983).

In Canada The Mack Training School at the General and Marine Hospital in St. Catharine's, Ontario was the first school of nursing patterned after the Nightingale school in 1874. In 1875 the board of directors of the Montreal General Hospital sought the assistance of Florence Nightingale in establishing a training school. However, it was not until 1890 under the direction of Nora Gertrude Livingstone, a graduate of New York Hospital, that the school began. In 1877 the Toronto General Hospital attempted to establish a training school but it did not become recognized until 1884 under the direction of Mary Agnes Snively, a graduate of Bellevue Hospital School of Nursing in New York. By 1909 seventy schools of nursing were established.

Early hospital diploma programs varied considerably in quality, length, and the clinical experience offered. Larger hospitals provided more exposure to a variety of clinical experiences. Some of these early diploma training schools were affiliated with universities that provided some of the courses in the natural and social sciences, such as physiology, psychology, and sociology. For example, Mercy Hospital in Chicago became affiliated with Northwestern University in 1889.

In 1918, the Rockefeller Foundation formed a committee to study nursing education. The committee's findings, which are referred to as the Goldmark Report published in 1923, revealed that

- Sciences, theory, and practice of nursing were frequently taught by unprepared instructors in poorly equipped basement classrooms.

- Hospitals controlled the total teaching hours. Content was minimal, and some subjects were omitted entirely.
- Lectures were often given to students at night after a long day's work.
- Students' practical experience was usually limited to those experiences found in the hospital.
- Students obtained their practical experience under the supervision of graduate nurses, who had neither preparation nor time to teach (Goldmark, 1923, pp. 310–312).

One of the recommendations of the Goldmark Report was that university schools of nursing be developed in an attempt to make nursing education programs independent of hospital needs—a concept recommended by Nightingale. It also recommended that a high school diploma be the minimum prerequisite for entry into schools of nursing. In response to the Goldmark Report, the Western Reserve University School of Nursing and the Yale University School of Nursing were established, many substandard schools closed, and high school graduation became the prerequisite for entry to a nursing program. In addition, the National League for Nursing Education (later known as the National League for Nursing) made an initial attempt to standardize diploma nursing programs. Standardization did not occur, however, until the late 1940s and early 1950s.

In 1925, the Committee on the Grading of Nursing Schools was organized and subsequently published two written reports: (a) *Nurses, Patients, and Pocketbooks* (1928), and (b) *Nursing Schools Today and Tomorrow* (1934). The 1928 report investigated the supply and demand of nurses; the 1934 report described the number of nursing schools and the type of educational experience they offered. The major recommendations of these reports were that nursing adopt a collegiate level of education, enrich the curriculum, and employ only faculty who had college degrees. This committee did not carry out the actual grading of nursing schools because of the large differences in programs throughout America.

At about the same time, a joint committee of the CNA and the Canadian Medical Association was established in 1929 to undertake a study of nursing education in Canada. This study was conducted by Dr. George M. Weir, a well-known educator and sociologist in the Department of Education of the University of British Columbia. Findings of this study, known as the *Survey of Nursing Education in Canada* (1932) and *the Weir Report*, reported serious weaknesses in hospital schools and recommended major reform. Recommendations of note were that (a) nurses needed a higher educational standard, (b) the system of nurse education needed to be removed from hospital control and brought into the general education system, and (c) that no hospital having fewer than 75 beds be recognized as competent to conduct an approved Training School (Weir, 1932). These findings, similar to those in the United States, led to a closing of a number of smaller training schools.

Another study on nursing service and education was conducted by Dr. Esther Lucille Brown in the 1940s. Dr. Brown, a sociologist, had previously conducted studies and published findings on the role of education in the professions of social work, engineering, medicine, and law. This landmark report, *Nursing for the Future*, published in 1948, viewed nursing service and education in terms of what was best to meet the needs of society. The purpose of the nursing education aspect of the study was to determine how a basic professional school of nursing should be organized, administered, controlled, and financed to prepare its graduates to meet community needs. Among Brown's 28 recommendations was a strong proposal supporting

> basic schools of nursing in universities and colleges, comparable in number to existing medical schools, that are sound in organizational and financial structure, adequate in facilities and faculty, and well-distributed to serve the needs of the entire country. (Brown, 1948, p. 178)

Diploma programs were the dominant nursing program from the late 1800s until the mid 1960s. Since that time, the number of these programs has continued to decline, even though most programs were associated with institutions of higher learning. In 1995 there were only 121 diploma programs in the United States (NLN 1995, p. 297). Some diploma programs have moved into nursing programs that grant baccalaureate degrees for nursing. These programs are referred to as "single purpose institutions."

Community College/Associate Degree Programs

Community college/associate degree nursing programs, which arose in the early 1950s, were the first and only educational programs for nursing that were systematically developed from planned research and controlled experimentation. Several trends and events influenced the development of these community college/associate degree programs in both the United States and Canada: (a) the Cadet Nurse Corps, (b) the community college movement, (c) earlier nursing studies, (d) the Canadian experiment, and (e) Dr. Montag's proposal for an associate degree.

The Cadet Nurse Corps of the United States was legislated and financed during World War II to provide additional nurses that would meet both military and home-based nursing needs. This Corps proved that qualified nurses could be educated in less time than the traditional 3 years. After World War II, the number of community colleges in the United States grew rapidly. The low tuition and "open door" policy of these colleges made higher education more accessible to all by offering the first 2 years of a 4-year college program. They also provided many vocational and adult education programs.

The studies conducted about nursing discussed earlier, such as the Goldmark Report, the Committee on Grading of Schools of Nursing, the Weir Report, and the Brown Report, also had a significant influence in the development of 2-year programs. The recommendations in all of these reports supported independent schools of nursing in institutions of higher learning separate from hospitals.

The Canadian experiment in nursing education also revealed that nurses could be equally prepared in 2 years instead of 3, provided that school authorities had complete control over the program. In 1948, the Canadian Nurses Association, with financing from the Red Cross, established the Metropolitan School of Nursing in Windsor, Ontario (CNA, 1968). This demonstration school was Canada's first independent school of nursing, separated financially and physically from a hospital. School authorities rather than hospital authorities directed the student's curriculum and clinical practice in the hospital. This pioneer project led to the establishment of the first nursing education program in an educational setting in Canada at the Ryerson Institute of Technology in 1963. The growth of similar independent schools of nursing in Canada was delayed until the community college system was developed in the 1970s and 1980s.

In the United States, associate degree programs were started after Mildred Montag published her doctoral dissertation in 1951, "The Education of Nursing Technicians," which proposed a 2-year education program for registered nurses (RNs) in the community college. Montag conceptualized a "nursing technician" or "bedside nurse" able to perform nursing functions broader than those of the practical nurse and smaller in scope than those of the professional nurse. The curriculum was to be an integrated one, half general education and half nursing, with careful selection of educational and clinical experiences. Emphasis was to be on education, not service. The program was intended to be complete in itself (terminal) and not a first step toward a baccalaureate degree. At the end of 2 years, the student was to be awarded an associate degree in nursing and be eligible to take the state board examination for registered nurse licensure. The first associate degree in nursing (ADN) program started at Columbia University Teachers' College in 1952 under the direction of Mildred Montag.

In 1952, an advisory committee was established by the American Association of Junior Colleges and the NLN to conduct cooperative research on nursing education in junior and community colleges. The objectives of this Cooperative Research Project were to describe the development of the associate degree nursing program, evaluate the graduates of these programs, and assess the future implications of the associate degree on nursing. This project, which included seven junior colleges and one hospital from six regions of the United States, was directed by Dr. Montag at Teachers College of Columbia University. Results of the project indicated (a) that 2-year nursing technicians could carry out the intended nursing functions, (b) that the program could be effectively set up in community colleges with the use of clinical facilities in the community, and (c) that the program attracted students. The success of this experiment and the rapid growth of community colleges encouraged the development of these programs. By 1965 there were 130 ADN programs; by 1996 there were 575 accredited programs (NLN, 1996, pp. 102–105).

Montag's original idea that these graduates be nursing technicians and that the degree become a terminal one did not materialize, however. In 1978, the ANA proposed a resolution about associate degree programs, stating that they were no longer to be considered terminal but part of a career upward mobility plan. Today many students enter an associate degree program with future intentions of continuing their education in nursing at the baccalaureate level.

Baccalaureate Programs

The first school of nursing in a university setting was established at the University of Minnesota in 1909. This program, however, differed little from the 3-year hospital program in curriculum and was therefore considered a superior diploma program. Students provided service to hospitals in exchange for education but received no higher education courses. Graduates were prepared for only the registered nurse certificate. It was not until 1919 that the University of Minnesota established its undergraduate baccalaureate degree in nursing. In the same year, the first baccalaureate degree program in nursing in the British Empire was established at the University of British Columbia in Vancouver, Canada (Street 1973, p. 115).

Most of the early baccalaureate programs were 5 years in length. They consisted of the basic 3-year diploma program in addition to 2 years of liberal arts. In 1919, there were eight baccalaureate programs in the United States. Growth of these programs was slow, in part because of prevailing attitudes about nursing and scholarly education for women. For example, nursing was considered a less-than-desirable vocation, and a liberal arts education and scholarship were thought to be incompatible for females, possibly posing problems for the marriage relationship. It must be remembered that not until 1920 were women granted the right to vote.

The eventual growth of baccalaureate education can be traced back to the Goldmark Report in 1923 and the Committee on the Grading of Nursing Schools in 1925. Both of these reports recommended that nursing schools be developed in institutions of higher learning. The Brown Report in 1948 added further impetus.

Today baccalaureate nursing programs are located in 4-year colleges and universities and are 4 to 5 years in length. The curriculum offers courses in the liberal arts, sciences, humanities, and nursing. Graduates must fulfill both the degree requirements of the college or university and the nursing program before being awarded a baccalaureate degree. The usual degree awarded in a bachelor of science in nursing (BSN).

It was not until the 1960s that the number of students enrolled in these programs increased markedly. By 1995, there were 581 baccalaureate programs of nursing in the United States (NLN 1995, 239–246).

Most baccalaureate programs admit registered nurses who have diplomas or associate degrees.

Some programs have special curricula to meet the needs of these students. Some universities also offer nursing students the opportunity to pursue a self-paced or independent study program. Many accept transfer credits from other accredited colleges and universities and offer students the opportunity to take challenge examinations when they believe they have the knowledge or skills taught in a course.

Now the baccalaureate degree is recommended as minimal preparation for entry into professional nursing practice. In 1965, the ANA recommended in a position paper that "Education for those who work in nursing should be placed in institutions of learning within the general system of education," that "minimal preparation for beginning professional nursing practice at the present time should be the baccalaureate degree education in nursing," and that "associate degree education in nursing should be the minimum preparation for beginning technical nursing practice" (ANA, 1966, p. 515). In Canada, the Canadian Nurses Association recommended the baccalaureate as entry level for professional practice in 1985. These recommendations arose out of concern for the increasing responsibilities nurses were expected to assume in response to the changing demands of health care and the need for nurses to keep pace with these changes to provide quality nursing.

Graduate Education

The earliest graduate nursing education programs originated in the late 1800s, at a time when any course work beyond the diploma was considered postgraduate education. Historical data about what is now considered graduate education (i.e., master's and doctoral preparation) is difficult to obtain because before the mid 1950s *all* postdiploma programs were grouped into the category of postgraduate education. Prior to that time, nursing instructors were under pressure to obtain advanced preparation in public health nursing, teaching, supervision, and in clinical nursing specialties. The first graduate courses and graduate program of study originated in 1899 at Columbia University Teachers' College (Donahue, 1985, p. 456).

Master's Programs The growth of university nursing programs encouraged the development of graduate study in nursing. In 1953 the newly established National League for Nursing encouraged educators to develop programs for master's degrees in nursing. The major emphasis of the programs was to be research and specialization for teaching and administration. In addition, regional planning for graduate education began in the 1950s with the creation of the NLN Subcommittee on Graduate Education (1954–1955), the Southern Regional Educational Board (SREB), and the Western Interstate Commission on Higher Education (WICHE).

The first *generic* master's programs were established at Yale and several other schools of nursing, which admitted students with a baccalaureate degree from a discipline other than nursing. These programs, leading to the graduate's initial professional degree in nursing and RN licensure, are now generally 2 years in length. Graduates of these programs demonstrate the same entry level competencies in nursing as do graduates from baccalaureate programs and are eligible to take the licensure examinations to become an RN. Today there are only a few generic master's programs. The first "clinical" master's degree (in psychiatric nursing) was offered at Rutger's University in New Jersey in 1954. By 1963, 32 master's programs were established. By the late 1960s, the master's degree in nursing had become widely recognized as significant for nurses in leadership roles. In Canada, the first master's program in nursing was established at the University of Western Ontario in London in 1959. This was followed by a program at McGill University in Montreal in 1961. By 1987, there were eleven master's programs in Canada.

In 1969, the ANA issued a *Statement on Graduate Education in Nursing* proclaiming that "the major purpose of graduate study in nursing should be the preparation of nurse clinicians capable of improving care through the advancement of nursing theory and science" (ANA, 1969). By the late 1970s, the proliferation of master's degree programs, which emphasized the preparation of clinical nurse specialists and nurse practitioners, had peaked.

In 1978, the ANA issued a new statement on graduate education that focused on "the preparation of highly competent individuals who can function in diverse roles, such as nurse generalists or specialists, researchers, theroreticians, teachers, administrators, consultants, public policy makers, system managers, and colleagues on multidisciplinary teams … prepared through master's, doctoral, and postdoctoral programs in nursing that subscribe to clearly defined standards of scholarships" (ANA, 1978, p. 8).

Today, master's programs vary considerably in admission requirements, length of program, curriculum, and costs. The degrees granted are the master of arts (MA), master in nursing (MN), master

of science in nursing (MSN), and master of science (MS). By 1995, there were about 234 nursing master's degree programs in the United States (NLN 1995, pp. 239–246).

In Canada, graduate education before 1965 stressed nursing education or administration as they related to "hospital" nursing or acute care. As a result, it was not unusual for public health nurses to obtain a master's degree in public health (MPH). By the 1970s there was a shift to a clinical specialization rather than a functional specialization. After 1980 the programs became less narrowly specialized (Field, Stinson & Thibodeaux, 1992, pp. 423–425).

Today master's degree programs may focus on an area of advanced clinical practice, such as psychiatric mental health nursing, or on areas such as administration or nursing management. See Chapter 23 for further information.

Doctoral Programs The historical development of doctoral education is also vague. It is thought that the first doctoral program for nurses was established at Columbia University Teachers College, offering an EdD in nursing in 1924. New York University started the first PhD nursing program in 1953, followed by the University of Pittsburgh in 1954 (Mataruzzo & Abdellah, 1971). In 1960 the first doctorate in nursing science (DNS) in psychiatric nursing was established at Boston University.

The first *generic* doctoral program in nursing was established at the Frances Payne Bolton School of Nursing at Case Western Reserve University in Chicago in 1979. This was a 3-year post non-nursing baccalaureate program. Other programs were established at Rush University in Chicago in 1988 and at the University of Colorado in 1990 (Forni, 1989). Because there were only a few doctoral programs in nursing before 1960, many nurses sought doctoral education in other fields, such as education and the behavioral and biologic sciences.

Development of doctoral programs in nursing was slow until the 1980s. Increased emphasis on nursing theory and research in the late 1980s provided impetus for the development of these programs. Doctoral programs in nursing award the degrees of doctor of nursing (DN), doctor of nursing science (DNS or DNSc), doctor of nursing education (DNEd), doctor of public health nursing (DPHN), doctor of education (EdD), and doctor of philosophy (PhD). Theoretically the PhD is a research degree, and the PhD candidate is expected to develop theory and to do basic research. The person with the professional doctorate (DNS, DNSc, DSN) is expected to use existing theory and engage in applied research (Meleis 1988, p. 436).

In Canada doctorate programs in nursing were not established until the late 1980s and early 1990s. The first nurse to obtain a PhD in nursing graduated from a conjoint program in 1990 offered by McGill University and the Université de Montréal (Field et al 1992).

CONSIDER...

- the pros and cons of the five levels of entry into registered nursing practice in the United States.
- your position in regard to the baccalaurcate degree as the entry to practice for registered nurses. Give your reasons.

Nursing Research

Although Florence Nightingale is generally considered the first "nurse researcher," her approach to and use of research had not been transmitted to America by the late 1800s. Research in nursing was hindered by the prevailing attitudes of rigid discipline and unquestioned obedience expected of nurses. Individualistic thought, creativity, and critical thinking or problem solving were discouraged. Nursing research in North America began in the 20th century with a 1912 research report, *The Educational Status of Nursing* by M. Adelaide Nutting. Since that time, the concept of research was introduced into nursing education programs, research journals in nursing were developed, and an Institute for Nursing Research was established. Nurses are now generating new knowledge and applying research in practice to improve client care. Details about the historical perspectives of nursing research are discussed in Chapter 11.

In the latter part of the 20th century, the development of nursing theories has also greatly increased the momentum toward nursing research (see Chapter 2).

SELECTED CONTEMPORARY ISSUES

Entry to Practice

In 1985, the ANA endorsed the baccalaureate degree (BSN) in nursing as the entry level for professional practice. According to the ANA's proposal, only the

baccalaureate graduate would be licensed under the legal title **registered nurse (RN).** The graduate with an associate degree in nursing would be considered a technical nurse and be licensed under the legal title **associate nurse (AN).** A timetable for implementation was established by the National Commission on Nursing Implementation Project (NCNIP, 1987).

This proposal has sparked vivid debates among graduates, students, and educators, some of whom perceive that it denigrates associate degree (AD) graduates. As a result, the National League for Nursing (NLN) has suggested that the title of *associate nurse* be replaced by *registered associate nurse*. However, this suggestion has not eliminated the controversy; many argue that AD graduates have held the title *registered nurse* since the inception of associate degree in nursing (ADN) programs and should retain that title.

As a professional organization, the ANA cannot legislate these changes. It is the responsibility of each state to define the legal boundaries of nursing practice and to designate the titles to be used by those practitioners who meet the individual state's criteria for licensure. If the ANA's proposal is to be accepted nationally, each state will need to adopt the proposal and implement its own changes in its licensure law. Some states have already initiated plans to implement these two levels of practice. Indeed, some states include the process of making nursing diagnoses and developing care plans in only the professional nurse's scope of practice. This has caused further concern to AD educators, who believe that 2-year graduates will be unable to obtain employment if these practices are not included in their practice acts.

If the ANA proposal is implemented, a grandfather clause would need to be considered for registered nurses who were educated in associate degree or diploma programs before the date of change. Under a grandfather clause, these nurses would retain the right to continue to be licensed and practice as registered nurses provided that their performance meets established standards. It should be noted, however, that a grandfather clause would protect only the nurse's license: If, for example, an institution required a minimum of a baccalaureate degree for the position of head nurse, an RN who is currently employed as a head nurse but who does not hold the baccalaureate degree would have no guarantee of retaining that position.

Licensure law changes also have major implications for diploma nurses and LPNs, because their status is not discussed in the proposal. In addition, this proposal entails that new standardized examinations must be developed to test the two levels of competence. This too has become a controversial issue in nursing, debated at state and national levels and among nurses of different educational backgrounds, nursing specialties, and clinical levels.

CONSIDER . . .

- the implications that implementing two levels of practice would have on titling and scope of practice. Does professionalism equate with baccalaureate education? What titles should be bestowed on the nonbaccalaureate graduate? Should terms such as *technical, associate,* or *professional* be used to describe nurses with RN licensure? Is the title *registered nurse associate* preferable to *associate nurse*?
- whether separate licensure and licensing examinations should be developed for BSN and AD graduates. Should separate licensing remain for LVNs or LPNs?
- how many categories of nursing practitioners there should be. Why?
- the position statements of your state/provincial nursing associations about nursing education and entry for practice.

Outcome-Based Education and Differentiated Practice

The need for delineating expectations of professional competency and differentiated educational preparation of nurses at all levels will be a challenge in years to come. Just as nursing practice is challenged to measure client outcomes, nursing education will be challenged to develop and refine graduate competencies of the associate degree, baccalaureate, master's, and doctoral programs.

Aydelotte (1992, p. 462) states that "the use of differences can be advantageous to all. The issue of differentiation deals with the preparation, roles, and relationship between professionals and paraprofessionals, the characteristics of each, and the need for both; the difference and interplay between generalists and specialists; the difference between careers and jobs; and the difference in the motivation of individuals and the career paths they choose." Differentiated competency statements that set clear practice expectations for all levels of nurses will enable nurses to practice as educated, encourage the

development of differentiated job descriptions, and may facilitate collaboration and mutual respect. Educators will be able to monitor the effectiveness of their programs more readily because the quality of education will be evaluated by what the graduates are actually able to do.

CONSIDER . . .

- how the functions of graduates from diploma, ADN, or BSN programs in your practice area differ or are similar.
- how you would differentiate the function of an AD or BSN nurse if you were the nurse manager of an acute care unit.
- the practice settings of ADNs and BSNs in your community. Do you think the practice settings of both kinds of nurses should be the same?
- how you would differentiate the functions of nurses with master's and doctoral degrees from those of the baccalaureate graduate.

Continuing Nursing Education and Continuing Competence

The major purpose of continuing education is to ensure continuing competence of practitioners and public safety. The major issues related to continuing education are whether it should be mandatory or voluntary and whether it guarantees continuing competence. Generally speaking, states and provincial (or territorial) associations do not impose specific requirements on licensed professionals to *demonstrate* their continuing competence to practice. However, in many states, continuing education is mandatory for licensees to renew their registration, licensure, or other qualification. (Mandatory continuing education was introduced in the United States in the 1970s, and now almost one-half of all state nursing boards require licensees to take continuing education courses). Opponents of mandatory continuing education argue that there is no evidence to support the effectiveness of mandatory education; that it cannot be assumed that participation in continuing education programs results in learning or competence; and that it violates adult learning principles, which emphasize self-directed, self-motivated learning. In addition, many continuing education programs are not available to all nurses, and there are no accreditation or approval mechanisms and tools to assess effectiveness. Because of these problems, many state nursing associations and Canadian nurses have chosen a voluntary approach. When a voluntary approach is used, incentives are often provided to motivate nurses who may be reluctant to participate in continuing education. Incentives include providing certificates of attendance to heighten nurses' portfolios and increasing the types of programs available. Several other factors may hinder or enhance participation in continuing education: (a) accessibility; (b) employer support that encourages time off with or without pay, permits alterations in work schedules, and offers financial help with registration fees; (c) family commitments; (d) type of credentials that increase opportunities for advancement on completion of the course; and (e) economic gains that nurses can receive by completing the course.

Effective means to evaluate nurses' competence remains an issue. McCrone (1995) states that "competence is knowledge, skills, judgment and the application of knowledge, skills and judgment. It is the application that is really important." However, evaluating nurses' competence is no easy task. Methods used include peer review (e.g., performance appraisals and chart audits), examinations, self-assessment tools, education and workplace accreditation, and quality assurance programs.

CONSIDER...

- previous continuing education courses you have attended. What motivated you to attend? What recognition did you receive for attending? How did the course influence your practice?
- your position on mandatory versus voluntary continuing education.
- factors that have hindered your attendance at a continuing education course. What could be done to eradicate these factors?
- whether health professionals should be tested periodically to demonstrate competence and to receive recertification or relicensure. What kind of testing would you recommend?
- whether mandatory refresher courses should be provided periodically to address new developments and new technologies.

Downsizing, Layoffs, and Restructuring

Changing trends in health care delivery are influencing patterns of nursing practice and nursing education. These trends include increasing costs, shortened lengths of hospital stay, increased acuity of clients in acute care hospitals, increased outpatient and community-based health care services, institutional downsizing, a changing skill mix with increased use of unlicensed assistive personnel (UAPs), and the rapid growth of informatives (use of knowledge technology).

Many hospitals have laid off nurses in the past few years. They are now decreasing their hiring of RNs and increasing the hiring of UAPs.

Layoffs are seriously affecting the employment opportunities for both practicing nurses whose employment is terminated and for new nursing graduates. Because more and more UAPs are being hired, most agencies are now looking for experienced nurses. Employment thus is becoming extremely competitive for experienced nurses. For new graduates, the question is how they can gain experience without a job.

In addition to downsizing, hospitals are also addressing their cost and quality care concerns by developing new delivery models, such as program management, patient-focused care, and case management (see Chapter 4); and by redefining job functions. Restructuring within agencies changes the role of nursing from the traditional department of nursing to teams of interdisciplinary delivery systems. As a result, job functions are also changing. For example, with loss of the traditional department of nursing, the role of senior nurse administrators or executives is being redefined. Restructuring gives rise to a number of concerns. First, there is concern that the voice of nursing will be overlooked. Second, as a result of decreases in middle management, caregiving staff will need to make more clinical and administrative decisions; do they have appropriate skills? Third, there will be a need to identify and monitor standards of nursing within a multidisciplinary context. Fourth, nurses will need to develop mechanisms to raise professional practice issues. New organizational supports will be necessary to help nurses meet their professional practice standards.

Additionally, many institutions have developed an integrated, cross-trained multifunctional worker who may or may not be licensed in a health care discipline (see page 22 for further information). The professional nurse, however, still retains responsibility and accountability for client care. Delegating functions and supervision of assistive personnel has thus become a major responsibility of the professional nurse. This responsibility can be troublesome for new inexperienced graduates who are still attempting to master skills themselves and often require assistance from the more experienced nurse.

Another major change in agencies is the use of management and nursing information systems to enhance nursing productivity and save dollars. Most hospitals are now using management information systems (MIS) for staffing, measuring acuity levels, and evaluating productivity. Nursing information systems (NIS) are programs that connect nurses with other departments, such as the pharmacy, the laboratory, the purchasing department, and other areas to obtain census data and to retrieve information. Many agencies, however, do not have systems that support nursing documentation (Manuel & Sorensen, 1995, p. 251). New programs are therefore needed to enhance nursing functions, and nurses themselves will need to be skilled in nursing informatics.

All of these changes in health care delivery have implications for nursing curricula of the future. Nurse educators need to prepare nurses who not only are able to provide health care in today's world but also are able to adapt to constant societal changes and needs while still providing quality care.

Changes recommended by the National League for Nursing in its 1993 publication "A Vision for Nursing Education" and by the Pew Health Professions Commission (1991), which advised nurse edu-

cators to shift away from acute-care-driven, institution-focused curricula because hospitals will need fewer nurses in the future (Shugars, O'Neil & Bader, 1991). The American Association of Colleges of Nursing (AACN) focused its recommendations for reform specifically on cognitive and interpersonal abilities (see the accompanying box).

CONSIDER...

- the pros and cons of increasing the numbers of unlicensed assistive personnel in your practice area. How will it affect your roles and functions?
- competencies you will need to become a leader within a multidisciplinary team. What continuing education programs or workshops would you recommend to help nurses meet these requirements?

Multiskilled Cross-Trained Practitioners

The multiskilled worker is an individual who can perform tasks or functions in more than one discipline. Multiskilling is a concept that is neither clearly defined nor evaluated. There are many interpretations of what multiskilling involves and many variations in the preparation of multiskilled workers. Some view multiskilling as "on the job training" for individuals to perform skills from several disciplines. For example, a trainee may be taught to obtain a 12-lead ECG and perform phlebotomy. Others say that individuals who are already certified in one profession can take on a second certification such as medical laboratory and X-ray technology, nursing and respiratory therapy, physical therapy and occupational therapy. Still others believe that a 4-year baccalaureate degree could be developed to prepare a multiskilled worker (Beachey, 1988, p. 319). Crissman and Jelsma (1990, p. 64A) suggest that cross-training can be used effectively in nursing departments to avoid layoffs and replace "floating practices"—periodic reassignments of nurses from an overstaffed area to an understaffed area. For example, intensive care unit (ICU) nurses may be cross-trained to function in the cardiac care unit (CCU), labor and delivery nurses to function in postpartum areas, or nurses in a newborn intensive care unit to function in the emergency department. Such cross-training broadens nurses' practice capacities and enhances their careers. Properly developed,

---

Essential Cognitive and Interpersonal Abilities

- Critical thinking
- Ethical decision making
- Information seeking, sorting, and selection
- Establishing and maintaining nurse-client relationships
- Therapeutic communication, including teaching and advocacy
- Coordination of care
- Interdisciplinary team participation
- Sensitivity to racial, ethical, and cultural diversity
- Critical self-assessment

SOURCE: Adapted from *Nursing Education's Agenda for the 21st Century* by the American Association of Colleges of Nursing, 1993, Washington, DC: ANA, p. 7.

cross-training programs can establish realistic expectations of cross-trained nurses. For example, using Benner's stages of expertise (see Chapter 7), a neonatal intensive care unit (NICU) nurse who is cross-trained for the emergency unit will be proficient or expert in the NICU, but in the emergency department, the nurse initially will be only a novice or advanced beginner and will require appropriate support.

Before training or education of multiskilled workers can begin, each discipline must delineate its professional competencies into tasks or skills, a process referred to as *quantification*. To some nurses, this process reduces caregiving to procedural tasks, turns nurses into technicians, and undermines the individualized needs of clients. From this perspective, multiskilling resembles multitasking.

According the MacIntyre (1981), one of the hallmarks of a professional practice is that "internal goods" are embedded in it. For example, to become excellent in the practice of nursing, the nurse must achieve certain standards of skilled practical knowledge, discretionary judgment, client advocacy, and moral agency. Jacques (1993, p. 4) refers to those internal goods as "invisible work." A nurse who administers medications or monitors an intravenous line (visible work), for example, is also at the same time performing invisible work such as gathering clinical assessment data, providing information or instructions for home care, communicating information to clients from others, and communicating in ways that establish a helping relationship. Benner (1991) emphasizes that professional practice requires

that nurses respond to the human concerns of the client in a particular situation. These caring responses involve preserving dignity, control, and autonomy and mobilizing hope in situations of fear and suffering. Such responses cannot be taught by rules; they are learned only within the overall tradition of nursing practice. It is for these reasons that some nurses oppose multiskilling.

Advocates of multiskilling suggest that if the objective is to optimize the RN's use of time, cross-training assistants will provide more support for the RN in nonprofessional tasks. They believe that the changing role of the nurse demands that nurses delegate more of their basic duties to health care assistants and auxiliary personnel. Delegation will enable nurses to take on functions normally associated with other health professionals. However, because of the potential for unsafe practice and ineffective or inappropriate use of nurses, appropriate staff education and follow-up must be provided for health care workers involved in multiskilling. Agencies need to identify and evaluate expected clinical outcomes of multiskilling. Its purpose should not be solely to provide a "quick fix" for rising costs.

CONSIDER . . .

- the pros and cons of multiskilled practitioners. In a practice setting you are familiar with, what activities would you consider for cross-training nonprofessional workers that would increase time for your professional functions?

READINGS FOR ENRICHMENT

Carnegie, M. E. (1995). *The path we tread: Blacks in nursing worldwide, 1854–1994* (3rd ed.). New York, NY: National League for Nursing.

This book chronicles the history of African Americans in nursing from 1854. African American nurses have made significant contributions to nursing and health care, forging paths for nurses of all cultural and racial heritages in all nations. The book is divided into eight sections, which describe the involvement of African American nurses in the Crimean War, the American Civil War, and the Spanish-American War; the development of education programs for African American

nurses; the involvement of African American nurses in professional nursing organizations and the U.S. military services; and nursing and health care in 17 African nations and 9 Caribbean nations. Dr. Carnegie provides a rich thread for the fabric of nursing history past and present, relating such little-known facts as (1) that Harriet Tubman and Sojourner Truth were nurses, (2) that a black nurse from Jamaica served with Florence Nightingale in the Crimea, (3) that Howard University, a school for African Americans in Washington, DC, established the first nursing program in a university setting in 1893.

→

READINGS FOR ENRICHMENT *continued*

Neidlinger, S. H., Bostrum, J., Stricker, A., Hild, J., & Zhang, J. Q. (1993, March). Incorporating nursing assistive personnel into a nursing professional practice model. *Journal of Nursing Administration, 23,* 29–37.

This article describes a pilot project in which nursing assistive personnel (NAP) were incorporated into the existing nursing professional practice model at a tertiary care university medical center. Each unit was given the responsibility of delineating the specific functions of its assistive personnel and the approach for integrating NAP into the existing model of practice. A plan to use permanent, unit-based NAP was developed, implemented, and evaluated. Researchers discovered that by redistributing selected nursing activities, the units were able to integrate NAP effectively to fulfill nonprofessional tasks and thus support the work of the registered nurse. The authors recommend that registered nurses receive more training in delegating tasks and supervising unlicensed assistive personnel.

Porter-O'Grady, T. (1994, Feb.). The real values of partnership: Preventing professional amorphism. *Journal of Nursing Administration, 24,* 11–15.

In response to cost constraints, many health care settings are implementing changes. "Multifunctional workers are being created, department walls are being torn down, service configurations are being redesigned, critical paths are being created, and new roles are emerging." Porter-O'Grady contends that the most disturbing trend in the redesigning and restructuring of the health care system is a deemphasis of the centrality of nursing. He discusses seven factors that limit the success of such efforts and provides eight principles to build real partnerships between nursing and other health care professions and create a positive integrated health care environment.

Schorr, T. M., & Zimmerman, A. (1988). *Making choices: Taking chances. Nurse leaders tell their stories.* St. Louis: Mosby.

This book includes autobiographies of over 40 contemporary nursing leaders, including Linda Aiken, Myrtle Aydelotte, Imogene King, Eleanor Lambertson, Madeleine Leininger, Mildred Montag, and Margretta Styles. These very personal stories written by the leaders themselves are rich in knowledge, history, and inspiration. Many write of the influence of nurses they had known; the support offered by parents, spouses, other family members, and close friends; their personal joys and heartaches; and their professional successes and failures. It is a remarkable account of career choices and chances.

Wilkinson, J. M. (1996, March/April). The C word. A curriculum for the future. *Nursing and Healthcare: Perspectives on Community* 17(2):72–77.

Wilkinson emphasizes that nursing education needs to be restructured to produce graduates who are prepared to assume a central role in helping to achieve cost-effective, quality health services. She believes that depth of content is lacking in current curriculums. "Differentiation and role specialization need to occur at the *undergraduate* level, a differentiation that occurs horizontally as well as vertically and at all levels." Wilkinson advocates a curriculum that offers a common core of studies for all nurses in the first year. A differentiated program would be offered in the second year; content would include either one of two tracks—intervention (illness care) or prevention (wellness care). Therefore, second-year students would choose to become licensed as either a registered nurse interventionist (RNI) or a registered nurse preventionist (RNP). Content for third-level studies (third and fourth years) and fourth-level studies (graduate education) is also discussed.

SUMMARY

Nursing is still evolving as a profession according to various criteria established by experts in the social sciences. Using Pavalko's eight criteria of a profession, certain characteristics of nursing, such as a code of ethics and relevance to social values, are highly developed; others, such as nursing theory, education, individual motivation, autonomy, commitment, and sense of community, are, to varying degrees, less developed.

Historical perspectives of nursing practice reveal recurring themes or influencing factors. For example, *women have traditionally cared for others but often in subservient roles. Religious orders left an imprint on nursing by instilling such values as compassion, devotion to duty, and hard work. Wars created an increased need for nurses and medical specialties. Science and technology have increased the complexity of care, necessitating change in the educational requirements of nursing and the need for specialization. Societal attitudes have influenced nursing's image. Visionary leaders have made notable contributions to improve the status of nursing.*

Nursing education has changed dramatically since the mid 1800s. Early apprenticeship programs established in the 1800s were designed to meet the service needs of the hospital, not the educational needs of the student. Today, nursing education is provided primarily in college and university settings independent of hospitals' needs—a concept proposed by Florence Nightingale. Growth of ADN programs in community colleges began in the 1950s after the demonstration school of nursing (Metropolitan School of Nursing) in Canada and Mildred Montag's proposal supported a 2-year education program for RNs. Although baccalaureate programs began in the early 1900s, baccalaureate education began to take hold only after the release of the 1923 Goldmark Report. The Brown, Weir, and other studies added further impetus. Master's and doctoral programs in nursing grew significantly in the latter part of the 20th century. Admission requirements, length of program, curriculum, and costs for these programs vary considerably.

Nursing research began in the early 1900s with M. Adelaide Nutting's research report, The Educational Status of Nursing. *Since that time, the concept of research has been introduced into nursing education programs, research journals in nursing have been developed, and the Institute for Nursing Research has been established. Nurses are now generating new knowledge and applying research in practice to improve client care. The development of nursing theories in the latter part of the 20th century has also greatly increased the momentum toward nursing research.*

Many controversial issues are affecting nursing. What should the entry level for practice be to prepare professional nurses for the future? Which nursing graduates should be entitled to licensure as an RN? If only baccalaureate nurses are eligible to be licensed as RNs, what should graduates of AD or 2-year community colleges and diploma programs be called? How do the functions of graduates from various nursing education programs differ? How many levels of nursing education should there be? Should all nurses be prepared to function in all practice areas? How can continuing competence of practitioners be ensured? Should nurse practice acts be standardized? Who should accredit and certify nursing education programs? How can nurses effectively deal with downsizing and restructuring to ensure quality care? Will multiskilled health care workers enhance or hinder professional nursing practice? These and other issues will require astute consideration and handling by nursing if it is to be truly effective in meeting the changing needs of society and, at the same time, further its development as a profession.

SELECTED REFERENCES

American Nurses Association. (1965, Dec.). ANA's first position on education for nursing. *American Journal of Nursing, 65,* 106–111.

American Nurses Association. (1969). *Statement on graduate education in nursing.* Kansas City, MO: Author.

American Nurses Association. (1973). *Standards of nursing practice.* Kansas City, MO: Author.

American Nurses Association. (1978). *Statement on graduate nursing education in nursing.* Kansas City, MO: Author.

American Nurses Association. (1979). First position paper on education for nursing. *American Journal of Nursing, 79,* 1231.

American Nurses Association. (1980). *Nursing: A social policy statement.* Kansas City, MO: Author.

American Nurses Association. (1984). *Standards for professional nursing education.* Washington, DC: Author.

American Nurses Association. (1985). *Facts about nursing 84–85.* Washington, DC: Author.

American Nurses Association. (1987). *Proceedings of the 1987 House of Delegates.* Washington, DC: Author.

American Nurses Association. (1991a). *Nursing and the American Nurses Association.* Washington, DC: Author.

American Nurses Association. (1991b). *Standards of clinical nursing practice.* Washington, DC: Author.

ANA delegates vote to limit RN title to BSN grads: "Associate nurse": wins vote for technical level. (1985, Sept.). *American Journal of Nursing, 85,* 1016, 1017, 1020, 1022, 1024, 1025.

Aydelotte, M. K. (1992). Nursing education: Shaping the future. In L. H. Aiken & C. M. Fagin, *Charting nursing's future: Agenda for the 1990s,* pp. 462–484. Philadelphia: Lippincott.

Barber, B. Some problems in the sociology of the professions. (1965). In K. S. Lynn, *The professions in America.* Boston: Houghton Mifflin.

Beachey, W. (1988, Nov.). Multicompetent health professionals: Needs, combinations, and curriculum development. *Journal of Allied Health, 17,* 319–329.

Bevis, E. O. (1989). *Curriculum building in nursing: A process* (3rd ed.). New York: National League for Nursing. Publication No. 15-2277.

Bixler, G. K., & Bixler, R. W. (1945, Sept.). The professional status of nursing. *American Journal of Nursing, 45,* 730.

Brown, E. L. (1948). *Nursing for the future: A report prepared for the National Nursing Council.* New York: Russell Sage Foundation.

Bullough, B., Bullough, V., & Soukup, M. (1983). *Nursing issues and strategies for the eighties.* New York: Springer.

Butter, I. H. (1989, March/April). Women's participation in health-care delivery: Recent changes and prospects. *Health Values,* 13:40–44.

Canadian Nurses Association. (1968). *The leaf and the lamp.* Ottawa: Author.

Canadian Nurses Association. (1985, Feb.). *CNA position statements.* Ottawa: Author.

Canadian Nurses Association. (1993). *Entrance requirements for nursing education programs in Canada.* Ottawa: Author.

Committee on the Grading of Nursing Schools. (1928). *Nurses, patients, and pocketbooks.* New York: NLNE.

Committee on the Grading of Nursing Schools. (1934). *Nursing schools today and tomorrow.* New York: NLNE.

Crissman, S., & Jelsma, N. (1990, March). Cross-training: Practicing effectively on two levels. *Nursing Management,* 21, 64A–64H.

Davis, J. (1966). *The nursing profession.* New York: Wiley.

Dickens, C. (1896). *Martin Chuzzlewit.* Boston: Estes and Lauriat.

Dolan, J. A., Fitzpatrick, M. L., & Herrmann, E. K. (1983). *Nursing in society: A historical perspective* (15th ed.). Philadelphia: W. B. Saunders.

Donahue, M. P. (1985). *Nursing: The finest art. An illustrated history.* St. Louis: Mosby.

Fahy, E. T. (1995, Jan./Feb.). If you don't know where you've been, how do you know where you are going? *Nursing and Health Care: Perspectives on Community,* 16, 5.

Field, P. A., Stinson, S. M., & Thibaudeau, M. F. (1992). Graduate education in nursing in Canada. In A. J. Baumgart & J. Larsen, *Canadian nursing faces the future* (2nd ed.) (pp. 421–445). St. Louis: Mosby-Year Book.

Fitzpatrick, M. (1983). *Prologue to professionalism.* Bowie, MD: Robert J. Brady.

Flexner, A. (1915). Is social work a profession? *Proceedings of the National Conference of Charities and Correction* (pp. 576–581). New York: New York School of Philanthropy.

Forni, P. R. (1987, Feb.). Nursing's diverse master's programs: The state of the art. *Nursing and Health Care,* 8, 70–75.

Forni, P. R. (1989, Oct.). Models for doctoral programs: First professional degree or terminal degree? *Nursing and Health Care,* 10, 428–434.

Goldmark, J. (1923). *Nursing and nursing education in the United States.* New York: Macmillan.

Hall-Long, B. A. (1995, Jan./Feb.). Nursing is past, present, and future political experiences. *Nursing and Health Care: Perspectives on Community,* 16, 24–28.

Henderson, V. (1966). *The nature of nursing: A definition and its implications for practice, research, and education.* New York: Macmillan.

Jacques, R. (1993, Winter). Untheorized dimensions of caring work: Caring as a structural practice and caring as a way of seeing. *Nursing Administrative Quarterly,* 17, 1–10.

Kalisch, P. A., & Kalisch, B. J. (1986). *The advance of American nursing* (2nd ed.). Boston: Little, Brown.

Kalisch, P. A., & Kalisch, B. J. (1987). *The changing image of the nurse.* Menlo Park, CA: Addison-Wesley Nursing.

Keeling, A. W., & Ramos, M. C. (1995, Jan./Feb.). The role of nursing history in preparing nursing for the future. *Nursing and Health Care: Perspectives on Community,* 16, 31–34.

Large, J. T. (1976, Oct.). Harriet Newton Phillips: The first trained nurse in America. *Image: Journal of Nursing Scholarship,* 8, 49–51.

Lenburg, C. (1984, June). Preparation for professionalism through regents external degrees. *Nursing and Health Care,* 5, 318–325.

Lewis, E. P. (1983, Sept./Oct.) News outlook: The issue that won't go away. A report on the 1983 NLN convention. *Nursing Outlook,* 31, 246–247.

MacIntyre, A. (1981). *After virtue.* Notre Dame, IN: University of Notre Dame Press.

Mataruzzo, J., & Abdellah, F. (1971). Doctoral education for nurses in the United States. *Nursing Research,* 20, 404–414.

McCrone, E. (1995, Sept. 6–9). Focusing on competence. Presentation at Council on Licensure, Enforcement and Regulation, 15th Annual Meeting, San Antonio, TX.

Meleis, A. (1988, Nov./Dec.). Doctoral education in nursing: Its present and its future. *Journal of Professional Nursing* 6:436–446.

Merton, R. K. (1958, Jan.). The function of the professional organization. *American Journal of Nursing,* 58, 50–54.

Miller, B. K. (1985, April). Just what is a profession? *Nursing Success Today,* 2, 21–27.

Moloney, M. M. (1986). *Professionalization of nursing: Current issues and trends.* Philadelphia: Lippincott.

Montag, M. L. (1951). *The education of nursing technicians.* New York: Putnam.

Montag, M. L. (1958). *Community college education for nursing.* New York: McGraw-Hill.

National Commission on Nursing Implementation Project (NCNIP). 1987. Timeline for transition into the future: Nursing education system for two categories of nurse. Milwaukee: National Commission on Nursing Implementation Project.

National Council of State Boards of Nursing. (1986). *A study of nursing practice and role delineation and job analysis of entry level performance of registered nurses.* Chicago: Author.

National League for Nursing. (1978). *Roles and competencies of graduates of diploma programs in nursing.* New York: Author.

National League for Nursing. (1979). *Competencies of graduates of nursing programs.* New York: Author.

National League for Nursing. (1990). *Competencies of the associate degree graduate on entry into practice* (2nd ed.). New York: Author.

National League for Nursing. (1993). *Vision for nursing education.* New York: NLN.

National League for Nursing. (1995). Baccalaureate and master's degree programs in nursing accredited by the National League for Nursing 1995–1996. *N&HC: Perspectives on Community, 16*(4):239–246.

National League for Nursing. (1995). Diploma programs in nursing accredited by the National League for Nursing 1995–1996. *N&HC: Perspectives on Community, 16*(5):297–298.

National League for Nursing. (1996). Associate degree programs accredited by the NLN 1996–1997. *N&HC: Perspectives on Community, 17*(2):102–108.

Nightingale, F. (1860). *Notes on nursing: What it is, and what it is not.* Commemorative Edition. Philadelphia: Lippincott.

NLN members agree to shelve entry issues and call for steps to spur career mobility. (1989, Aug.). *American Journal of Nursing, 89,* 1082–1083.

NLN seeks compromise on entry: ADNs hold out for RN licensure. (1987, Jan.). *American Journal of Nursing, 87,* 113, 124–125.

Pavalko, R. M. (1971). *Sociology of occupations and professions.* Itasca, IL: Peacock.

Pew Health Professions Commission. Report of the Taskforce on Health Care Workforce Regulation. (1995, Dec.). *Reforming health care workforce regulation: Policy considerations for the 21st century,* San Francisco: Author.

Phaneuf, M. C., & Lang, M. (1985). *Issues in professional nursing practice 7: Standards of nursing practice.* Washington, DC: ANA.

Primm, P. L. (1986, May/June). Entry into practice: Competency statements for BSNs and ADNs. *Nursing Outlook, 34,* 135–137.

Schuyler, C. B. (1992). Florence Nightingale. In F. Nightingale, *Notes on nursing: What it is, and what it is not.* Commemorative Edition. Philadelphia: Lippincott. pp. 3–17.

Schutzenhofer, K. K. (1987, Sep.-Oct.). The measurement of professional autonomy. *Journal of Professional Nursing, 3*(5): 278–283.

Shugars, D., O'Neil, E., & Bader, J. (1991). *Healthy America: Practitioners for 2005, an agenda for action for U.S. health professional schools.* Durham, NC: Pew Health Professions Commission.

Spence, J. T., Helmreich, R. L., & Stapp, L. L. (1974). The personal attribute questionnaire: A measure of sex-role stereotypes and masculinity-femininity. *JSAS Catalog of Selected Documents in Psychology, 4*:42, MS#617.

Strauss, A. (1966). The structure and ideology of American nursing: An interpretation. In J. Davis, *The nursing profession* (pp. 60–108). New York: Wiley.

Street, M. M. (1973). *Watch-fires on the mountains: The life and writings of Ethel Johns.* Toronto, Canada: University of Toronto Press.

Stull, M. K. (1986, May/June). Entry skills for BSNs. *Nursing Outlook, 34,* 138, 153.

Styles, M. M. (1982). *On nursing: Toward a new endowment.* St. Louis: Mosby.

Styles, M. M. (1983, Nov.). The anatomy of a profession. *Heart and Lung, 12,* 570–575.

Tracy, J. Samarel, N., & DeYoung, S. (1995, April). Professional role development in baccalaureate nursing education. *Journal of Nursing Education, 34,* 180–182.

Weir, G. M. (1932). *Survey of nursing education in Canada.* Toronto: University of Toronto Press.

Young, J. (1992, Feb./March). Changing nursing's image through professionalism. *Imprint: 39,* 50, 54–55.

2

CHAPTER

Nursing Theories and Conceptual Frameworks

OBJECTIVES

- Identify the purposes and essential elements of nursing theories.

- Differentiate the terms *concept, conceptual framework, concep-* *tual model, theory, construct, proposition,* and *hypothesis*.

- Discuss selected theories of nursing in terms of client, environment, health, and nursing.

- Describe the relationship of nursing theory to the nursing process and nursing research.

"There are two modes of acquiring knowledge, namely by reasoning and experience. Reasoning draws a conclusion and makes us grant the conclusion, but does not make the conclusion certain, nor does it remove doubt so that the mind may rest on the intuition of truth, unless the mind discovers it by the path of experience."

— Roger Bacon, 1928

Theory development is considered by many nurses to be one of the most crucial tasks facing the profession today. Historically, nurses have used knowledge derived from the physical and behavioral sciences, such as medicine, psychology, and sociology. As an increasingly emerging profession, nursing is now deeply involved in identifying its own unique knowledge base—that is, the body of knowledge essential to nursing practice, or a so-called nursing science. To identify this knowledge base, nurses must develop and recognize concepts and theories that are specific to nursing.

- Theories offer ways of looking at (conceptualizing) a discipline—such as nursing—in clear, explicit terms that can be communicated to others. Although most nurses have a clear idea of what nursing is, its uniqueness needs to be clearly stated to other health care workers and the public.
- Professionalism and a desire for collegial status with other health professionals have made the need for conceptual frameworks of nursing to be explicit. If nurses are to be considered health professionals, they must communicate exactly what makes their place in the interdisciplinary team unique and important.
- Theory development gained momentum in the 1960s and has progressed markedly since then through the work of several nurse theorists and the participation of nurses in theory conferences and in research to refine or validate the theories.
- Because opinions on the nature and structure of nursing vary, theories continue to be developed. Each theory bears the name of the person or group who developed it and reflects the beliefs of the developer.
- Nursing theories serve several essential purposes. See the accompanying box.

DEFINING TERMS

Before specific theories and conceptual frameworks can be understood, the terms *concept*, *conceptual*

Purposes of Nursing Theories and Conceptual Frameworks

Provide direction and guidance for (a) structuring professional nursing practice, education, and research; and (b) differentiating the focus of nursing from other professions.

In Practice

- Assist nurses to describe, explain, and predict everyday experiences.
- Serve to guide assessment, intervention, and evaluation of nursing care.
- Provide a rationale for collecting reliable and valid data about the health status of clients, which are essential for effective decision making and implementation.
- Help to establish criteria to measure the quality of nursing care.
- Help build a common nursing terminology to use in communicating with other health professionals. Ideas are developed and words defined.
- Enhance autonomy (independence and self-governance) of nursing through defining its own independent functions.

In Education

- Provide a general focus for curriculum design.
- Guide curricular decision making.

In Research

- Offer a framework for generating knowledge and new ideas.
- Assist in discovering knowledge gaps in the specific field of study.
- Offer a systematic approach to identify questions for study, select variables, interpret findings, and validate nursing interventions.

---

framework, *conceptual model*, and *theory* must be clarified. **Concepts,** the building blocks of theory, are abstract ideas or mental images of phenomena. Concepts are words that bring forth mental pictures of the properties and meanings of objects, events, or things. Concepts may be (a) readily observable, or *concrete*, ideas such as thermometer, rash, and lesion; (b) indirectly observable, or *inferential* ideas, such as pain and temperature; or (c) nonobservable, or *abstract* ideas, such as equilibrium, adaptation, stress, and powerlessness. Many concepts apply to nursing: concepts about human beings, health, helping relationships, and communication. Nursing theories address and specify relationships among four major abstract concepts referred to as the **metaparadigm** of nursing—the most global philosophical or conceptual framework of a profession. The term originates from two Greek words: *meta*, meaning *with*; and *paradigm*, meaning *pattern*.

There are four concepts considered to be central to nursing:

1. *Person* or *client*, the recipient of nursing care (includes individuals, families, groups, and communities).

2. *Environment*, the internal and external surroundings that affect the client. This includes people in the physical environment, such as families, friends, and significant others.

3. *Health*, the degree of wellness or well-being that the client experiences.

4. *Nursing*, the attributes, characteristics, and actions of the nurse providing care on behalf of, or in conjunction with, the client.

Each nurse theorist's definitions of these four major concepts vary in accordance with personal philosophy, scientific orientation, experience in nursing, and the effects of that experience on the theorist's view of nursing. See Table 2–1 for selected theorists' definitions and descriptions of person, environment, health, and nursing.

The terms *theory* and *conceptual framework* are often used interchangeably in nursing literature. Strictly speaking, they differ in their levels of abstraction; conceptual framework is more abstract than theory. A **conceptual framework,** viewed simply, is a group of related concepts. It provides an overall view or orientation to focus thoughts. A conceptual framework can be visualized as an umbrella under which many concepts can exist. A **conceptual model,** a term also used interchangeably with *conceptual framework*, is a graphic illustration or diagram of a conceptual framework. A **theory** is a supposition or system of ideas that is proposed to explain a given phenomenon. For example, Newton proposed his theory of gravity to explain why objects always fall from a tree to the ground. A *theory* goes one step beyond a *conceptual framework*; a theory relates concepts by using definitions that state significant relationships between concepts.

Theories generally include three elements:

1. A set of well-defined constructs or concepts. A **construct** is a concept that has been invented to suit a special purpose. It is measurable and can be observed in relation to other constructs. For example, "id," "ego," and "super ego" are constructs Sigmund Freud developed to explain the concept of personality. To use a nursing example, the constructs in Imogene King's (1981) theory of goal attainment include perception, communication, interaction, transaction, self, role, growth and development, stress, time, and space.

2. A set of **propositions,** statements that specify the relationships among the constructs. For example, one of the eight propositions King developed to describe the relationship among the concepts in her theory of goal attainment is that "if perceptual accuracy is present in nurse-client interactions, transactions (goal attainment) will occur" (King, 1981).

3. **Hypotheses,** conjectures that test the relationships between the constructs and propositions. Because theory is abstract, it cannot be applied to practice. Instead, hypotheses derived from the theory are tested. For example, a testable hypothesis derived from King's goal-attainment theory is that "perceptual accuracy in nurse-client interactions increases mutual goal setting" (King, 1981).

The major purpose of a conceptual framework is to give clear and explicit direction to the three areas of nursing: practice, education, and research. A theory, in contrast, is more limited in scope. Its primary purpose is to generate knowledge in a field. A theory explores phenomena, expresses relationships between facts, generates a hypothesis, and predicts future events and relationships.

Because the primary purpose of nursing theory is to generate scientific knowledge, nursing theory and nursing research are closely related. Scientific knowledge is derived from testing hypotheses (assumptions) generated by theories for nursing. Research determines the utility of those hypotheses, and research findings may be developed into theories for nursing. In the research process, comparisons are made between the observed outcomes of research and the relationship predicted by the hypotheses.

OVERVIEW OF SELECTED NURSING THEORIES

The nursing theories discussed in this chapter vary considerably (a) in their level of abstraction; (b) in their conceptualization of the client, health/illness, and nursing; and (c) in their ability to describe, explain, or predict. Some theories are broad in scope; others are limited. Only brief summaries of the theorist's central theme and basic assumptions are included here. For each theorist's definition and description of the client, environment, health, and nursing, see Table 2–1. The theories are presented in chronologic order according to dates of publication.

Theories and models can be viewed according to how they explain and relate the four concepts of the nursing metaparadigm (Wesley, 1995, p. 2).

1. *Developmental theories and models* focus on growth, development, and maturation. They emphasize *change* that occurs in specific stages, levels, or phases; are orderly and predictable; and occur in a particular direction. The goal is to maximize growth and development.

2. *Systems theories and models* focus on persons as open systems that receive input from the environment, process it, provide output to the environment, and receive feedback. During this process, the system strives for a balance between internal and external forces to maintain a dynamic tension of forces. The goal of systems theories and models is to view the whole rather than the sum of the parts.

3. *Interaction theories and models* emphasize the relationships among persons. They focus on the person as an active participant and on the person's perceptions, self-concept, and ability to communicate and perform roles. The goal is achievement through reciprocal interaction.

Nightingale's Environmental Theory

Florence Nightingale, often considered the first nurse theorist, defined nursing over 100 years ago as "the act of utilizing the environment of the patient to assist him in his recovery" (Nightingale, 1860). She linked health with five environmental factors: (1) pure or fresh air, (2) pure water, (3) efficient drainage, (4) cleanliness, and (5) light, especially direct sunlight. Deficiencies in these five factors produced lack of health or illness.

The above factors attain significance when one considers that sanitation conditions in hospitals of the mid 1800s were extremely poor and that women working in the hospitals were often unreliable, uneducated, and incompetent to care for the ill.

In addition to the factors above, Nightingale also stressed the importance of keeping the client warm, maintaining a noise-free environment, and attending to the client's diet in terms of assessing intake, timeliness of the food, and its effect on the person.

Nightingale set the stage for further work in the development of nursing theories. Her general concepts about ventilation, cleanliness, quiet, warmth, and diet remain integral parts of nursing and health care today.

TABLE 2–1 Theorists' Definitions/Descriptions of Four Major Concepts

Florence Nightingale (1860) Environmental theory

Person/Client	An individual with vital reparative processes to deal with disease and desirous of health but passive in terms of influencing the environment or nurse.
Environment	The major concepts for health are ventilation, warmth, light, diet, cleanliness, and absence of noise. Although the environment has social, emotional, and physical aspects, Nightingale emphasized the physical aspects.
Health	Being well and using one's powers to the fullest extent. Health is maintained through prevention of disease via environmental health factors. Disease is a reparative process nature institutes because of some want of attention.
Nursing	Provision of optimal conditions to enhance the person's reparative processes and prevent the reparative process from being interrupted.

TABLE 2–1 **Theorists' Definitions/Descriptions of Four Major Concepts** *continued*

Hildegard Peplau (1952, 1963, 1980) Interpersonal relations model

Person/Client	Focuses on the individual rather than families or communities. The individual is a developing organism living in an unstable equilibrium and striving to reduce anxiety.
Environment	Not specifically defined.
Health	Health means forward movement of the personality and other ongoing human processes in the direction of creative, constructive, productive, personal, and community living. It is promoted through the interpersonal process.
Nursing	A significant therapeutic and interpersonal process that functions with other human processes to make health possible. It is a human relationship between an individual who has a felt need or who is sick and a nurse who is educated to recognize and respond to the need for help.

Virginia Henderson (1955, 1966) Definition of nursing

Person/Client	A whole, complete and independent being who has 14 fundamental needs to breathe, eat and drink, eliminate, move and maintain posture, sleep and rest, dress and undress, maintain body temperature, keep clean, avoid danger, communicate, worship, work, play, and learn.
Environment	The aggregate of the external conditions and influences affecting the life and development of an organism.
Health	Viewed in terms of the individual's ability to perform 14 components of nursing care unaided (e.g., breathe normally, eat and drink adequately). Health is a quality of life basic to human functioning and requires independence and interdependence. It is the quality of health rather than life itself that allows people to work most effectively and to reach their highest potential level of satisfaction in life. Individuals will achieve or maintain health if they have the necessary strength, will, or knowledge.
Nursing	The unique function of the nurse is to assist clients, sick or well, in performing these activities contributing to health, its recovery, or peaceful death—activities that clients would perform unaided if they had the necessary strength, will, or knowledge. Also, to do so in such a way as to help clients gain independence as rapidly as possible.

Martha E. Rogers (1970, 1989) Science of unitary human beings

Person/Client	A unified whole possessing integrity and manifesting characteristics that are more than and different from the sum of its parts; an organized patterned energy field that continually exchanges matter and energy with the environmental energy field, resulting in continuous repatterning. The human being has the capacity for abstraction and imagery, language and thought, and sensation and emotion.
Environment	The irreducible, four-dimensional energy field identified by pattern and manifesting characteristics different from those of the parts. Each environmental field is specific to its given human field. They are identified by wave patterns manifesting continuous change, and both change continuously and creatively.
Health	Positive health symbolizes wellness. It is a value term defined by the culture or individual. Health and illness are considered "to denote behaviors that are of high value and low value."
Nursing	A humanistic science dedicated to compassionate concern with maintaining and promoting health, preventing illness, and caring for and rehabilitating the sick and disabled. Nursing seeks to promote symphonic interaction between the environment and the person, to strengthen the coherence and integrity of the human beings, and to direct and redirect patterns of interaction between the person and the environment for the realization of maximum health potential.

TABLE 2–1 *continued*

Dorothea E. Orem (1971, 1980, 1985, 1991, 1995) General theory of nursing

Person/Client	A unity who can be viewed as functioning biologically, symbolically, and socially and who initiates and performs self-care activities on own behalf in maintaining life, health, and well-being; self-care activities deal with air, water, food, elimination, activity and rest, solitude and social interaction, prevention of hazards to life and well-being, and promotion of human functioning.
Environment	The environment is linked to the individual, forming an integrated and interactive system.
Health	Health is a *state* that is characterized by soundness or wholeness of developed human structures and of bodily and mental functioning. It includes physical, psychologic, interpersonal, and social aspects. *Well-being* is used in the sense of individuals' perceived condition of existence. Well-being is a state characterized by experiences of contentment, pleasure, and certain kinds of happiness; by spiritual experiences; by movement toward fulfillment of one's self-ideal; and by continuing personalization. Well-being is associated with health, with success in personal endeavors, and with sufficiency of resources.
Nursing	A helping or assisting service to persons who are wholly or partly dependent—infants, children, and adults—when they, their parents, guardians, or other adults responsible for their care are no longer able to give or supervise their care. A creative effort of one human being to help another human being. Nursing is deliberate action, a function of the practical intelligence of nurses, and action to bring about humanely desirable conditions in persons and their environments. It is distinguished from other human services and other forms of care by its focus on human beings.

Imogene King (1971, 1981) Goal attainment theory

Person/Client	Three interacting systems: individuals (personal systems), groups (interpersonal systems), and society (social systems); the personal system is a unified, complex, whole self who perceives, thinks, desires, imagines, decides, identifies goals, and selects means to achieve them.
Environment	Adjustments to life and health are influenced by an individual's interactions with environment. The environment is constantly changing.
Health	A dynamic state in the life cycle; illness is an interference in the life cycle. Health implies continuous adaptation to stress in the internal and external environments through the use of one's resources to achieve maximum potential for daily living.
Nursing	A helping profession that assists individuals and groups in society to attain, maintain, and restore health. If this is not possible, nurses help individuals die with dignity. Nursing is perceiving, thinking, relating, judging, and acting vis-à-vis the behavior of individuals who come to a nursing situation. A nursing situation is the immediate environment, spatial and temporal reality, in which nurse and client establish a relationship to cope with health states and adjust to changes in activities of daily living if the situation demands adjustment. It is an interpersonal process of action, reaction, interaction, and transaction whereby nurse and client share information about their perceptions in the nursing situation.

Betty Neuman (1974, 1982, 1989, 1995) Systems model

Person/Client	Open system consisting of a basic structure or central core of survival factors surrounded by concentric rings that are bounded by lines of resistance, a normal line of defense, and a flexible line of defense. The total person is a composite of physiologic, psychologic, sociocultural, and developmental variables.

→

TABLE 2–1   Theorist's Definitions/Descriptions of Four Major Concepts *continued*

Betty Neuman *continued*

Environment	Both internal and external environments exist and a person maintains varying degrees of harmony and balance between them. It is all factors affecting and affected by the system.
Health	Wellness is the condition in which all parts and subparts of an individual are in harmony with the whole system. Wholeness is based on interrelationships of variables that determine the resistance of an individual to any stressor. Illness indicates lack of harmony among the parts and subparts of the system of the individual. Health is viewed as a point along a continuum from wellness to illness; health is dynamic (i.e., constantly subject to change). Optimal wellness or stability indicates that all a person's needs are being met. A reduced state of wellness is the result of unmet systemic needs. The individual is in a dynamic state of wellness-illness, in varying degrees, at any given time.
Nursing	A unique profession in that it is concerned with all of the variables affecting an individual's response to stressors, which are intra-, inter-, and extrapersonal in nature. The concern of nursing is to prevent stress invasion, or, following stress invasion, to protect the client's basic structure and obtain or maintain a maximum level of wellness. The nurse helps the client, through primary, secondary, and tertiary prevention modes, to adjust to environmental stressors and maintain client system stability.

Sister Callista Roy (1970, 1976, 1984, 1991) Adaptation model

Person/Client	A biopsychosocial being who is in constant interaction with the environment and who has four modes of adaptation, based on *physiologic needs*, *self-concept* (physical self, moral-ethical self, self-consistency, self-ideal and expectancy, and self-esteem), *role function*, and *interdependence relations*.
Environment	All the conditions, circumstances, and influences surrounding and affecting the development and behavior of persons or groups; the input into the person as an adaptive system involving both internal and external factors.
Health	A state and a process of being and becoming an integrated and whole person. Lack of integration represents lack of health.
Nursing	A theoretical system of knowledge that prescribes a process of analysis and action related to the care of the ill or potentially ill person. As a science, nursing is a developing system of knowledge about persons used to observe, classify, and relate the processes by which persons positively affect their health status. As a practice discipline, nursing's scientific body of knowledge is used to provide an essential service to people, that is, to promote ability to affect health positively.

Jean Watson (1979, 1985, 1988) Human caring theory

Person/Client	Viewed as greater than and different from the sum of the parts and to be valued, cared for, respected, nurtured, understood, and assisted. The individuality of each person is important.
Environment	Encompasses social, cultural, and spiritual aspects and all of the influences of society, which provides value to determine how a person should behave and the goals to strive toward.
Health	Encompasses a high level of overall physical, mental, and social functioning. It is a subjective state, one which each person defines.
Nursing	Combines the research process with the problem-solving approach and is concerned with promoting and restoring health, preventing illness, and caring for the sick. The nurse uses a caring process to help the individual achieve an optimal degree of inner harmony to promote self-knowledge, self-healing, and/or insight into the meaning of life.

TABLE 2–1 *continued*

Rosemarie Parse (1981, 1989, 1995) Human becoming theory

Person/Client An open being, more than and different from the sum of its parts, in mutual simultaneous interchange with the environment, who chooses from options (value priorities) and bears responsibility for choices. The person participates with the universe in creating patterns and is recognized by these patterns.

Environment Human beings and the "universe" (environment) are inseparable—interchanging energy, unfolding together for greater complexity and diversity and influencing one another's rhythmic patterns of relating. Humans and the environment interchange energy to create what is in the world, and each person chooses the meaning given to the situation he or she creates.

Health A lived experience, a synthesis of values, a way of living, and a rhythmic process of being and becoming.

Nursing A human science that focuses on the quality of the client's life from the client's perspective and involves innovation and creativity. The nurse is responsible for guiding individuals and families in choosing possibilities for changing the health process.

Madeleine Leininger (1985, 1988, 1991) Culture care diversity and universality theory

Person/Client Human beings are caring and capable of feeling concern for others; caring about human beings is universal, but ways of caring vary across cultures.

Environment Not specifically defined, but concepts of world view, social structure, and environmental context are closely related to the concept of culture.

Health A state of well-being that is culturally defined, valued, and practiced. Is universal across cultures but is defined differently by each culture. It includes health systems, health care practices, health patterns, and health maintenance and promotion.

Nursing A learned humanistic art and science that focuses on personalized behaviors, functions, and processes to promote and maintain health or recovery from illness. It has physical, psychosocial, and cultural significance for those being assisted. It uses a problem-solving approach, as depicted in the Sunrise Model, and uses three models of action: culture care preservation, culture care accommodation, and culture care repatterning.

Peplau's Interpersonal Relations Model

Hildegard Peplau, a psychiatric nurse, introduced her interpersonal concepts in 1952 and based them on available theories at the time: psychoanalytic theory, principles of social learning, and concepts of human motivation and personality development. *Psychodynamic nursing* is defined as understanding one's own behavior to help others identify felt difficulties and applying principles of human relations to problems arising during the experience.

Peplau views nursing as a maturing force that is realized as the personality develops through educational, therapeutic, and interpersonal processes.

Nurses enter into a personal relationship with an individual when a felt need is present. This nurse-client relationship evolves in four phases:

1. *Orientation.* During this phase, the client seeks help, and the nurse assists the client to understand the problem and the extent of need for help.

2. *Identification.* During this phase, the client assumes a posture of dependence, interdependence, or independence in relation to the nurse (relatedness). The nurse's focus is to assure the person that the nurse understands the interpersonal meaning of the client's situation.

3. *Exploitation.* In this phase, the client derives full value from what the nurse offers through the

relationship. The client uses available services on the basis of self-interest and needs. Power shifts from the nurse to the client.

4. *Resolution.* In this final phase, old needs and goals are put aside and new ones adopted. Once older needs are resolved, newer and more mature ones emerge.

During the nurse-client relationship, nurses assume many roles: stranger, teacher, resource person, surrogate, leader, and counselor. Today, Peplau's model continues to be used by clinicians when working with individuals who have psychologic problems.

Henderson's Definition of Nursing

Virginia Henderson is well known for her *Textbook on the Principles and Practice of Nursing* (1955), co-authored with Canadian nurse Bertha Harmer; her subsequent publications including *The Nature of Nursing* (1966); and numerous scholarly papers. She was motivated to develop her ideas because she was dissatisfied with the emphasis that nursing education programs placed on technical competence and mastery of nursing procedures; her experiences in psychiatric, pediatric, and community health nursing were other major influences.

In 1955, Henderson formulated a definition of the unique function of nursing. This definition was a major stepping-stone in the emergence of nursing as a discipline separate from medicine. She wrote, "The unique function of the nurse is to assist the individual, sick or well, in the performance of those activities contributing to health or its recovery (or to peaceful death) that he would perform unaided if he had the necessary strength, will, or knowledge, and to do this in such a way as to help him gain independence as rapidly as possible" (Henderson, 1966, p. 3). Like Nightingale, Henderson described nursing in relation to the client and the client's environment. Unlike Nightingale, Henderson saw the nurse as concerned with both well and ill individuals, acknowledged that nurses interact with clients even when recovery may not be feasible, and mentioned the teaching and advocacy roles of the nurse.

Basic to her definition are various assumptions about the individual: namely, that the individual (a) needs to maintain physiologic and emotional balance, (b) requires assistance to achieve health and independence or a peaceful death, and (c) needs the necessary strength, will, or knowledge to achieve or maintain health. These needs give direction to the nurse's role.

Henderson conceptualized the nurse's role as assisting sick or well individuals in a supplementary or complementary way. The nurse needs to be a partner with the client, a helper to the client, and, when necessary, a substitute for the client. The nurse's focus is to help individuals and families (which she viewed as a unit) to gain independence in meeting 14 fundamental needs (Henderson, 1966):

1. Breathing normally

2. Eating and drinking adequately

3. Eliminating body wastes

4. Moving and maintaining a desirable position

5. Sleeping and resting

6. Selecting suitable clothes

7. Maintaining body temperature within normal range by adjusting clothing and modifying the environment

8. Keeping the body clean and well-groomed to protect the integument

9. Avoiding dangers in the environment and avoiding injuring others

10. Communicating with others in expressing emotions, needs, fears, or opinions

11. Worshiping according to one's faith

12. Working in such a way that one feels a sense of accomplishment

13. Playing or participating in various forms of recreation

14. Learning, discovering, or satisfying the curiosity that leads to normal development and health, and using available health facilities

Henderson has published many works and continues to be cited in current nursing literature. Her emphasis on the importance of nursing's independence from, and interdependence with, other health care disciplines is well recognized.

Rogers' Science of Unitary Human Beings

Martha Rogers first presented her theory of unitary human beings in 1970. It contains complex conceptualizations related to multiple scientific disciplines. Her theory was influenced by Einstein's theory of relativity, which introduced the four coordinates of space-time; Burr and Northrop's electrodynamic theory of life, which revealed the pattern and organization of the electrodynamic field; von Bertalanffy's general systems theory; and many other disciplines, such as anthropology, psychology, sociology, astronomy, religion, philosophy, history, biology, and literature.

Rogers views the person as an irreducible whole, the whole being greater than the sum of its parts. *Whole* is differentiated from *holistic*, the latter often being used to mean only the sum of all the parts. She states that humans are dynamic energy fields in continuous exchange with environmental fields, both of which are infinite. Both human and environmental fields are characterized by pattern, a universe of open systems, and four-dimensionality. According to Rogers, *unitary man*

- Is an irreducible, four-dimensional energy field identified by pattern.
- Manifests characteristics different from the sum of the parts.
- Interacts continuously and creatively with the environment.
- Behaves as a totality.
- As a sentient being, participates creatively in change.

Key concepts Rogers uses to describe the individual and the environment are energy fields, openness, pattern and organization, and multidimensionality. *Energy fields* are the fundamental level of humans and the environment (all that is outside a given human field). Energy fields are dynamic, constantly exchanging energy from one to the other. The concept of *openness* holds that the energy fields of humans and the environment are open systems, that is, infinite, integral with one another, and in continuous process. *Pattern* refers to the unique identifying behaviors, qualities, and characteristics of the energy fields that change continuously and innovatively. Rogers defines *four-dimensionality* as a nonlinear domain without temporal or spiritual attributes. All reality is considered to be four-dimensional.

To Rogers, the life process in humans is homeodynamic, involving continuous and creative change. She provides three principles of homeodynamics to offer a way of perceiving how unitary human beings develop: integrality (formerly complementarity), resonance, and helicy. According to the principle of *integrality*, the human and environmental fields interact mutually and simultaneously. *Resonancy*

means the wave pattern in the fields change continuously and from lower- to higher-frequency patterns. *Helicy* postulates that the field changes are innovative, probabilistic, and characterized by increasing diversity of field patterns and repeating rhythmicities.

Nurses applying Rogers' theory in practice (a) focus on the person's wholeness, (b) seek to promote symphonic interaction between the two energy fields (human and environment) to strengthen the coherence and integrity of the person, (c) coordinate the human field with the rhythmicities of the environmental field, and (d) direct and redirect patterns of interaction between the two energy fields to promote maximum health potential.

Some find Rogers' concepts difficult to understand, but a specific example can help clarify them. Nurses' use of therapeutic touch is based on the concept of human energy fields (see Chapter 19). The human energy field is identified by pattern. The qualities of the field vary from person to person and are affected by pain and illness. Although the field is infinite, realistically it is most clearly "felt" within several feet of the body. The nurse trained in therapeutic touch can assess and feel the energy field and manipulate it to help a person manage pain.

Orem's General Theory of Nursing

Dorothea Orem's theory, first published in 1971, has been widely accepted by the nursing community. It includes three related concepts: self-care, self-care deficit, and nursing systems.

Self-Care

Self-care theory postulates that self-care and the self-care of dependents are learned behaviors that individuals initiate and perform on their own behalf to maintain life, health, and well-being. Self-care theory is based on four concepts: self-care, self-care agency, self-care requisites, and therapeutic self-care demand. *Self-care* refers to those activities an individual performs independently throughout life to promote and maintain personal well-being. *Self-care agency* is the individual's ability to perform self-care activities. It consists of two agents: a *self-care agent* (an individual who performs self-care independently) and a *dependent care agent* (a person other than the individual who provides the care). Adults care for themselves, whereas infants, the aged, the ill, and the disabled require assistance with self-care activities.

Self-care requisites, also called *self-care needs*, are measures or actions taken to provide self-care. There are three categories of self-care requisites:

1. *Universal requisites* are common to all people. They include maintaining intake and elimination of air, water, and food; balancing rest, solitude, and social interaction; preventing hazards to life and well-being; and promoting normal human functioning.

2. *Developmental requisites* result from maturation or are associated with conditions or events, such as adjusting to a change in body image or to the loss of a spouse.

3. *Health deviation requisites* result from illness, injury, or disease or its treatment. They include actions such as seeking health care assistance, carrying out prescribed therapies, and learning to live with the effects of illness or treatment.

Therapeutic self-care demand refers to all self-care activities required to meet existing self-care requisites or, in other words, the use of actions to maintain health and well-being (Figure 2–1).

Self-Care Deficit

Self-care deficit theory asserts that people benefit from nursing because they have health-related limitations in providing self-care. These limitations may result from illness, injury, or from the effects of medical tests or treatments. Two variables affect these deficits: self-care agency (ability) and therapeutic self-care demands (the measures of care required to meet existing requisites). *Self-care deficit* results when self-care agency is not adequate to meet the known self-care demand. Orem's self-care deficit theory explains not only when nursing is needed but also how people can be assisted through five methods of helping: acting or doing for, guiding, teaching, supporting, and providing an environment that promotes the individual's abilities to meet current and future demands.

Nursing Systems

Nursing systems theory postulates that nursing systems form when nurses prescribe, design, and provide nursing that regulates the individual's self-care capabilities and meets therapeutic self-care requirements. Orem identifies three types of nursing systems:

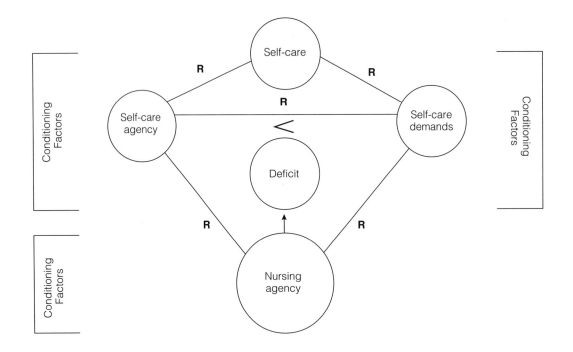

FIGURE 2–1 *The major components of Orem's self-care deficit theory. "R" indicates a relationship between components; "<" indicates a current or potential deficit where nursing would be required.*

SOURCE: From *Nursing Concepts of Practice* (4th ed.) by D. E. Orem, 1991, St. Louis, Mosby-Year Book, p. 64. Reprinted with permission.

1. *Wholly compensatory* systems are required for individuals who are unable to control and monitor their environment and process information.

2. *Partly compensatory* systems are designed for individuals who are unable to perform some (but not all) self-care activities.

3. *Supportive-educative (developmental)* systems are designed for persons who need to learn to perform self-care measures and need assistance to do so (Figure 2–2).

The five methods of helping discussed above can be used in each nursing system.

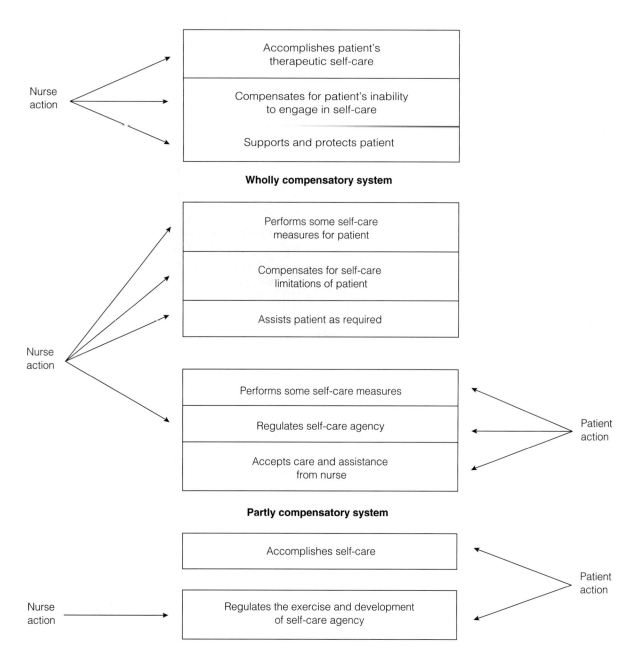

FIGURE 2–2 *Orem's basic nursing systems.*

Source: From *Nursing Concepts of Practice* (5th ed) by D. E. Orem, 1995, St. Louis: Mosby, p. 307. Used with permission.

King's Goal Attainment Theory

Imogene King's theory of goal attainment is based on systems theory, the behavioral sciences, and deductive and inductive reasoning. She first published *Toward a Theory for Nursing: General Concepts of Human Behavior* in 1971. Initially, King formulated her theory as a conceptual framework for nursing when, as an associate professor of nursing at Loyola University in Chicago, she developed a master's degree program in nursing. King refined her concepts in her 1981 publication, *A Theory for Nursing: Systems, Concepts, Process.*

King's theory consists of three dynamic interacting systems: (a) personal systems (individuals), (b) interpersonal systems (groups), and (c) social systems (society). Key concepts are identified for each system as follows:

1. Personal system concepts: perception, self, body image, growth and development, space and time

2. Interpersonal system concepts: interaction, communication, transaction, role, stress, and coping

3. Social system concepts: organization, authority, power, status, and decision making

The client and nurse are personal systems or subsystems within interpersonal and social systems. To identify problems and to establish goals, the nurse and client perceive one another, act and react, interact, and transact. *Transactions* are defined as purposeful interactions that lead to goal attainment. Transactions have the following characteristics:

- They are basic to goal attainment and include social exchange, bargaining and negotiating, and sharing a frame of reference toward mutual goal setting.
- They require perceptual accuracy in nurse-client interactions and congruence between role performance and role expectation for nurse and client.
- They lead to goal attainment, satisfaction, effective care, and enhanced growth and development.

King postulates seven hypotheses in goal attainment theory:

1. Perceptual congruence in nurse-client interactions increases mutual goal setting.

2. Communication increases mutual goal setting between nurses and clients and leads to satisfactions.

3. Satisfactions in nurses and clients increase goal attainment.

4. Goal attainment decreases stress and anxiety in nursing situations.

5. Goal attainment increases client learning and coping ability in nursing situations.

6. Role conflict experienced by clients, nurses, or both decreases transactions in nurse-client interactions.

7. Congruence in role expectations and role performance increases transactions in nurse-client interactions.

King's theory highlights the importance of the participation of all individuals in decision making and deals with the choices, alternatives, and outcomes of nursing care. The theory offers insight into nurses' interactions with individuals and groups within the environment.

Neuman's Systems Model

Betty Neuman, a community health nurse and clinical psychologist, began developing her model while lecturing in community health nursing at the University of California at Los Angeles. The model is based on Gestalt theory, Selye's stress theory, and general systems theory. Neuman's model was first published in 1972 in *Nursing Research* in an article co-authored by R. J. Young, "Model for Teaching Total Person Approach to Patient Problems." Refinements were published as the Neuman Systems Model in 1974, 1982, 1989, and 1995.

Neuman's systems model is based on the individual's relationship to stress, the reaction to it, and reconstitution factors that are dynamic in nature. *Reconstitution* is the state of adaptation to stressors.

Neuman views the client as an open system consisting of a basic structure or central core of energy resources (physiologic, psychologic, sociocultural, developmental, and spiritual) surrounded by two concentric boundaries or rings referred to as *lines of resistance* (Figure 2–3). The lines of resistance represent internal factors that help the client defend against a stressor; one example is an increase in the body's leukocyte count to combat an infection. Outside the lines of resistance are two lines of defense. The inner or *normal line of defense*, depicted as a solid line, represents the person's state of equilibrium or the state of adaptation developed and maintained over time and considered normal for that person. The *flexible line of defense*, depicted as a broken line, is dynamic and can be rapidly altered over a short period of time. It is a protective buffer

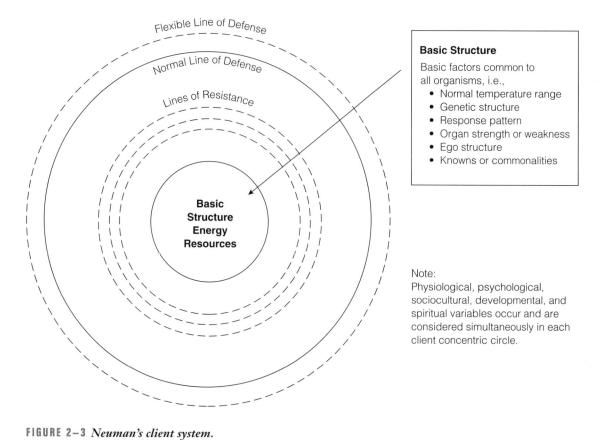

Basic Structure

Basic factors common to
all organisms, i.e.,

- Normal temperature range
- Genetic structure
- Response pattern
- Organ strength or weakness
- Ego structure
- Knowns or commonalities

Basic
Structure
Energy
Resources

Note:
Physiological, psychological,
sociocultural, developmental, and
spiritual variables occur and are
considered simultaneously in each
client concentric circle.

Flexible Line of Defense

Normal Line of Defense

Lines of Resistance

FIGURE 2–3 *Neuman's client system.*

SOURCE: From *The Neuman Systems Model* (3rd ed.) by B. Neuman, 1995, Norwalk, CT: Appleton & Lange, p. 26.
Used with permission.

that prevents stressors from penetrating the normal line of defense. Certain variables (e.g., sleep deprivation) can create rapid changes in the flexible line of defense.

Neuman describes a *stressor* as any environmental force that alters the system's stability. Stressors are categorized as *intrapersonal stressors*, those that occur within the individual (e.g., an infection); *interpersonal stressors*, those that occur between individuals (e.g., unrealistic role expectations); and *extrapersonal stressors*, those that occur outside the person (e.g., financial concerns). The individual's reaction to stressors depends on the strength of the lines of defense. When the lines of defense fail, the resulting reaction depends on the strength of the lines of resistance. As part of the reaction, a person's system can adapt to a stressor, an effect known as *reconstitution.*

Nursing interventions focus on retaining or maintaining system stability. These interventions are carried out on three preventive levels:

1. *Primary prevention* identifies risk factors, attempts to eliminate the stressor, and focuses on protecting the normal line of defense and strengthening the flexible line of defense. A reaction has not yet occurred, but the degree of risk is known.

2. *Secondary prevention* relates to interventions or active treatment initiated after symptoms have occurred. The focus is to strengthen internal lines of resistance, reduce the reaction, and increase resistance factors.

3. *Tertiary prevention* refers to intervention following that in the secondary stage. It focuses on readaptation and stability and protects reconstitution or return to wellness following treatment. The nurse emphasizes educating the client in strengthening resistance to stressors and ways to help prevent recurrence of reaction or regression.

Betty Neuman's model of nursing has been widely accepted by the nursing community, nationally and internationally. It is applicable to a variety of nursing practice settings involving individuals, families, groups, and communities.

Roy's Adaptation Model

Sister Callista Roy's adaptation model, widely used by nurse educators, researchers, and practitioners, was introduced in 1970 in *Nursing Outlook* as "Adaptation: A Conceptual Framework in Nursing." The model was published in book form in 1976 and 1984 as *Introduction to Nursing: An Adaptation Model* and in 1991 as *The Roy Adaptation Model: The Definitive Statement*. Roy, a nurse and sociologist, based her theory on Harry Helson's work in psychophysics and on her observations of the great resilience of children and their ability to adapt to major physical and psychologic changes.

Roy focuses on the individual as a biopsychosocial adaptive system that employs a feedback cycle of input, throughput, and output. Both the individual and the environment are sources of stimuli that require modification to promote adaptation, an ongoing purposive response. Adaptive responses contribute to health, which she defines as the process of being and becoming integrated; ineffective or maladaptive responses do not contribute to health. Each person's adaptation level is unique and constantly changing.

As an open system, an individual receives *input* or stimuli from both the self and the environment. Roy identifies three classes of stimuli:

1. *Focal stimuli:* the internal or external stimuli most immediately confronting the person and contributing to behavior

---

RESEARCH NOTE

How Do Nurses View the Usefulness of Roy's Adaptation Model in Practice?

In one study, a qualitative research methodology was used to investigate how 20 nurses viewed the use of the Roy adaptation model as a framework for nursing practice within a hospital setting. The study addressed three questions: (1) How do nurses use the Roy adaptation model in their daily practice? (2) What are the advantages and disadvantages of using the Roy model in practice? (3) What factors affect nurses' use of the Roy model in their practice?

In answer to the first question, the researchers found that nurses integrated the Roy adaptation model into their practice on four levels: (a) *conscious integration*, in which the nurses specifically identified the model as their personal framework for client care; (b) *unconscious integration*, in which the nurses used the model's concepts but did not specifically relate them to a guiding framework; (c) *directed integration*, in which the structure of existing documentation and care planning systems provided the impetus for implementing the concepts; and (d) *lack of integration*, in which the nurses had limited knowledge of the model.

Answers to the second question revealed that the model was generally found to be useful in focusing, organizing, and directing nurses' thoughts and actions regarding client care, resulting in a perception of improved

quality of nursing process and client outcomes. One perceived disadvantage was that a structured nursing process documentation system might tend to limit the need for critical thinking. Also, some nurses stated that the documentation system was time-consuming. Moreover, the language of the model was used only rarely in communicating with others.

Answers to the third question indicated that there were both facilitating and inhibiting factors to integrating the Roy model into the practice setting. Prior education on the Roy model and participation in professional advancement activities facilitated integration of the model, whereas lack of education and resistance to change inhibited implementation of model-based practice.

Implications: Although knowledge of Roy's model varied widely among the subjects in this study, the study's results indicated that the use of this nursing conceptual framework can provide structure for focusing, organizing, and directing thoughts and actions related to client care. However, it is not necessary that the language of the model be used in communicating with others.

SOURCE: "Using Roy's Adaptation Model in Practice: Nurses' Perspectives" by M. E. Weiss, W. J. Hastings, D. C. Holly, and D. I. Craig, Summer, 1994, *Nursing Science Quarterly*, 7(2), 80–86.

2. *Contextual stimuli:* all other internal or external stimuli present

3. *Residual stimuli:* beliefs, attitudes, or traits having an indeterminate effect on the person's behavior but whose effects are not validated

Throughput makes use of a person's (a) *processes*, which are control mechanisms that a person uses as an adaptive system and (b) *effectors*, which refer to the physiologic function, self-concept, and role function involved in adaptation. *Output* of the system refers to the individual's behaviors, which can be either adaptive responses promoting the system's integrity or ineffective responses, such as not following a prescribed therapy. These outputs or responses provide feedback for the system.

Roy's adaptive systems consists of two interrelated subsystems. The *primary subsystem* is a functional or internal control process that consists of the regulator and the cognator. The *regulator* processes input automatically through neural-chemical-endocrine channels. The *cognator* processes input through cognitive pathways, such as perception, information processing, learning, judgment, and emotion. Roy views the regulator and cognator as methods of coping.

The *secondary subsystem* is an effector system that manifests cognator and regulator activity. It consists of four adaptive modes:

1. The *physiologic mode* involves the body's basic physiologic needs and ways of adapting in regard to fluid and electrolytes, activity and rest, circulation and oxygen, nutrition and elimination, protection, the senses, and neurologic and endocrine function.

2. The *self-concept mode* includes two components: the *physical* self, which involves sensation and body image, and the *personal* self, which involves self-ideal, self-consistency, and the moral-ethical self.

3. The *role function mode* is determined by the need for social integrity and refers to the performance of duties based on given positions within society.

4. The *interdependence mode* involves one's relations with significant others and support systems that provide help, affection, and attention.

Watson's Human Caring Theory

Jean Watson was educated in psychiatric and mental health nursing and received her doctorate in educational psychology and counseling. Her theory of the science of caring was first published in *Nursing: The Philosophy and Science of Caring* in 1979. She refined her ideas in *Nursing: Human Science and Human Care* in 1985 and 1988.

Watson believes the practice of caring is central to nursing; it is the unifying focus for practice. Two major assumptions underlie human care values in nursing: (a) care and love constitute the primal and universal psychic energy, and (b) care and love are requisite for our survival and the nourishment of humanity. Watson's major assumptions about caring are shown in the accompanying box.

Watson's Assumptions of Caring

- Human caring in nursing is not just an emotion, concern, attitude, or benevolent desire. *Caring* connotes a personal response.

- Caring is an intersubjective human process and is the moral ideal of nursing.

- Caring can be effectively demonstrated only interpersonally.

- Effective caring promotes health and individual or family growth.

- Caring promotes health more than does curing.

- Caring responses accept a person not only as they are now, but also for what the person may become.

- A caring environment offers the development of potential while allowing the person to choose the best action for the self at a given point in time.

- Caring occasions involve action and choice by nurse and client. If the caring occasion is transpersonal, the limits of openness expand, as do human capacities.

- The most abstract characteristic of a caring person is that the person is somehow responsive to another person as a unique individual, perceives the other's feelings, and sets one person apart from another.

- Human caring involves values, a will and a commitment to care, knowledge, caring actions, and consequences.

- The ideal and value of caring is a starting point, a stance, and an attitude that has to become a will, an intention, a commitment, and a conscious judgment that manifests itself in concrete acts.

Nursing interventions related to human care are referred to as *carative factors*. Watson outlines the following ten factors:

1. Forming a *humanistic-altruistic system of values.* This factor relates to satisfaction through giving and extending the sense of self. Although the values are learned early in life, they can be greatly influenced by educators.

2. Instilling *faith and hope.* Feelings of faith and hope promote wellness by helping the client to adopt health-seeking behaviors. By developing an effective nurse-client relationship, the nurse facilitates feelings of optimism, hope, and trust.

3. Cultivating *sensitivity to one's self and others.* Nurses who are able to recognize and express their feelings are better able to allow others to express theirs.

4. Developing a *helping-trust (human care) relationship.* This kind of relationship involves effective communication, empathy, and nonpossessive warmth. It promotes and accepts the expression of positive and negative feelings.

5. Expressing *positive and negative feelings.* Sharing feelings of sorrow, love, and pain is a risk-taking experience. The nurse must be prepared for negative feelings.

6. Using a *creative problem-solving caring process.* Caring linked to the nursing process contributes to a creative problem-solving approach to nursing care.

7. Promoting *transpersonal teaching-learning.* This factor separates caring from curing and shifts responsibility for wellness to the client.

8. Providing a *supportive, protective, or corrective mental, physical, sociocultural, and spiritual environment.* Because the client can experience change in any aspect of the internal and external environments, the nurse must assess and facilitate the client's abilities to cope with mental, emotional, and physical changes.

9. Assisting with *gratification of human needs.* Caring is conveyed by recognizing and attending to the physical, emotional, social, and spiritual needs of the client.

10. Being sensitive to *existential-phenomenologic-spiritual force.* Phenomenology describes data of the immediate situation that help people understand the phenomenon in question. The *phenomenal field* is the individual's frame of reference; this field can be known only to the person. A phenomenal field involves many levels of consciousness, such as awareness, perceptions of self, body sensations, thoughts, values, feelings, intuitive insights, beliefs, and hopes. When nurse and client come together, two phenomenal fields come together. Both are in a process of being, becoming, and developing transpersonal understanding. Existential psychology is a science of human existence that employs the method of phenomenologic analysis. Persons possess three spheres of being: mind, body, and soul. Allowing for expression of these forces leads to a better understanding of self and others. See Chapter 19 for further information about holism and holistic nursing.

Parse's Human Becoming Theory

Rosemarie Rizzo Parse has broad experience in nursing theory, research, administration, and practice. She is the founder and president of Discovery International, Inc., an organization that promotes excellence in nursing science and provides health guidance services to individuals, families, and groups in Pittsburgh. Parse first published her theory in 1981 in *Man-Living-Health: A Theory for Nursing* and has since then retitled her theory as the human becoming theory, substituting the term *human* for *man* and *becoming* for *health.* Major factors motivating and influencing her theory development were her life experiences and interactions with others, the works of existential philosophers such as Martin Heidegger, Jean-Paul Sartre, and Maurice Merleau-Ponty; and specific concepts from Martha Rogers' *Science of Unitary Human Beings.*

Parse's theoretical assumptions blend Rogers' principles and concepts of integrality, resonancy, helicy, complementarity, energy field, openness, pattern and four-dimensionality (see page 36), with the following beliefs from existential-phenomenologic theory: human subjectivity, intentionality, coconstitution, coexistence, and situational freedom.

Human subjectivity means that people grow in a dialectic (reasoning) relationship with the world that gives meaning to what emerges in the process of becoming. *Intentionality* is involvement with the world through a fundamental nature of knowing, being present, and open.

Coconstitution refers to the idea that the meaning that emerges in any situation is related to the particular components or constituents of that situation.

Coexistence means that people as emerging beings are in the world with others. *Situational freedom* refers to the idea that people participate in choosing the situations in which they find themselves, as well as their attitudes toward the situation. Humans are therefore always choosing.

Parse's nine original key concepts or assumptions (1981) have been reduced to three principles (1995, p. 6):

1. Human becoming is freely choosing personal *meaning* in situations in the intersubjective process of relating value priorities.

2. Human becoming is cocreating *rhythmic patterns* or relating in open process with the universe.

3. Human becoming is *cotranscending* multidimensionally with emerging possibles.

These three principles focus on meaning, rhythmicity, and cotranscendence. Within each principle, succeeding concepts build on preceding ones:

- *Meaning* arises from a person's interrelationship with the world and refers to happenings to which the person attaches varying degrees of significance.
  a. Imaging—structuring the meaning of an experience
  b. Valuing—confirming cherished beliefs
  c. Languaging—expressing valued images

- *Rhythmicity* is the movement toward greater diversity.
  a. Revealing-concealing—simultaneously disclosing some aspects of self and hiding others
  b. Enabling-limiting—the result of making choices; in choosing, one is both enabled in some things and limited in others
  c. Connecting-separating—a simultaneous process: connecting with some phenomena results in separating from others

- *Cotranscendence* is the process of reaching out beyond the self.
  a. Powering—moving toward all future possibilities
  b. Originating—distinguishing self from others
  c. Transforming—an ongoing process of change; moving toward greater diversity by transcending the present

Parse's model of human becoming enables nurses to understand more clearly how individuals choose and bear responsibility for patterns of personal health. Parse contends that the client, not the nurse, is the authority figure and decision maker. The nurse's role involves helping individuals and families in choosing the possibilities for changing the health process. Specifically, the nurse's role consists of illuminating meaning (uncovering what was and what will be), synchronizing rhythms (leading through discussion to recognize harmony), and mobilizing transcendence (dreaming of possibilities and planning to reach them).

Leininger's Cultural Care Diversity and Universality Theory

Madeleine Leininger, a well-known nurse anthropologist, has written extensively on transcultural nursing concepts and is a proponent of the science of human caring. She first published her cultural care diversity and universality theory in 1985 in the journal *Nursing and Health Care*, explained it further in 1988 and then in 1991, in her book *Culture Care Diversity and Universality: A Theory of Nursing*. In this book she produced the Sunrise Model to depict her theory (see also Chapter 18).

Leininger postulates that caring and culture are inextricably linked. Educated in cultural and social anthropology, Leininger observed a marked number of differences between Western and non-Western cultures in caring and health practices. She defines *transcultural nursing* as a major area of nursing that focuses on comparative study and analysis of different cultures and subcultures in the world, with respect to their caring behavior, nursing care, and health values, beliefs, and patterns. The goal of transcultural nursing is to develop a scientific and humanistic body of knowledge in order to provide culture-specific and culture-universal nursing practices. She believes culture is the broadest and the most holistic means to conceptualize, understand, and be effective with people.

Leininger states that *care* is the essence of nursing and the dominant, distinctive, and unifying feature of nursing. She says that there can be no cure without caring, but that there may be caring without curing. She emphasizes that human caring, although a universal phenomenon, varies among cultures in its expressions, processes, and patterns; it is largely culturally derived. These differences in caring values and behaviors lead to differences in the expectations of those seeking care. For example, cultures that perceive illness primarily as a personal and internal body experience—caused by physical,

Leininger's Descriptions of Care and Caring

- Caring includes assistive, supportive, and facilitative acts toward or for another individual or group with evident or anticipated needs.

- Caring serves to ameliorate or to improve human conditions or life ways. It emphasizes healthful, enabling activities of individuals and groups that are based on culturally defined, ascribed, or sanctioned helping modes.

- Caring is essential to human development, growth, and survival.

- Caring behaviors include comfort, compassion, concern, coping behavior, empathy, enabling, facilitating, interest, involvement, health consultative acts, health instruction acts, health maintenance acts, helping behaviors, love, nurturance, presence, protective behaviors, restorative behaviors, sharing, stimulating behaviors, stress alleviation, succor, support, surveillance, tenderness, touching, and trust.

genetic, and intrabody stresses—tend to use more medications and physical techniques than cultures that view illness as an extrapersonal experience.

Leininger identifies many caring constructs (see the accompanying box). Leininger believes that the goal of health care personnel should be to work toward an understanding of care and the values, health beliefs, and life-styles of different cultures, which will form the basis for providing culture-specific care.

CONSIDER . . .

- ways in which the concepts of three nursing theorists you choose may be applied to clients in various practice settings: (1) a prenatal clinic, (2) a hospital unit, (3) a long-term care facility, (4) a mental health unit. Are the theorist's definitions of the client and other concepts applied readily in all of the above practice settings?
- which theories discussed in this chapter are applicable to clients of all age groups.
- whether the theories discussed in this chapter are applicable to individuals as clients, families as clients, and communities as clients.

ONE MODEL VERSUS SEVERAL MODELS

Many nurses believe that having a single, universal model for nursing would offer the following advantages:

- It would further the development of nursing as a profession.
- It would give all nurses a common framework, enhancing communication and research.
- It would promote understanding about the nurse's role in nontraditional nursing settings, such as independent nurse practitioner practice, self-help clinics, and health maintenance organizations (HMOs), correcting the common misconception that nurses provide care only for sick persons.

In contrast, advocates of several different conceptual models point out the following:

- Most disciplines have several conceptual models, which allow members to explore phenomena in different ways and from different viewpoints.
- Several models increase an understanding of the nature of nursing and its scope.
- Several models foster development of the full scope and potential of the discipline.

It is possible that in the 21st century more models for nursing will be developed and that existing ones will be refined in accordance with societal needs and with their tested usefulness.

RELATIONSHIP OF THEORIES TO THE NURSING PROCESS

Conceptual models for nursing are abstractions that are operationalized or made real by the use of the nursing process. See Chapter 14 for detailed information on the nursing process.

1. *Assessing.* The specific data collected about a client's health needs relate directly to the theorist's view of the client. For example, if the client is seen as having 14 fundamental needs, the nurse collects data about these 14 needs.

2. *Diagnosing.* In this step, the nurse analyzes assessment data to identify actual, potential, and possible nursing diagnoses. The nurse outlines or writes the client's actual or potential health prob-

lems as a nursing diagnostic statement in accordance with the nursing model used.

3. *Planning*. Planning also relates directly to the conceptual nursing model. The nurse establishes goals for resolution of client problems, nursing interventions aimed at achieving those goals, and outcome criteria by which the nurse can evaluate whether or not the goals are met. These goals, interventions, and criteria are established in accordance with the modes of intervention outlined in the conceptual model.

TABLE 2–2 Selected Nursing Theories and the Nursing Process

Theory	Application of the Nursing Process	
Orem's general theory of nursing	*Assessing*	Involves collecting data about the client's capacities (knowledge, skills, and motivation) to perform universal, developmental, and health-deviation self-care requisites. Determines self-care deficits.
	Diagnosing	Stated in terms of the client's limitations to maintain self-care (a deficit in self-care agency).
	Planning	Involves considering and designing, with the client's participation, an appropriate nursing system (wholly compensatory, partially compensatory, and/or supportive-educative) that will help the client achieve an optimal level of self-care (i.e., enhance the client's self-care agency).
	Implementing	Assisting the client by acting for or doing for, guiding, supporting, providing a developmental environment, and teaching.
	Evaluating	Determining the client's level of achievement in resolving self-care deficits and in performing self care.
Roy's adaptation model	*Assessing*	Involves two levels. *First-level assessment* includes collecting data about output behaviors related to the four adaptive modes (physiologic, self-concept, role function, and interdependence modes). *Second level assessment* includes collecting data about internal and external stimuli (focal, contextual, or residual) that are influencing the identified behaviors.
	Diagnosing	Focuses on adaptation problems and uses one of three alternative methods: 1. Stating behaviors within one mode with their most relevant influencing stimuli. 2. Clustering behavioral information and labeling it according to indicators of positive adaptation and a typology of common adaptation problems related to each mode. Roy provides a typology of indicators of positive adaptation and a typology of commonly recurring adaptation problems according to each of the four modes. 3. Labeling a behavioral pattern when more than one mode is being affected by the same stimuli.
	Planning	Setting goals in terms of behaviors the client is to achieve and planning nursing interventions to promote the effectiveness of the client's coping mechanisms and adaptive behaviors.
	Implementing	Altering and manipulating the focal, contextual, and residual stimuli by increasing, decreasing, or maintaining them.
	Evaluating	Determining the client's output behaviors with those identified in the goals.

4. *Implementing.* Implementing the planned interventions draws on scientific knowledge that is not part of the nursing model. The nursing model instructs the nurse what to do and directly influences what nursing interventions are planned, but it does not tell the nurse how to do it.

5. *Evaluating.* Evaluating is a continuous nursing function. How is the client adjusting and reacting? What does the client see as needs? How does the client see these needs changing? Has the client achieved the desired consequences? The answers to these questions help the nurse evaluate the effectiveness of the total nursing process and the nursing model.

Table 2–2 outlines how two selected nurse theorists have addressed the nursing process.

CONSIDER...

• using one nursing theory and applying its nursing process concepts to the following clients: (1) a healthy 10-month-old infant, (2) a woman in labor, (3) a hospitalized adolescent who has leukemia, (4) an older client in an extended care facility.

READINGS FOR ENRICHMENT

Arndt, M. J. (1995, Summer). Parse's theory of human becoming in practice with hospitalized adolescents. *Nursing Science Quarterly, 8*(2), 86–90.

This author applies Parse's theory of human becoming to the care of hospitalized adolescents and their families. Four scenarios are included to illustrate the practice methodology of this theory: an 18-year-old boy with Hirschsprung's disease; a 17-year-old boy with acute myelogenous leukemia; an 18-year-old girl with acute myeloblastic leukemia; and a 15-year-old girl admitted for surgery for an abdominal mass.

Gless, P. A. (1995, Jan./Feb.). Applying the Roy adaptation model to the care of clients with quadriplegia. *Rehabilitation Nursing, 20*(1), 11–16.

Gless states that clients with quadriplegia can benefit from a holistic approach to care that focuses on promoting positive coping and adaptation, an approach that the Roy adaptation model delineates. This article discusses major assumptions of Roy's adaptation model and offers a case study to show the effectiveness of using the nursing process within the model's guidelines to help a client with quadriplegia adapt to living in a long-term care facility. Roy's five steps of the nursing process (assessment of stimuli, nursing diagnosis, goal setting, nursing interventions, and evaluation) are applied to the physiologic, self-concept, role-function, and interdependent adaptive modes.

LaFerrier, R. H. (1995, Sept./Oct.). Orem's theory in practice: Hospice nursing care. *Home Healthcare Nurse, 13*(5), 50–54.

The author applies the six care concepts of Orem's theory—self-care, self-care agency, therapeutic self-care demand, self-care deficit, nursing agency, and nursing system—to hospice care. A case study is provided to illustrate clinical application of these concepts in palliative care.

Marckx, B. B. (1995, July). Watson's theory of caring: A model for implementation in practice. *Journal of Nursing Care Quality, 9*(4), 43–54.

Marckx introduces Jean Watson's theory of human caring in nursing as an innovative approach to improving care for residents in a special dementia unit. Specific examples of ways that Watson's model can be applied in typical nurse-client situations are presented. Implementation strategies with creative visual aids are included, and research tools for the evaluation of outcomes are described.

Russell, J., & Hezel, L. (1994, July). Role analysis of the advanced practice nurse using the Neuman health care systems model as a framework. *Clinical Nurse Specialist, 8*(4), 215–220.

Because the role of the advanced practitioner of nursing is perceived and operationalized differently from practice setting to practice setting, practitioners need to analyze and differentiate role expectations within specific practice situations. The Neuman systems model provides a systematic framework for role analysis, development, enactment, and evaluation. This article describes the general systems theory that is the basis of the Neuman model, outlines how the Neuman systems model provides a basis for role analysis, and provides a structure to analyze the role of the clinical nurse specialist. The benefit of a systematic micro-analysis of the role of the clinical nurse specialist will be to develop a template to be used in the analysis of a particular position in the real world.

Woods, F. C. (1994, Summer). King's theory in practice with elders. *Nursing Science Quarterly, 7*(2), 65–69.

Woods discusses the utilization of Imogene King's theory of goal attainment with a group of older adults living in a nursing home and experiencing many of the health problems associated with advanced age. Nurse participants met weekly for 10 weeks to explore methods to promote continuous health restoration. Wood designs an assessment tool based on King's conceptual framework and discusses the development of nursing diagnoses, client-centered goals, and interventions using interactions, transactions, perceptions, and expressions of self to achieve goal attainment.

Wright, P. S., Piazza, D., Holcombe, J., & Foote, A. (1994, Jan.). A comparison of three theories of nursing used as a guide for the nursing care of an 8-year-old child with leukemia. *Journal of Pediatric Oncology Nursing, 11*, 14–19.

These authors evaluate three nursing theories that can be used to provide a framework for holistic pediatric oncology nursing practice: the Roy adaptation model, the Neuman systems model, and the Orem general theory of nursing. The authors compare each theory in terms of the metaparadigm of nursing and present a critique. Four comparative tables are included. The decision of which theory to use is left to the individual nurse.

SUMMARY

As an increasingly emerging profession, nursing is now deeply involved in identifying its own unique knowledge base—that is, the body of knowledge essential to nursing practice, or a so-called nursing science. If nurses are to be considered health professionals, they must communicate exactly what makes their place in the interdisciplinary team unique and important. Theories offer ways of conceptualizing a discipline in clear, explicit terms that can be communicated to others.

Because opinions about the nature and structure of nursing vary, theories continue to be developed. Each nursing theory bears the name of the person or group who developed it and reflects the beliefs of the developer. The theories vary considerably in (a) their level of abstraction; (b) their conceptualization of the client, health/illness, and nursing; and (c) their ability to describe, explain, or predict. Some theories are broad in scope; others are limited.

Definitions and a clear understanding of the terms care *and* caring *are being developed. The major theorists involved to date are Leininger and Watson.*

Nursing theories serve several essential purposes, some of which are to differentiate the focus of nursing from other professions; to structure professional nursing practice, education, and research; to help build a common nursing terminology to use in communicating with other health professionals; and to enhance autonomy of nursing through defining its own independent functions. Because the primary purpose of nursing theory is to generate scientific knowledge, nursing theory and nursing research are closely related. Scientific knowledge is derived from testing hypotheses generated by the-

ories for nursing. Research determines the utility of those hypotheses, and research findings may be developed into theories for nursing.

The major distinction between a theory and a conceptual framework or model is the level of abstraction, with the conceptual framework being more abstract than the theory. A conceptual model is a system of related concepts or a conceptual diagram. Its major purpose is to give clear and explicit direction to the three areas of nursing: practice, education, and research. A theory generates knowledge in a field.

Nursing theories address and specify relationships among four major concepts, the building blocks of theory: person or client, environment, health/illness, and nursing. Each nurse theorist's definitions of these four major concepts vary in accordance with personal philosophy, scientific orientation, experience in nursing, and how that experience has affected the theorist's view of nursing.

Nursing theories included three elements: (a) a set of well-defined constructs, (b) a set of propositions, and (c) hypotheses. Concepts in a conceptual framework are linked together to form a proposition, a statement that expresses the relationship between concepts and is capable of being tested, believed, or denied.

Models for nursing relate to the nursing process in that they are operationalized or made real by the use of the nursing process. How nurses view human beings and the nurse's role influences how they assess and intervene.

It is possible that in the 21st century more models for nursing will be developed or that existing ones will be refined in accordance with societal needs and with their tested usefulness.

SELECTED REFERENCES

Boykin, A., & Schoenhofer, S. (1993). *Nursing as caring: A model for transforming practice.* New York: National League for Nursing Press. Pub. No. 15-2549.

Carboni, J. T. (1995, Spring). A Rogerian process of inquiry. *Nursing Science Quarterly, 8*(1), 22–37.

Carter, K. F., & Dufour, L. T. (1994, Fall). King's theory: A critique of the critiques. *Nursing Science Quarterly, 7*(3), 128–133.

Chin, P. L., & Kramer, M. K. (1991). *Theory and nursing: A systematic approach* (4th ed.). St. Louis: Mosby.

Harmer, B., & Henderson, V. (1955). *Textbook of the principles and practice of nursing* (5th ed.). Riverside, NJ: Macmillan.

Henderson, V. (1966). *The nature of nursing: A definition and its implications for practice, research, and education.* Riverside, NJ: Macmillan.

Henderson, V. A. (1991). *The nature of nursing: Reflections after 25 years.* New York: National League for Nursing Press. Pub. No. 15-2346.

King, I. M. (1971). *Toward a theory for nursing: General concepts of human behavior.* New York: Wiley.

King, I. M. (1981). *A theory for nursing: Systems, concepts, process.* New York: Wiley.

Leininger, M. M. (1978). *Transcultural nursing: Concepts, theories, and practices.* New York: Wiley.

Leininger, M. M. (1980, Oct.). Caring: A central focus of nursing and health care services. *Nursing and Health Care, 1*(3), 135–143.

Leininger, M. M. (1984). *Care: The essence of nursing and health.* Thorofare, NJ: Charles B. Slack.

Leininger, M. M. (1985, April). Transcultural care diversity and universality: A theory of nursing. *Nursing and Health Care, 6*(4), 208–212.

Leininger, M. M. (1988, Nov.). Leininger's theory of nursing: Cultural care, diversity and universality. *Nursing Science Quarterly, 1*(4), 152–160.

Leininger, M. M. (ed.). (1991). *Culture care diversity and universality: A theory of nursing.* New York: National League for Nursing Press. Pub. No. 15-2402.

Madrid, M., & Barrett, E. A. M. (Eds.). (1994). *Rogers' scientific art of nursing practice.* New York: National League for Nursing Press. Pub. No. 15-2610.

Neuman, B. (1974). The Betty Neuman health-care systems model: A total person approach to patient problems. In J. P. Riehl & C. Roy (Eds.), *Conceptual models for nursing practice.* New York: Appleton-Century-Crofts.

Neuman, B. (1982). *The Neuman systems model: Applications to nursing education and practice.* New York: Appleton-Century-Crofts.

Neuman, B. (1989). *The Neuman systems model: Applications to nursing education and practice* (2nd ed.). Norwalk, CT: Appleton & Lange.

Neuman, B. (1995). *The Neuman systems model* (3rd ed.). Norwalk, CT: Appleton & Lange.

Neuman, B. M., & Young, R. J. (1972, June). A model for teaching total person approach to patient problems. *Nursing Research, 21*, 264–269.

Nicoll, L. H. (1992). *Perspectives on nursing theory* (2nd ed.). Philadelphia: Lippincott.

Nightingale, F. (1957). *Notes on nursing.* Philadelphia: Lippincott. (Original work published 1860).

Orem, D. E. (1971). *Nursing: Concepts of practice.* Hightstown, NJ: McGraw-Hill.

Orem, D. (1980). *Nursing: Concepts of practice* (2nd ed.). Hightstown, NJ: McGraw Hill.

Orem, D. E. (1985). *Nursing: Concepts of practice* (3rd ed.). Hightstown, NJ: McGraw Hill.

Orem, D. E. (1991). *Nursing: Concepts of practice* (4th ed.). St. Louis: Mosby-Year Book.

Orem, D. E. (1995). *Nursing: Concepts of practice* (5th ed.). St. Louis: Mosby.

Orem, D. E., & Vardiman, E. M. (1995, Winter). Orem's theory and positive mental health: Practical considerations. *Nursing Science Quarterly, 8*(4), 165–173.

Parker, M. E. (Ed.). (1990). *Nursing theories in practice.* New York: National League for Nursing Press. Pub. No. 15-2350.

Parker, M. E. (Ed.). (1993). *Patterns of nursing theories in practice.* New York: National League for Nursing Press. Pub. No. 15-2548.

Parse, R. R. (1981). *Man-living-health: Theory of nursing.* New York: Wiley.

Parse, R. R. (1987). *Nursing science: Major paradigms, theories, and critiques.* Philadelphia: W. B. Saunders.

Parse, R. R. (1989). *Man-living-health: A theory of nursing.* In J. Riehl-Sisca (Ed.), *Conceptual models for nursing practice* (3rd ed.) (pp. 253–257). Norwalk, CT: Appleton-Lange.

Parse, R. R. (Ed.). (1995). *Illumination: The human becoming theory in practice and research.* New York: National League for Nursing Press. Pub. No. 15-2670.

Peplau, H. E. (1952). *Interpersonal relations in nursing.* New York: Putnam.

Peplau, H. E. (1963, Oct./Nov.). Interpersonal relations and the process of adaptations. *Nursing Science, 1*(4), 272–279.

Peplau, H. E. (1980). The Peplau developmental model for nursing practice. In J. P. Riehl & C. Roy (Eds.), *Conceptual models for nursing practice* (2nd ed.) (pp. 53–75). New York: Appleton-Century-Crofts.

Rogers, M. E. (1970). *An introduction to the theoretical basis of nursing.* Philadelphia: F. A. Davis.

Rogers, M. E. (1989). Nursing: A science of unitary human beings. In J. Riehl-Sisca (Ed.), *Conceptual models for nursing practice* (3rd ed.) (pp. 181–188). Norwalk, CT: Appleton & Lange.

Rogers, M. E. (1994, Spring). The science of unitary human beings: Current perspectives. *Nursing Science Quarterly, 7*(1), 33–35.

Roy, C. (1970, March). Adaptation: A conceptual framework in nursing. *Nursing Outlook, 18*, 42–45.

Roy, C. (1976). *Introduction to nursing: An adaptation model.* Englewood Cliffs, NJ: Prentice-Hall.

Roy, C. (1984). *Introduction to nursing: An adaptation model* (2nd ed.). Englewood Cliffs, NJ: Prentice Hall.

Roy, C., & Andrews, H. A. (1991).*The Roy adaptation model: The definitive statement.* Norwalk,CT: Appleton &Lange.

Sarter, B. (1988). *The stream of becoming: A study of Martha Rogers' theory.* New York: National League for Nursing Press. Pub. No. 15-2205.

Watson, J. (1979). *Nursing: The philosophy and science of caring.* Boston: Little, Brown.

Watson, J. (1985). *Nursing: Human science and human care: A theory of nursing.* Norwalk, CT: Appleton-Century-Crofts.

Watson, J. (1988). *Nursing: Human science and human care. A theory of nursing.* New York: National League for Nursing Press. Pub. No. 15-2236.

Wesley, R. L. (1995). *Nursing theories and models* (2nd ed.). Springhouse, PA: Springhouse.

3

Health and Wellness

OBJECTIVES

- Differentiate health, wellness, and well-being.

- Compare various models of health outlined in this chapter.

- Identify factors affecting health status, beliefs, and practices.

- Describe factors affecting health care compliance.

- Discuss three broad goals stated by the U.S. Department of Health and Human Services to meet the health challenges of the 1990s.

> "[Health] goes beyond the condition of the flesh, it's also a condition of the spirit…. It also involves the whole way we live, the way we think, our social responsibility, our attitude toward the world, our enthusiasm for life.
>
> — George Leonard

Nurses need to clarify their understanding of health and wellness because their definitions largely determine the scope and nature of nursing practice. Clients' health beliefs also influence their health practices.

- Some people think of health and wellness (or well-being) as the same thing or, at the very least, as accompanying one another. However, health may not always accompany well-being: A person who has a terminal illness may have a sense of well-being; conversely, another person may lack a sense of well-being yet be in a state of good health.
- For many years, the concept of disease was the yardstick by which health was measured. In the late 19th century, the "how" of disease (pathogenesis) was the major concern of health professionals.
- Currently, the emphasis on health and wellness (salutogenesis) is increasing.

CONCEPTS OF HEALTH, WELLNESS, AND WELL-BEING

Health

There is no consensus about any definition of health. There is knowledge of how to attain a certain level of health, but health itself cannot be measured.

Traditionally, **health** has been defined in terms of the presence or absence of disease. Nightingale defined health as a state of "being well and using every power the individual possesses to the fullest extent" (Nightingale, 1969 [1860], p. 334). The World Health Organization (WHO) takes a more holistic view of health. It defines health as "a state of complete physical, mental, and social well-being, and not merely the absence of disease or infirmity" (WHO, 1947, p. 1). This definition

- Reflects concern for the individual as a total person functioning physically, psychologically, and socially. Mental processes determine people's relationship with their physical and social sur-

roundings, their attitudes about life, and their interaction with others.
- Places health in the context of environment. People's lives, and therefore their health, are affected by everything they interact with—not only environmental influences such as climate and the availability of nutritious food, comfortable shelter, clean air to breathe, and pure water to drink but also other people, including family, lovers, employers, co-workers, friends, and associates of various kinds.
- Equates health with productive and creative living. It focuses on the living state rather than on categories of disease that may cause illness or death.

In 1953 the (United States) President's Commission on Health Needs of the Nation made the following statement about health:

> "*Health* is not a condition; it is an adjustment. It is not a state but a process. The process adapts the individual not only to our physical, but also our social environments." (President's Commission, 1953, p. 4)

This definition emphasizes health as an adaptive process rather than a state.

Health has also been defined in terms of role and performance. Parsons (1972, p. 107) wrote that health is "the state of optimum capacity of an individual for effective performance of his roles and tasks." Parsons further explained that when people feel well, they assume the health role; when they feel ill, in contrast, they assume the sick role. He describes four aspects of the sick role:

- The person is not held responsible for the illness.
- The person is exempt from the usual social tasks.
- The person has an obligation to get well.
- The person has an obligation to seek competent help to treat the illness.

Dubos (1978) views health as a creative process. Individuals are actively and continually adapting to their environments. In Dubos's view, the individual must have sufficient knowledge to make informed choices about his or her health and also the income and resources to act on choices. Dubos believes that complete well-being is unobtainable, thus contradicting the 1947 definition by the World Health Organization.

In 1980, the American Nurses Association (ANA) defined health in their social policy as "a dynamic state of being in which the developmental and behavioral potential of an individual is realized to the fullest extent possible" (ANA, 1980, p. 5). In this definition, health is more than a state or the absence of disease; it includes striving toward optimal functioning.

In the past few decades, a number of health professionals, including nurse theorists, have provided definitions of health and wellness. See Table 2–1 on page 31.

Personal Definitions of Health

Health is a highly individual perception. Nevertheless, most people define and describe health as the following:

- Being free from symptoms of disease and pain as much as possible
- Being able to be active and to do what they want or must
- Being in good spirits most of the time

Developing a Personal Definition of Health

The following questions can help nurses develop a personal definition of health.

- Is a person more than a biophysiologic system?
- Is health more than the absence of disease symptoms?
- Is health the ability of an individual to perform work?
- Is health the ability of an individual to adapt to the environment?
- Is health a condition of a person's actualization?
- Is health a state or a process?
- Is health the effective functioning of self-care activities?
- Is health static or changing?
- Are health and wellness the same?
- Are disease and illness different?
- Are there levels of health?
- Are wellness, health, and illness separate entities or points along a continuum?
- Is health socially determined?
- How do you rate your health, and why?

These characteristics indicate that health is not something that a person achieves suddenly at a specific time. It is an ongoing *process*—a way of life—through which a person develops and encourages every aspect of the body, mind, and feelings to interrelate harmoniously as much as possible.

Many factors affect individual definitions of health. Definitions vary according to an individual's previous experiences, expectations of self, age, and sociocultural influences (see page 59).

Nurses should be aware of their own personal definitions of health and should appreciate that other people have their own individual definitions as well. The person's definition of health influences behavior related to health and illness. By understanding clients' perceptions of health and illness, nurses can provide more meaningful assistance to help clients regain or attain a state of health. To facilitate development of a personal definition of health, see the box at the left below.

Wellness and Well-Being

Wellness is a state of well-being. It means engaging in attitudes and behaviors that enhance quality of life and maximize personal potential (Anspaugh, Hamrick & Rosata, 1991, p. 2). Basic concepts of wellness

---

Concepts of Wellness

- Wellness is a choice—a decision you make to move toward optimal health.
- Wellness is a way of life—a life-style you design to achieve your highest potential for well-being.
- Wellness is a process—a developing awareness that there is no end point, but that health and happiness are possible in each moment, here and now.
- Wellness is an efficient channeling of energy—energy received from the environment, transformed within you, and sent on to affect the world outside.
- Wellness is the integration of body, mind, and spirit—the appreciation that everything you do, and think, and feel, and believe has an impact on your state of health.
- Wellness is the loving acceptance of yourself.

SOURCE: Reprinted with permission, *Wellness Workbook*, Travis & Ryan, Ten Speed Press, Berkeley, CA. © 1981, 1988 by John W. Travis, MD.

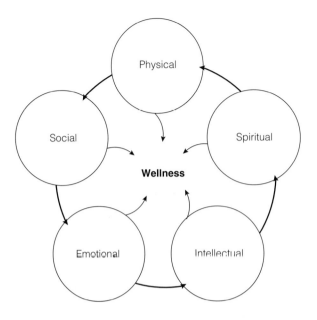

FIGURE 3-1 *The dimensions of wellness.*

include self-responsibility; an ultimate goal; a dynamic, growing process; daily decision making in the areas of nutrition, stress management, physical fitness, preventive health care, emotional health, and other aspects of health; and most importantly, the whole being of the individual.

Leddy and Pepper (1993, p. 221) contend that people confuse the *process* of health with the *status* of well-being. **Well-being** is a *subjective* perception of balance, harmony, and vitality. It is a state that can be described objectively, occurs in levels, and can be plotted on a continuum.

Travis and Ryan (1988, p. xiv) state that wellness is a choice; a way of life; a process; efficient handling of energy; integration of body, mind, and spirit; and loving acceptance of self. See the box on page 54.

Anspaugh et al. (1991, p. 3) propose five dimensions of wellness (Figure 3–1). To realize optimal health and wellness, people must deal with the factors within each dimension:

- *Physical.* The ability to carry out daily tasks, achieve fitness (e.g., pulmonary, cardiovascular, gastrointestinal), maintain adequate nutrition and proper body fat, avoid abusing drugs and alcohol or using tobacco products, and generally to practice positive life-style habits.
- *Social.* The ability to interact successfully with people and within the environment of which each person is a part, to develop and maintain

intimacy with significant others, and to develop respect and tolerance for those with different opinions and beliefs.
- *Emotional.* The ability to manage stress and to express emotions appropriately. Emotional wellness involves the ability to recognize, accept, and express feelings and to accept one's limitations.
- *Intellectual.* The ability to learn and use information effectively for personal, family, and career development. Intellectual wellness involves striving for continued growth and learning to deal with new challenges effectively.
- *Spiritual.* The belief in some force (nature, science, religion, or a higher power) that serves to unite human beings and provide meaning and purpose to life. It includes a person's own morals, values, and ethics.

Each of the five components overlap to some extent, and factors in one component often directly affect factors in another. For example, a person who learns to control daily stress levels from a physiologic perspective is also helping to maintain the emotional stamina needed to cope with a crisis. Wellness involves working on *all* aspects of the model.

Illness and Disease

People may view illness and disease as the same entity; however, health professionals generally view them as completely separate. Emotions are not believed to cause disease, but they may create an environment in which disease can develop through their effect upon the immune system.

Illness is a highly personal state in which the person feels unhealthy or ill. Illness may or may not be related to disease. An individual could have a disease, for example, a growth in the stomach, and not feel ill. By the same token, a person can feel ill, that is, feel uncomfortable, yet have no discernible disease. Illness is highly subjective; only the individual person can say he or she is ill.

Disease is a term that can be described as an alteration in body functions resulting in a reduction of capacities or a shortening of the normal life span. Traditionally, intervention by physicians has the goal of eliminating or ameliorating disease processes. Primitive people thought disease was caused by "forces" or spirits. Later, this belief was replaced by the single-causation theory. Today, multiple factors are considered to interact in causing disease and determining an individual's response to treatment.

Another distinction needs to be made between disease and deviance. **Deviance** is behavior that goes against social norms. Some deviant behaviors may be considered diseases according to the earlier definition of disease. For example, alcoholism can result in an alteration of body functioning, a reduction in capacities, and a shortening of the life span. Other deviant behavior can be considered a disease, not because it alters the function of a body organ, but because it disrupts a family or a community. An example is drug addiction. However, differentiation between disease and deviance is not always clear and often depends on the perspective of the person observing the behavior.

CONSIDER...

- what behaviors of others indicate to you that they are healthy or unhealthy.
- your own definition of health.
- whether your own definition of health changes from year to year.
- whether you believe that your clients should agree with your definition of health.
- which factors you believe most affect your own sense of wellness.

MODELS OF HEALTH AND WELLNESS

Because health is such a complex concept, various researchers have developed models or paradigms to explain health and in some instances its relationship to illness or injury. Models can be helpful in assisting health professionals to meet the health and wellness needs of individuals. Nurses need to clarify their understanding of health, wellness, and illness for the following reasons:

- Nurses' definitions of health largely determine the scope and nature of nursing practice. For example, when health is defined narrowly as a physiologic phenomenon, nurses confine themselves to assisting clients regain normal physiologic functioning. When health is defined more broadly, the scope of nursing practice increases correspondingly.
- People's health beliefs influence their health practices. Thus, a nurse's health values and practices may differ from those of a client. Nurses need to ensure that plans of care developed for individuals relate to the client's conception of

health. Otherwise, clients may fail to respond to a health care regimen.

Smith's Models of Health

Judith Smith (1981, p. 47) describes four models of health: (1) the clinical model, (2) the role performance model, (3) the adaptive model, and (4) the eudaemonistic model.

Clinical Model

The narrowest interpretation of health occurs in the clinical model. People are viewed as physiologic systems with related functions, and health is identified by the absence of signs and symptoms of disease or injury. To laypersons, it is considered the state of not being "sick." In this model, the opposite of health is disease or injury.

Many medical practitioners use the clinical model. The focus of many medical practices is the relief of signs and symptoms of disease and the elimination of malfunctioning and pain. When the signs and symptoms of disease are no longer present in a person, the medical practitioner often considers that the individual's health is restored.

Role Performance Model

Health is defined in terms of the individual's ability to fulfill societal roles, that is, to perform work. According to this model, people who can fulfill their roles are healthy even if they appear clinically ill. For example, a man who works all day at his job as expected is healthy even though an X-ray film of his lung indicates a tumor.

It is assumed in this model that sickness is the inability to perform one's work. A problem with this model is the assumption that a person's most important role is the work role. People usually fulfill several roles (e.g., mother, daughter, friend), and certain individuals may consider nonwork roles paramount in their lives.

Adaptive Model

The focus of the adaptive model is adaptation. In the adaptive model, health is a creative process; disease is a failure in adaptation, or *maladaption*. The aim of treatment is to restore the ability of the person to adapt, that is, to cope. According to this model, extreme good health is flexible adaptation to the environment and interaction with the environment to maximum advantage (Smith, 1981, p. 45). Sister

Callista Roy's adaptation model of nursing (Roy & Andrews, 1991) views the person as an adaptive system (see page 42). The focus of this model is stability, although there is also an element of growth and change.

Murray and Zentner (1989, p. 570) indicate this growth and change in their definition of health: "a state of well-being in which the person is able to use purposeful, adaptive responses and processes, physically, mentally, emotionally, spiritually, and socially, in response to internal and external stimuli (stressors) in order to maintain relative stability and comfort and to strive for personal objectives and cultural goals."

Eudaemonistic Model

The eudaemonistic model incorporates the most comprehensive view of health (Smith, 1981, p. 44). Health is seen as a condition of actualization or realization of a person's potential. Actualization is the apex of the fully developed personality. (Maslow presents this concept of health.) In this model, the highest aspiration of people is fulfillment and complete development, i.e., actualization. Illness, in this model, is a condition that prevents self-actualization.

Pender includes stabilizing and actualizing tendencies in her definition of health: "Health is the actualization of inherent and acquired human potential through satisfying relationships with others while adjustments are made as needed to maintain structural integrity and harmony with the environment" (1987, p. 27).

Leavell and Clark's Agent-Host-Environment Model

The *agent-host-environment model* of health and illness, also called the *ecologic model*, originated in the community health work of Leavell and Clark (1965) and has been expanded into a general theory of the multiple causes of disease. The model is used primarily in predicting illness rather than in promoting wellness, although identification of risk factors that result from the interaction of agent-host-environment are helpful in promoting and maintaining health.

The model has three dynamic interactive elements:

1. *Agent.* Any environmental factor or stressor (biologic, chemical, mechanical, physical, or psychosocial) that by its presence or absence (e.g., lack of essential nutrients) can lead to illness or disease.

2. *Host.* Person(s) who may or may not be at risk of acquiring a disease. Family history, age, and lifestyle habits influence the host's reaction.

3. *Environment.* All factors external to the host that may or may not predispose the person to the development of disease. Physical environment includes climate, living conditions, sound (noise) levels, and economic level. Social environment includes interactions with others and life events, such as the death of a spouse.

Because each of the agent-host-environment factors constantly interacts with the others, health is an ever-changing state. When the variables are in balance, health is maintained; when variables are not in balance, disease occurs.

Health-Illness Continua

Health-illness continua (grids or graduated scales) can be used to measure a person's perceived level of wellness.

Dunn's High-Level Wellness Grid

Dunn describes a health grid in which a health axis and an environmental axis intersect (1959a, p. 786). It demonstrates the interaction of the environment with the illness-wellness continuum (Figure 3–2).

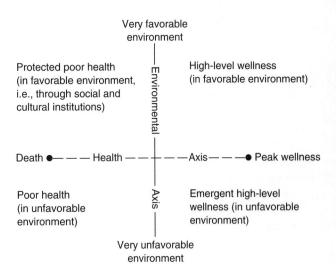

FIGURE 3–2 *Dunn's health grid: its axes and quadrants.*

SOURCE: "High-Level Wellness for Man and Society" by H. L. Dunn, June 1959, *American Journal of Public Health, 49,* p. 788. Used with permission of the American Public Health Association.

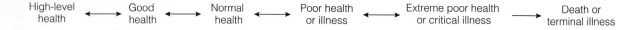

FIGURE 3–3 *The health continuum, from high-level health to death.*

The health axis extends from peak wellness to death, and the environmental axis extends from very favorable to very unfavorable. The intersection of the two axes forms four health/wellness quadrants:

1. *High-level wellness in a favorable environment.* An example of this is a person who implements healthy life-style behaviors and has the biopsychosocial, spiritual, and economic resources to support this life-style.

2. *Emergent high-level wellness in an unfavorable environment.* An example of this is a woman who has the knowledge to implement healthy life-style practices but does not implement adequate self-care practices because of family responsibilities, job demands, or other factors.

3. *Protected poor health in a favorable environment.* An example of this is an ill person (e.g., one with multiple fractures or severe hypertension) whose needs are met by the health care system and who has access to appropriate medications, diet, and health care instruction.

4. *Poor health in an unfavorable environment.* An example of this is a young child who is starving in a drought-stricken country.

In his book about high-level wellness in the individual, Dunn (1973) explores the concept of wellness as it relates to family, community, environment, and society. He believes that family wellness enhances wellness in individuals. In a well family that offers trust, love, and support, the individual does not have to expend energy to meet basic needs and can move forward on the wellness continuum. By providing effective sanitation and safe water, disposing of sewage safely, and preserving beauty and wildlife, the community enhances both family and individual wellness. Environmental wellness is related to the premise that humans must be at peace with and guard the environment. Societal wellness is significant because the status of the larger, social group affects the status of smaller groups. Dunn believes that social wellness must be considered on a worldwide basis.

Health and illness or disease can be viewed as the opposite ends of a health continuum. From the high level of health on the left side of the continuum, a person's condition can move through good health, normal health, poor health, and extremely poor health, eventually to death. Persons move back and forth within this continuum day by day. There is no distinct boundary across which people move from health to illness or from illness back to health. How persons perceive themselves and how others see them vis-a-vis health and illness will also affect their placement on the continuum. There is considerable range in which people can be considered healthy or ill (Figure 3–3).

CONSIDER . . .

- which model of health you are most comfortable with. Why?
- whether a nurse who believes in the adaptive model of health can assist a client who believes in a role performance model.
- how a clinical model differs from an adaptive model.

HEALTH STATUS, BELIEFS, AND BEHAVIORS

The *health status* (state) of an individual is the health of that person at a given time. In its general meaning, the term may refer to anxiety, depression, or acute illness and thus describes the individual's problem in general. Health status can also describe such specifics as pulse rate and body temperature. The *health beliefs* of an individual are those concepts about health that an individual believes true. Such beliefs may or may not be founded on fact. Some of these are influenced by culture, such as the "hot-cold" system of some Hispanic Americans. In this system, health is viewed as a balance of hot and cold qualities within a person. Citrus fruits and some fowl are considered cold foods, and meats and bread are hot foods. In this context, hot and cold do not denote temperature or spiciness but innate qualities of the food. For example, a fever is said to be caused by an excess of hot foods. Another example of a culturally related health belief is the belief that health and illness are closely associated with the amount and quality of blood in the body. For example, among some people in the South, "high blood," caused by too much blood in the body, causes headaches and dizziness (Mitchell & Loustau, 1981, pp. 41–42). For additional information about ethnic views of health and illness, see Chapter 18.

Health behaviors are the actions people take to understand their health state, maintain an optimal state of health, prevent illness and injury, and reach their maximum physical and mental potential. Behaviors such as eating wisely, exercising, paying attention to signs of illness, following treatment advice, and avoiding known health hazards such as smoking are all examples. The ability to relax, emotional maturity, productivity, and self-expression also affect one's health (McCann/Flynn & Heffron, 1988, pp. 37–38).

Health behavior is intended to prevent illness or disease or to provide for early detection of disease. Nurses preparing a plan of care with an individual need to consider the person's health beliefs before they suggest a change in health behaviors.

Many variables influence a person's health status, beliefs, and behaviors or practices. These factors may or may not be under conscious control. People can usually control their health behaviors and can choose healthy or unhealthy activities. In contrast, people have little or no choice over their genetic makeup, age, sex, physical environments, culture, or areas of residence.

Biologic Dimension

Genetic makeup, race, sex, age, and developmental level all significantly influence a person's health.

Genetic makeup influences biologic characteristics, innate temperament, activity level, and intellectual potential. It has been related to susceptibility to specific disease, such as diabetes and breast cancer.

Race is associated with predisposition to certain diseases. For example, people of African heritage have a higher incidence of sickle-cell anemia and hypertension than the general population, and Native Americans have a higher rate of diabetes.

Sex influences the distribution of disease. Certain acquired and genetic diseases are more common in one sex than in the other. Disorders more common among females include osteoporosis and autoim-

mune diseases such as rheumatoid arthritis. Those more common among males are stomach ulcers, abdominal hernias, and respiratory diseases.

Age and developmental level are also significant factors. The distribution of disease varies with age. For example, arteriosclerotic heart disease is common in middle-aged males but occurs infrequently in younger persons; such communicable diseases such as whooping cough and measles are common in children but rare in older persons, who have acquired immunity to them.

Psychologic Dimension

Psychologic (emotional) factors influencing health include mind-body interactions, self-concept, and job satisfaction.

Mind-body interactions can affect health status positively or negatively. Emotional responses to stress affect body function. For example, a person worried about the outcome of surgery may chain-smoke. Prolonged emotional distress may increase susceptibility to organic disease or precipitate it. Emotional distress may influence the immune system through central nervous system and endocrine alterations. Alterations in the immune system are related to the incidence of infections, cancer, and autoimmune diseases.

Emotional reactions also occur in response to body conditions. For example, a person diagnosed with a terminal illness may experience fear and

---

RESEARCH NOTE

Does the Public Believe There Is a Connection Between Positive Mental Attitude and Health?

The authors of one study researched what people believe "positive mental attitude" (PMA) means. The researchers analyzed responses from 167 people. The majority indicated that PMA means optimism or hope: 77% of the respondents agreed that PMA can prevent illness, and 94% agreed that PMA can assist in recovery from illness.

Implications: Nurses should include data about the mental attitude of clients when planning care.

SOURCE: "Positive Mental Attitude and Health: What the Public Believes" by E. Bruckbauer and S. E. Ward, Winter 1993, *Image: Journal of Nursing Scholarship, 25*, 311–315.

depression. *Self-concept* is how a person feels about self (self-esteem) and perceives the physical self (body image), needs, roles, and abilities. Self-concept affects how people view and handle situations. Such attitudes can affect health practices, responses to stress and illness, and the times when treatment is sought.

Cognitive Dimension

Cognitive or intellectual factors influencing health include life-style choices and spiritual and religious beliefs.

Life-style choices include patterns of eating; exercise; use of tobacco, drugs, and alcohol; and methods of coping with stress. Overeating, getting insufficient exercise, and being overweight are closely related to the incidence of heart disease, arteriosclerosis, diabetes, and hypertension. Excessive use of tobacco is clearly implicated in lung cancer, emphysema, and cardiovascular diseases.

Spiritual and religious beliefs can significantly affect health behavior. For example, Jehovah's Witnesses oppose blood transfusions; some fundamentalists believe that a serious illness is a punishment from God; some religious groups are strict vegetarians; and Orthodox Jews perform circumcision on the eighth day of a male baby's life.

Geography

Geography determines climate, and climate affects health. For instance, malaria and malaria-related conditions occur more frequently in tropical than temperate climates.

Environment

People are becoming increasingly aware of their environment and how it affects their health and level of wellness. Pollution of the water, air, and soil can affect the support of life. Pollution can occur naturally (e.g., lightning-caused fires produce smoke, which pollutes the air). Other substances in the environment, such as asbestos, are considered carcinogenic (i.e., they cause cancer). Cigarette smoke is now considered "hazardous to one's health," with rates of all types of cancer higher among smokers.

Another environmental hazard is radiation. Two sources of radiation that can be hazardous to health are machines and drugs that emit radiation. The improper use of X rays, for example, can harm many of the body's organs. Another common source of radiation is the sun's ultraviolet rays. Light-skinned people are more susceptible to the harmful effects of the sun than are dark-skinned people.

The main component of acid rain is sulfur dioxide, produced by ore smelters and related industries. The other components are nitrogen oxides. These emissions are thought by scientists to damage forests, lakes, and rivers. As a result, fish and fish eggs are damaged by the increasingly acidic water.

Another environmental hazard that is receiving increasing attention is the "greenhouse effect." The glass roof of a greenhouse permits the sun's radiation to penetrate, but the resulting heat does not escape back through the glass. Carbon dioxide in the earth's atmosphere acts very much like the glass roof of a greenhouse, hence the surface temperature of the earth is increasing.

Other sources of environmental contamination are pesticides and chemicals used to control weeds and plant diseases. These contaminants can be found in some animals and plants that are subsequently ingested by people. In excessive levels, they are harmful to health.

Standards of Living

An individual's standard of living (reflecting occupation, income, and education) is related to health, morbidity, and mortality. Hygiene, food habits, and the propensity to seek health care advice and follow health regimens vary among high-income and low-income groups.

Low-income families often define health in terms of work; if people can work they are healthy. They tend to be fatalistic and believe that illness is not preventable. Because their present problems are so great and all efforts are exerted toward survival, an orientation to the future may be lacking.

The environmental conditions of poverty-stricken areas also have a bearing on overall health. Slum neighborhoods are overcrowded and in a state of deterioration. Sanitation services tend to be inadequate. Many streets are strewn with garbage, and alleys are overrun by rats. Fires and crime are constant threats. Recreational facilities are almost nonexistent, forcing children to play in streets and alleys.

Occupational roles also predispose people to certain illnesses. For instance, some industrial workers may be exposed to carcinogenic agents. More affluent people may fulfill stressful social or occupational roles that predispose them to stress-related diseases. Such roles may also encourage overeating or social use of drugs or alcohol.

Family and Cultural Beliefs

The family passes on patterns of daily living and life-styles to offspring. For example, a woman who was abused as a child may physically abuse her small son. Physical or emotional abuse may cause long-term health problems. Emotional health depends on a social environment that is free of excessive tension and does not isolate the person from others. A climate of open communication, sharing, and love fosters the fulfillment of the person's optimum potential.

Culture and social interactions also influence how a person perceives, experiences, and copes with health and illness. Each culture has ideas about health, and often these are transmitted from parents to children. For example, in some traditional Chinese families health is defined as a balance of energy (yin and yang). Yin is dark, cold, wet, negative, and female; yang is light, warm, dry, positive, and male. An imbalance of yin and yang results in disease. Ethnic and cultural influences on health are discussed in detail in Chapter 18.

People of certain cultures may perceive home remedies or tribal health customs as superior and more dependable than the health care practices of North American society. For example, a person of Asian origin may prefer to use herbal remedies and acupuncture to treat pain rather than analgesic medications. Cultural rules, values, and beliefs give people a sense of being stable and able to predict outcomes. The challenging of old beliefs and values by second-generation ethnic groups may give rise to conflict, instability, and insecurity, in turn contributing to illness.

Social Support Networks

Social support networks are closely related to an individual's internal factors of self-concept, cognition, and psychologic make-up; these influence the person's motivation and ability to develop supportive networks. Having a support network (family, friends, or a confidant) and job satisfaction helps people avoid illness. Support people also help the person confirm that illness exists. Persons with inadequate support networks sometimes allow themselves to become increasingly ill before confirming the illness and seeking therapy. Support people also provide the stimulus for an ill person to become well again.

CONSIDER...

- what behaviors you consider to be the most likely to affect your own health.
- how you would respond to a client who holds health beliefs that are contrary to the treatment that is prescribed.

HEALTH BELIEF MODELS

Several theories or health belief/behavior models have been developed to help determine whether an individual is likely to participate in disease prevention and health promotion activities. These models can be useful tools in the development of programs for helping people change to healthier life-styles and develop a more positive attitude to preventive health measures. See also Chapter 8.

Health Locus of Control Model

Locus of control is a concept from social learning theory that nurses may consider when determining who is most likely to take action regarding health, that is, whether clients believe that their health status is under their own or others' control. People who believe that they have a major influence on their own health status, that is, who believe health is largely self-determined, are called *internals*. Persons who are internally controlled are more likely than others to take the initiative in their own health care, be more knowledgeable about their health, and adhere to prescribed health care regimens, such as taking medication, making and keeping appointments with physicians, maintaining diets, and giving up smoking. By contrast, people who believe their health is largely controlled by outside forces (e.g., chance, luck, or powerful others) and is beyond their control are referred to as *externals*. Externally controlled people may need assistance to become more internally controlled if behavior changes are to be successful. Locus of control is a measurable concept that can be used to predict which people are most likely to change their behavior. Measurement instruments are shown in Chapter 16.

The results of a study by Lewis suggest that greater personal control over one's life is associated with higher levels of self-esteem, greater purpose in life, and decreased self-report of anxiety (Lewis, 1982, p. 113). Nurses can use this information about a client's locus of control to plan internal reinforcement training if necessary in order to improve client compliance.

Rosenstock's and Becker's Health Belief Models

In the 1950s, Rosenstock (1974) proposed a health belief model (HBM) intended to predict which individuals would or would not use such preventive measures as screening for early detection of cancer. Becker (1974) modified the health belief model to include these components: *individual perceptions, modifying factors,* and *variables likely to affect initiating action.*

The health belief model (Figure 3–4) is based on motivational theory. Rosenstock assumed that good health is an objective common to all people. Becker added "positive health motivation" as a consideration.

Individual Perceptions

Individual perceptions include the following:

- *Perceived susceptibility.* A family history of a certain disorder, such as diabetes or heart disease, may make the individual feel at high risk.
- *Perceived seriousness.* The question here is: In the perception of the individual, does the illness cause death or have serious consequences? Concern about the spread of acquired immune deficiency syndrome (AIDS) reflects the general public's perception of the seriousness of this illness.
- *Perceived threat.* According to Becker, perceived susceptibility and perceived seriousness combine to determine the total perceived threat of an illness to a specific individual. For example, a person who perceives that many individuals in the community have AIDS may not necessarily per-

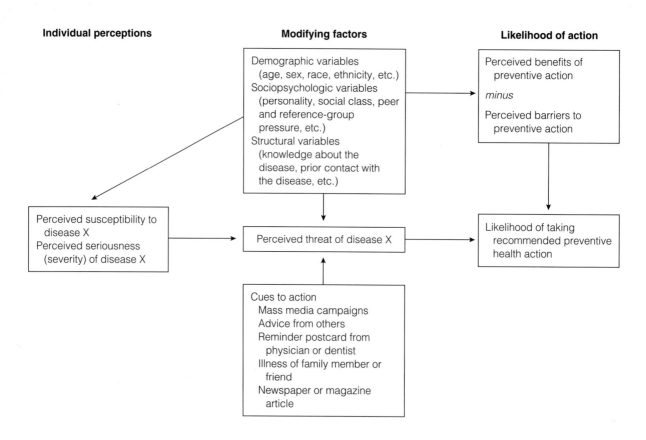

FIGURE 3–4 *The health belief model.*

SOURCE: "Selected Psychosocial Models and Correlates of Individual Health-Related Behaviors" by M. H. Becker, D. P. Haefner, S. V. Kasi, et al., 1977, *Medical Care, 15,* pp. 27–46. Used with permission.

ceive a threat of the disease; if the person is a drug addict or a homosexual, however, the perceived threat of illness is likely to increase because of the combined susceptibility and seriousness.

Modifying Factors

Factors that modify a person's perceptions include the following:

- *Demographic variables.* Demographic variables include age, sex, race, and ethnicity. An infant, for example, does not perceive the importance of a healthy diet; an adolescent may perceive peer approval as more important than family approval and participate as a consequence in hazardous activities or adopt unhealthy eating and sleeping patterns.
- *Sociopsychologic variables.* Social pressure or influence from peers or other reference groups (e.g., self-help or vocational groups) may encourage preventive health behaviors even when individual motivation is low. Expectations of others may motivate people, for example, not to drive an automobile after drinking alcohol.
- *Structural variables.* Structural variables that are presumed to influence preventive behavior are knowledge about the target disease and prior contact with it. Becker found higher compliance rates with prescribed treatments among mothers whose children had frequent ear infections and occurrences of asthma.
- *Cues to action.* Cues can be either internal or external. Internal cues include feelings of fatigue, uncomfortable symptoms, or thoughts about the condition of an ill person who is close. External cues are listed in Figure 3–4.

Likelihood of Action

The likelihood of a person's taking recommended preventive health action depends on the perceived benefits of the action minus the perceived barriers to the action.

- *Perceived benefits of the action.* Examples include refraining from smoking to prevent lung cancer, and eating nutritious foods and avoiding snacks to maintain weight.
- *Perceived barriers to action.* Examples include cost, inconvenience, unpleasantness, and life-style changes.

Nurses play a major role in helping clients implement healthy behaviors. They help clients monitor health, supply anticipatory guidance, and impart knowledge about health. Nurses can also reduce barriers to action (e.g., by minimizing inconvenience or discomfort) and can support positive actions.

CONSIDER...

- whether your own health beliefs have changed in the past 10 years.
- which factors you believe most affect health practices.

HEALTH CARE COMPLIANCE

Compliance, also referred to as adherence, is the extent to which an individual's behavior (for example, taking medications, following diets, or making life-style changes) coincides with medical or health advice. Degree of compliance may range from disregarding every aspect of the recommendations to following the total therapeutic plan. There are many reasons why some people comply and others do not. See the accompanying box.

To enhance compliance, nurses need to ensure that the client is able to perform the prescribed therapy, understands the necessary instructions, is a willing participant in establishing goals of therapy, and values the planned outcomes of behavior changes.

Factors Influencing Compliance

- Client motivation to become well
- Degree of life-style change necessary
- Perceived severity of the health care problem
- Value placed on reducing the threat of illness
- Difficulty in understanding and performing specific behaviors
- Degree of inconvenience of the illness itself or of the regimens
- Belief that the prescribed therapy or regimen will or will not help
- Complexity, side-effects, and duration of the proposed therapy
- Specific cultural heritage that may make compliance difficult
- Degree of satisfaction and quality and type of relationship with the health care providers
- Overall cost of prescribed therapy

When a nurse identifies noncompliance, it is important to find out why and, by taking the following steps, assist the client to comply:

- *Establish why the client is not following the regimen.* Where indicated, the nurse can, for example, provide information, correct misconceptions, attempt to decrease expense, or suggest counseling if psychologic problems are interfering with compliance. It is also essential that the nurse reevaluate the suitability of the health advice provided.
- *Demonstrate caring.* Show sincere concern about the client's problems and decisions and at the same time accepting the client's right to a course of action. For example, a nurse might tell a client who is not taking his heart medication, "I can appreciate how you feel about this, but I am very concerned about your heart."
- *Encourage healthy behaviors through positive reinforcement.* If the man who is not taking his heart medication is walking every day, the nurse might say, "You are really doing well with your walking."
- *Use aids to reinforce teaching.* For instance, the nurse can leave pamphlets for the client to read later or make a "pill calendar," a paper with the date and number of pills to be taken.
- *Establish a therapeutic relationship of freedom, mutual understanding, and mutual responsibility with the client and support persons.* By providing knowledge, skills, and information, the nurse gives clients control over their health and establishes a cooperative relationship, which results in greater compliance.

CONSIDER...

- your response to a client who fails to follow your health care advice.
- the reasons why a client may fail to follow health care instructions about taking medications.

"HEALTHY PEOPLE 2000" GOALS

Health People 2000, a report by the U.S. Department of Health and Human Services (USDHHS, 1990, p. 43) outlines three broad goals to meet the health challenge of the 1990s:

1. Increase the span of healthy life for Americans.
2. Reduce health disparities among Americans.

3. Achieve access to preventive services for all Americans.

A central purpose of *Healthy People 2000* is to increase the proportion of Americans who live long and healthy lives. Healthy life means a full range of functional capacity at each life stage. It extends into the final quarter of a person's life and focuses on freedom from chronic, disabling disease and conditions, from preventable infection, and from serious injury.

Health disparities occur among certain population groups in terms of life expectancy, infant mortality rate, years of healthy life, and potential years of life lost before age 65 (USDHHS, 1990, pp. 46–48). For example

- Years of healthy life for European Americans is 63 years compared to only 56 for African Americans and 62 for Hispanics (1990).
- Infant mortality rates are greater among African Americans than European Americans (17.9 deaths per 1000 live births compared to 8.6 in 1987).
- Compared to European-American males, African-American males have higher percentages of lost years of life before age 65: 55% higher for cancer, 180% higher for stroke, 100% higher for lung disease, and 630% higher for homicide (1987).

Achievement of the second goal of *Healthy People 2000* depends on significant improvements in the health of populations (e.g., African Americans) that are at the highest risk of disease, disability, and premature death.

Access to preventive services for all Americans means more than the availability of services. Preventive services must be integrated with basic primary health care. Approximately 18% of all Americans and 31% of those who lack private or public health insurance have no source of primary health care. Over the next decade, particular attention needs to be given to increasing the number of people who have a primary source of health care and who have adequate insurance coverage. Health care systems need to cover preventive services such as the following:

- Providing health care services that ensure the health of pregnant women and the birth of healthy babies
- Monitoring of child growth and development
- Immunizing children against childhood diseases and immunizing adults who are vulnerable to influenza and pneumonia

READINGS FOR ENRICHMENT

Health desk for Windows: The complete personal wellness software program. (1994, May/June). *Computers in Nursing, 12*(3), 177–178.

Health Desk for Windows: The Complete Personal Wellness Program is a computer software program offered by Health Desk Corporation in Berkeley, California. This software is available for self-use by health-minded individuals or as a teaching tool for nurses to use with their clients in the home setting. *Health Desk* is an information management and educational tool to help people take a more active role in managing their health. It provides general information about the human body and helps the user explore health topics, track health-related activities and medical history, and manage personal medical records. The program includes (a) a Personal Conditions option, where the use can enter a description of medical conditions with date and commentary; (b) a Symptoms screen, which enables the user to describe a condition by checking off items in a list; (c) a Medication screen to enter medication details; and (d) a Health Managers option for obtaining and recording information about exercise, weight, stress, heart health, and women's health. Data provided in the program for instruction are accepted by the American Academy of Family Physicians Foundation.

Jensen, L., & Allen, M. (1993, Fall). Wellness: The dialectic of illness. *Image: Journal of Nursing Scholarship, 25*, 220–223.

The authors describe a generic paradigm describing the relationship of health, disease, wellness, and illness. According to the authors, these four can be thought of as one in the same process, reflecting the changing person in a changing world.

U.S. Department of Health and Human Services, Public Health Service. (1990). *Healthy People 2000: National health promotion and disease prevention objectives.* DHHS Pub no. (PHS) 91-50212. Washington, DC: U.S. Government Printing Office.

This 700-page document presents specific data to achieve the three *Healthy People 2000* goals: (a) increasing the span of a healthy life for Americans, (b) reducing health disparities among Americans, and (c) allowing all Americans access to preventive services. Measurable targets or objectives to be achieved by the year 2000 are organized into 22 priority areas. The first 21 of these are grouped into three broad categories: health promotion, health protection, and preventive services. The 22nd area deals with surveillance and data systems. A section of the end of the document deals with age-related objectives for children, adolescents and young adults, adults, and older adults.

- Adequate screening to detect high blood pressure, high blood cholesterol, and cancer, (e.g., breast, cervical, oropharyngeal, and colorectal)
- Counseling on injury prevention, nutrition, and smoking cessation

These three goals can serve as basic values that underlie all health promotion, health protection, and disease prevention services. See Chapters 8 and 16 for additional information.

SUMMARY

The perspective from which health is viewed has changed; instead of merely the absence of disease, health has come to mean a high level of wellness or the fulfillment of one's maximum potential for physical, psychosocial, and spiritual functioning. Wellness is an active, five-dimensional process of becoming aware of and making choices toward a higher level of well-being. The five dimensions of wellness are the physical, social, emotional, intellectual, and spiritual dimensions. Well-being is considered a subjective perception of balance, harmony, and vitality. It is a state rather than a process. Illness is usually associated with disease but may occur independently of it. Illness is a highly personal state in which the person feels unhealthy or ill. Disease alters body functions and results in a reduction of capacities or a shortened life span.

Because notions of health are highly individual, the nurse must determine each client's perception of health to provide meaningful assistance. This involves well-developed communication skills. Nurses need to be aware of their own personal definitions of health. Most people describe health as freedom from symptoms of disease, the ability to be active, and a state of being in good spirits.

Various models have been developed to explain health. These include Smith's clinical, role performance, adaptive, and eudaemonistic models; Leavell and Clark's agent-host-environment model; Dunn's high-level wellness grid; and Rosenstock's health belief model.

The health status of an individual is affected by many variables over which the person has varying degrees of control: biologic factors (genetic make-up, race, sex, age, and developmental level); psychologic factors (mind-body interactions, self-concept, and job satisfaction); cognitive factors (life-style choices and spiritual and religious beliefs); and external factors (geography, physical environment, standards of living, family and cultural beliefs, and social support networks).

A person's decision to implement health behaviors or to take action to improve health depends on such factors as the importance of health to the person, perceived threat of a particular disease or severity of the health care problems, perceived benefits of preventive or therapeutic actions, inconvenience and unpleasantness involved, degree of life-style change necessary, cultural ramifications, and cost.

Nurses can enhance health care compliance by identifying the reasons for noncompliance if it occurs, demonstrating caring, using positive reinforcement to encourage healthy behaviors, using aids to reinforce teaching, and establishing a therapeutic relationship of freedom, mutual understanding, and mutual responsibility with the client and support persons.

SELECTED REFERENCES

American Nurses Association. (1980). *Nursing: A social policy statement.* Kansas City, MO: Author.

Anspaugh, D. J., Hamrick, M. H., & Rosata, F. D. (1991). *Wellness: Concepts and applications.* St. Louis: Mosby-Year Book.

Becker, M. H. (Ed.). (1974). *The health belief model and personal health behavior.* Thorofare, NJ: Charles B. Slack.

Dubos, R. (1978). Health and creative adaptation. *Human Nature, 74*(1), entire issue.

Dunn, H. L. (1959a, June.) High-level wellness in man and society. *American Journal of Public Health, 49,* 786.

Dunn, H. L. (1959b, Nov.). What high-level wellness means. *Canadian Journal of Public Health, 50,* 447.

Dunn, H. L. (1973). *High-level wellness.* Arlington, VA: Beatty.

Edlin, G, & Golanty, E. (1992). *Health and wellness: A holistic approach* (4th ed.). Boston: Jones and Bartlett.

Jensen, L., & Allen, M. (1993, Fall). Wellness: The dialectic of illness. *Image: Journal of Nursing Scholarship, 25,* 220–223.

Leavell, H. R., & Clark, E. G. (1965) *Preventive medicine for the doctor in his community* (3rd ed.). New York: McGraw-Hill.

Leddy, S., & Pepper, J. M. (1993). *Conceptual bases of professional nursing* (3rd ed.). Philadelphia: Lippincott.

Lewis, F. M. (1982, March/April). Experienced personal control and quality of life in late-stage cancer patients. *Nursing Research, 31,* 113–118.

McAllister, G., & Farquhar, M. (1992, Dec.). Health beliefs: A cultural division? *Journal of Advanced Nursing, 17,* 1447–1454.

McCann/Flynn, J. B., & Heffron, P. B. (1988). *Nursing: From concept to practice* (2nd ed.). East Norwalk, CT: Appleton & Lange.

Mitchell, P. H., & Loustau, A. (1981). *Concepts basic to nursing* (3rd ed.). New York: McGraw-Hill.

Murray, R. B., & Zentner, J. P. (1989). *Nursing concepts for health promotion* (4th ed.). Norwalk, CT: Appleton & Lange.

Nightingale, F. (1969). *Notes on nursing: What it is and what it is not.* New York: Dover Books. (Original work published in 1860)

Parsons, T. (1972). Definitions of health and illness in the light of American values and social structure. In E. G. Jaco (Ed.), *Patients, physicians, and illness* (2nd ed.). New York: Free Press.

Pender, N. J. (1987). *Health promotion in nursing practice* (2nd ed.). Norwalk, CT: Appleton & Lange.

President's Commission on Health Needs of the Nation. (1953). *Building Americans' Health.* Vol. 2 Washington, D.C.: U.S. Government Printing Office.

Rosenstock, I. M. (1974). Historical origins of the health belief model. In M. H. Becker (Ed.), *The health belief model and personal health behavior.* Thorofare, NJ: Charles B. Slack.

Roy, C., & Andrews, H. A. (1991). *The Roy adaptation model: The definitive statement.* Norwalk, CT: Appleton & Lange.

Smith, J. A. (1981, April). The idea of health: A philosophical inquiry. *Advanced Nursing Science, 3,* 43–50.

Travis, J. W., & Ryan, R. S. (1988). *Wellness workbook* (2nd ed.). Berkeley, CA: Ten Speed Press.

U.S. Department of Health and Human Services, Public Health Service. (1990). *Healthy People 2000: National health promotion and disease prevention objectives.* DHHS Pub no. (PHS) 91-50212. Washington, D.C.: U.S. Government Printing Office.

World Health Organization. (1947). *Constitution of the World Health Organization: Chronicle of the World Health Organization I.* Geneva: Author.

4

CHAPTER

Collaboration in Health Care

by Suzanne Beyea

OBJECTIVES

- Discuss factors affecting current health care delivery.

- Compare various billing and payment methods for health care services.

- Discuss strategies to minimize health care costs.

- Explain essential aspects of collaborative health care: definitions, objectives, and benefits.

- Discuss the nurse's collaborative role.

"The boundaries of each health care profession are constantly changing, and members of various professions cooperate by exchanging knowledge and ideas about how to deliver high quality health care. Collaboration among health care professionals involves recognition of the expertise of others within and outside one's profession and referral to those providers when appropriate. Collaboration also involves some shared functions and a common focus on the same overall mission."
—The American Nurses Association, 1995

Health care reform is a major issue today because of rising costs of health care, concerns about the quality of care provided, uneven distribution of services, and inequities in access to care.

- Traditionally, models of health care have shown a one-sided distribution of power in provider-client relationships. The system has been physician dominated and has focused on cure of illness.
- Recently, however, the health care system has moved toward more collaborative efforts and initiatives in which the provider and client become partners in the health care experience. Many advocate client-centered and client-directed collaborative care. "Collaboration in health care should lead to comprehensive, holistic care that is client-centered. It can offer a solution to the seemingly insoluble problems in the current health care system" (Miccolo & Spanier, 1993, p. 443).
- To reduce health care costs and, at the same time, provide quality care is a challenge. Restructuring health care delivery involves redesigning systems, processes, practices, and peoples' jobs in ways that improve outcomes for clients.
- Health care restructuring has significant implications for nursing, which is a critical component of the health care system.

COLLABORATIVE HEALTH CARE

Collaboration is an evolving concept both in theory and practice. In 1992 the ANA Congress on Nursing Practice adopted the following operational definition of the concept of collaboration:

"**Collaboration** means a collegial working relationship with another health care provider in the provision of (to supply) patient care. Collaborative practice requires (may include) the discussion of patient diagnosis and cooperation in the management and delivery of care. Each collaborator is available to the other for consultation either in person or by communication device, but need not be physically present on the premises at the time the actions are performed. The patient-designated health care provider is responsible for the overall direction and management of patient care" (ANA, 1992).

Virginia Henderson (1991, p. 44) defines collaborative care as "a partnership relationship between doctors, nurses, and other health care providers with patients and their families." It is a process by which health care professionals work together with clients to achieve quality health care outcomes. Mutual respect and a true sharing of both power and control are essential elements. Ideally, collaboration becomes a dynamic, interactive process in which clients (individuals, groups, or communities) confer with physicians, nurses, and other health care providers to meet their health objectives. Effective collaboration requires cooperation and coordination between client(s) and various health care providers across the continuum of care.

When reviewing the nursing literature about the construct of collaboration, Baggs and Schmitt (1988, p. 145) found the following critical attributes for collaboration:

- Sharing in planning, decision-making, problem solving, goal setting, and responsibility
- Working together cooperatively
- Coordinating
- Communicating openly

Certain beliefs and characteristics common to collaborative care practices are shown in the accompanying box.

The overall objectives of collaborative initiatives are high-quality client care and client satisfaction. In addition, many health care professionals believe that a multidisciplinary, collaborative framework can limit costs as well as enhance quality. Collaborative practice models propose to achieve several objectives:

- Provide client-directed and client-centered care using a multidisciplinary, integrated, participative framework.
- Enhance continuity across the continuum of care, from prehospitalization through an acute episode of illness to transfer or discharge and recuperation.
- Improve client(s) and family satisfaction with care.

Characteristics and Beliefs Basic to Collaborative Health Care

- Clients have a right to self-determination: that is, the right to choose to participate or not to participate in health care decision making.

- Clients and health care professionals interact in a reciprocal relationship. Instead of making decisions about the client's health care, health care professionals foster joint decision making. Client dependence and professional dominance are minimized; client participation in the health care process is maximized.

- Equality among human beings is desired in health care relationships. The ideas of both clients and health care professionals receive an equal hearing.

- Responsibility for health falls on the client rather than on health care professionals.

- Each individual's concept of health is important and legitimate for that individual. Although clients lack expert knowledge, they have their own ideas about health and illness. Health care professionals need to understand these ideas to be able to effectively help the client.

- Collaboration involves negotiation and consensus seeking rather than questioning and ordering.

- Provide quality, cost-effective, research-based care that is outcome driven.
- Promote mutual respect, communication, and understanding between client(s) and members of the health care team.
- Create a synergy among clients and providers, in which the sum of their efforts is greater than the parts.
- Provide opportunities to address and solve system-related issues and problems.
- Develop interdependent relationships and understanding among providers and clients.

Collaborative practice can include nurse-physician interaction in joint practice, nurse-physician collaboration in care giving, or interdisciplinary teams or committees.

Interdisciplinary collaborative practice teams may consist of a single unit or a group of units with similar client populations. Most committees consist of physicians, nurses, social workers, pharmacists, and other health care professionals (Velianoff, Neely, and Hall, 1993, p. 27). Such multidisciplinary

teams address clinical practice guidelines and clinical issues so as to ensure cost-effective, quality outcomes. Committees such as these may provide the foundation for establishing a truly collaborative practice setting.

The Nurse as a Collaborator

Nurses collaborate with clients, peers, and other health care professionals. They frequently collaborate about client care but may also be involved, for example, in collaborating on bioethical issues, on legislation, on health-related research, and with professional organizations. The box on page 70 outlines selected aspects of the nurse's role as a collaborator.

Prescott and her co-authors (1987, 1991) view collaboration as important in the development of professional nursing practice and as a way to improve client outcomes. To fulfill a collaborative role, nurses need to assume accountability and increased authority in practice areas. Education is integral to ensuring that the members of each professional group understand the collaborative nature of their roles, specific contributions, and the importance of working together. Each professional needs to understand how an integrated delivery system centers on the client's health care needs rather than on the particular care given by one group.

Collaboration in practice is not yet a reality for most nurses. However, because nurses are now more highly educated and have a defined area of expertise, nurses increasingly are functioning more as autonomous health professionals.

Benefits of Collaborative Care

A collaborative approach to health care ideally benefits clients, professionals, and the health care delivery system. Care becomes client centered and, most important, client directed. Clients become informed consumers and actively participate with the health care team in the decision-making process. When clients are empowered to participate actively and professionals share mutually set goals with clients, everyone—including the organization and health care system—ultimately benefit. When quality improves, adherence to therapeutic regimens increases, lengths of stay decrease, and overall costs to the system decline. When professional interdependence develops, collegial relationships emerge, and overall satisfaction increases. The work environment becomes more supportive and acknowledges

---

The Nurse as a Collaborator

With Clients:

- Acknowledges, supports, and encourages clients' active involvement in health care decisions.
- Encourages a sense of client autonomy and an equal position with other members of the health care team.
- Helps clients set mutually agreed-upon goals and objectives for health care.
- Provides client consultation in a collaborative fashion.

With Peers:

- Shares personal expertise with other nurses and elicits the expertise of others to ensure quality client care.
- Develops a sense of trust and mutual respect with peers that recognizes their unique contributions.

With Other Health Care Professionals:

- Recognizes the contribution that each member of the interdisciplinary team can make by virtue of his or her expertise and view of the situation.
- Listens to each individual's views.
- Shares health care responsibilities in exploring options, setting goals, and making decisions with clients and families.
- Participates in collaborative interdisciplinary research to increase knowledge of a clinical problem or situation.

With Professional Nursing Organizations:

- Seeks out opportunities to collaborate with and within professional organizations.
- Serves on committees in state (or provincial) and national nursing organizations or specialty groups.
- Supports professional organizations in political action to create solutions for professional and health care concerns.

With Legislators:

- Offers expert opinions on legislative initiatives related to health care.
- Collaborates with other health care providers and consumers on health care legislation to best serve the needs of the public.

---

the contributions of each team member. "Because authority is shared, this effort results in more integrated and comprehensive care, as well as shared control of costs and liability" (Miccolo & Spanier, 1993, p. 447).

Competencies Basic to Collaboration

Key features necessary for collaboration include effective communication skills, mutual respect, trust, giving and receiving feedback, decision making, and conflict management.

Communication

Collaborating to solve complex problems requires effective communication skills. Initially the health care team needs to define collaboration clearly, establish its goals and objectives, and specify role expectations.

Effective communication can occur only if the involved parties are committed to understanding each other's professional roles and appreciating each other as individuals. Additionally, they must be sensitive to differences among communication styles (Tannen, 1990, p. 48). Instead of focusing on distinctions, each professional group needs to center on their common ground: the client's needs.

Currently, there is little research that provides an understanding of interprofessional communication behaviors. Coeling and Wilcox (1994, p. 49) studied 270 physicians and nurses to assess their elements of communication. They found that physicians placed more emphasis on the content of communication than did nurses, whereas nurses placed more importance on relationship-related factors than did their physician peers. Both groups reported a greater need for collaboration. They also expressed concern about having adequate time and an appropriate environment to communicate effectively.

Mutual Respect and Trust

Mutual respect occurs when two or more people show or feel honor or esteem toward one another. **Trust** occurs when a person is confident in the actions of another person. Both mutual respect and trust imply a mutual process and outcome. They must be expressed both verbally and nonverbally. Sometimes professionals may verbalize respect or trust of others but demonstrate by their actions a lack of trust and respect. The health care system itself has not always created an environment that promotes respect or trust of the various health care providers. Although progress has been made toward creating more collegial relationships, past attitudes may continue to impede efforts toward collaborative practice.

Giving and Receiving Feedback

One of the most difficult challenges for professionals is giving and receiving timely, relevant, and helpful **feedback** to and from each other and their clients. When professionals work closely together, it may be appropriate to address attitudes or actions that affect the collaborative relationship. Feedback may be affected by each person's perceptions, personal space, roles, relationships, self-esteem, confidence, beliefs, emotions, environment, and time.

Negative feedback implies not negative content but rather a negative communication style, such as an attitude of condescension; positive feedback is characterized by a communication style that is warm, caring, and respectful. A review of basic communication skills and an opportunity to practice listening and giving and receiving feedback can enhance any professional's ability to communicate effectively (Ferguson, Howell & Batalden, 1993, p. 5). Giving and receiving feedback helps individuals acquire self-awareness, while assisting the collaborative team to develop an understanding and effective working relationship.

Decision Making

The decision-making process at the team level involves shared responsibility for the outcome. Obviously, to create a solution, the team must follow each step of the decision-making process beginning with a clear definition of the problem. See decision-making in Chapter 12. Team decision making must be directed at the objectives of the specific effort. Factors that enhance the process include mutual respect and constructive and timely feedback (Mariano, 1989, p. 287).

Decision making at the team level requires full consideration and respect of diverse viewpoints. Members must be able to verbalize their perspectives in a nonthreatening environment. Group members effectively use communication skills and give and receive feedback in the decision-making process. Interdependent relationships are actualized as members focus on client care issues (Velianoff, et al., 1993, p. 28).

An important aspect of decision making is the interdisciplinary team focusing on the client's priority needs and organizing interventions accordingly. The discipline best able to address the client's needs is given priority in planning and is responsible for providing its interventions in a timely manner. For example, a social worker may first direct attention to a client's social needs when these needs interfere with the client's ability to respond to therapy. Nurses, by the nature of their holistic practice, are often able to help the team identify priorities and areas requiring further attention.

Conflict Management

Role conflict can occur in any situation where individuals work together. **Role conflict** arises when people are called on to carry out roles that have opposing or incompatible expectations. In an interpersonal conflict, different people have different expectations about a particular role. Interrole conflict exists when one person's or group's expectations differ from the expectations of another person or group. Any one of these types of conflict can affect interdisciplinary collaboration.

Team members may reduce role conflict by clarifying role perceptions and expectations, identifying professional competencies, exploring how roles may overlap, and negotiating role-related responsibilities (Ducanis & Golin, 1981, p. 181). To reduce role conflict, team members can also conduct interdisciplinary conferences, take part in interdisciplinary education in basic programs, and most important, accept personal responsibility for team work (Benson & Ducanis, 1995, p. 211). Ongoing research exploring how professionals relate and how teams function will help professionals better understand ways to reduce role conflict when they collaborate with others.

CONSIDER...

- what barriers to collaborative care you experience in your practice setting.
- what characteristics support collaborative practice in your practice setting.
- approaches you might implement to enhance collaboration.
- how your values, beliefs, and work experiences influence your abilities to be a collaborative member of a health care team.
- how nurses can promote collaborative practice.
- situations where collaborative practice may be impossible or impractical.

FACTORS IMPACTING CURRENT HEALTH CARE DELIVERY

Worldwide, there are a number of significant influences on health and health care. The World Health

Organization (WHO) has set an objective that all persons will achieve by the year 2000 a level of health that will permit them to lead socially and economically productive lives. The report *Healthy People 2000* (1990) focuses on national health promotion and disease prevention goals for U.S. citizens. Increasingly, governments and society are striving to reduce health risks, minimize the incidence of chronic illness, and improve the health and quality of life for all. The overall goal is to provide health care for all individuals, but health and health care are not guaranteed. Today, the most pressing question for the health care system remains how to provide quality health care that is in line with the socioeconomic realities of society. A number of factors influence the provision of health care; they are described below.

Consumer Needs and Wants

Although the diagnosis and treatment of illness are still necessities, the focus of health care is changing. Health care consumers are demanding comprehensive, holistic, and compassionate health care that is also affordable. Clients expect that health care providers will view each person as a biopsychosocial whole and respond to his or her individual needs. They want wellness-related care that focuses on the quality of life, not the quantity of life. They want expert care that humanistically integrates the available technology and provides information and services related to health promotion and illness prevention.

Today's health care consumers have greater knowledge about their health than in previous years and they are increasingly influencing health care delivery. Formerly, people expected a physician to make decisions about their care; today, however, consumers expect to be involved in making any decisions.

Consumers have also become aware of how lifestyle affects health. As a result, they desire more information and services related to health promotion and illness prevention.

Increasingly people are actively assuming responsibility for their level of health and are willing to participate in health-promoting activities. They are beginning to view health care professionals as a resource to guide these activities. Many health plans already provide participants with memberships to physical fitness clubs and nutrition classes or offer free attendance at smoking cessation classes.

Detailed information about health and wellness, the nurse's role as health promoter, and the health promotion of individuals and families is provided in Chapters 3, 8, and 16.

Self-Help Initiatives

Responsibility for the self is a major belief underlying holistic health that recognizes the interdependency of body, mind, and spirit. Increasingly people are adopting the view that the self is empowered with the ability to create or maintain health or disease. For further information about holistic health, see Chapter 19.

Today many individuals seek answers for acute and chronic health problems through nontraditional approaches to health care. Alternative medicine and support groups are among two of the most popular self-help choices. Each year, more adults are using alternative or unconventional therapies to treat numerous health problems. The most commonly used therapies include relaxation techniques, chiropractic treatments, massage, imagery, spiritual healing, weight loss programs, and herbal medicine. Back problems, fibromyalgia, cancer, allergies, arthritis, insomnia, chronic fatigue syndrome, strains or sprains, headache, high blood pressure, digestive problems, anxiety, and depression are the most common conditions for which individuals seek unconventional therapy.

In addition to alternative therapies, many adults participate in one or more self-help groups during their lifetime. In North America, there are more than 500 different mutual support or self-help groups that focus on nearly every major health problem or life crisis people experience. These groups developed, in part, because people felt such organizations could meet needs not addressed by the traditional health care system. Alcoholics Anonymous (AA), which formed in 1935, serves as a model for many of these groups. The National Self-Help Clearinghouse in the United States provides information on current support groups and guidelines about how to start a self-help group. Groups vary in effectiveness, but most provide education to encourage self-care as well as offering social and emotional support.

Changing Demographics and Epidemiology

Among the problems facing the health care system are the unmet needs of low-income individuals and families and the special needs of older adults, people who have AIDS, and the homeless. In both the United States and Canada, there has been tremendous increase in the number of older adults, which has exerted a significant impact on the health care system. Experts predict that by the year 2020, there will be over 50 million adults over the age of 65 years in the United States (Abrams, Beers & Berkow, 1995, p. 1351). The growing numbers of older adults, combined with the fact that the average older adult has three or more chronic health conditions, will greatly impact the health care system and insurers in the future.

A major epidemiologic influence on the health care system is the increasing numbers of individuals infected with the human immunodeficiency virus (HIV) or acquired immune deficiency syndrome (AIDS). The AIDS epidemic is growing each year, and the survival rate for individuals with AIDS is low. The Centers for Disease Control and Prevention report that a total of 501,310 Americans have been diagnosed with AIDS and 62% of that group have died. Worldwide, it is estimated that 18 million adults and 1.5 million children have been infected with HIV, and of that group, 4.5 million individuals have developed AIDS (Centers for Disease Control and Prevention, 1995, pp. 849, 851).

The growing number of homeless individuals is a major health problem. It has been estimated that in a 5-year period from 1985 to 1990, 5.7 million Americans were homeless and lacked some type of permanent residence. (Link, Susser, Stueve, Phelan, Moore & Struening, 1994, p. 1911).

Factors contributing to homelessness include: the high cost of housing, reduced federal subsidies for low-income housing, alcohol and drug abuse, and the deinstitutionalization of mental health facilities. The homeless population has physical, mental, social, and emotional problems. Limited access to health care services significantly contributes to the general poor health of the homeless in the United States.

Health Care Costs

Expenditures for health care in the United States were approximately $940 billion in 1993 (Smith, 1993, p. 73). Despite these tremendous expenses, a number of Americans have limited access to health care. In fact, experts estimate that as many as 37 million Americans have inadequate or no insurance (Smith, 1993, p. 71). However, in the United States

there are no accurate data about how many individuals are underinsured or uninsured.

The health care system in the United States is thought to be in financial distress. For example, since its inception, Medicare has repeatedly increased monthly premiums, deductibles, and related taxes.

Several alternative health delivery systems have been implemented to control costs. These include health maintenance organizations (HMOs), preferred provider organizations (PPOs), physician/hospital organizations (PHOs) and so on (see page 75 for further information). Additionally, the development of prospective payment systems significantly influenced the health care system. See cost-containment strategies next. Concerns remain, however, about ways to further reduce health care costs and at the same time achieve the desired goal of improving the quality of health care delivery.

Employers, legislators, insurers, and health care providers continue to collaborate in efforts to resolve these concerns. Ethical issues such as rationing of health care, access to health care, the use of health care technology and extraordinary interventions, and organ transplantation can be resolved only through collaboration.

Technologic Advances

Technology has had a major influence on health care costs and services. In fact, available technology often influences decisions about the level of care and intervention. With advances in medicine and technology, an individual's life span can in many cases be extended. However, that same technology may result in fragmentation of care and acceleration of health care costs. New medical devices, technologic advances, and new medications frequently are introduced with limited consideration to the associated costs or the efficacy of their use. For example, the vital functions of circulation and breathing of a client who has no measurable brain activity can be maintained through advanced life support. In the United States, it is estimated that over 25% of Medicare dollars are expended for the last year of life (Abrams, et al., 1995, p. 1365). At the societal level, the difficult questions of when and how life should be extended through use of technology have not been answered.

CONSIDER...

- which demographic factors most affect your practice setting.

- how you feel about the use of alternative medicine versus the use of traditional medicine.
- which self-help or alternative health care strategies you view as effective.
- what self-help groups are available in your community that you have found to be effective.
- how you would advise a client who asks you about the use of a nontraditional approach to health care.
- changes you would recommend in the health care system to improve health care for older adults, the homeless, and people with AIDS.

COST-CONTAINMENT STRATEGIES

Efforts have been made for many years to control health care costs, yet they continue to rise. Some of the main cost-containment strategies are competition, price controls, alternative insurance delivery systems, managed care, health promotion and illness prevention, and alternative care providers.

Competition

In the 1970s in the United States, regulations were changed to permit competition among the agencies that deliver health care and provide insurance. Currently, there appears to be little reduction in costs that can be attributed to competition. Competition has, however, led to the establishment of walk-in clinics, urgent care clinics, and alternative health care providers, for example, which offer additional care choices for clients.

Price Controls

Price controls for health care services have been established in various ways. Freezes on physicians' fees have been imposed at various times for short periods and many states limit reimbursement to physicians and hospitals for services provided to Medicaid clients. **Group self-insurance** plans are another means to reduce costs. These plans involve a designated group, such as employees in a large company, a group of companies, or a union, for example. The designated group assumes all or part of the costs of health care for its members. They can often provide coverage at a lower cost than insurance companies because they are exempt from certain taxes and fees.

The passage of the Tax Equity and Fiscal Responsibility Act (TEFRA) in 1982 brought about a dramatic restructuring of health care delivery in the United States. Through this act, the federal government changed the payment method for Medicare from a retrospective system to a **prospective payment system.** This legislation limits the amount paid to hospitals that are reimbursed by Medicare. Reimbursement is made according to a classification system known as **diagnosis-related groups** (DRGs). The system establishes pretreatment diagnosis billing categories and a payment schedule.

Using DRGs, a hospital is paid a predetermined amount for clients with a specific diagnosis. For example, a hospital that admits a client with a diagnosis of cholelithiasis is reimbursed with a specific dollar amount, regardless of the cost of services, the length of stay, or the acuity or complexity of the client's illness. Prior to the DRG system, hospitals billed retrospectively, that is, after services were rendered. In contrast, prospective payment or billing is determined *before* the client is ever admitted to the hospital. DRG rates are set in advance of the year during which they apply and are considered fixed unless major, uncontrollable events occur. The Health Care Financing Administration (HCFA) is authorized to administer and enforce this system.

This legislation has had a tremendous impact on health care delivery in the United States because hospitals and providers, rather than Medicare or other third-party payors, run the risk of monetary losses. If a hospital's cost per case exceeds the defined limit, it incurs a loss; if the cost is less than the defined limit, it makes a profit. Thus, this type of prospective payment system offers financial incentives for withholding unnecessary tests or procedures and avoiding prolonged hospital stays and excessive expenditures.

Notable effects of prospective payment systems include the earlier discharge of clients, a decline in admissions, a rise in the number and type of outpatient services, and an increased focus on the costs of care. One result of the decline in admissions is that most of those clients who are admitted to acute care hospitals are seriously ill and have complex health care needs. The earlier discharge of clients has led to an expansion of home care services and an increased use of technology and specialists.

To protect clients from DRG abuses, Medicare introduced state **peer review organizations** (PROs). Made up of physicians, nurses, and other health care professionals, PROs are intended to monitor the hospitals and ensure high-quality care under DRGs. PROs have developed screening guidelines that determine whether admissions should occur or procedures should be performed. PROs also review health care records, render payment decisions, and handle related problems, such as admission criteria.

Alternative Delivery Systems

With the advent of increased costs, alternative delivery systems were created. Private insurers created new programs, such as the health maintenance organization (HMO) and the preferred provider organization (PPO), as strategies to control costs. Insurers also encouraged outpatient diagnostic testing and surgery, required second opinions for surgery, and implemented a variety of other cost-cutting initiatives.

Health maintenance organizations are group health care agencies that provide basic and supplemental health maintenance and treatment services to voluntary enrollees. The enrollees or their employers prepay a fixed periodic fee that is set without regard to the amount or kind of services provided. To receive federal funds, an HMO must offer physician services, hospital and outpatient services, emergency services, short-term mental health services, treatment and referral for drug and alcohol problems, laboratory and radiologic services, and preventive health services. By encouraging preventive and wellness services and by offering ambulatory services, HMOs have reduced the cost of health insurance to the consumer.

The **preferred provider organization** emerged as another alternative health care delivery system. It consists of a group of physicians or a hospital that provides companies with health services at a discounted rate. Hospitals, physicians, and insurance companies are major sponsors of PPOs. Physicians can belong to one or more PPO, and the client chooses a primary care provider among the physicians who belong to a particular PPO.

Physician/hospital organizations (PHOs) are joint ventures between a group of private practice physicians and a hospital. PHOs combine both resources and personnel to provide managed care alternatives and medical services. PHOs work with a variety of insurers to provide services. A typical PHO will include primary care providers and specialists.

A PHO may be part of an **integrated delivery system** (IDS). Such a system incorporates acute care services, home health care, extended and skilled care facilities, and outpatient services. Most integrated delivery systems provide care throughout the life span. Insurers can contract with IDSs to provide all required services, rather than the insurer contracting with multiple agencies for the same services. Ideally, an IDS enhances continuity of care and communication between professionals and various agencies providing managed care.

Managed Care

Managed care describes a health care system whose goals are to provide cost-effective, quality care that focuses on improved outcomes for groups of clients. In managed care, health care providers and agencies collaborate so as to render the most appropriate, fiscally responsible care possible. Managed care denotes an emphasis on cost controls, customer satisfaction, health promotion, and preventive services. Health maintenance organizations (HMOs) and preferred provider organizations (PPOs) are examples of provider systems committed to managed care.

Hospitals and other health care agencies have adopted many of the principles of managed care. Hospitals have developed strategies to reduce costs and ensure quality outcomes for groups of clients. They have not only developed PHOs and IDSs but also have adopted practice innovations, including case management, critical pathways, and patient-focused care. These models require nurses, physicians, and ancillary providers to collaborate as they develop and implement health care.

Case management describes a model of integrating health care services for individuals or groups. Various case management models exist that strive to provide cost-effective care and ensure quality outcomes. Generally, case management involves nurse-physician teams that assume collaborative responsibility for planning, assessing needs, and coordinating, implementing, and evaluating care for groups of clients from preadmission to discharge or transfer and recuperation. Case managers, however, may be a social worker or other appropriate professional.

Case managers generally coordinate care for a specific client population, such as clients with AIDS, in a particular setting. A critical component of their role is collaboration with other health care professionals and the client to achieve established

---

Key Responsibilities of Case Managers

Assessing clients and their homes and communities

Coordinating and planning client care

Collaborating with other health professionals

Monitoring clients' progress

Evaluating client outcomes

---

outcomes. Key responsibilities for case managers are shown in the accompanying box.

Critical pathways are interdisciplinary plans for managed care of a client that specify interdisciplinary assessments, interventions, treatments, and outcomes for specific health-related conditions across a time line. Critical pathways are also called critical paths, interdisciplinary plans, anticipated recovery plans, interdisciplinary action plans, and action plans. These plans can be developed for surgical procedures, medical diagnoses, emergency care, trauma care, and health-related interventions. They are usually used for high-volume case types or situations that have relatively predictable outcomes. The pathways are designed in collaboration with members of the health care team who are involved in managing the case type. See Figure 4–1 for a sample critical pathway.

Critical pathways establish the sequence and timing of interdisciplinary interventions and incorporate education, discharge planning, assessments, consultations, nutrition, medications, activities, diagnostic testing, therapeutic measures, and so on.

Critical pathways strive to meet several goals: to achieve realistic, expected client and family outcomes; to promote professional, collaborative practice and care; to ensure the continuity of care; to guarantee the appropriate use of resources; to reduce costs and length of stay; and to provide the framework for continuous quality improvement.

When agencies use critical pathways, members of the health care team work together to set client goals and delineate professional roles, functions, and responsibilities. Once the critical pathway is developed, the collaborative team pilots the tool and revises it as indicated. If care for a specific case type is delivered using a critical pathway, a case manager may be assigned to the case type. Critical pathways may be used in managed care settings, tra-

ditional delivery systems, or patient-focused care models.

Patient-focused care describes a delivery model that provides services to clients in their particular setting. Care activities center on the client, and clients leave the unit only for services that cannot be provided on the unit. Laboratory, pharmacy, and radiologic services, for example, may be located on or adjacent to hospital units. *Cross-training*, development of multiskilled workers who can perform tasks or functions in more than one discipline, is an essential element of patient-focused care. For further information about multiskilled cross-trained practitioners, see Chapter 1.

Because patient-focused care may result in the blurring of roles, collaboration is vital during the design and implementation process. Efficiency, decreased costs, and the increased use of paraprofessionals may all be integral to the managed care system in the future. Many hospitals have adopted some components of patient-focused care in efforts to improve client and staff satisfaction and to reduce costs.

Partners in practice is another system associated with managed care. The partners-in-practice system is a partnership established between an experienced senior registered nurse and an individual who supports the nurse as a technical assistant. The technical assistant is assigned to the nurse, not to a case load of clients. By delegating tasks to the technical assistant, the registered nurse is therefore able to concentrate on providing professional client care.

The registered nurse is responsible for defining the role, standards, and nursing care activities. By providing direction and supervision, the registered nurse is also accountable for the overall care delivered in the partnership. An official contract is used to confirm the relationship, and both members are paired on the same time schedule.

Health Promotion and Illness Prevention

Health promotion and preventive care can maximize a client's well-being, speed recovery from illness, and decrease complications from long-term illness. Preventive care and health education have become increasingly important parts of the health care delivery system. Many hospitals and community clinics offer health education on life-style changes to promote health.

Critical Pathway for Client Following
Myocardial Infarction (Uncomplicated)

Expected Length of stay: 6 days

	Date _____ Day 1: Admission to Coronary Care Unit	Date _____ Day 2	Date _____ Day 3: Transfer to Stepdown Unit
Daily outcomes	Client will: • have stabilizing vital signs and hemodynamic measures • remain alert and oriented • verbalize pain or discomfort using a 0–10 scale • verbalize control of chest pain • verbalize understanding of ongoing treatment and need for hospitalization • demonstrate ability to adhere to activity restrictions • have lungs clear to auscultation • maintain urine output >30 mL/hr • verbalize feelings regarding ongoing stressors • verbalize/demonstrate ability to cope	Client will: • have stable vital signs and hemodynamic measures • remain alert and oriented • verbalize control of chest pain • verbalize presence or absence of pain or discomfort on a 0–10 scale • verbalize understanding of ongoing treatment and need for hospitalization • demonstrate ability to adhere to activity restrictions • have lungs clear to auscultation • maintain urine output >30 mL/hr • verbalize feelings regarding ongoing stressors and illness • verbalize/demonstrate ability to cope	Client will: • be afebrile, with stable vital signs • remain alert and oriented • verbalize presence or absence of pain or discomfort • be free of chest pain • verbalize understanding of ongoing treatment and need for hospitalization • demonstrate ability to adhere to activity restrictions • tolerate activity level without dyspnea, shortness of breath, or chest pain • have lungs clear to auscultation • maintain urine output >30 mL/hr • verbalize feelings regarding ongoing stressors and illness • verbalize ability to cope • verbalize understanding of transfer to stepdown unit • verbalize beginning understanding of home care instructions
Assessments, tests, and treatments	CBC EKG PA and lateral chest x-ray ABGs PT/PTT Cardiac enzymes q8hr x 3 Cardiovascular assessment q4hr and prn Continuous cardiac monitoring Vital signs and O_2 saturation, q4hr and prn Incentive spirometer q2hr Oxygen to maintain O_2 saturation >95% Assist with ADLs Monitor arterial blood gases Weight	Vital signs and O_2 saturation, q4hr and prn Cardiovascular assessment q4hr and prn Continuous cardiac monitoring Intake and output every shift Oxygen to maintain O_2 saturation >95% Weight	Vital signs and O_2 saturation q4hr and prn Cardiovascular assessment q4hr and prn Continuous cardiac monitoring Intake and output every shift Oxygen to maintain O_2 saturation >96% Assist with ADLs Transfer to stepdown unit as ordered Weight
Knowledge deficit	Orient to room and hospital routine Review plan of care Include family in teaching Evaluate understanding of teaching	Review plan of care Brief MI teaching Include family in teaching Evaluate understanding of teaching	Reinforce earlier teaching regarding ongoing care Begin discharge teaching using MI teaching packet regarding rest, activity, and diet Include family in teaching Evaluate understanding of teaching

FIGURE 4–1 *Critical pathway for client following myocardial infarction (uncomplicated).*

➤

Myocardial Infarction (Uncomplicated) (continued)

	Date _____ Day 1: Admission to Coronary Care Unit	Date _____ Day 2	Date _____ Day 3: Transfer to Stepdown Unit
Psychosocial	Assess level of anxiety Encourage verbalization of concerns Provide information and ongoing support and encouragement to client and family	Assess level of anxiety Encourage verbalization of concerns Provide information and ongoing support and encouragement to client and family	Encourage verbalization of concerns Provide ongoing support and encouragement to client and family
Diet	American Heart Association diet as tolerated, providing small, frequent, nutritious feedings Avoid extremes in temperatures	American Heart Association diet as tolerated, providing small, frequent, nutritious feedings Avoid extremes in temperatures	American Heart Association diet as tolerated, providing small, frequent, nutritious feedings Avoid extremes in temperatures
Activity	Assess safety needs and provide appropriate precautions Bed rest Assist with ADLs Provide rest periods Monitor responses to visitors and limit accordingly	Maintain safety precautions Bed rest with commode privileges Assist with ADLs Transfer to chair, as tolerated Provide rest periods Monitor responses to visitors and limit accordingly	Maintain safety precautions Chair, ambulate in room Assist with ADLs Provide rest periods Monitor responses to activity
Medications	IV KVO Consider thrombolytics IV heparin as ordered Aspirin as ordered IV nitro as ordered IV beta blockers as ordered Sleeping medication if ordered	IV KVO IV heparin as ordered Aspirin as ordered IV nitro as ordered and then begin weaning per order IV beta blockers as ordered Sleeping medication if ordered Stool softener	Intermittent IV device IV heparin as ordered Aspirin as ordered Cardiac meds as ordered Sleeping medication if ordered Stool softener Laxative if no BM in 3 days
Transfer/discharge plans	Establish discharge goals with client and family Consult with social service regarding VNA projected needs for home health care (if any)	Review progress toward discharge goals with client and family Referral to cardiac rehab	Review progress toward discharge goals with client and family Cardiac rehab evaluation completed

	Date _____ Day 4	Date _____ Day 5	Date _____ Day 6
Psychosocial	Encourage verbalization of concerns Provide ongoing support and encouragement to client and family	Encourage verbalization of concerns Provide ongoing support and encouragement to client and family	Encourage verbalization of concerns Provide ongoing support and encouragement to client and family
Diet	American Heart Association diet as tolerated, providing small, frequent, nutritious feedings	American Heart Association diet as tolerated, providing small, frequent, nutritious feedings	American Heart Association diet as tolerated, providing small, frequent, nutritious feedings

	Date _____ Day 4	Date _____ Day 5	Date _____ Day 6
Activity	Ambulate in room 3–4 times/day Ambulate in hallway Maintain safety precautions Monitor responses to activity	Ambulate in room 3–4 times/day Ambulate in hallway Start stair walking Maintain safety precautions Monitor responses to activity	Ambulate in room 3–4 times/day Ambulate in hallway Maintain safety precautions Monitor responses to activity
Medications	Intermittent IV device D/C heparin Aspirin as ordered Sleeping medication if ordered Stool softener Cardiac meds as ordered	D/C intermittent IV device Aspirin as ordered Sleeping medication if ordered Stool softener Cardiac meds as ordered	Aspirin as ordered Sleeping medication if ordered Stool softener Cardiac meds as ordered

Transfer/discharge plans	Continue to review progress
	  toward discharge goals
	Finalize discharge plans
	Finalize referral to cardiac
	  rehab
	Continue discharge teaching
		Finalize plans for home care
		  if needed
		Make any other appropriate
		  referrals
		Continue discharge teaching
			Finalize plans for home care
			  if needed
			Make any appropriate referrals
			Complete discharge teaching

Potential Client Variances

Myocardial Infarction (Uncomplicated)

	Possible Complications	**Health Conditions**	**Nursing Diagnoses**

	• Dysrhythmias
	• Congestive heart failure
	• Pericarditis
	• Extension of MI
		• Diabetes
		• Hypertension
		• Kidney failure
		• Pre-existing coronary or
		  respiratory disease
			• Acute pain
			• Anxiety
			• Fear
			• Ineffective individual coping
			• Decreased cardiac output
			• Activity intolerance
			• Ineffective management of
			  therapeutic regimen

FIGURE 4–1 *Critical pathway for client following myocardial infarction (uncomplicated).*

SOURCE: *Critical Pathways for Collaborative Care* by S. C. Beyea, 1996. Menlo Park, CA: Addison-Wesley Nursing, pp. 63–66. Reprinted with permission.

Wellness centers are receiving greater recognition as legitimate components of the health care system. Employer-sponsored wellness programs have also indicated that they are cost-effective because they reduce absenteeism and illness.

Alternative Care Providers

Many of the primary services traditionally provided by physicians are now offered by advanced practice nurses such as nurse practitioners, nurse midwives, and clinical nurse specialists. When provided by nurses the service costs less and provides a perspective on health promotion and wellness.

CONSIDER . . .

- whether managed care has improved people's access to care.
- whether managed care solves or creates problems for the health care system.
- how decisions regarding early discharge programs should be made. Should they be made by health care professionals or by legislators?

- how decisions about allocation of resources should be made.

HEALTH CARE ECONOMICS

Because health care is an exceedingly expensive entity in contemporary society, many approaches have been developed to finance it and, at the same time, maintain quality.

Billing Methods

There are three main types of billing for health care services: fee-for-service, capitation, and fee-for-diagnosis.

Fee-for-Service

In the fee-for-service method, clients pay the practitioner for each health service they receive rather than the professional receiving a fixed amount of compensation. Ideally, clients choose the service they need and each pays for this service. In reality, not all clients are willing or able to choose the service they require and not all health care providers are willing to relinquish their prescriptive power or work for a fixed amount. Therefore, collaboration is required to select mutually acceptable health services in the fee-for-service billing.

Capitation

Under **capitation,** health care providers are paid a fixed dollar amount per person, for providing an agreed-upon set of health services to a defined population for a specific period of time. If the costs of providing service are lower than the fixed dollar amount, the provider organization makes a profit. If costs exceed payment, however, then the provider organization takes a financial loss.

Health maintenance organizations (HMOs), preferred provider organizations (PPOs), and physician/hospital organizations (PHOs) discussed earlier are managed care systems and thus subject to capitation. In other words, payors negotiate health care costs, and the providers take both the potential financial risks and benefits.

Fee-for-Diagnosis

Fee-for-diagnosis is a type of prospective payment system (PPS). Agencies are provided with a fixed dollar amount for the care of a client based on the client's main and secondary diagnoses, demographic information (e.g., age and sex), and the usual treatment provided for the health problems. The diagnosis-related group (DRG) system is an example of a fee-for-diagnosis system. See page 74.

Because a diagnosis is needed to establish a fee for the health care provider, the fee-for-diagnosis system does not provide incentives for reducing costs by providing preventive care.

Payment Sources

United States

In the United States, there are three main sources of payment: government health plans, private insurance, and personal payment.

Government Health Plans The federal government, through Social Security, has in place a number of health care programs, including Medicare and Medicaid.

Medicare Medicare is designed to provide health care to people 65 years and older.

Medicare clients pay a deductible and coinsurance. **Coinsurance** is the 20% share of a payment that is paid by the client; the other 80% is paid by the government.

Medicare is divided into two parts: Part A is available to the disabled and to people 65 years and over. It provides insurance toward hospitalization, home care, and hospice care. Part B is voluntary and provides partial coverage of physician services to people eligible for Part A. Clients pay a monthly premium for this coverage.

Medicare does not cover dental care, dentures, eyeglasses, hearing aids, or examinations to prescribe and fit hearing aids. Most preventive care, including routine physical examinations and associated diagnostic test, is not included.

Medicaid Medicaid is a public assistance program paid out of general taxes for people who require financial assistance (i.e., low-income groups). Medicaid is paid by federal and state governments. Each state program is distinct. Some states provide very limited coverage, whereas others pay for dental care, eyeglasses, and prescription drugs.

Private Insurance In the United States, numerous commercial health insurance carriers offer a wide range of coverage plans. There are two types of private health insurance: not-for-profit (e.g., Blue Cross-Blue Shield) and for-profit (e.g., commercial companies such as Metropolitan Life, Travelers, and

Aetna). Private health insurance pays either the entire bill or, more often, 80% of the costs.

With these plans, insurance may be purchased either as an individual plan or as part of a group plan through a person's employer, union, student association, or similar organization. The individual usually pays a monthly premium to obtain this protection. Group plans offer premiums at lower costs. Some employers share the costs of the premiums, and this benefit is often a major item in labor contracts.

Personal Payment Direct personal payment is the payment of money for services not covered by insurance. The percentage of health care costs paid personally by an individual is higher in the United States than that paid by people in England, Germany, or Canada, for example.

Canada

In Canada, the Canadian National Hospital Insurance Program was started in 1958, and the National Medical Care Insurance Program (Medicare) began in 1968. These plans provide universal coverage through a single-payor system that is regionally controlled. Enacted in 1984, the Canada Health Act (CHA) penalizes provinces that permit extra billing of clients and creates incentives for home care, community health clinics, and health promotion services. In addition, many provincial initiatives are currently under way to improve quality and efficiency and decrease health care costs. As in the United States, hospital beds are decreasing and community resources are increasing. However, there are serious concerns about increasing health care costs.

Australia

Australia's Medicare system provides health care for all who are legally permanent residents of Australia or are visitors from countries with which Australia has a health care agreement. The Medicare system consists of three parts: (1) free or subsidized treatment by a general practitioner, medical specialist, or optometrist; (2) free treatment as public patients in a public hospital; and (3) subsidized prescription medicines. Clients may choose their own general practitioner; however, treatment by a specialist requires referral by a general practitioner.

The Medicare system is funded through the Australian tax system and pays 85% of the Schedule fee, which is set by the government. If a client or client family spends in excess of the government-set amount on health care costs within a given year

(A\$247.90 in 1993), the Medicare system will pay 100% of Schedule fees for the remainder of that year through the Medicare Safety Net. This entitlement is designed to protect individuals and families from high medical expenses.

Australia's public hospital system is funded jointly by the Commonwealth, State, and Territory governments and is administered by the State/Territory Health Departments. Medicare does not pay for private accommodation in either a public or private hospital, so individuals who choose to be treated as private patients must pay the difference between the amount Medicare subsidizes and the cost of service. Medicare pays 75% of the Schedule fee for private physician services. Private patient services can also be paid for through private insurance such as Medibank Private.

CONSIDER...
- whether the government or employers should provide health insurance benefits.
- how capitation affects nursing care.

NURSING ECONOMICS

Few efforts have been made to determine the actual costs of nursing care. Traditionally, the cost of nursing services has been included in the average hospital bill within the general category of "room rate." Often, the number of clients determined the number of nurses needed. However, when the prospective payment system was introduced, it became necessary for hospitals to determine their staffing needs more efficiently. In the early 1960s, a *patient classification system* (PCS) was developed at Johns Hopkins Hospital that identified the needs for nursing care in quantitative terms. Since that time, various PCSs have been developed that assess the acuity of illness and the corresponding complexity and amount of nursing care required.

Quality care and cost tradeoffs in hospitals dominate the literature of the past decade. Both consumers and health care professionals are expressing concerns about diminished quality of care resulting from cost constraints, early discharge, nursing shortages, and the increased use of unlicensed assistive personnel (UAPs). Determining the precise cost of nursing services is a major challenge for nursing. What are the exact costs of high-quality nursing care? How many nursing care hours are required for each DRG? What is the best *skill mix*—that is, ratio

Nursing's Agenda for Health Care Reform (Executive Summary)

The basic components of nursing's "core of care" include

- A restructured health care system which
  - Enhances consumer access to services by delivering primary health care in community-based settings.
  - Fosters consumer responsibility for personal health, self-care, and informed decision making in selecting health care services.
  - Facilitates utilization of the most cost-effective providers and therapeutic options in the most appropriate settings.

- A federally defined standard package of essential health care services available to all citizens and residents of the United States, provided and financed through an integration of public and private plans and sources:
  - A public plan, based on federal guidelines and eligibility requirements, will provide coverage for the poor and create the opportunity for small businesses and individuals, particularly those at risk because of preexisting conditions and those potentially medically indigent, to buy into the plan.
  - A private plan will offer, at a minimum, the nationally standardized package of essential services. This standard package could be enriched as a benefit of employment, or individuals could purchase additional services if they so choose. If employers do not offer private coverage, they must pay into the public plan for their employees.

- A phase-in of essential services, in order to be fiscally responsible:
  - Coverage of pregnant women and children is critical. This first step represents a cost-effective investment in the future health and prosperity of the nation.
  - One early step will be to design services specifically to assist vulnerable populations who have had limited access to our nation's health care system. A "Healthstart Plan" is proposed to improve the health status of these individuals.

- Planned change to anticipate health service needs that correlate with changing national demographics.

- Steps to reduce health care costs include
  - Required usage of managed care in the public plan and encouraged in private plans.

- Incentives for consumers and providers to utilize managed care arrangements.
- Controlled growth of the health care system by planning and prudent resource allocation.
- Incentives for consumers and providers to be cost efficient in exercising health care options.
- Development of health care policies based on effectiveness and outcomes research.
- Assurance of direct access to a full range of qualified providers.
- Elimination of unnecessary bureaucratic controls and administrative procedures.

- Case management will be required for those with continuing health care needs. This will reduce the fragmentation of the present system, promote consumers' active participation in decisions about their health, and create an advocate on their behalf.

- Provisions for long-term care, which include
  - Public and private funding for services of short duration to prevent personal impoverishment.
  - Public funding for extended care if consumer resources are exhausted.
  - Emphasis on the consumers' responsibility to financially plan for their long-term care needs, including new personal financial alternatives and strengthened private insurance arrangements.

- Insurance reforms to improve access to coverage, including affordable premiums, reinsurance pools for catastrophic coverage, and steps to protect both insurers and individuals against excessive costs.

- Access to services assured by no payment at the point of service and elimination of balance billing in both public and private plans.

- Establishment of public/private sector review—operating under the federal guidelines and including payers, providers, and consumers—to determine resource allocation, cost reduction approaches, allowable insurance premiums, and fair and consistent reimbursement levels for providers. This review would progress in a climate sensitive to ethical issues.

SOURCE: *Nursing's Agenda for Health Care Reform*, American Nurses Association, 1991, Washington, DC: Author. PR-3 22M 6/91. Reprinted with permission.

of registered nurses to licensed practical nurses and nursing assistants—on each hospital unit? Since 1983, many studies have been undertaken to determine the actual costs of nursing care and the cost-effectiveness of nursing care. Researchers have investigated such topics as the impact of nurse-physician collaboration; new cost-effective interventions; cost benefits of primary nursing, nurse practitioners, and nursing midwives; cost-effectiveness of home care; and so on. The quality of the nursing care of the future will rely on ongoing research.

CONSIDER...

- whether cost-containment programs implemented in your agency have influenced nursing care.
- measures that have been implemented in your agency to relieve nurses of non-nursing tasks.
- the role nurses play in maintaining quality nursing care in your agency.
- what cost-effective care nurses could provide that may substitute for physicians' services in your community.
- who should reimburse the nurse for services.

NURSING'S AGENDA FOR HEALTH CARE REFORM

In 1991, the American Nurses Association (ANA) published *Nursing's Agenda for Health Care Reform*, which sets forth recommendations for health care reform. This agenda was a joint effort of the ANA, the National League for Nursing (NLN), and the American Association of Colleges of Nursing (AACN). The American Organization of Nurse Executives (AONE) also participated.

A central objective of this reform is to provide a basic "core" of essential health care services to everyone. The statement calls for a restructuring of the health care system to focus on consumers and their health needs. It also recommends that health care be delivered in such diverse settings as schools, workplaces, and homes and that the health care system shift its focus from illness and cure to wellness and care. See the box on page 82.

The AONE (1992, p. 42) writes that effective health care must

1. Encourage consumer partnerships so that consumers can take an active role in their health and their care and in decisions about their care.

2. Allow all U.S. citizens and residents access to basic health care services.

3. Increase health care access by the use of physician and nonphysician providers.

4. Create incentives that promote health, wellness, and prevention; individuals with chronic illnesses will not be penalized.

5. Promote affordable, safe, and effective health care.

6. Make provisions for skilled and long-term care.

7. Make provisions for catastrophic care, with some limitation on extraordinary procedures.

8. Finance health care through a combination of public- and private-sector funding.

READINGS FOR ENRICHMENT

Flarey, D. L. (1995). *Redesigning nursing care delivery: Transforming our future.* Philadelphia: Lippincott.

This book describes the transformation of nursing and redesigning the health care system. Twenty chapters offer information on a variety of subjects from the theory to the practice of health care delivery.

Kasch, C. R. (1986, Summer). Establishing a collaborative nurse-patient relationship: A distinct focus of nursing action in primary care. *Image: Journal of Nursing Scholarship, 18,* 44–47.

Kasch points out that the changing patterns of disease and illness and the movement toward a health-oriented health care system are reshaping primary care. Kasch points out that nurses are making a distinct contribution to primary care, that they provide qualitatively different care in some situations, and that nurses and physicians working collaboratively provide a higher quality of care than either group working independently.

Trofino, J. (1995, March). The brave new world of health care. *Canadian Nurse,* 28–32.

This author takes a futuristic look at health care, identifying forces that are effecting change. She discussed trends, including the emergence of the multi-skilled worker, new roles for nurses, case management, and new models for leadership. She proposes that in the future, health care consumers will "direct" their relationships with health care providers. Prospective roles and career opportunities for nurses are considered and promise an exciting future for nursing practice.

SUMMARY

Collaborative health care is a concept that addresses many existing problems in the health care system. Its multidisciplinary, integrated, and participative approach focuses on client-centered and client-directed care. Collaborative care involves mutual goal setting and care planning between the client, physicians, nurses, and other involved health care providers.

Key competencies necessary for collaborative practice include effective communication skills, mutual respect and trust, giving and receiving feedback, decision-making ability, and conflict management. In addition, each health team member needs knowledge about the roles, views, and unique contributions of the other team members.

Several factors are currently impacting health care delivery. These include (a) the World Health Organization's objective for all people to achieve by the year 2000 a level of health that will permit them to lead socially and economically productive lives; (b) consumers of health care, who are insisting on comprehensive, holistic, compassionate, and affordable health care that includes services related to health promotion and illness prevention; (c) increasing recognition by consumers of self-help initiatives such as alternative or nontraditional health care and self-help groups; (d) changing demographics, such as an increase in the older, homeless, and AIDS populations; (e) economic issues related to health care, in particular, the exorbitant costs of health care and inequities in people covered by insurance in the United States; and (f) technologic advances.

Several cost-containment strategies have been implemented in past years, including competition, price controls, alternative delivery systems, managed care, health promotion and illness prevention, and alternative care providers. Despite these measures, however, health care costs continue to rise.

Various billing and payment methods are used for health care services rendered. Billing methods include fee-for-service, capitation, and fee-for-diagnosis. Payment sources include government health plans (e.g., Medicare and Medicaid in the United States), private insurance (e.g., Blue Cross), and personal payment.

Health care systems remain challenged to provide cost-efficient care and, at the same time, to ensure quality care to all. Nursing's Agenda for Health Care Reform *emphasizes a basic "core" of essential health care services for everyone and a restructuring of the health care system to focus on consumers and their health needs.*

SELECTED REFERENCES

Abbott, J., Young, A., Haxton, R., & Van Dyke, P. (1994). Collaborative care: A professional model that influences job satisfaction. *Nursing Economics, 12,* 167–174.

Abrams, W. B., Beers, M. H., & Berkow, R. (Eds.). (1995). *The Merck manual of geriatrics* (2nd ed.). Whitehouse Station, NJ: Merck.

Alpert, H. B., Goldman, L. D., Kilroy, C. M., & Pike, A. W. (1992). 7 Grysmish: Toward an understanding of collaboration. *Nursing Clinics of North America, 27,* 47–59.

American Nurses Association. (1988). *Case management: A challenge for nurses.* Kansas City, MO: Author.

American Nurses Association. (1991). *Nursing's agenda for health care reform.* Washington, DC: Author. PR-3 22M 6/91

American Nurses Association. (1992). *House of delegates report: 1992 convention, Las Vegas, Nev.* (pp. 104–120). Kansas City, MO: Author.

American Nurses Association. (1995). *Nursing's policy statement.* Washington, DC: Author.

American Organization of Nurse Executives. (1992, Nov.). Eight premises for a reformed American health-care system. *Nursing Management, 23,* 42, 44.

Baggs, J. G., & Schmitt, M. H. (1988). Collaboration between nurses and physicians. *Image: The Journal of Nursing Scholarship, 20,* 145–149.

Benson, L., & Ducanis, A. (1995). Nurses' perceptions of their role and role conflicts. *Rehabilitation Nursing, 20,* 204–211.

Beyea, S. C. (1996). *Critical pathways for collaborative care.* Menlo Park, CA: Addison-Wesley Nursing.

Centers for Disease Control and Prevention. (1995). First 500,000 AIDS cases—United States, 1995. *Morbidity and Mortality Weekly Report, 44*(46). 849–853.

Chimmer, N. E., & Easterling, A. (1993). Collaborative practice through nursing case management. *Rehabilitation Nursing, 18,* 226–229.

Coeling, H. V., & Wilcox, J. R. (1991). Professional recognition and high-quality patient care through collaboration: Two sides of the same coin. *AACN, 18,* 230–237.

Coeling, H. V., & Wilcox, J. R. (1994). Steps to collaboration. *Nursing Administration Quarterly, 18,* 44–55.

Ducanis, A., & Golin, A. (1981). *The interdisciplinary health care team.* Rockville, MD: Aspen.

Eisen, D. M., Kessler, R. C., Foster, C., Norlock, F. E., Calkins, D. R., & Delbanco, T. L. (1993). Unconventional medicine in the United States: Prevalence, costs, and patterns of use. *New England Journal of Medicine, 328,* 246–252.

Fagin, C. M. (1992). Collaboration between nurses and physicians: No longer a choice. *Academic Medicine, 67,* 295–303.

Ferguson, S., Howell, T., & Batalden, P. (1993). Knowledge and skills needed for collaborative work. *Quality Management in Health Care, 1,* 1–11.

Flarey, D. L. (1995). *Redesigning nursing care delivery: Transforming our future.* Philadelphia: Lippincott.

Fonner, E. (1993). Five practical steps for improving collaboration in health care. *Health Care Strategic Management, 11,* 14–18.

Forbes, E. J., & Fitzsimons, V. (1993). Education: The key for holistic interdisciplinary collaboration. *Holistic Nursing Practice, 7,* 1–10.

Henderson, V. A. (1991). *The nature of nursing: Reflections after 25 years.* New York: National League for Nursing.

Henneman, E. A., Lee, J. L., & Cohen, J. I. (1995). Collaboration: A concept analysis. *Journal of Advanced Nursing, 21,* 103–109.

Jones, R. A. P. (1994a). Conceptual development of nurse-physician collaboration. *Holistic Nursing Practice, 8,* 1–11.

Jones, R. A. P. (1994b). Nurse-physician collaboration: A descriptive study. *Holistic Nursing Practice, 8,* 38–53.

Larson, E. L. (1995). New rules for the game: Interdisciplinary education for health professionals. *Nursing Outlook, 43,* 180–185.

Lee, P. R., & Estes, C. L. (Eds.). (1990). *The nation's health.* Boston: Jones and Bartlett.

Link, B. G., Susser, E., Stueve, A., Phelan, J., Moore, R. E., & Struening, E. (1994). Lifetime and five-year prevalence of homelessness in the United States. *American Journal of Public Health, 84*(12), 1907–1912.

Lott, T. F., Blazey, M. E., & West, M. G. (1992). Patient participation in health care: An underused resource. *Nursing Clinics of North America, 27,* 61–75.

Mariano, C. (1989). The case for interdisciplinary collaboration. *Nursing Outlook, 37,* 285–288.

Marosy, J. P. (1994). Collaboration: A key to future success in long-term home care. *Journal of Home Health Care Practice, 6,* 42–48.

McEwen, M. (1994). Promoting interdisciplinary collaboration. *Nursing and Health Care, 15,* 304–307.

Meadors, A. C. (1993). The United States healthcare system and quality of care. In A. F. Al-Assaf & J. A. Schmele (Eds.), *The textbook of total quality in healthcare.* Delray Beach, FL: St. Lucie Press.

Miccolo, M. A., & Spanier, A. H. (1993). Critical care management in the 1990s. *Critical Care Unit Management, 9*(3), 443–453.

Molloy, S. P. (1994). Defining case management. *Home Healthcare Nurse, 12,* 51–54.

Murphy, G. T. & Stern, P. N. (1994). Joining forces to collaborate: The essence of critical care practice. *The Official Journal of the Canadian Association of Critical Care Nurses, 5,* 17–21.

Prescott, P. A., Dennis, K. E., & Jacox, A. K. (1987). Clinical decision making of staff nurses. *Image: The Journal of Nursing Scholarship, 19,* 56–62.

Prescott, P. A., Phillips, C. Y., Ryan, J. W., & Thompson, K. O. (1991). Changing how nurses spend their time. *Image: The Journal of Nursing Scholarship, 23,* 23–28.

Smith, L. (1993). The coming health care shakeout. *Fortune,* 70–75.

Tannen, D. (1990). *You just don't understand.* New York: Ballantine Books.

US Department of Health and Human Services, Public Health Service. 1990. *Healthy People 2000: National Health Promotion and Disease Prevention Objectives.* DHHS Pub no. (PHS) 91-50212. Washington, DC: US Government Printing Office.

Velianoff, G. D., Neely, C., & Hall, S. (1993). Development levels of interdisciplinary collaborative practice Committees. *Journal of Nursing Administration, 23,* 26–29.

Winstead-Fry, P., Bormolini, S., & Keech, R. R. (1995). Clinical care coordination: A working partnership. *Journal of Nursing Administration, 7,* 46–51.

Zander, K. (1988). Nursing case management: Strategic management of cost and quality outcomes. *Journal of Nursing Administration, 18,* 23–39.

5

Values, Ethics, and Advocacy

OBJECTIVES

- Explain how nurses can help clients clarify their values to facilitate ethical decision making.

- Explain the uses and limitations of professional codes of ethics.

- Explain how cognitive development, values, moral frameworks, and codes of ethics affect moral decisions.

- Discuss common bioethical issues currently facing health care professionals.

- Discuss ways in which nurses can enhance their ethical decision-making abilities.

- When presented with an ethical situation, identify the moral principles involved.

- Discuss the advocacy role of the nurse.

> "My belief is that no human being or society composed of human beings ever did or ever will come to much unless their conduct was governed and guided by the love of some ethical ideal."
>
> —Thomas H. Huxley

Today's nurses are focusing more attention on their ethical responsibilities and conflicts they may experience as a result of their unique relationships in professional practice.

- Advances in medical and reproductive technology, clients' rights, social and legal changes, and a growing concern with the allocation of scarce resources have given rise to increasing concerns about ethical issues.
- Professionals are governed by standards of conduct set forth by their respective professions. Nursing codes of ethics are established by international, national, and state or provincial nursing associations.
- Nurses need to consider certain ethical principles or rules when examining an ethical situation and making ethical decisions. When ethical decisions are made many factors come into play, including the values and beliefs of clients, of the profession, and of other professionals; the nurse's own values and beliefs; and the rights and responsibilities of all parties.
- Nurses have a major responsibility to protect the rights of clients, that is, to act as client advocates. Advocacy derives from the ethical principles of beneficence, the duty to "do good," and nonmaleficence, the duty to do no harm.

VALUES

Values are freely chosen, enduring beliefs or attitudes about the worth of a person, object, idea, or action. Freedom, courage, family, and dignity are examples of values. Values frequently derive from a person's cultural, ethnic, and religious background; from societal traditions; and from the values held by peer group and family.

Values form a basis for behavior. Once a person becomes aware of his or her values, they become an internal control for behavior; thus, a person's real values are manifested in consistent patterns of behavior.

Values exist within a person in relationship to one another. A **value system** is the organization of a person's values along a continuum, that is, from most important to least important. Values form the basis of **purposive behavior,** which refers to actions that a person performs "on purpose" with the intention of reaching some goal or bringing about a certain result. Thus, purposive behavior is based on a person's decisions or choices, and these decisions or choices are based on the person's underlying values.

Values Transmission

Values are learned and are greatly influenced by a person's sociocultural environment. For example, if a parent consistently demonstrates honesty in dealing with others, the child will probably begin to value honesty. Acquiring values is a gradual process, usually occurring at an unconscious level. Because values are learned through observation and experience, they are heavily influenced by a person's sociocultural environment. For example, some cultures value the treatment of a folk healer over that of a physician. For additional information about cultural values relative to health and illness, see Chapter 18.

Personal Values

Most people derive some values from the society or subgroup of society in which they live. A person may

---

Examples of Societal and Personal Values

Societal Values	Personal Values
• Human life	• Family unity
• Individual rights	• Worth of others
• Individual autonomy	• Independence
• Liberty	• Religion
• Democracy	• Honesty
• Equal opportunity	• Fairness
• Power	• Love
• Health	• Sense of humor
• Wealth	• Safety
• Youth	• Peace
• Vigor	• Beauty
• Intelligence	• Harmony
• Imagination	• Financial security
• Education	• Material things
• Technology	• Property of others
• Conformity	• Leisure time
• Friendship	• Work
• Courage	• Travel
• Compassion	• Physical activity
• Family	• Intellectual activity

internalize some or all of these values and perceive them as *personal values*. People need societal values to feel accepted, and they need personal values to produce a sense of individuality. See the box on page 87 for examples of personal and societal values.

Professional Values

Professional values often reflect and expand on personal values. Nurses acquire professional values during socialization into nursing—from codes of ethics, nursing experiences, teachers, and peers. As members of a caring profession, nurses hold values that relate to both competence and compassion. Watson outlined four important values of nursing (1981, pp. 20–21).

1. *Strong commitment to service.* Nursing is a helping, humanistic service. Because they are responsible for assessing and promoting health, nurses should value the caring aspect of nursing as well as their contribution to the health and well-being of people.

2. *Belief in the dignity and worth of each person.* This value means that the nurse acts in the best interest of the client regardless of nationality, race, creed, color, age, sex, politics, social class, or health status.

3. *Commitment to education.* This reflects a societal value of lifelong learning. In nursing, continuing education is needed to maintain and expand the nurse's level of competence and to increase the body of professional knowledge.

4. *Autonomy.* Nurses need to become more assertive in promoting nursing care and developing the ability to assume independent functions.

In a sense, nurses should be "value-neutral." This does not mean that nurses can or should divorce themselves from their personal and professional values; it does mean that nurses should be aware of the client's values and not assume that their own are superior. A "value-neutral" attitude permits a nurse to establish effective relationships with clients who have differing values.

CONSIDER...

- what values you hold about life, health, illness, and death. How do your values influence the nursing care you provide?
- whether a nurse who smokes can effectively help a client stop smoking or whether a nurse

who is overweight can effectively help a client who needs to lose weight.
- whether a nurse whose religious beliefs oppose the use of contraceptives can effectively teach a client about family planning.
- how your values influence the career choices you make (e.g., your initial choice to become a nurse, your choice of practice setting, and your choice of specialty).

Values Clarification

Values clarification is a process by which people identify, examine, and develop their own individual values. A principle of values clarification is that no one set of values is right for everyone. When people are able to identify their values, they can retain or change them and thus act on the basis of freely chosen, rather than unconscious, values. Values clarification promotes personal growth by fostering awareness, empathy, and insight.

A widely used theory of values clarification was developed in 1966 by Raths, Harmin, and Simon (cited in Fowler & Levine-Ariff, 1987, p. 143). This "valuing process" includes cognitive, affective, and behavioral components, referred to as "choosing," "prizing," and "acting." See the accompanying box.

Identifying Personal Values

Nurses need to know specifically what values they hold about life, health, illness, and death. Nursing

---

Values Clarification

Choosing (cognitive)	Beliefs are chosen
	• Freely, without outside pressure.
	• From among alternatives.
	• After reflecting and considering consequences.
Prizing (affective)	Chosen beliefs are prized and cherished.
Acting (behavioral)	Chosen beliefs are
	• Affirmed to others.
	• Incorporated into one's behavior.
	• Repeated consistently in one's life.

SOURCE: Adapted from *Values and Teaching* (2nd ed.) by L. Raths, M. Harmin, and S. Simon, 1978, Columbus, OH: Merrill, p. 47. Used with permission of authors.

students should explore their own values and beliefs regarding situations such as

- Individual's right to make decisions for self
- Abortion
- Passive euthanasia
- Active euthanasia
- Blood transfusion
- Acquired immune deficiency syndrome (AIDS)
- Withholding fluids and nutrition

When considering these issues, the nurse should ask: "Can I accept this or live with this?" "Why does this bother me?" "What would I do or want done in this situation?" (Corey, Corey & Callahan, 1984, pp. 57–94).

Helping Clients Identify Values

Nurses need to help clients identify values as they influence and relate to a particular health problem. Examples of behaviors that may indicate the need for values clarification are listed in the accompanying box.

The following process may help clients clarify their values.

1. *List alternatives.* Make sure that the client is aware of all alternative actions and has thought about the consequences of each. Ask, "Are you considering other courses of action?"

2. *Examine possible consequences of choices.* Ask, "What do you think you will gain by doing that?" "What benefits do you foresee from doing that?"

3. *Choose freely.* To determine whether the client chose freely, ask: "Did you have any say in that decision?" "Did you have a choice?"

4. *Feel good about the choice.* To determine how the client feels, ask, "How do you feel about that decision (or action)?" Because some clients may not feel satisfied with their decision, a more sensitive question may be "Some people feel good after a decision is made; others feel bad. How do you feel?"

5. *Affirm the choice.* Ask, "What will you say to others (family, friends) about this?"

6. *Act on the choice.* To determine whether the client is prepared to act on the decision, ask, for example, "Will it be difficult to tell your wife about this?"

7. *Act with a pattern.* To determine whether the client consistently behaves in a pattern, ask, "How many times have you done that before?" or "Would you act that way again?"

When implementing these seven steps, the nurse assists the client to think each question through, never imposing personal values. When clarifying values, the nurse never offers an opinion (e.g., "It would be better to do it this way") or offers a judgment (e.g., "That's not the right thing to do"). The nurse offers an opinion only when the client asks the nurse for it, and then only with care.

MORALS

Morality (morals) is similar to ethics and many people use the two words interchangeably. Morality usually refers to an individual's personal standards of what is right and wrong in conduct, character, and attitude. Ethics usually refers to the moral standards of a particular group such as nurses. (See Table 5–1 for a comparison of morals and ethics.)

Sometimes the first clue to the moral nature of a situation is an aroused conscience, or an awareness of feelings such as guilt, hope, or shame. The tendency to respond to the situation with words such as *ought, should, right, wrong, good,* and *bad* is another indicator. Finally, moral issues are concerned with important social values and norms: they are not about trivial things.

Behaviors That May Indicate Unclear Values

Behavior	Example
Ignoring a health professional's advice	A client with heart disease who values hard work ignores advice to exercise regularly.
Inconsistent communication or behavior	A pregnant woman says she wants a healthy baby but continues to drink alcohol and smoke tobacco.
Numerous admissions to a health agency for the same problem	A middle-aged, obese woman repeatedly seeks help for back pain but does not lose weight.
Confusion or uncertainty about which course of action to take	A woman wants to obtain a job to meet financial obligations but also wants to stay at home to care for an ailing husband.

TABLE 5–1 Comparison of Morals and Ethics

Morals	Principles and rules of right conduct
	Private, personal
	Commitment to principles and values is usually defended in daily life
Ethics	Formal responding process used to determine right conduct
	Professionally and publicly stated
	Inquiry or study of principles and values
	Process of questioning, and perhaps changing, one's morals

Moral Development

Moral development is a complex process that is not fully understood. It is more than the imprinting of parents' rules and virtues or values upon children; rather, moral development is the process of learning what ought to be done and what ought not to be done. The terms *morality, moral behavior,* and *moral development* need to be distinguished. **Morality** refers to the requirements necessary for people to live together in society; **moral behavior** is the way a person perceives those requirements and responds to them; **moral development** is the pattern of change in moral behavior with age.

Kohlberg

Kohlberg's theory specifically addresses moral development in children and adults (Berkowitz & Oser, 1985). The morality of an individual's decision is not Kohlberg's concern; rather, he focuses on the reasons why an individual makes a decision. According to Kohlberg, moral development progresses through three levels and six stages. Levels and stages are not always linked to a certain developmental stage, because some persons progress to a higher level of moral development than others.

At Kohlberg's first level, called the *premoral* or *preconventional level*, children are responsive to cultural rules and labels of good and bad, right and wrong. However, children interpret these in terms of the physical consequences of their actions, that is, punishment or reward. At the second level, the *conventional level*, the individual is concerned about maintaining the expectations of the family, group, or nation and sees this as right. The emphasis at this level is conformity and loyalty to one's own expectations as well as society's. The third level is called the *postconventional, autonomous,* or *principled level*. At this level, people make an effort to define valid values and principles without regard to outside authority or to the expectations of others. For additional information about Kohlberg's levels, see Table 5–2.

With reference to Kohlberg's six stages, Munhall (1982, p. 14) writes that stage four, the "law and order" orientation, is the dominant stage of most adults. It is recognized that there is a difference is action between nurses who act at the conventional level (level II) and those who act at the postconventional or principled level (level III): Refer to examples in Table 5–2.

Gilligan

Carol Gilligan (1982), after more than 10 years of research with women subjects, found that women often considered the situations that Kohlberg used in his research to be irrelevant. Women scored consistently lower on his scale of moral development, in spite of the fact that they approached moral situations with considerable sophistication. Gilligan maintains that most frameworks do not include the concepts of caring and responsibility.

In contrast to Kohlberg's theory of moral development, which emphasizes fairness, rights, and autonomy in a *justice framework*, Gilligan focuses on a *care perspective*, which is organized around the notions of responsibility, compassion (care), and relationships. Gilligan contends that for women, moral maturity is less a matter of abstract, impersonal justice and more an ethic of caring relationships.

The ethic of *justice*, or fairness, is based on the idea of equality: that everyone should receive the same treatment. This is the development path usually followed by men. It is widely accepted by the theorists in the field. By contrast, the ethic of *care* is based on a premise of nonviolence: that no one should be harmed or abandoned. This is the path typically followed by women. It is an approach that has been given very little attention in the literature. Distinctions between a justice orientation and a caring orientation are shown in the accompanying box.

Gilligan feels that a blend of justice and care perspectives is necessary for a person to reach maturity. The blending of these two perspectives could give

TABLE 5-2 Kohlberg's Stages of Moral Development

Level and Stage	Definition	Example
Level I Preconventional		
Stage 1: Punishment and obedience orientation	The activity is wrong if one is punished, and the activity is right if one is not punished.	A nurse follows a physician's order so as not to be fired.
Stage 2: Instrumental-relativist orientation	Action is taken to satisfy one's needs.	A client in hospital agrees to stay in bed if the nurse will buy the client a newspaper.
Level II Conventional		
Stage 3: Interpersonal concordance (good boy, nice girl)	Action is taken to please another and gain approval.	A nurse gives older clients in hospital sedatives at bedtime because the night nurse wants all clients to sleep at night.
Stage 4: Law and order orientation	Right behavior is obeying the law and following the rules.	A nurse does not permit a worried client to phone home because hospital rules stipulate no phone calls after 9:00 P.M.
Level III Postconventional		
Stage 5: Social contract, legalistic orientation	Standard of behavior is based on adhering to laws that protect the welfare and rights of others. Personal values and opinions are recognized, and violating the rights of others is avoided.	A nurse arranges for an East Indian client to have privacy for prayer each evening.
Stage 6: Universal-ethical principles	Universal moral principles are internalized. Person respects other humans and believes that relationships are based on mutual trust.	A nurse becomes an advocate for a hospitalized client by reporting to the nursing supervisor a conversation in which a physician threatened to withhold assistance unless the client agreed to surgery.

SOURCE: Adapted from *Moral Development: A Guide to Piaget and Kohlberg* by Ronald Duska and Mariaellen Whelan. Copyright © 1975 by The Missionary Society of St. Paul the Apostle in the State of New York. Used by permission of Paulist Press.

Comparison of Moral Justice and Care Orientations

Justice Orientation	*Care Orientation*
Focuses on the moral vision of "not to treat others unfairly."	Focuses on the moral vision of "not to turn away from someone in need."
Requires understanding of what "fairness" means.	Requires understanding of what constitutes "care."
Draws attention to problems of inequality and oppression.	Draws attention to problems of detachment or abandonment.
Holds up an ideal of reciprocal rights and equal respect for individuals.	Holds up an ideal of attention and response to need.

rise to a new view of human development and a better understanding of human relations. To Gilligan, two intersecting dimensions characterize human relationships: equality and attachment. All relationships can be described as unequal or equal and as attached or detached. Most people have been vulnerable both to oppression and to abandonment. Thus, two moral visions—one of justice and one of care—recur in human experience.

Gilligan describes three stages in the process of developing an "ethic of care" (1982, p. 74). Each stage ends with a transitional period. A *transitional period* is a time when the individual recognizes a conflict or discomfort with some present behavior and considers new approaches.

- *Stage 1. Caring for oneself.* In this first stage of development, the person is concerned only with caring for the self. The individual feels isolated, alone, and unconnected to others. There is no concern or conflict with the needs of others because the self is the most important. The focus of this stage is survival. The end of this stage occurs when the individual begins to view this approach as selfish. At this time, the person also begins to see a need for relationships and connections with other people.
- *Stage 2. Caring for others.* During this stage, the individual recognizes the selfishness of earlier behavior and begins to understand the need for caring relationships with others. Caring relationships bring with them responsibility. The definition of *responsibility* includes self-sacrifice, where "good" is considered to be "caring for others." The individual now approaches relationships with a focus of not hurting others. This approach causes the individual to be more responsive and submissive to others' needs, excluding any thoughts of meeting one's own. A transition occurs when the individual recognizes that this

approach can cause difficulties with relationships because of the lack of balance between caring for oneself and caring for others.
- *Stage 3. Caring for oneself and others.* During this last stage, a person sees that there is a need for a balance between caring for others and caring for the self. One's concept of responsibility is now defined as including both responsibility for the self and for other people. In this final stage, care still remains the focus on which decisions are made. However, the person now recognizes the interconnections between the self and others and thus realizes that it is important to take care of one's own needs, because if those needs are not met, other people may also suffer.

CONSIDER . . .

- what you think of as moral and immoral. For example, what motives or traits of character and actions do you consider as being moral and/or immoral?
- how society's values affect the meaning of morality to people.

RESEARCH NOTE

How Do Nurses Resolve Moral/Ethical Situations?

Millette conducted a qualitative descriptive study that examined the moral decision-making processes used by 24 nurses. Each participant was asked to describe an actual experience that involved a moral choice. The researcher explored the perspectives of each nurse and used Gilligan's framework to determine whether a justice or caring orientation prevailed in the situation. Three stories are presented as exemplars: one reveals a mostly caring orientation; another reveals a mostly justice orientation; and the third reveals a pure caring orientation. These exemplars also indicate the institutional forces and recurring themes that were active.

Findings indicated that the majority of the 24 stories had a caring orientation. In 7 narratives the justice orientation predominated. However, there were no situations of a pure justice perspective indicating that in every case, the caring perspective was present.

Nurses' perceived lack of power is the most common recurring theme. Many participants reported feeling powerless to intervene in the preferred manner for the client's

well-being. Financial security was another factor in the nurse's decision-making process. Several nurses who had some degree of financial security felt freer to act on their client's behalf. Another common theme related to relationships with administration. As a group, these nurses did not express confidence or trust in their supervisors, and in some situations, nurses expressed a sense of betrayal and abandonment.

Implications: The nurses' ability to act on their convictions appears to be directly related to the autonomy or power that the nurses have in a given situation. In many health care settings, nurses are not free to act as moral agents. Nurses need to learn to cooperate effectively with each other in order to increase their power and their capacity to influence their own practice.

SOURCE: Using Gilligan's Framework to Analyze Nurses' Stories of Moral Choice, by B. E. Millette, *Western Journal of Nursing Research*, December 1994, 16:660–674.

Moral Frameworks

Four general moral frameworks are teleology, deontology, intuitionism, and the ethic of caring. **Teleology** looks to the consequences of an action in judging whether that action is right or wrong. **Utilitarianism,** one specific teleologic theory, is summarized in the ideas, "the greatest good for the greatest number" and "the end justifies the means."

Deontology proposes that the morality of a decision is not determined by its consequences. It emphasizes duty, rationality, and obedience to rules. For instance, a nurse might believe it is necessary to tell the truth no matter who is hurt. There are many deontologic theories; each justifies the rules of acceptable behavior differently. For example, some state that the rules are known by divine revelation; others refer to a natural law or social contract; still others propose both of these as sources.

The difference between teleology and deontology can be seen when each approach is applied to the issue of abortion. A person taking a teleologic approach might consider that saving the mother's life (the end, or consequence) justifies the abortion (the means, or act). A person taking a deontologic approach might consider any termination of life as a violation of the rule "Do not kill" and, therefore, would not abort the fetus, regardless of the consequences to the mother. It is important to note that the approach, or framework, guides making the moral decision; it does not determine the outcome (e.g., the person taking a teleologic approach might have considered that saving the life of the fetus justified the death of the mother).

A third framework is **intuitionism,** summarized as the notion that people inherently know what is right or wrong; determining what is right is not a matter of rational thought or learning. For example, a nurse inherently knows it is wrong to strike a client; the nurse does not need to be taught this or to reason it out.

Benner and Wrubel (1989) proposed **caring** as the central goal of nursing as well as a basis for nursing ethics. Unlike the preceding theories which are based on the concept of fairness (justice), an ethic of caring is based on relationships. Caring theories stress courage, generosity, commitment, and responsibility. Caring is a force for protecting and enhancing client dignity. Caring is of central importance in the client-nurse relationship. For example, guided by this ethic, nurses use touch and truth-telling to affirm clients as persons rather than objects and to assist them to make choices and find meaning in their illness experiences.

Moral Principles

Moral principles are statements about broad, general philosophic concepts such as autonomy and justice. They provide the foundation for **moral rules,** which are specific prescriptions for actions. For example, "People should not lie" (rule) is based on the moral principle of respect of autonomy for people. Principles are useful in ethical discussions because even people who do not agree on which action to take may be able to agree on the principles that apply. That agreement can serve as the basis for an acceptable solution. For example, most people would agree that nurses are obligated to respect their clients (a principle), even if they disagree about whether a nurse should deceive a client about the client's prognosis (action).

Autonomy refers to the right to make one's own decisions. Respect for autonomy means that nurses recognize the individual's uniqueness, the right to be what that person is, and the right to choose personal goals. People have "inward autonomy" if they have the faculty and ability to make choices. People have "outward autonomy" if their choices are not limited or imposed by others.

Nurses who follow the principle of autonomy respect a client's right to make decisions even when those choices seem not to be in the client's best interest. Respect for people also means treating others with consideration. In a health care setting, this principle is violated when a nurse disregards clients' subjective accounts of their symptoms (e.g., pain). Finally, respect for autonomy means that people should not be treated as "a means to an end"; this principle comes into play, for example, in the requirement that clients give informed consent before tests and procedures are carried out. (See Informed Consent in Chapter 6.)

Nonmaleficence means the duty to do no harm. This principle is the basis of most codes of nursing ethics. Although this would seem to be a simple principle to follow in nursing practice, in reality it is complex. Harm can mean deliberate harm, risk of harm, and unintentional harm. In nursing, intentional harm is always unacceptable. However, the risk of harm is not always clear. A client may be at risk of harm during a nursing intervention that is intended to be helpful. For example, a client may react adversely to a medication. Sometimes, the degree to which a risk is morally permissible can be in dispute.

Beneficence means "doing good." Nurses are obligated to "do good," that is, to implement actions that benefit clients and their support persons. However, in an increasingly technologic health care system, "doing good" can also pose a risk of doing harm. For example, a nurse may advise a client about an intensive exercise program to improve general health but should not do so if the client is at risk of heart attack.

Justice is often referred to as fairness. Nurses frequently face decisions in which a sense of justice should prevail. For example, a nurse is alone on a hospital unit, and one client arrives to be admitted at the same time another client requires a medication for pain. Instead of running from one client to the other, the nurse weighs the situation and then acts based on the principle of justice.

Fidelity means to be faithful to agreements and responsibilities one has undertaken. Nurses have responsibilities to clients, employers, government, society, the profession, and to themselves. Circumstances often affect which responsibilities take precedence at a particular time.

Veracity refers to telling the truth. Most children are taught always to tell the truth, but for adults, the choice is often less clear. Does a nurse tell the truth when it is known that doing so will cause harm? Does a nurse tell a lie when it is known that the lie will relieve anxiety and fear? Bok (1992) concludes that lying to sick and dying people is rarely justified. The loss of trust in the nurse and the anxiety caused by not knowing the truth, for example, usually outweigh any benefits derived from lying.

ETHICS

The term **ethics** derives from the Greek *ethos*, meaning custom or character. It has several meanings in common usage. First, it refers to a method of inquiry that assists people to understand the morality of human behavior; that is, ethics is the study of morality. When used in this sense, ethics is an activity; it is a way of looking at or investigating certain issues about human behavior. Second, ethics refers to the practices, beliefs, and standards of behavior of a certain group (e.g., physicians' ethics, nursing ethics). These standards are described in the group's code of professional conduct. **Bioethics** is ethics as

applied to life (i.e., to life and death decision making). Because of technologic advances, bioethics is receiving increased prominence in literature and discussions. Nursing ethics refers to ethical issues involved in nursing practice.

Nurses are accountable for their ethical conduct. In 1991, the American Nurses Association (ANA) revised *Standards of Clinical Nursing Practice*. Professional Performance Standard V relates to ethics; see the accompanying box.

Nurses need to understand their own values related to moral matters and to use ethical reasoning to determine and explain their moral positions. Sometimes it is not enough for nurses to be aware of an ethical issue; they also need moral principles and reasoning skills to explain their position. Otherwise they may give emotional responses, which often are not helpful.

Nursing Codes of Ethics

A **code of ethics** is a formal statement of a group's ideals and values. It is a set of ethical principles that is shared by members of the group, reflects their moral judgments over time, and serves as a standard for their professional actions. Codes of ethics are usually

---

ANA Standards of Professional Performance

Standard V: Ethics

The nurse's decisions and actions on behalf of clients are determined in an ethical manner.

Measurement Criteria

1. The nurse's practice is guided by the *Code for Nurses*.
2. The nurse maintains client confidentiality.
3. The nurse acts as a client advocate.
4. The nurse delivers care in a nonjudgmental and nondiscriminatory manner that is sensitive to client diversity.
5. The nurse delivers care in a manner that preserves/protects client autonomy, dignity, and rights.
6. The nurse seeks available resources to help formulate ethical decisions.

SOURCE: *Standards of Clinical Nursing Practice*, American Nurses Association, 1991, Washington, DC: Author, p. 15. Used by permission.

higher than legal standards, and they can never be less than the legal standards of the profession.

International, national, state, and provincial nursing associations have established codes of ethics. The International Council of Nurses (ICN) developed and adopted their first code of ethics in 1953. The ICN Code was revised in 1965 and again in 1973. The ANA first adopted a code of ethics in 1950; it was revised in 1968, 1976, and 1985 and is simply referred to as the *Code for Nurses.* (see the inside back cover). In 1980, the Canadian Nurses Association (CNA) adopted a code of ethics; it was revised in 1991. Increasingly, professional nursing associations are taking an active part in improving and enforcing standards. Nurses are responsible for being familiar with the code that governs their practice.

Nursing codes of ethics have the following purposes:

1. To inform the public about the minimum standards of the profession and to help them understand professional nursing conduct

2. To provide a sign of the profession's commitment to the public it serves

3. To outline the major ethical considerations of the profession

4. To provide general guidelines for professional behavior

5. To guide the profession in self-regulation

6. To remind nurses of the special responsibility they assume when caring for clients

Because the wording in a code of ethics is intentionally vague, such codes can serve as general guides. They do not give direction for actions to take in specific cases. For example, the first item in the ANA *Code for Nurses* refers to respect for human dignity and states that in caring for clients, nurses should be "unrestricted by considerations of the nature of health problems." Does that mean that it is wrong for a pregnant nurse to refuse to care for a client with active herpes? Or that it is wrong to refuse to care for a client who uses rude language? When making ethical decisions, nurses should consider their code of ethics together with a more unified ethical theory, ethical principles, and the relevant data about each situation.

CONSIDER . . .

- how your code of ethics affects your daily practice.

- obstacles you have encountered related to the professional code of ethics.

- who you would expect to support you in a clinical setting when you face an ethical problem.

Types of Ethical Problems

Nurses encounter two broad types of problems: decision-focused problems and action-focused problems. Each requires a different approach (Wilkinson, 1993, p. 4).

In **decision-focused problems,** the difficulty lies in deciding what to do. The question is, What *should* I do? For example:

> Because Leon is committed to the sanctity of life, he wishes his client to have artificial nutrition and hydration. As a nurse, Leon also believes in relieving suffering, so when he sees that the tube-feedings are prolonging the client's pain, and even contributing to her discomfort, he wishes to have the feedings discontinued. He is not comfortable with either choice.

In this case, two principles clearly apply, so no matter what the nurse does, an important value must be sacrificed. This is the typical **ethical dilemma** that people commonly refer to as "being between a rock and a hard place." The nature of a dilemma dictates that there are no easy solutions. However, because the difficulty is personal and internal, nurses can address decision-focused problems by learning to make better decisions by, for example, reviewing their own personal value systems, taking advantage of staff development offerings, and attending ethics rounds.

In **action-focused problems,** the difficulty lies not in making the decision, but in implementing it. In these situations, nurses usually feel secure in their judgment about what is right but act on their judgment only at personal risk. The central question is, What *can* I do? or What risks am I willing to take to do what is right? **Moral distress,** one type of action-focused problem, occurs when the nurse knows the right course of action but cannot carry it out because of institutional policies or other constraints (Jameton, 1984, p. 6). This results in feelings of anger, guilt, and loss of integrity on the part of the nurse and can impact client care. For example:

> A resident physician has told the nurses to order complete blood count (CBC) and urinalysis on all clients and to get the results before calling him to the emergency room to examine the

clients. The nurses believe this is unethical because it is wasteful and poses unnecessary discomfort and possible risks for clients. However, they do not have the authority or the access to decision-making channels needed to change the situation. So they order the tests, but they feel guilty and upset because they believe what they are doing is wrong.

Unlike decision-focused problems, action-focused problems cannot be resolved by improving one's decision-making skills. Even after a nurse decides what is *right* to do, the issue becomes what the nurse actually can do given the conditions of practice. Research indicates that nurses' actions are influenced by such constraints as verbal threats, fear of losing their jobs or their nursing licenses, fear of physicians, fear of the law or lawsuits, and lack of support from both peers and administrators (Wilkinson, 1987/88, p. 21). Action-focused problems require knowledge, experience, communication, and the ability to make integrity-preserving compromises. To deal successfully with these problems, nurses must shift their attention away from "making the right decision" and focus on the factors that are preventing the "right action" (Wilkinson, 1993, p. 5).

Conflicts Within Nursing

Ethical conflicts also arise from nurses' unresolved questions about the nature and scope of their practice. High-technology and specialty roles (intensive care nurses, advanced practice nurses) have expanded the scope of nursing practice, often causing nursing and medical activities to overlap. This creates value conflicts for nurses. For example:

- Although nurses value health promotion and wellness, many still work in hospitals, and many are involved in high-tech treatment of illness.
- Although the profession values a humanistic, caring approach and emphasizes nurse-client relationships, many nurses spend much of their time attending to the client's machines.

Conflicting Loyalties and Obligations

Because of their unique position in the health care system, nurses experience conflicting loyalties and obligations to clients, families, physicians, employing institutions, and licensing bodies. The client's needs may conflict with institutional policies, physician preferences, needs of the client's family, or even laws of the state. According to the nursing code of

ethics, the nurse's first allegiance is to the client. However, it is not always easy to determine which action best serves the client's needs. For instance, a nurse may believe that the client's interests require telling the client a truth that others have been withholding. But this might damage the client-physician relationship, in the long run causing harm to the client rather than the intended good.

Making Ethical Decisions

Responsible ethical reasoning is rational thinking. It is also systematic and based on ethical principles and civil law. It should *not* be based on emotions, intuition, fixed policies, or precedent. (A *precedent* is an earlier similar occurrence. For example, "We have always done it this way" is a statement reflecting a decision based on precedent.)

Several decision-making models have been proposed to help nurses make ethical decisions. Two of these are shown in the accompanying box. Thompson and Thompson (1985, p. 99) propose a ten-step bioethical decision model to help nurses examine ethical issues and make a decision. Cassels and Redman (1989, pp. 465–466) identify 11 skills thought to be necessary for nurses to function as **moral agents**—that is, to participate in ethical decision making. Professional nurses should be responsible for acquiring these skills either as a part of their basic or as part of their continuing education. Regardless of which model the nurse chooses, many components enter into the decision-making process. These include the following:

- Facts of the specific situation
- Ethical theories and principles
- Nursing codes of ethics
- The client's rights
- Personal values
- Factors that contribute to or hinder one's ability to make or enact a choice, such as cultural values, societal expectations, degree of commitment, lack of time, lack of experience, ignorance or fear of the law, and conflicting loyalties

Ethical decision making that entails a person's choices, values, and actions begins in desire: People are inspired by a desire to pursue the good as they each see it. However, to know that what they are pursuing truly is good, people must rely on reason. Ethical choices, values, and actions then become a *reasoned* desire (Husted & Husted, 1995, pp. 178–183).

Ethical Decision-Making Models

Thompson and Thompson (1985)

- Review the situation to determine health problems, decision needs, ethical components, and key individuals.
- Gather additional information to clarify situation.
- Identify the ethical issues in the situation.
- Define personal and professional moral positions.
- Identify moral positions of key individuals involved.
- Identify value conflicts, if any.
- Determine who should make the decision.
- Identify range of actions with anticipated outcomes.
- Decide on a course of action and carry it out.
- Evaluate/review results of decision/action.

Cassells and Redman (1989)

- Identify the moral aspects of nursing care.
- Gather relevant facts related to a moral issue.
- Clarify and apply personal values.
- Understand ethical theories and principles (e.g., autonomy and justice).
- Utilize competent interdisciplinary resources (e.g., clergy, literature, family, other caregivers, and consultants).
- Propose alternative actions.
- Apply nursing codes of ethics to help guide actions.
- Choose and implement resolutive action.
- Participate actively in resolving the issue.
- Apply state/federal laws governing nursing practice.
- Evaluate the action taken.

SOURCES: *Bioethical Decision-Making for Nurses* by J. B. Thompson and H. O. Thompson, 1985, Norwalk, CT: Appleton-Century Crofts, p. 99; and "Preparing Students to Be Moral Agents in Clinical Nursing Practice" by J. Cassells and B. Redman, June 1989, *Nursing Clinics of North America*, 24(2), pp. 463–473. Used with permission.

Examples of Nurses' Obligations in Ethical Decisions

- Maximizing the client's well-being
- Balancing the client's need for autonomy with family members' responsibilities for the client's well-being
- Supporting each family member and enhancing the family support system
- Carrying out hospital policies
- Protecting other clients' well-being
- Protecting the nurse's own standards of care

same time preserves the integrity of all involved. Nurses have multiple obligations to balance in moral situations. See the box above for examples.

An important first step in ethical decision making is to ensure that the problem has ethical or moral content. Not all nursing problems have moral content. The following criteria may be used to determine whether a moral situation exists (Fry, 1989b, p. 491):

- There is a need to choose between alternative actions that conflict with human needs or the welfare of others.
- The choice to be made is guided by universal moral principles or theories, which can be used to provide some kind of justification for the action.
- The choice is guided by a process of weighing reasons.
- The decision must be freely and consciously chosen.
- The choice is affected by personal feelings and by the particular context of the situation.

In some cases, the most important question is *who* should make the decision. When the decision maker is the client, the nurse functions in a supportive role. Clients need knowledge about the probability and nature of consequences attending various courses of action. Nurses share their special knowledge and expertise with clients to enable them to make informed decisions.

The following questions may help the nurse determine who owns a problem:

- For whom is the decision being made?
- Who should be involved in making the decision, and why?

Nurses are responsible for deciding on their own actions and for supporting clients who are making ethical decisions or coping with the results of decisions that other people have made. A good decision is one that is in the client's best interest and at the

- What criteria (social, economic, psychologic, physiologic, or legal) should be used in deciding who makes the decision?
- What degree of consent is needed by the subject?

The accompanying box shows an example using a bioethical decision-making model proposed by Cassels and Redman (1989, pp. 465–466).

Because they have ethical obligations to their clients, to the agency that employs them, and to the physician, nurses must weigh competing factors when making ethical decisions. In many health care settings, nurses do not always have the autonomy to act on their moral or ethical choices.

Integrity-preserving moral compromise is the settling of differences in which the conflicting values of all parties are respected and concessions are made. The compromises preserve each person's integrity because no one is forced to give up self-interests, principles, or moral integrity. All parties are encouraged to discuss personal values, their assessment of the situation, and the perceived "best

---

Clinical Application
Bioethical Decision-Making Model

Situation

Mrs. LaVesque, a 67-year-old woman, is hospitalized with multiple fractures and lacerations caused by an automobile accident. Her husband, who was killed in the accident, was taken to the same hospital. Mrs. LaVesque, who had been driving the automobile, constantly questions Kate Murillo, her primary nurse, about her husband. The surgeon, Dr. Mario Gonzales, has told the nurse not to tell Mrs. LaVesque about the death of her husband; however, he does not give the nurse any reason for these instructions. Ms. Murillo expresses concern to the charge nurse, who says the surgeon's orders must be followed. Ms. Murillo is not comfortable with this and wonders what she should do.

Nursing Actions	Considerations
1. Identify the moral aspects. See the criteria provided on page 97 to determine whether a moral situation exists.	In this situation, the ethical dilemma is either to tell the truth or to withhold it. There is conflict between the values of honesty and loyalty: The primary nurse wants to be honest with Mrs. LaVesque without being disloyal to the surgeon and the charge nurse. Her choice will probably be affected by her concern for Mrs. LaVesque and perhaps by the surgeon's incomplete communication with her.
2. Gather relevant facts related to the issue.	Data should include information about the client's health problems. Determine who is involved, the nature of their involvement, and their motives for acting. In this case, the people involved are the client (who is concerned about her husband), the husband (who is deceased), the surgeon, the charge nurse, and the primary nurse. Motives are not known. Perhaps the nurse wishes to protect her therapeutic relationship with Mrs. LaVesque; possibly the physician believes he is protecting Mrs. LaVesque from psychologic trauma and consequent physical deterioration.
3. Determine ownership of the decision.	In this case, the decision is being made for Mrs. LaVesque. The surgeon obviously believes that he should be the one to decide, and the charge nurse agrees. It would be helpful if caregivers agreed on criteria for deciding who the decision maker should be.
4. Clarify and apply personal values.	We can infer from this situation that Mrs. LaVesque values her husband's welfare, that the charge nurse val-

Bioethical Decision-Making Model *continued*

ues policy and procedure, and that Ms. Murillo seems to value a client's right to have information. Ms. Murillo needs to clarify her own and the surgeon's values, as well as confirm the values of Mrs. LaVesque and the charge nurse.

5. Identify ethical theories and principles.

For example, failing to tell Mrs. LaVesque the truth can negate her autonomy. The nurse would uphold the principle of honesty by telling Mrs. LaVesque. The principles of beneficence and nonmaleficence are also involved because of the possible effects of the alternative actions on Mrs. LaVesque's physical and psychologic well-being.

6. Identify applicable laws or agency policies.

Because Dr. Gonzales simply "gave instructions" rather than an actual order, agency policies might not require Ms. Murillo to do as he says. She should clarify this with the charge nurse. She should also be familiar with the nurse practice act in her state or province.

7. Use competent interdisciplinary resources.

In this case, Ms. Murillo might consult literature to find out whether clients are harmed by receiving bad news when they are injured. She might also consult with the chaplain.

8. Develop alternative actions and project their outcomes on the client and family. Possibly because of the limited time available for ethical deliberations in the clinical setting, nurses tend to identify two opposing, either-or alternatives (e.g., to tell or not to tell) instead of generating multiple options (DeWolf, 1989, p. 80). This creates a dilemma even when none exists.

Two alternative actions, with possible outcomes, follow:
1. Follow the charge nurse's advice and do as the surgeon says. Possible outcomes: (a) Mrs. LaVesque might become increasingly anxious and angry when she finds out that information has been withheld from her; or (b) by waiting until Mrs. LaVesque is stronger to give her the bad news, the health care team avoids harming Mrs. LaVesque's health.
2. Discuss the situation further with the charge nurse and surgeon, pointing out Mrs. LaVesque's right to autonomy and information. Possible outcomes: (a) The surgeon acknowledges Mrs. LaVesque's right to be informed, or (b) he states that Mrs. LaVesque's health is at risk and insists that she not be informed until a later time.

Regardless of whether the action is congruent with Ms. Murillo's personal value system, Mrs. LaVesque's best interests take precedence.

9. Apply nursing codes of ethics to help guide actions. Codes of nursing usually support autonomy and nursing advocacy.

If Ms. Murillo believes strongly that Mrs. LaVesque should hear the truth, then as a client advocate, she should choose to confer again with the charge nurse and surgeon.

10. For each alternative action, identify the risk and seriousness of consequences for the nurse.

If Ms. Murillo tells Mrs. LaVesque the truth without the agreement of the charge nurse and surgeon, she risks the surgeon's anger and a reprimand from the charge nurse. If Ms. Murillo follows the charge nurse's advice, she will receive approval from the charge nurse and surgeon; however, she risks being seen as unassertive, and she violates her personal value of truthfulness. If Ms. Murillo requests a conference, she may gain respect for her assertiveness and professionalism, but

→

Bioethical Decision-Making Model *continued*	she risks the surgeon's annoyance at having his instructions questioned.
11. Participate actively in resolving the issue.	The appropriate degree of nursing input varies with the situation. Sometimes nurses participate in choosing what will be done; sometimes they merely support a client who is making the decision. In this situation, if an action cannot be agreed upon, Ms. Murillo must decide whether this issue is important enough to merit the personal risks involved.
12. Implement the action.	
13. Evaluate the action taken.	Ms. Murillo can begin by asking, "Did I do the right thing?" Involve the client, family, and other health members in the evaluation, if possible. Ms. Murillo can ask herself whether she would make the same decisions again if the situation were repeated. If she is not satisfied, she can review other alternatives and work through the process again.

SOURCE: Model adapted from "Preparing Students to Be Moral Agents in Clinical Nursing Practice" by J. Cassells and B. Redman, June 1989, *Nursing Clinics of North America, 24*(2), 463–473.

decision" for the client (Fry, 1989a, p. 152). For example, a nurse with a profound moral conviction against abortion might agree to care for an abortion client if there were no other way for the client to receive adequate care (Fry, 1989a, p. 152). The outcome of integrity-preserving moral compromise is for the parties involved to reach a decision that respects the values held by the decision makers; the outcome does not necessarily fall in line with what any one person thinks ought to be done. Each participant needs to recognize reasonable differences of opinion, see things from others' points of view, and reach an agreement that is mutual and peaceful for all concerned.

According to Winslow and Winslow (1991, pp. 309, 315–320), an integrity-preserving moral compromise is one in which the following elements are present:

1. *Some basic moral language must be shared.* Currently, moral and ethical issues are expressed in the language of client care, client rights, autonomy, and client advocacy. One task of institutional ethics committees is to provide a setting in which a mutual moral language can be built.

2. *A context of mutual respect must exist.* All parties must listen with respect to those with whom they differ. Coercive measures are not used. Without mutual respect, compromise becomes capitulation or persuasion. Everyone's views must be considered.

3. *The moral perplexity of the situation must be honestly acknowledged.* Each person should retain a sense of humility, remembering that there are elements of uncertainty and that he or she could be wrong.

4. *Legitimate limits to compromise must be admitted.* There are times when one cannot compromise. Compromise is more likely when there is factual uncertainty, ambiguity, and an extremely complex situation. The more certain a person is of the facts and the more clearly convinced he or she is about the morality of a course of action, the less room there is for compromise. The limits of compromise are reached when a person is so certain about a particular course of action that to compromise on that point would be to compromise the sense of self as a moral agent.

Specific Ethical Issues

The changing scope of nursing practice has led to an increasing incidence of conflicts between clients' needs and expectations and nurses' professional values. Some of these conflicts center on life-and-death issues, such as abortion, organ transplantation, and euthanasia; AIDS; and the allocation of health care resources. With the development of sophisticated technology that impacts the course and outcome of illness, nurses and clients face more complex ethical decisions. Because today's public is better informed about medical advances and issues, it is important that nurses become comfortable in dealing with clients, families, and peers facing ethical decisions. Nurses are ethically obligated to maintain a non-judgmental attitude, be honest, and protect the client's right to privacy and confidentiality.

Life-and-Death Issues

Abortion Abortion is a highly publicized issue about which many people, including nurses, feel very strongly. Debate continues, pitting the principle of the sanctity of life against the principle of autonomy and the woman's right to control her own body. This is an especially volatile issue because no public consensus has yet been reached.

Most state and provincial laws have provisions known as *conscience clauses* that permit individual physicians and nurses, as well as institutions, to refuse to assist with an abortion if doing so violates their religious or moral principles. However, nurses have no right to impose their values on a client, and nursing codes of ethics support clients' rights to information and counseling regarding abortion. For example, the CNA's *Code of Ethics for Nursing* (1991) states, "Based upon respect for clients and regard for their right to control their own care, nursing care reflects respect for the right of choice held by clients."

Organ Transplantation Organs for transplantation may come from living donors or from donors who have just died. Many living people choose to become donors by giving consent under the Uniform Anatomical Gift Act (see Chapter 6).

Ethical issues related to organ transplantation include allocation of organs, selling of body parts, involvement of children as potential donors, consent, clear definition of death, and conflicts of interest between potential donors and recipients. In some situations, a person's religious beliefs may also present conflict. For example, certain religions forbid the mutilation of the body, even for the benefit of another person.

Euthanasia, a Greek word meaning "good death," is popularly known as "mercy killing." Advances in technology have allowed many people who would

not have survived only a few years ago to be kept alive by extraordinary means. Euthanasia can be classified as either active or passive. **Active euthanasia** involves the administration of a lethal agent to end life and alleviate suffering. Regardless of the intent to end suffering, active euthanasia is regarded as contemplated murder, is forbidden by law, and can result in criminal charges of murder. **Passive euthanasia** involves the withdrawal of extraordinary means of life support, such as removing a ventilator or withholding special attempts to revive a client (e.g., giving the client "no code" status).

The concept of *death with dignity* and concerns about *quality of life* have brought about "right to die" statutes and living wills or Advance Directives. These are now accepted in several States. (Chapter 6 provides additional information.) These statutes absolve health care personnel from possible liability when they support a client's wishes not to prolong life unduly. However, such statutes are complex and nurses are advised to familiarize themselves with the statutes in their particular state or province.

Decisions to withdraw nutrition and hydration and to terminate or withhold sustaining treatment are complex.

Withdrawing or Withholding Food and Fluids It is generally accepted that providing food and fluids is part of nursing practice and, therefore, a moral duty. A nurse is morally obligated, however, to withhold food and fluids when it is more harmful to administer them than to withhold them (ANA, 1988a, p. 2). In addition, "It is morally as well as legally permissible for nurses to honor the refusal of food and fluids by competent patients in their care" (ANA, 1988a, p. 3). The *Code for Nurses* supports this statement through the nurse's role as a client advocate and through the moral principle of autonomy.

Termination of Life-Sustaining Treatment Antibiotics, organ transplants, and technologic advances have helped prolong life. However, the ability to restore health has not kept pace with the capacity to prolong life. Clients may specify that they wish to have life-sustaining measures withdrawn, they may have advance directives on this matter, or they may specify a surrogate decision maker. When these decisions are made, the nurse, as the primary caregiver, must ensure that sensitive care and comfort measures are given as the client's illness progresses. A decision to withdraw treatment is not a decision to withdraw care.

CONSIDER . . .

- how you would help a client who is contemplating an abortion but has moral distress about doing so. She tells you her boyfriend is strongly opposed to an abortion. She, however, "feels too young to be a mother," and yet feels guilty about terminating the pregnancy.
- your views about asking a client under the age of 18 to donate a kidney for a sibling.
- the meaning of "extraordinary care." Can it include providing food and fluids?
- the concept of "death with dignity." Is passive euthanasia justifiable, and should it be legalized?

Acquired Immune Deficiency Syndrome (AIDS)

Because of its assumed association with homosexual and bisexual behavior, prostitution, and illicit drug use, AIDS bears a social stigma. In a recent study, nurses caring for AIDS clients reported conflicting feelings of anger, fear, sympathy, fatigue, helplessness, and self-enhancement (Breault & Polifroni, 1992). According to ANA, the moral obligation to care for an HIV-infected client cannot be set aside unless the risk exceeds the responsibility. "Not only must nursing care be readily available,… but nurses must also be advised of the risks and the responsibilities they face in providing care.… Accepting personal risk which exceeds the limits of duty is not morally obligatory; it is a moral option" (ANA, 1988b, p. 31).

Other ethical issues center on testing for HIV status and for the presence of AIDS in health care professionals and clients. Questions arise as to whether testing should be mandatory or voluntary and to whom test results should be given. Most people are opposed to mandatory testing. The U.S. Public Health Service (CDC, 1987, p. 509) provides recommendations as to which persons should be considered for HIV antibody counseling and testing (see the accompanying box). It also recommends that voluntary testing be made available to anyone, including all health care professionals. In addition, the CDC recommends that HIV-positive health care professionals avoid performing "exposure prone procedures."

CONSIDER . . .

- whether a nurse who is HIV positive should continue to practice nursing.

Recommendations for Persons to Be Counseled and Tested for HIV Antibody

- Persons who have a sexually transmitted disease*
- IV-drug abusers†
- Persons who consider themselves at risk
- Persons who received a transfusion of blood or blood components from 1978–1985‡
- Women of childbearing age with risk of HIV infection: Includes those who
  a. Have used IV drugs
  b. Have engaged in prostitution
  c. Have sexual partners who are infected or at risk (e.g., bisexual, IV-drug abusers, or hemophiliacs)
  d. Are living in communities or were born in countries where there is a high prevalence of infection among women (e.g., Haiti, Central Africa)
  e. Received a transfusion between 1978 and 1985
- Persons planning marriage§
- Prostitutes (male and female)
- Persons in correctional systems
- Persons undergoing medical evaluation or treatment for conditions that might be suggestive of AIDS

* Includes all persons seeking treatment for STD in all health care settings.
† Includes all persons in IV-drug abuse treatment and outreach programs.
‡ The risk of infection is greatest for persons receiving large numbers of units of blood collected from areas with high incidence of AIDS.
§ Decisions about routine premarital testing should take into consideration the prevalence in that area or population and the cost-effectiveness of such testing.

SOURCE: "Public Health Service Guidelines for Counseling and Antibody Testing to Prevent HIV Infection and AIDS, Centers for Disease Control, 1987, *MMWR, 36,* 509–515.

- whether clients have a right to know about the HIV status of their health care providers and whether health care professionals have a right to know about the HIV status of their clients.
- the pros and cons of testing all clients for HIV when they enter a health care facility.

Allocation of Health Resources

Allocation of health care goods and services, including organ transplants, artificial joints, and the services of specialists, has become an especially urgent issue as medical costs continue to rise and more stringent cost-containment measures are implemented. For example, the number of office visits and the length of hospital stay are decisions that are increasingly being influenced not by medical considerations but by administrative policies of health care facilities and funding entities, such as insurance companies, HMOs, and Medicare.

Some critics dispute that health care is a scarce resource in North America; instead, they contend that it is people's access to health care that is scarce for many people. Increasing people's access to health care is costly, however, and makes decisions about providing and financing health care difficult.

CONSIDER...

- whether people of all ages have the right to the same health care or whether health care is a privilege and right for those who have the ability to pay. Consider the homeless, the unemployed, older adults, the uninsured.
- whether there should be a level of "essential" care that is provided for all individuals and a higher level that must be financed privately.
- whether preventive care services should receive the same financing as illness services.

STRATEGIES TO ENHANCE ETHICAL DECISION MAKING

Rodney and Starzomski (1993, p. 24) and Davis and Aroskar (1991, p. 65) describe several strategies to help nurses overcome possible organizational and social constraints that may hinder the ethical practice of nursing and create moral distress for nurses. These strategies encompass areas of education, administration, practice, and research.

Become aware of one's own values and the ethical aspects of nursing situations. Much of this chapter has been devoted to discussions of nursing values and ethical situations. Most nursing programs include courses at the undergraduate and graduate levels. Continuing education, in the form of inservice programs or other activities, also helps practicing professionals learn more about ethics.

Be familiar with nursing codes of ethics. The content and intent of codes center on supporting nursing practice based on ethical principles.

Understand the values of other health care professionals. An understanding of the values that other health

care professionals hold enables nurses to appreciate and respect values, opinions, and responsibilities similar to and different from their own. For example, nurses may find it helpful to know that the American Medical Association considers it morally permissible to refrain from exercising or to discontinue extraordinary efforts to prolong life. In this context, the choice of action is decided on the basis of doing good and avoiding harm.

Some educational institutions now include interdisciplinary ethics education at both undergraduate and graduate levels to enhance the understanding of beliefs, responsibilities, and values among various members of the health care team. For example, nurses and medical students together take classes on bioethics, professional ethics, and business ethics. The goal of this type of interdisciplinary education is to bring about better team communication in the practice setting.

Participate on ethics committees. Because nurses have more contact with the client and family than other members of the health care team, they know the client better and have access to special kinds of information not available to other health care professionals (Mahon, 1990, p. 266). Nurses offer unique perspectives that can greatly improve the quality of the ethical decisions made in health care settings. One important way for nurses to provide input is to serve on institutional ethics committees. Standards established by the Joint Commission on Accreditation of Healthcare Organizations (JCAHO) support this involvement (see the accompanying box).

Ethics committees typically review cases, write guidelines and policies, and provide education and counseling. They ensure that relevant facts are brought out; provide a forum in which diverse

---

JCAHO Standards Related to Ethics

Nursing Care Standard 3.2. Nursing staff members have a defined mechanism for addressing ethical issues in patient care.

Nursing Care Standard 3.2.1. When the hospital has an ethics committee or other defined structures for addressing ethical issues in patient care, nursing staff members participate.

SOURCE: *Accreditation Manual for Hospitals* by the Joint Commission on Accreditation of Healthcare Organizations, 1992, Oakbrook Terrace, IL: Author, p. 37.

views, such as views on resource allocation, can be expressed; reduce stress for caregivers; and can reduce legal risks. These factors tend to produce better decisions than would otherwise be made (Hosford, 1986, p. 15).

Institutional policies and guidelines about such issues as informed consent, the withdrawal or withholding of life-sustaining treatment, and do-not-resuscitate (DNR) orders provide direction for all health care practitioners to resolve ethical conflicts. To encourage the most effective functioning, ethics committees need to include representatives of all parties involved—consumers, hospital administrators, nurses, physicians, attorneys, hospital chaplains, social workers, and bioethicists.

Participate in or establish a nursing ethics group. A nursing ethics group can address the specific ethical issues of nursing practice and explore ethical choices nurses consider on a daily basis. Nurses are most commonly involved in issues of client's refusal of treatment, informed consent, discontinuation of life-saving treatment, withholding of information from clients, confidentiality, client competence, and allocation of resources (Cassells & Redman, 1989, pp. 467–469).

Nursing ethics committees can also provide an opportunity for nurse-to-nurse collaboration, facilitating effective cooperation among nurses and increasing nurses' power or capacity to produce change and to implement the care they believe to be most beneficial to their clients (Millette 1994, pp. 671–672). For nurses to act freely as moral agents within any institution, collaboration among and support of peers are essential. Discussions with peers during difficult ethical situations helps to reduce nurses' moral distress.

Participate in or establish educational ethics rounds. Ethics rounds using hypothetical or real cases can be used to explore ethical principles and discuss ethical dilemmas. Ethics rounds incorporate the traditional teaching approach for clinical rounds, but the focus is on the ethical dimensions of client care rather than the client's clinical diagnosis and treatment. Discussions may be held at the bedside, where health care professionals can speak directly to the client. Consent from the client must first be obtained.

Ethics rounds help all those involved to articulate their own views, encourage discussion of value conflicts, and help individuals apply decision-making skills. There are various formats. The clients and issues to be discussed may be presented by staff nurses, advanced nursing students, clinical nurse specialists, or ethics consultants, among others. Rounds serve as examples for future situations the nurse may confront. Each health care facility establishes the format and procedure of ethics rounds to fit its particular situation.

Help to establish an ethical research base. Research is needed to establish effective ways to develop ethical health policies and to evaluate the effectiveness of specific strategies in enhancing the moral agency of health care professionals.

ADVOCACY

An **advocate** is one who pleads the cause of another, and a **client advocate** is an advocate for clients' rights. The origin of the word *advocate* derives from the Latin *advocatus*, meaning "one summoned to give evidence." The focus of the client advocacy role is to respect client decisions and enhance client autonomy. Values basic to client advocacy are shown in the accompanying box.

Levels and Types of Advocacy

Kohnke (1982) identifies three levels of advocacy: (1) advocacy for self, (2) advocacy for the client, and (3) advocacy for the community of which the nurse

---

Nursing Values Basic to Client Advocacy

- The client is a holistic, autonomous being who has the right to make choices and decisions.

- Clients have the right to expect a nurse-client relationship that is based on shared respect, trust, collaboration in solving problems related to health and health care needs, and consideration of their thoughts and feelings.

- Clients are responsible for their health.

- Nurses are responsible for helping clients' use their strengths to achieve the highest level of health possible.

- It is the nurse's responsibility to ensure the client has access to health care services that meet health needs.

- The nurse and client are equally able and responsible for the outcomes of care.

TABLE 5–3 Types of Advocacy

Type	Description	Example
Legal advocacy	Related to various tribunals and other court case work.	Limited to the work of attorneys or other court-appointed agents.
Self-advocacy	Individual people or groups speaking or acting on behalf of other people on issues that are of mutual interest. Individuals are encouraged to speak for themselves in order to encourage an element of self-empowerment.	Individual clients or family members telling the physician their own requirements related to treatment. Nurses behaving assertively in describing their own needs to administrators.
Collective or class advocacy	Refers to relatively large organizations that pursue the interests of a category of people. Such organizations usually have a national resource that provides full-time officers, as well as volunteers who are able to act as advocates.	American Association for Retired Persons (AARP), National Association for the Advancement of Colored People (NAACP). Professional organizations: American Nurses Association (ANA), Canadian Nurses Association (CNA).
Citizen or client advocacy	Concerned primarily with empowering people through an individual relationship. One person represents, as if they were his or her own, the interests of another person who has needs that are unmet and are likely to remain unmet without special intervention.	Nurse, social worker, court appointed temporary guardian.

is a part. Kohnke postulates that one cannot be an advocate for others if one is unable to advocate for oneself. The nurse needs self-knowledge as well as professional knowledge about nursing and health care or needs to know where to obtain such knowledge to assist clients in their decision making. Nurses as knowledgeable professionals have an obligation and a right to share their unique knowledge with the community when needed (Kohnke, 1982, pp. 8–11). Today's health care crises of AIDS, homelessness, teenage pregnancy, child and spouse abuse, drug and alcohol abuse, and increasing health care costs all demand the nurse to fulfill the role of advocate in the community.

Gates (1995, p. 32) states that advocacy encompasses a range of approaches including legal, self, collective (class), and citizen advocacy. Citizen advocacy may be likened to client advocacy. See Table 5–3.

The Advocate's Role

The primary goal of the client advocate is to protect the rights of clients. The role of client advocate has three major components (Nelson, 1988, p. 126): protector of the client's self-determination, mediator, and actor.

As a *protector*, the nurse assists the client to make informed decisions. As a *mediator*, the nurse acts as an intermediary between the client and other people in the environment. As an *actor*, the nurse directly intervenes on the client's behalf.

According to Kohnke (1982, p. 5) the actions of an advocate are to *inform* and *support*. An advocate informs clients about their rights in a situation, and provides them with the information they need to make an informed decision. The first step in informing is to make sure the client agrees to receiving the information. In addition, an advocate must (a) either have the necessary information or know how to get it, (b) want the client to have the information, (c) present information in a way that is meaningful to the client, and (d) deal with the fact that there may be those who do not wish the client to be informed.

An advocate supports clients in their decisions. Support can involve action or nonaction. An advocate must know how to provide support in an objective manner, being careful not to convey approval or disapproval of the client's choices. Advocacy involves accepting and respecting the client's right to decide, even if the nurse believes the decision is wrong. As advocates, nurses do not make decisions for clients; clients must make their own decisions freely. For example: After being fully informed about the chemotherapy treatment, the alternative treatments, and the possible consequences of the available choices, Mr. Rae decides against further chemotherapy for his cancer. The client advocate supports Mr. Rae in his decision. Underlying client advocacy are the beliefs that individuals have the following rights (Donahue, 1985, p. 1037):

- The right to select values they deem necessary to sustain their lives
- The right to decide which course of action will best achieve the chosen values
- The right to dispose of values in a way they choose without coercion by others

According to Leddy and Pepper (1993, p. 437), the role of the advocate involves influencing others. Nurses implement the advocacy role in two supportive ways: acting on behalf of the client, and giving the client full or at least mutual responsibility in decision making. An example of acting on behalf of a client is asking a physician to review with the client the reasons for and the expected duration of combined chemotherapy and radiation therapy because the client says he always forgets to ask the physician. An example of mutual responsibility for decision making is nurse-client collaboration in planning an exercise schedule.

There are many occasions when the nurse may speak up for clients. Examples include issues of resuscitation status, inadequate pain control, lack of information, or the client's desire to refuse a treatment. It is often stated that nurses are in a unique position to be client advocates because they spend more time with clients and their families than any other health care professionals. However, a number of challenges face nurses who wish to act as client advocates. To be a client advocate involves

- Being assertive.
- Recognizing that the rights and values of their clients and families must take precedence when they conflict with those of health care providers.
- Ensuring that clients and families are adequately informed to make decisions about their own health and health care.

Characteristics of Responsible Client Advocacy

- Conveying concern for the client's total situation
- Recognizing that what the client really wants may not be what the client verbalizes under stress
- Recognizing the effect a change in a client's situation may have on others
- Balancing the client's needs against others' needs and recognizing that change must come slowly
- Recognizing the importance of good working relationships and communication with others

---

Source: Adapted from "Want Some Good Advice? Think Twice About Being a Patient Advocate" by J. Zusman, November/December 1982, *Nursing Life, 6*, pp. 48–50.

- Being aware that potential conflicts may arise over issues that require consultation, confrontation, or negotiation between the nurses and administrative personnel or between the nurse and physician.
- Working with unfamiliar community agencies, or lay practitioners.

Advocacy may also require political action—communicating a client's health care needs to government and other officials who have the authority to do something about these needs.

Zusman (1982, p. 49) offers guidelines characteristic of responsible advocacy. These are shown in the accompanying box. Although Zusman says nurses should "think twice about being a patient advocate," Leddy and Pepper (1993, p. 44) comment that "the choice of the nurse is not really between being or not being an advocate; rather it is between assuming the advocate role by using a collaborative process or operating as an adversary to those with whom conflict occurs." Collaboration is the obvious choice.

Professional/Public Advocacy

Advocacy is needed for the nursing profession as well as for the public. Gains that nursing makes in developing and improving health policy at the institutional and government levels help both the public and the nursing profession to achieve better health care. Professional advocacy involves the following broad concerns (Leddy & Pepper, 1993, p. 445):

- Shaping policies aimed at removing financial barriers to health care
- Improving the quality of nursing care available
- Ending the shortage of nurses
- Improving nurses' economic rewards
- Expanding nurses' independent roles within the delivery system
- Developing new roles outside the hospital

Nurses who function responsibly as advocates for themselves, their clients, and the community in which they reside are in a position to effect change. To act as an advocate, the nurse needs an objective understanding of the ethical issues in nursing and health care. The nurse also needs knowledge of the laws and regulations that affect nursing practice and the health of society (see Chapter 6).

CONSIDER . . .

- whether nurses need autonomy to act as client advocates. What risks does the nurse take when assuming an advocacy role? What bene-fits might the nurse realize when acting as an advocate?
- factors that would make the nurse an appropriate or inappropriate advocate for a client. In what situations might you feel personally compromised as the client's advocate?
- what client advocacy needs may be required as a result of changes in technology.
- what societal situations require professional nursing advocacy.

SUMMARY

Values give direction and meaning to life and guide a person's behavior. They are freely chosen, prized and cherished, affirmed to others, and consistently incorporated into one's behavior. Most people derive some values from the society or subgroup of society in which they live. A person may internalize some or all of these values and perceive them as personal values. *Professional values* often reflect and expand on personal values. They are acquired during socialization into*

READINGS FOR ENRICHMENT

Bandman, E. L., & Bandman, B. (1990). *Nursing ethics through the life span* (2nd ed.). Norwalk, CT: Appleton & Lange.

Part 1 of this book provides general information on ethics. Part 2 focuses on nursing ethics through the life span. It discusses ethical issues in the procreative family, the problem of abortion, and separate chapters about the ethical issues in the nursing care of infants, children, adolescents, adults, the aged, and the dying. A section at the end of each chapter provides thought-provoking discussion questions.

Fox, A. E. (1994, Sept.). Ethical issues … Confronting the use of placebos for pain. *American Journal of Nursing, 94,* 42–45.

The author, a nurse, explains how she initiated a policy change that discontinued the unethical use of placebos. What seemed initially to be a simple process turned out to be a lengthy process involving considerable data collection: In addition to consulting with health care professionals within the agency, she obtained opinions from the American Medical Association, the JCAHO, the Agency for Health Care Policy and Research, and four attorneys. At issue was the matter of informed consent versus the therapeutic privileges of physicians.

Holleran, C. A. (1990). What are the ethical issues from a world-wide viewpoint? In J. C. McCloskey & H. K. Grace, *Current issues in nursing* (3rd ed.) (pp. 623–626). St. Louis: Mosby.

This author believes that nurses have a responsibility to speak out on several types of issues of concern to nurses worldwide. The issues include the export of outdated drugs, the promotion and aggressive sale of nonessential drugs to financially poor countries, aggressive promotion of costly commercially prepared infant formula in poor countries, disreputable sources of organs for transplants, prison nurses performing body searches for drugs or weapons, the handling of confidential information about a prisoner that could be important for others to know, and female circumcision.

Salladay, S. A., & McDonnel, M. M. (1992, Feb.). Facing ethical conflicts. *Nursing 92, 22,* 44–47.

A diabetic client who is acutely but not terminally ill wants all treatments discontinued. Caregivers wonder whether they would be assisting a suicide if they comply with her wishes. Two nurse ethicists, a nurse lawyer, and a nurse theologian discuss the case. A "what do you think" section encourages readers to explore this ethical dilemma further.

nursing—from codes of ethics, nursing experiences, teachers, and peers.

Values clarification is a process in which people identify, examine, and develop their own values. Nurses need to help clients clarify their values as they influence and relate to a particular health problem or to life-and-death issues.

Morality refers to what is right and wrong in conduct, character, or attitude—that is, the requirements necessary for people to live together in society. Moral behavior is the way a person perceives those requirements and responds to them. Moral development is the pattern of change in moral behavior that occurs with age. According to Kohlberg, moral development progresses through three levels: the premoral, or preconventional level; the conventional level; and the postconventional, autonomous, or principled level. Each level has two stages. Gilligan describes three stages in the process of developing an "ethic of care": caring for oneself, caring for others, and caring for self and others.

There are four general moral frameworks: teleology, deontology, intuitionism, and caring. Moral principles, such as autonomy, beneficence, nonmaleficence, justice, fidelity, and veracity, are broad, general philosophical concepts. Moral rules, by contrast, are specific prescriptions for actions. Moral issues are those that arouse conscience, are concerned with important values and norms, and evoke words such as good, bad, right, wrong, should, and ought.

Nursing codes of ethics are formal statements of the profession's ideals and values that serve as a standard for professional actions and inform the public of its commitment.

Ethical problems are created as a result of changes in society, advances in technology, conflicts within the nursing role itself, and nurses' conflicting loyalties and obligations to clients, families, employees, physicians, and other nurses. Decision-focused problems are those in which it is difficult to arrive at a decision; they can be relieved by improving one's decision-making skills. Action-focused problems arise when nurses believe they know the right action but cannot act on their judgment without great personal risk; improved decision-making skills will not relieve the effects of these problems. Nurses' ethical decisions are influenced by their role perceptions, moral theories and principles, nursing codes of ethics, level of cognitive development, and personal and professional values. The goal of ethical reasoning, in the context of nursing, is to reach a mutual, peaceful agreement that is in the best interests of the client; reaching the agreement may require compromise. Integrity-preserving moral compromise requires shared moral language, a context of mutual respect, and acknowledgment of a situation's moral complexity.

In all situations, nurses are ethically obligated to maintain a nonjudgmental attitude, be honest, and protect the client's right of privacy and confidentiality. To enhance their ethical decision making, nurses can gain a better understanding of their own values and those of other health care professionals; participate on ethics committees, nursing ethics groups, and educational rounds; and help establish an ethical research base. Ethics committees are multidisciplinary bodies that review cases, write guidelines and policies, and provide education and counseling.

The focus of client advocacy is to respect client decisions and enhance client autonomy. Its goal is to protect the rights of clients. Various levels and types of client advocacy include advocacy for self, advocacy for the client, and advocacy for the community of which the nurse is a part. Advocacy is also needed for the profession, which benefits not only nursing but also the public. Its goal is to achieve better health care. A number of challenges face nurses who assume the role of client advocacy.

SELECTED REFERENCES

American Nurses Association (1985a). *Code for nurses with interpretive statements.* Kansas City, MO: Author.

American Nurses Association. (1985b). *Ethical dilemmas confronting nurses.* Kansas City, MO: Author.

American Nurses Association. (1988a). *Ethics in nursing: Position statements and guidelines.* Kansas City, MO: Author.

American Nurses Association. (1988b). *Nursing and the human immunodeficiency virus: A guide for nursing's response to AIDS.* Kansas City, MO: Author.

American Nurses Association. (1991). *Standards of clinical nursing practice.* Washington, DC: Author.

Bandman, E. L., & Bandman, B. (1990). *Nursing ethics through the life span* (2nd ed.). Norwalk, CT: Appleton & Lange.

Belenky, M. F., Clinchy, B. M., Goldberger, N. R., & Tarule, J. M. (1986). *Women's ways of knowing: The development of self, voice, and mind.* New York: Basic Books.

Benner, P., & Wrubel, J. (1989). *The primacy of caring.* Redwood City, CA: Addison-Wesley Nursing.

Berkowitz, M. W., & Oser, F. (Eds.). (1985). *Moral education: Theory and application.* Hillsdale, NJ: Lawrence Erlbaum.

Bishop, A., & Scudder, J. (1987, April). Nursing ethics in an age of controversy. *Advances in Nursing Science, 9*(3), 34–43.

Bok, S. (1992). *Moral choice in public and private life.* New York: Pantheon Books. As cited in J. R. Ellis & C. L. Hartley, 1992, *Nursing in today's world* (4th ed.). Philadelphia: Lippincott.

Breault, A. J., and Polifroni, E. C. (1992, Jan.). Caring for people with AIDS: Nurses' attitudes and feelings. *Journal of Advanced Nursing, 17,* 21–27.

Canadian Nurses' Association. (1991). *Code of ethics for nursing.* Ottawa: Author.

Cassells, J., & Redman, B. (1989, June). Preparing students to be moral agents in clinical nursing practice. *Nursing Clinics of North America, 24,* 463–473.

Centers for Disease Control. (1987) Public Health Service guidelines for counseling and antibody testing to prevent HIV infection and AIDS. *MMWR, 36,* 509–515.

Corey, G., Corey, M., & Callahan, P. (1984). *Issues and ethics in the helping professions* (2nd ed.). Monterey, CA: Brooks/Cole.

Corcoran, S. (1988, July/Aug.). Toward operationalizing an advocacy role … helping another person to decide. *Journal of Professional Nursing, 4*(4), 242–248.

Curtin, L. L. (1993, Nov.). Ethics and economic pressures: A case in point … ethics in management. *Nursing Management, 24,* 17–18, 20.

Curtin, L. L. (1994a, Jan.). Ethical concerns of nutritional life support. *Nursing Management, 25,* 14–16.

Curtin, L. L. (1994b, Feb.). DNR in the OR: Ethical concerns and hospital policies. *Nursing Management, 25,* 29–31.

Czerwinski, B. (1990, June). An autopsy of an ethical dilemma. *Journal of Nursing Administration* 20:25–29.

Davis, A., & Aroskar, M. (1991). *Ethical dilemmas and nursing practice* (3rd ed.). Norwalk, CT: Appleton & Lange.

DeWolf, M. (1989, May). Ethical decision-making. *Seminars in Oncology Nursing* 5:77–81.

Duska, R., & Whelan, M. (1975). *Moral development: A guide to Piaget and Kohlberg.* New York: Paulist Press.

Edwards, B. S. (1994, Jan.). Ethical issues: When the family can't let go. *American Journal of Nursing, 94,* 52–56.

Eliason, M. J. (1993, Sept./Oct.). Ethics and transcultural nursing care. *Nursing Outlook, 41,* 225–228.

Ericksen, J., Rodney, P., & Starzomski, R. (1995, Sept.). When is it right to die? *Canadian Nurse, 91,* 29–33.

Erien, J. A. (1994, Feb.). Ethical dilemmas in the high-risk nursery: Wilderness experiences. *Journal of Pediatric Nursing, 9,* 21–26.

Fowler, M. D. M., & Levine-Ariff, J. (1987). *Ethics at the bedside.* Philadelphia: Lippincott.

Fry, S. (1989a, May/June). The ethics of compromise. *Nursing Outlook, 37,* 152.

Fry, S. (1989b, June). Teaching ethics in nursing curricula. *Nursing Clinics of North America, 24,* 485–497.

Fry, S. (1989c, July). Toward a theory of nursing. *Advanced Nursing Science, 11,* 9–22.

Gadow, S. (1990). Existential advocacy: Philosophical foundations of nursing. In T. Pence & J. Cantrall (Eds.), *Ethics in nursing: An anthology* (pp. 41–51). Pub. no. 20-2294. New York: National League for Nursing.

Gates, B. (1995, Jan. 25). Advocacy: Whose best interest? *Nursing Times, 91*(4), 31–32.

Gearhart, S., & Young, S. (1990, April). Intuition, ethical decision making, and the nurse manager. *Health Care Supervisor, 8,* 45–52.

Gibson, C. H. (1993, Dec.). Underpinnings of ethical reasoning in nursing. *Journal of Advanced Nursing, 18,* 2003–2007.

Gilligan, C. (1982). *In a different voice.* Cambridge, MA: Harvard University Press.

Gilligan, C., & Attanucci, J. (1988, July). Two moral orientations: Gender differences and similarities. *Merrill-Palmer Quarterly, 34*(3), 223–237.

Haddad, A. M. (1993, Fall). Problematic ethical experiences: Stories from nursing practice. *Bioethics Forum, 9,* 5–10.

Haddad, A. (1994, Jan.). Acute care decisions: Ethics in action … terminally ill patient's pain … increased doses of morphine might directly cause the patient's death. *RN, 57,* 20, 22–23.

Hawkey, M., & Steel, A. (1994, Sept. 14). Moral decisions. *Nursing Times, 90,* 58–59.

Hosford, B. (1986). *Bioethics committees.* Rockville, MD: Aspen Publishers.

Husted, G. L., & Husted, J. H. (1995). *Ethical decision-making in nursing* (2nd ed.). St. Louis: Mosby-Year Book.

International Council of Nurses. (1973). *ICN code for nurses: Ethical concepts applied to nursing.* Geneva: Imprimeries Populaires.

Jameton, A. (1984). *Nursing practice: The ethical issues.* Englewood Cliffs, NJ: Prentice-Hall.

Joint Commission on Accreditation of Healthcare Organizations. (1992). *Accreditation manual for hospitals.* Oakbrook Terrace, IL: Author.

Kohnke, M. F. (1980, Nov.). The nurse as advocate. *American Journal of Nursing, 80,* 2038–2040.

Kohnke, M. F. (1982). *Advocacy: Risk and reality.* St. Louis: Mosby.

Leddy, S., & Pepper, J. M. (1993). *Conceptual bases of professional nursing* (3rd ed.). Philadelphia: Lippincott.

Mahon, M. (1990). The nurse's role in treatment decisionmaking for the child with disabilities. *Issues in Law and Medicine, 6*(3), 247–268.

Mallick, M., & McHale, J. (1995, Jan. 25). Support for advocacy. *Nursing Times, 91*(4), 28–30.

Milholland, D. K. (1994, Feb.). Privacy and confidentiality of patient information: Challenges for nursing. *Journal of Nursing Administration, 24,* 19–24.

Millette, B. E. (1994, Dec.). Using Gilligan's framework to analyze nurses' stories of moral choices. *Western Journal of Nursing Research, 16*(6), 660–674.

Miya, P. A. (1994, Jan.). Ethical dilemmas: On camera … A little white lie. *American Journal of Nursing, 94,* 16.

Moore, S., & Fowler, G. A. (1993, Oct.). Twelve nurses tell their ethical stories. *Nursing Management, 24,* 63, 66.

Munhall, P. L. (1982, June). Moral development: A prerequisite. *Journal of Nursing Education, 21,* 11–15.

Nelson, M. L. (1988, May/June). Advocacy in nursing: How has it evolved and what are its implications for practice? *Nursing Outlook, 36*(3), 136–141.

Parker, R. S. (1990, Sept.). Nurses' stories: The search for a relational ethic of care. *Advances in Nursing Science, 13,* 31–40.

Pearson, C. (1994, April). Facing ethical dilemmas in the neonatal intensive care unit. *Journal of Pediatric Nursing, 9,* 131–132.

Raths, L., Harmin, M., & Simon, S. (1966). Values clarification. In M. D. M. Fowler & J. Levine-Ariff. (1987). *Ethics at the Bedside.* Philadelphia: Lippincott.

Raths, L., Harmin, M., & Simon, S. (1978). *Values and teaching* (2nd ed.). Columbus, OH: Merrill.

Rich, S. (1995, Jan. 25.). Meeting the challenges: Advocacy/ethics. *Nursing Times, 91*(4), 34–35.

Rodney, P., & Starzomski, R. (1993, Oct.). Constraints on the moral agency of nurses. *Canadian Nurse, 89,* 23–26.

Salladay, S. A. (1994a, Aug.). H.I.V. Status: Co-worker confidentiality. *Nursing94, 24,* 30.

Salladay, S. A. (1994b, Aug.). Organ donation: Family affair. *Nursing94, 24,* 28–29.

Salladay, S. A. (1994c, Sept.). Patient self-determination: Assessing competence. *Nursing94, 24,* 22.

Salladay, S. A. (1994d, Nov.). Terminal illness: Withholding the truth. *Nursing94, 24,* 30.

Salladay, S. A., & McDonnell, M. M. (1989, June). Spiritual care, ethical choices, and patient advocacy. *Nursing Clinics of North America, 24,* 543–549.

Salladay, S. A., & McDonnell, M. M. (1992, Feb.). Facing ethical conflicts. *Nursing 92, 22,* 44–47.

Steel, A., & Hawkey, M. (1994, Sept. 14). Moral dimensions. *Nursing Times, 90,* 58–59.

Steele, S. M., & Harmon, V. M. (1983). *Values clarification in nursing* (2nd ed.). Norwalk, CT: Appleton-Century-Crofts.

Thompson, J. E., & Thompson, H. O. (1985). *Bioethical decision-making for nurses.* Norwalk, CT: Appleton-Century-Crofts.

Thompson, J., & Thompson, H. (1990, June). Moral development. *Neonatal Network* 8:77–78.

Tschudin, V. (1994). *Deciding ethically: A practical approach to nursing challenges.* London: Baillière Tindall.

Uustal, D. (1990, Sept.). Enhancing your ethical reasoning. *Critical Care Nursing Clinics of North America, 2,* 437–442.

van Hooft, S. (1990, Feb.). Moral education for nursing decisions. *Journal of Advanced Nursing* 15:210–215.

Van Weel, H. (1995, Sept.). Euthanasia: Mercy, morals and medicine. *Canadian Nurse, 91,* 35–40.

Vergara, M., & Lynn-McHale, D. J. (1995, Nov.). Ethical issues. Withdrawing life support: Who decides? *American Journal of Nursing* 95:47–49.

Watson, J. (1981, Summer). Socialization of the nursing student in a professional nursing education programme. *Nursing Papers, 13,* 19–24.

Watson, J. (1985). *Nursing: Human science and human care.* Norwalk, CT: Appleton-Century-Crofts.

Wilkinson, J. (1987/88). Moral distress in nursing practice: Experience and effect. *Nursing Forum, 23,* 16–29.

Wilkinson, J. (1993, Jan.). All ethics problems are not created equal. *The Kansas Nurse, 68*(1), 4–6.

Winslow, B. J., & Winslow, G. R. (1991, June). Integrity and compromise in nursing ethics. *The Journal of Medicine and Philosophy, 16,* 307–323.

Zusman, J. (1982, Nov./Dec.) Want some good advice? Think twice about being a patient advocate. *Nursing Life, 6,* 49.

6

Legal Rights and Responsibilities

OBJECTIVES

- Describe primary sources of law and types of legal actions.

- Describe how nurse practice acts affect nursing.

- Discuss essential legal aspects of malpractice, informed consent, incident reports, DNR orders, euthanasia, and death-related issues.

- Discuss the problems of sexual harrassment in nursing and the chemically impaired nurse.

- Describe collective bargaining as it applies to nursing.

"The law is not an end in itself, nor does it provide ends. It is preeminently a means to serve what we think is right."

—William J. Brennan, 1957

Knowledge of legal rights and responsibilities related to nursing practice is essential to the nurse.

- Laws prohibit extremes of behavior so that individuals can live without fear for their person and their property (Hall, 1990, p. 35).
- In the past, nurses were not considered responsible for their actions. In fact, the hospital, physician, or clinic assumed responsibility for a nurse's actions. However, as nursing practice has become more autonomous, nurses have held increasing responsibility for their actions.
- Understanding one's own rights and responsibilities as well as those of others is essential for competent and safe nursing practice.
- In 1938, New York State passed the first nurse practice act. By 1952, all states had nurse practice acts. Nurse practice acts control the practice of nursing through licensing. They legally define the practice of nursing, thereby describing the scope of nursing and protecting the public. They also set the requirements for licensure, including educational requirements, and they describe the legal titles and abbreviations that a nurse may use.

THE JUDICIAL SYSTEM

The judicial systems in both the United States and Canada have their origins in the English common law system. Three primary sources of law are constitutions, statutes, and decisions of court (common law).

Constitutions

The constitution of a country constitutes the supreme laws of the country. The Constitution of the United States, for example, establishes the general organization of the federal government, grants certain powers to them, and places limits on what federal and state governments may do. Constitutions create legal rights and responsibilities and are the foundation for a system of justice.

Legislation (Statutes)

Laws enacted by any legislative body are called **statutory laws.** When federal and state laws (or, in Canada, provincial laws) conflict, federal law supersedes. Likewise, state or provincial laws supersede local laws.

The regulation of nursing is a function of state or provincial law. State or provincial legislatures pass statutes that define and regulate nursing; these statutes are known as nurse practice acts. These acts, however, must be consistent with constitutional and federal provisions. The Patient Self-Determination Act of 1991 enables clients to participate in decisions about their care, including the right to refuse treatment, even if such treatment is necessary to preserve life. This act requires that hospitals and other health care organizations receiving payment through Medicare and Medicaid do the following:

- Tell clients that they have the right to declare their personal wishes regarding treatment decisions, including the right to refuse medical treatment.
- Inform the client regarding the hospital's policy on how advance directives are honored.
- Provide a written statement on the client's chart indicating whether the client has an advance directive. A copy of the advance directive should be included on the client's chart.
- Provide staff and community education on advance directives.

Nurse practice acts, Good Samaritan laws, and laws regarding spouse or child abuse are other examples of statutes that affect nurses.

Common Law

The body of principles that evolves from court decisions is referred to as **common law** or *decisional law.* Common law is continually being adapted and expanded. To arrive at a ruling in a particular case, a court applies the same rules and principles applied in previous, similar cases; this practice is known as following precedent. Courts may depart from precedent when slight differences are noted between cases or when it is thought that a particular common law rule no longer applies to the needs of society.

See Table 6–1 for types of laws that affect nurses.

Types of Legal Actions

There are two kinds of legal actions: civil, or private, actions and criminal actions. **Civil actions** deal with issues between individuals; for example, a man may file a suit against a person who he believes cheated him. **Criminal actions** deal with disputes between

TABLE 6-1 **Types of Laws Affecting Nurses**

Category	Examples
Constitutional	Due process
	Equal protection
Statutory (legislative)	Nurse practice acts
	Good Samaritan acts
	Child and adult abuse laws
	Living wills
	Sexual harassment laws
	Americans with Disabilities Act
Criminal (public)	Homicide, manslaughter
	Theft
	Arson
	Active euthanasia
	Sexual assault
	Illegal possession of controlled drugs
Contracts (private/civil)	Nurse and client
	Nurse and employer
	Nurse and insurance
	Client and agency
Torts (private/civil)	Negligence
	Libel and slander
	Invasion of privacy
	Assault and battery
	False imprisonment
	Abandonment

an individual and the society as a whole; for example, if a man shoots a person, society brings him to trial.

SAFEGUARDING THE PUBLIC

The first laws applicable to nursing in the United States were passed in the 1890s. These were "permissive" laws because they placed no restrictions on nursing practice, stating that the registered nurse (RN) title could be used by individuals who were registered and paid the required fee. By 1923 all states had nurse registration laws.

In 1981, the ANA described nursing practice as including but not limited to "administration, teaching, counseling, supervision, delegation, and evaluation of practice and execution of the medical regimen, including the administration of medications and treatments prescribed by any person authorized by state law to prescribe" (ANA, 1981, p. 6).

In 1990, the ANA published *A Guideline for Suggested State Legislation* to help state nurses' associations revise their nurse practice acts. This guide suggests that a nurse practice act contain the following:

- A distinct differentiation between professional and technical nursing practice
- Authority for boards of nursing to regulate advanced nursing practice, including the authority to write prescriptions
- Clarification of nurses' responsibilities for supervising and delegating other personnel
- Authority of nursing boards to oversee unlicensed assistive personnel

Nurse practice acts are administered by state boards of nursing by authority of the governor of the state. The boards are appointed by the governor and usually consist of RNs, licensed practical nurses (LPNs) and consumers of nursing. State boards may be independent agencies of the state government or part of a bureau or department, such as the department of licensure and regulation.

State nursing practice acts permit professional nurses to delegate, but they do not permit delegating by licensed vocational/practical nurses. An important aspect of the delegating process is the ethical responsibility of delegatees to refuse any responsibilities for activities that they do not have the expertise to carry out safely and competently. This applies even if hospital policies, physicians, and other nurses request these activities be carried out.

Credentialing is the process of determining and maintaining competence in nursing practice. The credentialing process is one way in which the nursing profession maintains standards of practice and accountability for the educational preparation of its members. Credentialing includes licensure, registration, certification, and accreditation.

Licensure

Licenses are legal permits a government agency grants to individuals to engage in the practice of a profession and to use a particular title. A particular jurisdiction or area is covered by the license.

There are two types of licensure: mandatory and permissive. Under *mandatory licensure*, anyone who practices nursing *must* be licensed. Under *permissive licensure*, the title RN is reserved for licensed or, in Canada, registered practitioners, but the practice of nursing is not prohibited to others who are not licensed or registered. In the United States, nursing licensure is mandatory in all states. In Canada, most provinces and territories have mandatory registration.

In each state there is a mechanism by which licenses (or registration in Canada) can be revoked for just cause, for example, incompetent nursing practice, professional misconduct, or conviction of crime, such as using illegal drugs or selling drugs illegally. In each situation, all the facts are generally reviewed by a committee at a hearing. Nurses are entitled to be represented by legal counsel at such a hearing. If the nurse's license is revoked as a result of the hearing, either the nurse can appeal the decision to a court of law, or, in some states, an agency is designed to review the decision before any court action is initiated.

For advanced nursing practice, many states require a different license or have an additional clause that pertains to actions that may be performed only by nurses with advanced education. For example, an additional license may be required to practice as a nurse midwife, nurse anesthesiologist, or nurse practitioner. The advanced practice nurse also requires a license to be able to prescribe medication or order treatment from physical therapists or other health professionals. There is some controversy about the requirement for additional licensure for advanced practice. The ANA's position is that it is the function of the professional association, not the law, to establish the scope of practice for advanced nursing practice and that the state boards of nursing can regulate advanced nursing practice within each state (ANA, 1993b).

Registration

Registration is the listing of an individual's name and other information on the official roster of a governmental or nongovernmental agency. Nurses who are registered are permitted to use the title "Registered Nurse."

In the United States, all registered nurses are licensed by the board of nursing of the state; in Canada, they are licensed or registered by the provincial nursing association or college of nursing. The requirements for licensure vary by state and province. In the United States, all nursing candidates write the National Council Licensure Examinations. (NCLEX) for registered nursing or practical nursing.

Canada has a national comprehensive registered nurse examination, offered in both French and English. Nurses from other countries are granted registration by endorsement after successfully completing these examinations. Both licensure and registration must be renewed on an annual basis (in some states, every 2 years) to remain valid.

Certification

Certification is the voluntary practice of validating that an individual nurse has met minimum standards of nursing competence in advanced practice areas, such as maternal-child health, pediatrics, mental health, gerontology, and school nursing. Certification programs are conducted by the ANA and by specialty nursing organizations. In Canada, the Canadian Nurses Association (CNA) certifies nurses in a number of specialized fields of nursing. See Chapter 23 for additional information.

Accreditation

Accreditation is a process by which a voluntary organization, such as the National League for Nursing (NLN), or governmental agency, such as the state board of nursing, appraises and grants accredited status to institutions and/or programs or services that meet predetermined structure, process, and outcome criteria (ANA, 1979). Minimum standards for basic nursing education programs are established in each state of the United States and in each province in Canada. State accreditation or provincial approval is granted to schools of nursing meeting the minimum criteria.

According to the NLN, "accreditation reflects a program that is flexible and progressive, meeting the changing needs of the society it serves through sound educational methods and a humanistic approach" (NLN, 1991, p. vii). Unlike state approval or provincial accreditation, NLN accreditation is not a legal requirement. Some states, however, require NLN accreditation for any school wishing to maintain state accreditation.

Standards of Care

Another way the nursing profession attempts to ensure that its practitioners are competent and safe

Nursing Measures That Protect Nurses and Clients

- Know your job description.

- Follow the policies and procedures of the agency in which you are employed.

- Always identify clients before implementing nursing activities.

- Report all incidents or accidents involving clients.

- Maintain your clinical competence.

- Know your own strengths and weaknesses.

- Question any order a client questions.

- Question any order if a client's condition has changed since it was written.

- Question and record verbal orders to avoid miscommunication.

- Question standing orders if you are inexperienced in the particular area.

to practice is through the establishment of standards of practice. These standards are often used to evaluate the quality of care nurses provide. In addition to this basic set of standards, which are applicable in any practice setting, the ANA has developed standards of nursing practice for specific areas such as maternal-child, medical-surgical, geriatric, psychiatric, and community health nursing.

Standards have also been developed for Medicare and Medicaid clients. In addition, the Joint Commission for Accreditation of Healthcare Organizations (JCAHO) has developed accreditation standards that help ensure specific levels of care. In addition, individual health care agencies have developed standard care plans intended to reflect a standard of care. Specific nursing measures that promote safe nursing practice are shown in the accompanying box.

POTENTIAL LIABILITY AREAS

Malpractice

Malpractice refers "to the negligent acts of persons engaged in professions or occupations in which highly technical or professional skills are employed" (Bernzweig, 1990, p. 26). The elements of proof for nursing malpractice are (a) a duty of the nurse to the client, (b) a breach of the duty on the part of the nurse, (c) an injury to the client, and (d) a causal relationship between the breach of the duty and the client's subsequent injury. A nurse could be liable for malpractice if the nurse injured a client while performing a procedure differently from the way other nurses would have done it.

Nurses are responsible for their own actions, whether they are independent practitioners or employees of a health agency. The descriptions of malpractice do not mention good intentions; it is not pertinent that the nurse did not intend to be negligent. If a nurse administers an incorrect medication, even in good faith, the fact that the nurse failed to read the label correctly indicates malpractice if all of the conditions of negligence are met.

Another significant aspect of malpractice is that it encompasses both omissions and commissions; that is, a nurse can be negligent by forgetting to give a medication as well as by giving the wrong medication.

To avoid charges of malpractice, nurses need to recognize nursing situations in which negligent actions are most likely to occur and to take measures to prevent them. The most common situations are medication errors, burning a client, client falls, and failure to assess and take appropriate action.

Because of the increase in the number of malpractice lawsuits against health professionals, nurses are advised in many areas to carry their own liability insurance. Most hospitals have liability insurance that covers all employees, including all nurses. However, some smaller facilities, such as "walk-in" clinics, may not. Thus the nurse should always check with the employer at the time of hiring to see what coverage the facility provides. A physician or a hospital can be sued because of the negligent conduct of a nurse, and the nurse can also be sued and held liable for negligence or malpractice. Because hospitals have been known to countersue nurses when they have been found negligent and the hospital was required to pay, nurses are advised to provide their own insurance coverage and not rely on hospital-provided insurance.

Liability insurance coverage usually defrays all costs of defending a nurse, including the costs of retaining an attorney. The insurance also covers all costs incurred by the nurse up to the face value of the policy, including a settlement made out of court. In return, the insurance company may have the right to make the decisions about the claim and the settlement.

In the United States, insurance can be obtained through the ANA or private insurance companies; in Canada, it can usually be obtained through provincial nurses' associations. Nursing students in the United States can also obtain insurance through the National Student Nurses Association. In some states, hospitals do not allow nursing students to provide nursing care without liability insurance.

Documentation

The client's medical record is a legal document and can be produced in court as evidence. Often, the record is used to remind a witness of events surrounding a lawsuit, because several months or years usually elapse before the suit goes to trial. The effectiveness of a witness's testimony can depend on the accuracy of such records. Nurses, therefore, need to keep accurate and complete records of nursing care provided to clients. Failure to keep proper records can constitute negligence and be the basis for tort liability. Insufficient or inaccurate assessments and documentation can hinder proper diagnosis and treatment and result in injury to the client.

Informed Consent

Informed consent is an agreement by a client to accept a course of treatment or a procedure after complete information, including the risks of treatment and facts relating to it, has been provided by the physician. Informed consent, then, is an exchange between a client and a physician. Usually, the client signs a form provided by the agency. The form is a record of the informed consent, not the informed consent itself.

Obtaining informed consent for specific medical and surgical treatments is the responsibility of a physician (Bernzweig, 1990, p. 194; Maher, 1989, p. 38; Creighton, 1986, p. 36). Although this responsibility is delegated to nurses in some agencies and there are no laws that prohibit the nurse from being part of the information-giving process, the practice nevertheless is highly undesirable (Maher, 1989, p. 38). Often, the nurse's responsibility is to witness the giving of informed consent. This involves the following:

- Witnessing the exchange between the client and the physician
- Establishing that the client really did understand, that is, was really informed
- Witnessing the client's signature

If a nurse witnesses only the client's signature and not the exchange between the client and the physician, the nurse should write "witnessing signature only" on the form (Northrop & Kelly, 1987). If the nurse finds that the client really does not understand the physician's explanation, then the physician must be notified.

There are three major elements of informed consent:

1. The consent must be given voluntarily.
2. The consent must be given by an individual with the capacity and competence to understand.
3. The client must be given enough information to be the ultimate decision maker.

To give informed consent voluntarily, the client must not feel coerced. Sometimes fear of disapproval by a health professional can be the motivation for giving consent; such consent is not voluntarily given.

To give informed consent, the client must receive sufficient information to make a decision; otherwise, the client's right to decide has been usurped. Information needs to include benefits, risks, and alternative procedures. It is also important that the client understand. Technical words and language barriers can inhibit understanding. If a client cannot read, the consent form must be read to the client before it is signed. If the client does not speak the same language as the health professional who is providing the information, an interpreter must be acquired.

If given sufficient information, the client can make decisions regarding health. To do so, the client must be competent and an adult. A competent adult is a person over 18 years of age who is conscious and oriented. A person under 18 years who is considered "an emancipated minor" (i.e., self-supporting or married) can also give consent. A client who is confused, disoriented, or sedated is not considered functionally competent at that time.

There are three groups of people who cannot provide consent. The first is *minors*. In most areas, a parent or guardian must give consent before minors can obtain treatment. The same is true of an adult who has the mental capacity of a child and who has an appointed guardian. In some states, however, minors are allowed to give consent for such procedures as blood donations, treatment for drug dependence and sexually transmitted disease, and procedures for obstetric care. The second group is *persons who are unconscious or injured* in such a way that they are unable to give consent. In these situations, consent is usually obtained from the closest adult relative if existing statutes permit. In a life-threatening emergency, if consent cannot be obtained from the client or a relative, then the law generally agrees that consent is assumed. This is referred to as **implied consent.** The third group is *mentally ill persons* who have been judged to be incompetent. State and provincial mental health acts or similar statutes generally provide definitions of mental illness and specify the rights of the mentally ill under the law as well as the rights of the staff caring for such clients.

Accidents and Incidents

An incident report is an agency record of an accident or incident. This report is used to make all the facts about an accident available to agency personnel, to contribute to statistical data about accidents or incidents, and to help health personnel prevent future accidents. All accidents are usually reported on incident forms. Some agencies also report other incidents, such as the occurrence of client infection or the loss of personal effects. The accompanying box lists the information to be included in an incident report. The report should be completed as soon as possible, always within 24 hours of the incident, and filed according to agency policy. As incident reports are not part of the client's medical record, the facts of the incident should also be noted in the medical record.

Incident reports are often reviewed by an agency committee, which decides whether to investigate the incident further. The nurse may be required upon further investigation to answer such questions as what the nurse believes precipitated the accident, how it could have been prevented, and whether any equipment should be adjusted. Nurses who believe they may be dismissed or that suit may be brought should obtain legal advice. Even if the agency clears the nurse of responsibility, the client or the client's family may file suit. The plaintiff, however, bears the burden of proving that the accident occurred because reasonable care was not taken. Even if the accepted standard of care was not met, the plaintiff must prove that the accident was the direct result of failure to meet the acceptable standards of care and that the accident caused physical, emotional, or financial injury.

When an accident occurs, the nurse should first assess the client and intervene to prevent injury. If a client is injured, nurses must take steps to protect the client, themselves, and their employer. Most agencies have policies regarding accidents. It is important to follow these policies and not to assume one is negligent. Although negligence may be involved, accidents can and do happen even when every precaution has been taken to prevent them.

Wills

A **will** is a declaration by a person about how the person's property is to be disposed of after death. In order for a will to be valid the following conditions must be met:

- The person making the will must be of sound mind, that is, able to understand and retain mentally the general nature and extent of the person's property, the relationship of the beneficiaries and of relatives to whom none of the estate will be left, and the disposition being made of the property. A person, therefore, who is seriously ill and unable to carry out usual roles may be still able to direct preparation of a will.
- The person must not be unduly influenced by anyone else. Sometimes a client may be persuaded by someone who is close at that particular time to make that person a beneficiary. Clients sometimes are persuaded to leave their estates to persons looking after them rather than to their relatives. Frequently, the relatives contest the will in such situations and take the matter to court, claiming undue influence.

Nurses may be requested from time to time to witness a will, although most agencies have policies

---

> **Information to Include in an Incident Report**
>
> - Identify the client by name, initials, and hospital or identification number.
> - Give the date, time, and place of the incident.
> - Describe the facts of the incident. Avoid any conclusions or blame. Describe the incident as you saw it even if your impressions differ from those of others.
> - Identify all witnesses to the incident.
> - Identify any equipment by number and any medication by name and number.
> - Document any circumstance surrounding the incident, for example, that another client was experiencing cardiac arrest.

that nurses not do so. In most states and provinces, a will must be signed in the presence of two witnesses. In some situations, a mark can suffice if the person making the will cannot write a signature. When witnessing a will, the nurse (a) attests that the client signed a document that is stated to be the client's last will and (b) attests that the client appears to be mentally sound and appreciates the significance of their actions (Bernzweig, 1990, p. 372).

If a nurse witnesses a will, the nurse should note on the client's chart the fact that a will was made and the nurse's perception of the physical and mental condition of the client. This record provides the nurse with accurate information if the nurse is called as a witness later. The record may also be helpful if the will is contested. If a nurse does not wish to act as a witness—for example, if in the nurse's opinion undue influence has been brought on the client—then it is the nurse's right to refuse to act in this capacity.

Do-Not-Resuscitate Orders

Physicians may order "no code" or **do-not-resuscitate (DNR)** for clients who are in a stage of terminal, irreversible illness or expected death. DNR orders require that no effort be made to resuscitate the client in the event of a respiratory or cardiac arrest. The ANA believes that "the appropriate use of DNR orders can prevent suffering for many clients who choose not to extend their lives after experiencing cardiac arrest (ANA, 1992a, p. 2)." The ANA makes the following recommendations related to DNR orders:

- The competent client's values and choices should always be given highest priority, even when these wishes conflict with those of the family or health care providers.
- When the client is incompetent, an advance directive or the surrogate decision makers acting for the client should make health care treatment decisions.
- A DNR decision should always be the subject of explicit discussion between the client, family, any designated surrogate decision maker acting on the client's behalf, and the health care team.
- DNR orders must be clearly documented, reviewed, and updated periodically to reflect changes in the client's condition. Such documentation is required to meet standards of the Joint Commission on Accreditation of Healthcare Organizations (JCAHO, 1992).

- A DNR order is separate from other aspects of a client's care and does not imply that other types of care should be withdrawn, for example, nursing care to ensure comfort or medical treatment for chronic but non-life-threatening illnesses.
- If it is contrary to a nurse's personal beliefs to carry out a DNR order, the nurse should consult the nurse-manager for a change in assignment.

The ANA also recommends that each health care organization put into place mechanisms to resolve conflicts between clients, their families, and health care professionals, or between different health care professionals. Institutional ethics committees usually deal with such conflicts. It is important that nurses be represented on these institutional ethics committees, so that nursing perspectives can be heard and nurses can be involved in developing DNR policies.

An **advance medical directive** is a statement the client makes prior to receiving health care, specifying the client's wishes regarding health care decisions. There are three types of advance medical directives, the **living will,** the **health care proxy** or **surrogate,** and the **durable power of attorney for health care.** The living will states what medical treatment the client chooses to omit or refuse in the event that the client is unable to make those decisions and is terminally ill. For example, the client can indicate a wish not to be kept alive by artificial means such as cardiopulmonary resuscitation (CPR), respiratory ventilation, or tube feeding. With a health care proxy, the client appoints a proxy, usually a relative or trusted friend, to make medical decisions on the client's behalf in the event that the client is unable to do so. The health care proxy is not limited to terminal situations but can apply to any illness or injury in which the client is incapacitated. A durable power of attorney is a notarized statement appointing someone else to manage health care treatment decisions when the client is unable to do so.

The specific requirements of advance medical directives are directed by individual state legislation. In most states, advance directives must be witnessed by two people but do not require review by an attorney. Some states do not permit relatives, heirs, or physicians to witness advance directives.

The ANA (1991) supports the client's right to self-determination and believes that nurses must play a primary role in implementation of the law. The nurse is often the facilitator of discussions between clients and their families about health care and end-of-life decisions. The ANA recommends that the following questions be part of the nursing admission assessment regarding advance directives:

- Does the client have basic information about advance care directives, including living wills and durable power of attorney?
- Does the client wish to initiate an advance care directive?
- If the client has prepared an advance care directive, did the client bring it to the health care agency?
- Has the client discussed end-of-life choices with the family and/or designated surrogate, physician, or other health care team worker?

Nurses should learn the law regarding client self-determination for the state in which they practice, as well as the policy and procedures for implementation in the institution where they work.

Euthanasia

Euthanasia is the act of painlessly putting to death persons suffering from incurable or distressing disease. It is commonly referred to as "mercy killing." Regardless of compassion and good intentions or moral convictions, euthanasia is *legally wrong* in both Canada and the United States and can lead to criminal charges of homicide or to a civil lawsuit for withholding treatment or providing an unacceptable standard of care. Because advanced technology has enabled the medical profession to sustain life almost indefinitely, people are increasingly considering the meaning of quality of life. For some people, the withholding of artificial life-support measures or even the withdrawal of life support is a desired and acceptable practice for clients who are terminally ill or who are incurably disabled and believed unable to live their lives with some happiness and meaning.

Voluntary euthanasia refers to situations in which the dying individual desires some control over the time and manner of death. All forms of euthanasia are illegal except in states where right-to-die statutes and living wills exist. Currently, the legality of assisted suicide in the United States is being tested in the court of law. Right-to-die statutes legally recognize the client's right to refuse treatment.

Death and Related Issues

Legal issues surrounding death include issuing the death certificate, labeling of the deceased, autopsy, organ donation, and inquest. By law, a death certificate must be made out when a person dies. It is usually signed by the attending physician and filed with a local health or other government office. The family is usually given a copy to use for legal matters, such as insurance claims.

Nurses have a duty to handle the deceased with dignity and label the corpse appropriately. Mishandling can cause emotional distress to survivors. Mislabeling can create legal problems if the body is inappropriately identified and prepared incorrectly for burial or a funeral. Usually, the deceased's wrist identification tag is left on, and another tag is tied to the client's ankles, in case one of the tags becomes detached. Tags tied to the ankles are preferred, since any tissue damage they cause will be concealed by bed linen or clothing. A third tag is attached to the shroud. All identification tags should include the client's name, hospital number, and physician's name.

An **autopsy** or **postmortem examination** is an examination of the body after death. It is performed only in certain cases. The law describes under what circumstances an autopsy must be performed, for example, when death is sudden or occurs within 48 hours of admission to a hospital. The organs and tissues of the body are examined to establish the exact cause of death, to learn more about a disease, and to assist in the accumulation of statistical data.

It is the responsibility of the physician or, in some instances, of a designated person in the hospital to obtain consent for autopsy. Consent must be given by the decedent (before death) or by the next of kin. Laws in many states and provinces prioritize the family members who can provide consent as follows: surviving spouse, adult children, parents, siblings. After autopsy, hospitals cannot retain any tissues or organs without the permission of the person who consented to the autopsy.

Organ Donation

Under the Uniform Anatomical Gift Act in the United States or the Human Tissue Act in Canada, any person 18 years or older and of sound mind may make a gift of all or any part of the body for the following purposes: for medical or dental education, research, advancement of medical or dental science, therapy, or transplantation. The donation can be made by a provision in a will or by signing a cardlike form in the presence of two witnesses. This card is usually carried at all times by the person who signed it. In most states and provinces, the gift can be revoked, either by destroying the card or by revoking the gift orally in the presence of two witnesses. Nurses may serve as witnesses for persons consenting to donate organs. In some states (e.g., California), health care workers are required to ask survivors for consent to donate the deceased's organs.

Inquest

An **inquest** is a legal inquiry into the cause or manner of a death. When a death is the result of an accident, for example, an inquest is held into the circumstances of the accident to determine any blame. The inquest is conducted under the jurisdiction of a coroner or medical examiner. A *coroner* is a public official, not necessarily a physician, appointed or elected to inquire into the causes of death, when appropriate. A *medical examiner* is a physician who usually has advanced education in pathology or forensic medicine. Agency policy dictates who is responsible for reporting deaths to the coroner or medical examiner.

The Impaired Nurse

The impaired nurse refers to a nurse "whose practice has deteriorated because of chemical abuse, specifically the use of alcohol and drugs" (Ellis & Hartley, 1992, p. 234). Chemical dependence in health care workers has become a problem because of the high levels of stress involved in many health care settings and the easy access to addictive drugs.

In 1981, the ANA appointed a Task Force on Addiction and Psychological Disturbance to develop guidelines for identifying, treating, and assisting nurses impaired by alcohol or drug abuse or psychologic disturbance ("New ANA Task Force Will Seek Answers for Impaired RNs," 1982, p. 242). Ellis & Hartley (1992, p. 236) cite two reasons for concern for the chemically impaired nurse: "the first concern is for the nurse whose illness may go undetected and untreated for years; the second concern is for the client, whose care may be jeopardized by the nurse whose judgment and skills are impaired." The accompanying box lists behaviors that may be seen in the impaired nurse.

Several programs have been developed to assist impaired nurses to recovery. In many states, impaired nurses who enter an intervention program for treatment do not have their nursing license revoked, but their practice is closely supervised within the limitations placed by the intervention program.

Behavioral Indicators of Chemical Abuse

- Increasing isolation from colleagues, friends, and family
- Frequent reports of illness, minor accidents, and emergencies
- Complaints about poor work performance
- Inability to meet schedules and deadlines
- Tendency to avoid new and challenging assignments
- Mood swings, irritability, and depression
- Request for night shifts
- Social avoidance of staff
- Illogical and sloppy charting
- Excessive errors
- Increasing carelessness about personal appearance
- Medication "errors" that require many changes in charting
- Arriving on duty early or staying late for no reason
- Volunteering to administer client medications, especially pain medications

---

SOURCE: Adapted from *Chemical dependency in nursing: The deadly diversion* by E. Sullivan, L. Bissell, and E. Williams, 1988, Redwood City, CA: Addison-Wesley Nursing, pp. 30–32.

Sexual Harassment

Sexual harassment is a violation of the individual's rights and a form of discrimination. The Equal Employment Opportunity Commission (EEOC) defines sexual harassment as "unwelcome sexual advances, requests for sexual favors, and other verbal or physical conduct of a sexual nature" occurring in the following circumstances (EEOC, 1980, sections 3950.10–3950.11):

- When submission to such conduct is considered, either explicitly or implicitly, a condition of an individual's employment
- When submission to or rejection of such conduct is used as the basis for employment decisions affecting the individual
- When such conduct interferes with an individual's work performance or creates an "intimidating, hostile, or offensive working environment"

Strategies to Deter Sexual Harassment

- Confront the harasser, repeatedly if necessary, and clearly ask that the behavior stop.

- Report the harassment to authorities, using the "chain of command" and whatever formal complaint channels are available.

- Document the harassment, recording in detail the "who," "what," "where," and "when" of the situation and how you responded. Include witnesses if any.

- Seek support from others, such as friends, colleagues, relatives or an organized support group.

SOURCE: Reprinted with permission from *Sexual Harassment: It's Against the Law,* © 1992 American Nurses Association, Washington, D.C.

In health care, both clients and health care professionals may experience sexual harassment. Because sexual harassment is generally related to a power imbalance, female nurses are more likely to experience sexual harassment from male physicians or administrators. Diaz and McMillin (1991, p. 100) reported that 30% of the nurses studied experienced sexual harassment in the form of having been "sexually propositioned," "suggestively touched," or "sexually insulted" by physicians during their career. Such behavior is considered sexual harassment and can negatively affect client care. For example, to avoid uncomfortable situations, the nurse may refuse to care for the clients of a particular offensive physician or work on a unit with an offensive administrator, or the nurse may avoid calling a physician to report changes in client status or to suggest changes to improve client care.

The victim or the harasser may be male or female. The victim does not have to be of the opposite sex. Moreover, the victim does not have to be the person harassed; anyone who is affected by the offensive conduct may be considered a victim (ANA, 1992b, p. 2). Nurses must develop skills of assertiveness to deter sexual harassment in the workplace. See the accompanying box.

NURSES AS WITNESSES

A nurse may be called to testify in a legal action for a variety of reasons. The nurse may be a defendant in a malpractice or negligence action or may have been a health professional that provided care to the plaintiff. It is advisable that any nurse who is asked to testify in such a situation seek the advice of an attorney before providing testimony. In most cases, the attorney for the institution will provide support and counsel during the legal case. If the nurse is the defendant, however, it is advisable for the nurse to retain an attorney to protect the nurse's own interests.

A nurse may also be asked to provide testimony as an expert witness. An **expert witness** is one who has special training, experience, or skill in a relevant area and who is allowed by the court to offer an opinion on some issue within that nurse's area of expertise (Bernzweig, 1990, p. 431). Such a witness is usually called to help a judge or jury understand evidence pertaining to the extent of damage and the standard of care.

When called into court as a witness, the nurse has a duty to assist justice as far as possible. The nurse should always respond directly and truthfully to the questions asked. The nurse is not expected to volunteer additional information, nor is the nurse expected to remember completely all the details of a situation that may have occurred months or even years prior to the legal action. The nurse may ask to refer to the client record or to personal notes related to the incident. If the nurse does not remember the details of the incident, it is advisable to say so rather than to report an inaccurate recollection. In any case, it is the nurse's professional responsibility to provide accurate testimony, both during the pretrial discovery phase and the trial phase of a legal action.

COLLECTIVE BARGAINING

Collective bargaining is the formalized decision-making process between representatives of management and representatives of labor to negotiate wages and conditions of employment, including work hours, working environment, and fringe benefits of employment (e.g., vacation time, sick leave, and personal leave). Through a written agreement, both employer and employees legally commit themselves to observe the terms and conditions of employment. Collective bargaining is a controversial issue among nurses. Some nurses consider collective bargaining to be unprofessional and contrary to the altruistic nature of nursing. Others argue that collective bargaining is necessary to obtain control of nursing practice and economic security.

TABLE 6–2 Categories and Examples of Grievances

Category	Examples
Contract violations	Shift or weekend work is assigned inequitably.
	A nurse is dismissed without cause.
Violations of federal and state law	A female nurse is paid less than a male nurse for the same work.
	Appropriate payment is not given for overtime work.
	Minority group nurses are not promoted.
Management responsibilities	Appropriate locker room facilities are not provided.
	Safe client care is jeopardized by inadequate staffing.
Violation of agency rules	Performance evaluations are conducted only at termination of employment, but the contract requires annual evaluations.
	A vacation period is assigned without the nurse's agreement, as required in personnel policies.

SOURCE: *The grievance procedure*, American Nurses Association, 1985, Kansas City, MO: Author, pp. 2–4. Used by permission.

The collective bargaining process involves the recognition of a certified bargaining agent for the employees. This agent can be a union, a trade association, or a professional organization. The agent represents the employees in negotiating a contract with management.

In 1991, the United States Supreme Court clarified the composition of collective bargaining units in acute care facilities. They define eight bargaining units: registered nurses, physicians, professionals except for registered nurses and physicians, technical employees, skilled maintenance employees, business office and clerical employees, and guards (Blouin & Brent, 1994, p. 9).

When collective bargaining breaks down because an agreement cannot be reached, the employees usually call a strike. A **strike** is an organized work stoppage by a group of employees to express a grievance, enforce a demand for changes in conditions of employment or solve a dispute with management.

Because nursing practice is a service to people (often ill people), striking presents a moral dilemma to many nurses. Actions taken by nurses can affect the safety of people. When faced with a strike, each nurse must make an individual decision to cross or not to cross a picket line. Nursing students may also be faced with decisions about crossing picket lines in the event of a strike at a clinical agency used for learning experiences. The ANA supports striking as a means of achieving economic and general welfare.

Collective bargaining is more than the negotiation of salary terms and hours of work; it is a continuous process in which day-to-day working problems and relationships can be handled in an orderly and democratic manner. Day-to-day difficulties or grievances are handled through the grievance procedure, a formal plan established in the contract that outlines the channels for handling and settling grievances through progressively higher levels of administration. A **grievance** is any dispute, difference, controversy, or disagreement arising out of the terms and conditions of employment. Grievances fall into four main categories, outlined in Table 6–2.

READINGS FOR ENRICHMENT

Coker, L. H., & Johns, A. F. (1994, Dec.). Guardianship for elders: Process and issues. *Journal of Gerontological Nursing, 20,* 25–32.

Guardianship is described as a process through which one person or entity (guardian) acquires legal responsibility for another person (ward) who is unable to manage his or her affairs because of mental or physical incapacity. The authors describe the process of appointing a guardian, provide specific information regarding mental health law, including the concept of least restrictive management, and discuss the ways in which nurses can assist older clients and their families.

Smith, K. (1995, Sept./Oct.). The legislative process. *Orthopaedic Nursing, 14,* 58–63.

Smith presents an overview of the structure of the federal government and the legislative process and provides information to help people become involved in politics and policy making. For example, Smith offers general guidelines for presenting an issue to a legislator. Lobbying is described as an attempt to legitimately influence legislators to promote or suppress specific legislation.

SUMMARY

Accountability is an essential concept of professional nursing practice under the law. Nurses need to understand laws that regulate and affect practice to ensure that their actions are consistent with current legal principles and to protect themselves from liability. Nurse practice acts legally define and describe the scope of nursing practice that the law seeks to regulate. Competence in nursing practice is determined and maintained by various credentialing methods, such as licensure, registration, certification, and accreditation, which protect the public's welfare and safety. Standards of practice published by national and state or provincial nursing associations and agency policies, procedures, and job descriptions further delineate the scope of a nurse's practice.

Negligence or malpractice of nurses can be established when (a) the nurse (defendant) owed a duty to the client, (b) the nurse failed to carry out that duty, (c) the client (plaintiff) was injured, and (d) the client's injury was caused by the nurse's failure to carry out that duty. When a client is accidentally injured or involved in an unusual situation, the nurse's first responsibility is to take steps to protect the client and then to notify appropriate agency personnel.

The nurse is responsible for ensuring that informed consent from clients (or from the closest relative in emergencies or from parents or guardians when the client is a minor) are in the medical record before treatment regimens and procedures being. Informed consent implies that (a) the consent was given voluntarily, (b) the client was of age and had the capacity and competence to understand; and (c) the client was given enough information on which to make an informed decision.

Nurses must be knowledgeable about their responsibilities in regard to legal issues surrounding death: ensuring completion of the death certificate, labeling of the deceased, autopsy, organ donation, and inquest. Physicians may order no-code or do-not-resuscitate (DNR) for clients who are in a stage of terminal, irreversible illness or expected death. Nurses need to know their responsibility to clients who have a DNR order.

SELECTED REFERENCES

American Nurses Association. (1961). *Legal definition of nursing.* Kansas City, MO: Author.

American Nurses Association. (1976). *The code for nurses.* Kansas City, MO: Author.

American Nurses Association. (1979, April). Credentialing in nursing: A new approach. Report of the Committee for the Study of Credentialing in Nursing. *American Journal of Nursing, 79,* 674–683.

American Nurses Association. (1981). The Nursing Practice Act: Suggested state legislation. Kansas City, MO: Author.

American Nurses Association. (1985). *The grievance procedure.* Kansas City, MO: Author.

American Nurses Association. (1987). *Credentialing in nursing: Contemporary developments and trends.* Kansas City, MO: Author.

American Nurses Association. (1990). *A guideline for suggested state legislation.* Kansas City, MO: Author.

American Nurses Association. (1991). Position statement on nursing and the Patient Self-Determination Act. Washington, DC: Author.

American Nurses Association. (1992a). Position statement on nursing care and do-not-resuscitate decisions. Washington, DC: Author.

American Nurses Association. (1992b). Report to the Constituent Assembly on Sexual Harassment in the Workplace. Washington, DC: Author.

American Nurses Association. (1993a). *Sexual harassment: It's against the law.* Washington, DC: Author.

American Nurses Association. (1993b). Regulation of advanced nursing practice. In *Summary of Proceedings, 1993, House of Delegates.* Washington, DC: Author.

Bernzweig, E. P. (1990). *The nurse's liability for malpractice: A programmed course* (5th ed.). St Louis: Mosby.

Blouin, A. S., & Brent, N. J. (1994, Sept.) Revisiting collective bargaining. *Journal of Nursing Administration, 24,* 9–10, 36.

Calfee, B. E. (1991, Dec.). Protecting yourself—nursing negligence. *Nursing91, 21,* 34–39.

Creighton, H. (1986). *Law every nurse should know* (5th ed.). Philadelphia: W. B. Saunders.

Diaz, A. L., & McMillin, F. D. (1991, Feb.). A definition and description of nurse abuse. *Western Journal of Nursing Research* 13:97–109.

Ellis, J. B., & Hartley, C. L. (1992). *Nursing in today's world* (4th ed.). Philadelphia: Lippincott.

Equal Employment Opportunity Commission. (1980). Sex discrimination guideline. In *EEOC Rules and Regulations.* Chicago: Commerce Clearing House.

Hall, J. K. (1990, Oct.). Understanding the fine line between law and ethics. *Nursing90, 20,* 34–39.

Idemoto, B. K., Daly, B. J., Eger, D. L., Lombardo, B. A., Matthews, T., Morris, M., and Youngner, S. J. (1993, Jan.). Implementing the Patient Self-Determination Act. *American Journal of Nursing, 93,* 20–25.

Joint Commission on the Accreditation of Healthcare Organizations (JCAHO). (1992). *Nursing care standards: Accreditation manual for hospitals.* Oak Bluffs Terrace, IL: Author.

Maher, V. F. (1989, Nov.). Your legal guide to safe nursing practice. *Nursing89, 19,* 34–41.

Mezey, M., & Latimer, B. (1993, Jan./Feb.). The Patient Self-Determination Act: An early look at implementation. *The Hastings Center Report, 23,* 16–20.

New ANA task force will seek answers for impaired RNs. (1982). *American Journal of Nursing, 82*(2), 242.

Northrup, C., & Kelly, M. (1987). *Legal issues in nursing.* St. Louis: Mosby.

Sullivan, G. H. (1995, Sept.). Legally speaking: Giving a deposition. *RN, 58,* 57–61.

Sullivan, E., Bissell, L., & Williams, E. (1988). *Chemical dependency in nursing: The deadly diversion.* Redwood City, CA: Addison-Wesley Nursing.

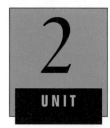

2

UNIT

Professional Nursing Roles

CHAPTER

Socialization to Professional Nursing Roles

OBJECTIVES

- Identify elements and boundaries of nursing roles.
- Describe selected roles that the professional nurse commonly assumes.
- Compare the socialization models of Simpson, Hinshaw, and Davis.
- Discuss Dalton's, Kramer's, and Benner's models of career stages.
- Discuss ways to manage role stress and role strain.

"Individuals enact roles mainly according to their personal knowledge of the role, the behavior modeling they have witnessed, the sets of expectations of others interacting with the role, and the social structure in which the role is being expressed. The boundaries for role enactment allow some liberties of expression, but for all roles there are limits."

—Luther Christman, Dean Emeritus, Rush University College of Nursing

Nurses assume a number of roles and responsibilities when they provide care to clients. Clients also assume a number of roles that may be influenced by the state of their health or illness.

- The term **"role"** can have many meanings, depending on the context in which it is used. In drama, the term *role* refers to a part in the play. In sociology, *role* can be defined as "the behavior oriented to the patterned expectation of others" (Merton 1968, p. 110).
- Role and status are closely linked concepts. Merton describes **status** as "a position in a social system involving designated rights and obligations" (1968 p. 110). Therefore, *status* refers to a position within a particular social structure; the charge nurse in a hospital nursing structure is one example. In the same example, role is the behavior associated with the position of charge nurse. Thus, status is the position, and role is the behavior relative to that position.
- A **status set** is the group of positions an individual holds.
- A **role set** is the various relationships that a person has in a particular position.

ROLE THEORY

Each person in society assumes a number of positions, such as student, parent, child, spouse, worker, and so on. Some positions are *ascribed*, that is, beyond the control of the person; gender, age, and race are examples of ascribed positions. Other positions are achieved, that is, earned; examples include nurse, president, and school principal. Of the many positions (statuses) a person assumes, one position is usually considered to be the most important source of that person's identity. This status is called the **salient** or **master status.** In earlier, rural society, a person's salient status often was membership in a

family, a religious group, or a village. In industrialized society, a man's professional or business occupation was frequently his salient status. Through the early 1900s, a woman's salient status was usually that of wife or mother. A woman often used her husband's name to indicate her own identity, introducing herself as, for example, Mrs. Dr. Wilson or Mrs. John Wilson. In contemporary society, the salient status for many women is their professional or business occupation and/or their position as wife or mother; for most men, the salient status is still their professional or business occupation.

Associated with statuses and roles are sets of *responsibilities* and *rights.* These apply to all social structures, including nursing. Most people learn through a process of socialization which sets of behaviors are expected of nurses and the responsibilities and rights that society associates with the nursing role. (See "Professional Socialization," later in this chapter.) These responsibilities, which can be considered promises, form the basis of the nursing profession's contract with society and outline the role obligations of nurses. These responsibilities also delineate the scope of nursing practice and formulate the structure of nurse-client relationships. Nurses assume four broad responsibilities (DeYoung, 1985): "(a) to help the ill regain their health, (b) to help the healthy maintain their health, (c) to help those who cannot be cured to realize their potential, and (d) to help the dying to live as fully as possible until their deaths" (p. 149).

Elements of Roles

Any role has three elements: the ideal role, the perceived role, and the performed role.

The *ideal role* refers to the socially prescribed or agreed-upon rights and responsibilities associated with the role. Persons who assume a certain role are provided with sets of expectations and obligations or norms that can be identified and used as criteria to judge the adequacy of performance in the role. The ideal role concept provides a relatively stable view of roles and role requirements, because the society at large is assumed to have the same or similar expectations about the pattern of behaviors that a person in a particular role should carry out. Although changes may occur in the prescribed rights and responsibilities associated with the ideal role, this ideal role tends to support a static view of role behaviors.

Role expectations are the norms specific to a position that identify the attitudes, cognitions, and behaviors required and anticipated of a person in a particular role. Ideal role expectations may also be determined by culture and education.

The *perceived role* refers to how a role incumbent (a person who assumes the role) believes he or she should behave in the role. A role incumbent's perceptions of the expected patterns of behavior may differ from the conventional ideal role expectations: Not every person may accept all the norms about a role or perceive them in the same way.

The *performed role* refers to what the role incumbent actually does. **Role performance** is defined as the behaviors of or actions taken by a person in relation to the expected behaviors of a particular position. **Role mastery** is the term used to indicate that a person demonstrates behaviors that meet the societal or cultural expectations associated with the specific role.

The person's perceptions and beliefs about what ought to be done is not the only factor influencing role performance. Other factors include health status, personal and professional values, needs of the client and support persons, and politics of the employing agency. A healthy nurse, for example, may provide care associated with prescribed and perceived roles more effectively than an unhealthy nurse. A nurse who values the client's right to participate in care planning will elicit the client's thoughts and feelings before planning care. A nurse who must work in a situation in which several of the staff are absent may be required to defer basic aspects of care (e.g., bath, changing bed linen) for some clients in order to meet more critical needs of other clients.

Role transition is a process in which a person assumes or develops a new role. In the new role, the person moves to a new set of responsibilities and, often, to new values as well. Role transition is influenced by many factors, such as the people associated with the new role, interpersonal factors in the organization, and the new role incumbents themselves.

CONSIDER...

- the many roles you have assumed. How successfully do you feel you fulfill the obligations of your various roles? How do your various roles create conflict in your life? What satisfactions do you experience in relation to your various roles?

- how your role as a nurse relates to your other life roles. Why did you choose to become a nurse? In what ways does your choice of nursing as a career enhance or interfere with your other life roles?

- your perceived roles of the nurse. What is the basis for your beliefs about the role of nursing?

Boundaries for Nursing Roles

Five determinants currently form the boundaries for nursing roles:

1. The consensus that nursing is concerned with four broad concepts: person, health, environment, and nursing. All broad descriptions of nursing involve these four major concepts and specify relationships among them (see "Conceptual Frameworks and Theories of Nursing" in Chapter 2). Conceptual frameworks provide the nurse with an understanding of the recipient of nursing care, what constitutes health and environment, and how these influence nursing goals and actions.

2. The *nursing process*, or standard scientific problem-solving method that nurses use in the clinical setting. The nursing process determines nursing actions appropriate for each client. The nursing process consists of five components: assessing, diagnosing, planning, implementing, and evaluating. (This process is described in detail in Chapter 14.)

3. Standards of nursing practice established by the nursing profession. Standards of practice outline nursing functions and the level of excellence required of the nurse. These standards also define the nurse's ethical and legal obligations to clients and their support persons, to employers, and to society (see Chapters 5 and 6.)

4. Nurse practice acts or nursing licensure laws of the specific jurisdiction that legally define the scope of nursing practice. Although nurse practice acts differ in various jurisdictions, they all have a common purpose: to protect the public (see Chapter 6).

5. National and international codes of ethics for nurses are fundamental to the practice of nursing. Codes of ethics describe the nurse's relationships to clients, support persons, colleagues, employers, and society (see Chapter 5.)

CONSIDER...

- how nursing models, the nursing process, standards of nursing practice, nurse practice acts, and nursing codes of ethics delineate the roles of nursing.
- Roy's model of nursing, specifically as it describes one's role function and self-concept. How might you view your various roles in relation to the Roy model?

PROFESSIONAL NURSING ROLES

Nurses assume a number of roles when they provide care to clients. Often, nurses carry out these roles concurrently, not exclusively of one another. For example, the nurse may act as a counselor while providing physical care and teaching aspects of that care. The roles required at a specific time depend on the needs of the client and the environment. Nurses are fulfilling expanded nursing roles, such as those of advanced nurse practitioner, nurse generalist, clinical nurse specialist, nurse clinician, and nurse anesthetist, that allow greater independence and autonomy (see Chapter 23).

Caregiver

The caregiver role has traditionally included those activities that assist the client physically and psychologically while preserving the client's dignity. The required nursing actions may involve full care for the completely dependent client, partial care for the partially dependent client, and supportive-educative care to assist clients in attaining their highest possible level of health and wellness.

Caregiving encompasses the physical, psychosocial, developmental, and spiritual realms. The quality of care is greatly influenced by the nurse's attitudes. The nurse supports the client by attitudes and actions that show concern for the client's welfare and a holistic view of the client as a person, not merely a mechanical being.

Benner and Wrubel (1989, p. 4) state that "caring is central to effective nursing practice.... Nursing can never be reduced to mere technique and scientific knowledge because humor, anger, 'tough love,' administering medications, and even client teaching have different effects in a caring con-

text than a noncaring one." Caring is central to most nursing interventions and an essential attribute of the expert nurse.

The nursing process provides nurses with a framework for providing care (see Chapter 14). A nurse may provide care directly or delegate it to other caregivers. Effective communication is an essential element of nursing.

Teacher

Teaching refers to activities by which one person (the teacher) helps another (the student or learner) learn new knowledge, attitudes, and behaviors. It is an interactive process between a teacher and one or more learners in which specific learning objectives or desired behavior changes are achieved (Redman, 1993, p. 8). The focus of the behavior change is usually the acquiring of new knowledge or technical skills.

The teaching process has four components—assessing, planning, implementing, and evaluating—which can be viewed as parallel to the parts of the nursing process. In the assessment phase, the nurse determines the client's learning needs and readiness to learn; during planning, sets specific learning goals and teaching strategies; during implementation, enacts teaching strategies; and, during evaluation, measures learning. See Chapter 9 for details about the teaching/learning process.

Many factors have increased the need for health teaching by nurses. Today, there is a new emphasis on health promotion and health maintenance rather than on treatment alone; as a result, people desire and require more knowledge. Shortened hospital stays mean that the clients must be prepared to manage convalescence at home. The increase in long-term illnesses and disabilities often requires that both the client and the family understand the illness and its treatment.

Counselor

Counseling is the process of helping a client recognize and cope with stressful psychologic or social problems, to develop improved interpersonal relationships, and to promote personal growth. It involves providing emotional, intellectual, and psychologic support. In contrast to the psychotherapist, who counsels individuals with identified problems, the nurse counsels primarily healthy individuals with normal adjustment difficulties. The nurse focuses on helping the person develop new attitudes, feelings, and behaviors rather than on promoting intellectual growth. The nurse encourages the client to look at alternative behaviors, recognize the choices, and develop a sense of control.

Counseling can be provided on a one-to-one basis or in groups. Often nurses lead group counseling sessions. For example, on the individual level, the nurse counsels clients who need to decrease activity levels, stop smoking, lose weight, accept changes in body image, or cope with impending death. At the group level, the nurse may be a leader, member, or resource person in any self-help group in which the nurse may assume the role of structuring activities and fostering a climate conducive to group interaction and productive work.

Obviously, counseling requires therapeutic communication skills. In addition, the nurse must be a skilled leader able to analyze a situation, synthesize information and experiences, and evaluate the progress and productivity of the individual or group. The nurse must also be willing to model and teach desired behaviors, to be sincere when dealing with people, and to demonstrate interest and caring in the welfare of others. The nurse-leader needs an inventive mind, a flexible attitude, and a sense of humor to deal with the varied experiences of people. Essential to leadership abilities are self-awareness, self-assurance, and self-understanding.

Client Advocate

An **advocate** pleads the cause of another or argues or pleads for a cause or proposal. Advocacy involves concern for and defined actions on behalf of another person or organization to bring about a change. A *client advocate* is an advocate of clients' rights. According to Disparti (1988, p. 140), advocacy involves promoting what is best for the client, ensuring that the client's needs are met, and protecting the client's rights. Some nurses believe client advocacy is an essential nursing function. Others believe that a client advocate need not be a nurse. All, however, recognize that many clients need an advocate to protect their rights and to help them speak up for themselves. See Chapter 5 for further discussion of the nurse as client advocate.

Change Agent

A *change agent* is a person or group who initiates changes or who assists others in making modifications in themselves or in the system (Kemp, 1986).

Brooten, Hayman, and Naylor (1978) describe a change agent as a professional who relies on a systematic body of knowledge about change to guide the change process. Types, theories, and the process of change are discussed in Chapter 13.

Leader

The leadership role can be applied at many different levels: individual, family, groups of clients, professional colleagues, or the larger society. At the client level, *nursing leadership* is defined as a mutual process of interpersonal influence through which a client is assisted to make decisions in establishing and achieving goals toward improved well-being and the professional nurse's practice is validated and professional growth enhanced (Leddy & Pepper, 1993, p. 384).

On a larger scale, leadership can be defined as translating innovative ideas into action or as influencing individuals or groups to take an active part in the process of achieving agreed-upon goals (Epstein, 1982, p. 2).

Effective leadership is a learned process requiring an understanding of the needs and goals that motivate people, the knowledge to apply the leadership skills, and the interpersonal skills to influence others. The leadership role of the nurse is discussed in Chapter 10.

Manager

The terms *management* and *leadership* are often confused because in much of the literature, leadership is associated with group interaction within an organizational setting. *Management* is defined as "the use of delegated authority within the formal organization to organize, direct, or control responsible subordinates ... so that all service contributions are coordinated to attain a goal" (Yura, Ozimek & Walsh, 1981, p. 5). Leadership, by contrast, may or may not require delegated authority within a formal organization.

The nurse manages the nursing care of individuals, families, and communities. The nurse-manager also delegates nursing activities to ancillary workers and other nurses, and supervises and evaluates their performance. Managing requires knowledge about organizational structure and dynamics, authority and accountability, leadership, change theory, advocacy, delegation, and supervision and evaluation. The role of the nurse as manager is discussed in Chapter 10.

Researcher

The majority of researchers in nursing are prepared at the doctoral and postdoctoral level, although an increasing number of clinicians with master's degrees are beginning to participate in research activity as part of their nursing role. However, "if nursing is to emerge in society as a socially significant, credible, scientific, and learned profession with a commitment to high-quality patient care, then research (for all nurses) is a necessity" (Starzomski, 1983, p. 34). It may be unrealistic to expect each nurse to conduct a study in the clinical setting. Many constraints in clinical settings must be reckoned with before research can become a legitimate and comfortable activity. However, if nursing is to develop as a research-based practice, it is not unreasonable to expect the nurse in the clinical area to (a) have some awareness of the process and language of research, (b) be sensitive to issues related to protecting the rights of human subjects, (c) participate in the identification of significant researchable problems, and (d) be a discriminating consumer of research findings.

Nursing students learn these investigative functions early in their careers to establish the connection that "knowing how we know is fundamental to doing what we do" (Wilson, 1985, p. viii). See Chapter 11 for more detailed information about the role of the researcher in nursing.

Consultant

A nurse consultant has an area of nursing expertise to share with other nurses and/or health professionals. *Consulting* is a process in which two people deliberate with one another. It is frequently done in all phases of the nursing process. Consulting implies that one person seeks advice or clarification from another. Lippitt and Lippitt write that the ultimate goal of consultation is "learning, growth, change" (1977, p. 130).

Nurse consultants are generally asked to verify findings, assist with change, or provide special nursing expertise. The person seeking the assistance is a consultee.

Collaborator

Nurses collaborate with clients, support persons, other nurses, and other health professionals. Basic to the collaboration process are sharing ideas, providing support to others, and sharing expertise.

Case Manager

Case management emerged in response to a number of changes in reimbursement programs and the need to manage clinical outcomes so as to limit costs.

Nurse case managers work with the multidisciplinary health care team to measure the effectiveness of the case management plan and monitor outcomes. Each agency or unit specifies the role of the nurse case manager. In some institutions, the case manager works with primary/staff nurses to oversee the care of a specific caseload. In other agencies, the case manager is the primary nurse or provides some level of direct care to the client and family. Insurance companies have also developed a number of roles for nurse case managers, and responsibilities may vary from managing acute hospitalizations to managing high-cost clients or case types.

Nursing case management requires effective communication skills and a clinical background in specific case type. The nurse case manager in a hospital is responsible for developing case management plans with the health care team and then evaluating outcomes. Commonly used tools include critical pathways and variance analysis. **Critical pathways** are versions of the case management plan that clearly describe interventions and outcomes for a specific case type. **Variances** are departures from the expected pathway. See Chapter 4 for additional information.

Regardless of the setting, case managers help ensure that care is oriented to the client, while at the same time controlling costs. Case managers may also be social workers, physicians, or paraprofessionals in any number of settings. Case managers are also in private practice, offering their services to families and individuals. With the ongoing need to limit costs and ensure quality, managed care and case management are increasingly important approaches to health care.

Quality Care Evaluator

Over the past 30 years, there has been considerable work on how to evaluate the quality of nursing care to determine what good care is, whether the care nurses give is appropriate and effective, and whether the quality of care provided is good. Evaluating the quality of nursing care is an essential part of professional accountability. Other terms used for this measurement are quality assessment and quality assurance. Quality assessment is an examination of services only; quality assurance implies that efforts are made to evaluate *and* ensure quality health care.

Some health care organizations have established a position for quality assurance coordinator. The responsibilities of the position include designing and implementing studies, reviewing findings, making recommendations for improvement, and coordinating the reevaluation process. However, nurses in a health organization assume the responsibilities of quality care evaluator.

In 1991, the American Nurses Association (ANA) published *Standards of Clinical Nursing Practice,* which provides the nursing profession with a framework for the delivery and evaluation of care.

CONSIDER...

- the ideal role of the nurse as presented in nursing mythology (literature, art, media). How does this relate to the "real" world of nursing?
- the various roles of the nurse. How successful are you in fulfilling the various roles of the nurse? Are there nursing roles that you need more knowledge of or experience with to become a better nurse? How will you go about obtaining this knowledge and experience?

PROFESSIONAL SOCIALIZATION

Socialization can be defined simply as the process by which people (a) learn to become members of groups and society, and (b) learn the social rules defining relationships into which they will enter. Socialization involves learning to behave, feel, and see the world in a similar manner as other persons occupying the same role as oneself (Hardy & Conway, 1988, p. 261). The goal of professional socialization is to instill in individuals the norms, values, attitudes, and behaviors deemed essential for the survival of the profession.

An intrinsic aspect of the socialization process is *social control*—the capacity of a social group to regulate itself through conformity and adherence to group norms to maintain the group's social order and organization. Sanctions are used to enforce norms. Positive sanctions reward conformity to norms; negative sanctions punish nonconformity. Sanctions may be either externally employed by a

source outside the individual (e.g., disciplinary action by a committee) or internally employed from within the individual (e.g., self-congratulations for a job well done). Socialization implies that the individual is induced to conform *willingly* to the ways of the group. Norms therefore become internalized standards. Professions require both a relatively long period of formal schooling and an informal, internalized system of ethics that guides practice of the professional role.

Professional socialization involves exposure to multiple agents of socialization. Agents of socialization are the people who initiate the socialization process, such as family members, teachers, child-care workers, peers, and the mass media. For children, the primary agents of socialization are the family, teachers, peers, and the mass media. In one-parent families, surrogate parents, such as child-care workers and baby-sitters, may also be major socialization agents. For adults, the influence of these agents continues but other agents arise, such as superiors and subordinates in the workplace, peers, and people in various other kinds of social groups. Socialization agents that nursing students encounter include clients, faculty, professional colleagues, other health care professionals, family (e.g., a nurse relative) and friends who occupy roles within or outside the formal institutional structure. The degree of congruence between the expectations of these multiple agents may either facilitate or hinder socialization.

One of the most powerful mechanisms of professional socialization is interaction with fellow students (Hardy & Conway, 1988, p. 267). Within this student culture, students collectively set the level and direction of their scholastic efforts, develop perspectives about the situation in which they are involved, the goals they are trying to achieve, kinds of activities that are expedient and proper, and a set of practices congruent with all of these. Students become bound together by feelings of mutual cooperation, support, and solidarity.

CONSIDER...

- the agents of professional socialization in your own experience. Is there a specific person who influenced your decision to become a nurse? How have other nurses influenced your development as a nurse?
- the sources of sanctions for the professional nurse. What legal, institutional, societal, and

professional sanctions (positive and negative) exist for nursing, both in your own practice and in the larger profession? How might these sanctions differ based on specialty area, geographic area, or level of practice?

Critical Values of Professional Nursing

It is within the nursing educational program that the nurse develops, clarifies, and internalizes professional values. Specific professional nursing values are stated in nursing codes of ethics (see Chapter 5), in standards of nursing practice (see Chapter 1), and in the legal system itself (see Chapter 6). Watson (1981, pp. 20–21) outlines four values critical for the profession of nursing:

1. A strong commitment to the service that nursing provides for the public
2. Belief in the dignity and worth of each person
3. A commitment to education
4. Autonomy

The first value, a strong commitment to the service that nursing provides for the public, is considered essential. Nursing is a helping, humanistic service directed to the health needs of individuals, families, and communities. The nurse's role is therefore focused on *health* and *care*. Nurses, being responsible for assessing and promoting the health status of all humans, need to value their contribution to the health and well-being of people. Since "care and caring is the central core and essence of nursing" (Watson, 1979), nurses also need to value the caring aspect of nursing.

The second value—the dignity and worth of each person—is based on Judeo-Christian philosophy of the sacredness of human life and the worth of the individual. Because nursing is a person-oriented profession, a basic belief in the worth of each person regardless of nationality, race, creed, color, age, sex, politics, social class, and health status is basic to nursing. Applied to nursing practice, this value means that the nurse always acts in the best interest of the client.

Commitment to education, the third value, reflects the lifelong value of learning in North American society. In terms of professional nursing, graduates need continuous education to maintain and expand their level of competencies to meet professional criteria, to anticipate the role of the nurse in the future, and to expand the body of professional knowledge. Nurses need to question nursing knowledge and practice critically, to contribute to nursing's theoretical base, and to test theories in nursing practice.

The fourth value—autonomy, or the right of self-determination as a profession—is "the one where the greatest emphasis should be placed at this time" (Watson, 1981, p. 21). Watson states that "nurses must have freedom to use their knowledge and skills for human betterment and the authority and ability to see that nursing service is delivered safely and effectively." A future challenge for nurses is to become more assertive in promoting nursing care and to develop the ability for independent behavior.

CONSIDER . . .

- Watson's four values of professional nursing, and identify behaviors that represent these values. What nurses in your experience embody these values? How do these nurses influence your own professional socialization?
- whether socialization is an outcome or a process.

Initial Process of Professional Socialization

Initial socialization prepares the student for the work setting. Several models have been developed to explain the initial process of socialization into professional roles. The models described here include those of Simpson, Davis, and Hinshaw. Each model outlines a sequential set of phases or "chain of events" beginning at the role of a lay person and ending at the role of a professional. Table 7–1 summarizes each model.

Simpson Model

Ida Harper Simpson (1967) outlines three distinct phases of professional socialization. In the first phase, the person concentrates on becoming proficient in specific work tasks. In the second phase, the person becomes attached to significant others in the work or reference group. In the third and final phase, the person internalizes the values of the professional group and adopts the prescribed behaviors.

Hinshaw Model

Ada Sue Hinshaw (1986) provides a three-phase general model of socialization that is an adaptation of

TABLE 7–1   Models of Initial Socialization into Professional Roles

Simpson (1967) Model	Hinshaw (1986) Model	Davis (1966) Doctrinal Conversion Model
Stage 1 Proficiency in specific work tasks	*Phase I* Transition of anticipated role expectations to the role expectations of societal group	*Stage 1* Initial innocence
		Stage 2 Labeled recognition of incongruity
Stage 2 Attachment to significant others in the work environment	*Phase II* Attachment to significant others/labeling incongruencies	*Stage 3* "Psyching out" and role simulation
		Stage 4 Increasing role simulation
		Stage 5 Provisional internalization
Stage 3 Internalization of the values of the professional group and adoption of the behaviors it prescribes	*Phase III* Internalization of role values/behaviors	*Stage 6* Stable internalization

SOURCES: Adapted from "Patterns of Socialization into Professions: The Case of Student Nurses" by I. H. Simpson, Winter 1967, *Sociological Inquiry, 37,* pp. 47–54; "Socialization and Resocialization of Nurses for Professional Nursing Practice" by A.S. Hinshaw, 1986, in E. C. Hein and M. J. Nicholson, Eds., *Contemporary Leadership Behavior: Selected Readings* (2nd ed.), Boston: Little, Brown; and "Professional Socialization as Subjective Experiences: The Process of Doctrinal Conversion among Student Nurses" by F. Davis, September 1966, Evian, France: Sixth World Congress of Sociology.

Simpson's model. During the *first* phase, individuals change their images of the role from anticipated concepts to the expectations of the persons who are setting the standards for them. Hinshaw states that (a) adults entering a profession have already learned a number of roles and values that help them to evaluate new roles and (b) these individuals are actively involved in the socialization process, having chosen to learn the new role expectations and enter the socialization process.

The *second* phase has two components: (a) learners attach themselves to significant others in the system, and at the same time (b) they label situations that are incongruent between their anticipated roles and those presented by the significant others. In the initial professional socialization, significant others are usually a group of faculty; in the work setting, they are selected colleagues or immediate supervisors. Hinshaw emphasizes the importance of appropriate role models in both educational programs and work settings. At this stage, individuals are able to verbalize that the expected role behaviors are not what they anticipated. It is a stage that often involves strong emotional reactions to conflicting sets of expectations. Successful resolution of conflicts depends on the existence of role models who demonstrate appropriate behaviors and who show how conflicting systems of standards and values can be integrated.

In the *third* phase, the student internalizes the values and standards of the new role. The degree to which values and standards are internalized and the extent to which incongruencies in role expectations are resolved is variable.

Kelman (1961, p. 57) defines three levels of value orientation. Individuals may demonstrate one or a blend of three levels:

- *Compliance.* The person demonstrates the expected behavior to get positive reactions from others but has not internalized the values. Compliance behavior can be dismissed when it no longer elicits positive responses.
- *Identification.* The person selectively adopts specific role behaviors that are acceptable to that person. The person may accept only expected behaviors rather than values. Identification behavior usually changes as role models change.
- *Internalization.* The person believes in and accepts the standards of the new role. The standards are a part of the person's own value system.

Davis Model

Fred Davis (1966) describes a six-stage doctrinal conversion process among nursing students.

Stage 1: Initial Innocence
When students enter a professional program, they

have an image of what they expect to become and how they should act or behave. Nursing students usually enter a nursing program with a service orientation and expect to look after sick people. However, educational experiences often differ from what the students expect. During this phase, students may express disappointment and frustration at the experiences they undergo and may question their value.

Stage 2: Labeled Recognition of Incongruity
In this phase students begin to identify, articulate, and share their concerns. They learn that they are not alone in their value incongruencies: Peers share the same concerns.

Stages 3 and 4: "Psyching Out" and Role Simulation
At this point, the basic cognitive framework for the internalization of professional nursing values begins to take shape. Students begin to identify the behaviors they are expected to demonstrate and through role modeling begin to practice the behaviors. In Davis's terms, this process becomes a matter of "psyching out" the faculty. The more effectively the role simulation is done, the more authentic the person believes the behavior to be, and it becomes part of the person. However, students may feel they are "playing a game" and are being "untrue to oneself," resulting in feelings of guilt and estrangement.

Stage 5: Provisional Internalization
In stage 5, students vacillate between commitment to their former image of nursing and performance of new behaviors attached to the professional image. Factors that enhance the students' new image are an increasing ability to use professional language and an increasing identification with professional role models, such as nursing faculty.

Stage 6: Stable Internalization
During stage 6, the student's behavior reflects the educationally and professionally approved model. However, preparation of the student for the work setting is only the initial process in socialization. New values and behaviors continue to be formed in the work setting.

Various factors facilitate the socialization process. Absence of these factors interferes with it. See the accompanying box.

Ongoing Professional Socialization and Resocialization

The process of socialization does not terminate with graduation from a program of study. It continues as

Factors that Facilitate the Socialization Process

- Clarity and consensus with which the occupants and aspirants (learners) perceive the roles and positions.
- Degree of compatibility of expectations within role sets—that is, all others who are involved with the learner, such as staff nurses, nurse managers, physicians, clients, and their families or significant others.
- Learning that has occurred before an entry to a position.
- Capability of socialization agents to manage the socialization process.
- Role models who demonstrate the desired characteristics and can enhance internalization of admired qualities.
- A well-developed and extended orientation or internship program that may include preceptors (people who act as teachers).
- Group support from others new to the position to share concerns.

SOURCES: Adapted from *Role Transition to Patient Care Management* by M. K. Strader and P. J. Decker, 1995, Norwalk, CT: Appleton & Lange, pp. 64–66; and *Role Theory: Perspectives for Health Professionals* (2nd ed.) by M. E. Hardy and M. E. Conway, 1988, Norwalk, CT: Appleton & Lange, p. 262.

the graduate begins a professional career and, in fact, continues throughout life. In school, the nursing student assimilates a central core of values emphasized by the faculty and the profession. In the work setting, the nurse faces the need to put the values of the profession into operation. The transition of the graduate to a full-fledged professional is facilitated if there is congruence between the norms, values, and expectations of the educational program and the realities of the work setting. However, practice settings are often bureaucratic and may be nonsupportive of professional career development. Three models of career stages or development—those of Kramer (1974); Dalton, Thompson, and Price (1977); and Benner (1984)—follow.

Kramer's Postgraduate Resocialization Model

Kramer (1974) introduced the concept of *reality shock* to explain discrepancies that arise between the behavioral expectations and values of the educational setting and those of the work setting. Reality shock results when the new graduate is unprepared (ineffectively socialized) to function effectively in the workplace. Kramer describes a four-stage postgraduate resocialization model for the transition of graduates from educational setting to work setting. See the accompanying box.

Dalton's Career Stages Model

Dalton, Thompson, and Price describe a four-stage model that emphasizes the development of competence derived from experience. As the individual's career progresses throughout each stage, activities, relationships, and psychological issues change in focus. For example, the individual's *major activities* progress from helping, learning, and following directions (stage 1) to shaping direction of the organization (stage 4). The *primary relationships* progress from that of an apprentice (stage 1) to that of sponsor (stage 4). The *major psychological issues* progress from a feeling of dependence (stage 1) to a feeling of comfort in exercising power (stage 4). These four stages are summarized in Table 7–2. Only a small percentage of nurses achieve the fourth stage because there are few stage-4 positions available.

Kramer's Postgraduate Resocialization Model

Stage I Skill and Routine Mastery
The nurse focuses on developing technical expertise and mastering specific skills to overcome feelings of frustration and inadequacy. May not focus on other important aspects of nursing care.

Stage II Social Integration
The nurse's major concern is having peers recognize the nurse's competence and accept the nurse into the group.

Stage III Moral Outrage
The nurse recognizes incongruities between conceptions of the *bureaucratic* role, which is associated with the rules and regulations and loyalty to agency administration; the *professional* role, which is committed to continued learning and loyalty to the profession; and the *service* role, which is concerned with compassion and loyalty to the client as a person.

Stage IV Conflict Resolution
The nurse resolves conflicts of stage III by surrendering behaviors and/or values or by learning to use both the values and behaviors of the professional and bureaucratic system in a politically astute manner.

SOURCE: *Reality Shock: Why Nurses Leave Nursing*, by M. Kramer, 1974, St. Louis: Mosby.

TABLE 7–2   Dalton, Thompson, and Price Career Stages

Stages	Central Activity	Primary Relationship	Major Psychologic Issue
Stage I	Helping and learning: performs fairly routine duties under the direction of a mentor	Apprentice, subordinate	Dependence
Stage II	Works independently as a competent peer	Colleague	Independence
Stage III	Influences, guides, directs, and helps others to develop	Informal mentor, role model	Assuming responsibility for others
Stage IV	Influences the direction of the organization or a segment of it; has one of three roles: manager, internal entrepreneur, or idea innovator	Sponsor	Exercising power

SOURCES: Adapted from "The Four Stages of Professional Careers—A New Look at Performance by Professionals" by G. W. Dalton, P. H. Thompson, and R. L. Price, Summer 1977, *Organizational Dynamics*, 19–42.

Benner's Stages of Nursing Expertise

Stage I Novice

No experience (e.g., nursing student). Performance is limited, inflexible, and governed by context-free rules and regulations rather than experience.

Stage II Advanced Beginner

Demonstrates marginally accepted performance. Recognizes the meaningful "aspects" of a real situation. Has experienced enough real situations to make judgments about them.

Stage III Competent Practitioner

Has 2 or 3 years of experience. Demonstrates organizational and planning abilities. Differentiates important factors from less important aspects of care. Coordinates multiple complex care demands.

Stage IV Proficient Practitioner

Has 3 to 5 years of experience. Perceives situations as wholes rather than in terms of parts, as in stage II. Uses maxims as guides for what to consider in a situation. Has holistic understanding of the client, which improves decision making. Focuses on long-term goals.

Stage V Expert Practitioner

Performance is fluid, flexible, and highly proficient; no longer requires rules, guidelines, or maxims to connect an understanding of the situation to appropriate action. Demonstrates highly skilled intuitive and analytic ability in new situations. Is inclined to take a certain action because "it felt right."

SOURCE: *From Novice to Expert: Excellence and Power in Clinical Nursing Practice*, by P. Benner, 1984, Menlo Park, CA: Addison-Wesley Nursing, pp. 21–34. Reprinted with permission.

Benner's Stages from Novice to Expert

Benner (1984) describes five levels of proficiency in nursing based on the Dreyfus model of skill acquisition derived from a study of chess players and airline pilots (Dreyfus & Dreyfus, 1980). The five stages, which have implications for teaching and learning, are novice, advanced beginner, competent, proficient, and expert. Benner believes that experience is essential for the development of professional expertise. See the box above.

CONSIDER...

- Benner's stages from novice to expert. Where are you on Benner's continuum in relation to your current area of practice? During your nursing career, what feelings have you experienced as you have moved along Benner's continuum? How might you assist a novice nurse to progress successfully to higher levels of practice?
- issues influencing the socialization process of RNs who return to school for baccalaureate education in nursing. What factors influenced your own decision to return to school?

ROLE STRESS AND ROLE STRAIN

Role stress is probably more prevalent now than ever before because of prevailing social conditions, such as inadequate adult socialization, rapid organizational change, and accelerated technology (Hardy & Hardy, 1988, p. 170). **Role stress** occurs when role obligations are unrealistic, vague, conflicting, or irritating. It is generated by the social structure or system; the source is primarily external to the person. Role stress may create **role strain,** an emotional reaction accompanied by psychologic responses, such as anxiety, tension, irritation, resentment, and depression; physiologic responses, such as diaphoresis, increased heart rate, increased blood pressure, increased rate and depth of respirations, and increased muscle tension; and social responses, such as withdrawal from interaction, job dissatisfaction, and reduced involvement with colleagues and organizations (Hardy & Hardy, 1988, p. 190). Common role stress problems and descriptions are shown in the box on page 138.

Role ambiguity is a characteristic of all positions occupied by professionals who often deal with uncertainty, the unexpected, and unpredictable activities and behavior (Hardy & Hardy, 1988, p. 201). Nurses in particular often experience role ambiguity because of the diversity of their role partners and multiple subroles of the nursing role. (In contrast, a technician's role expectations are explicit, and work can often be routinized.) Ambiguity can significantly affect a person's role performance, satisfaction, and commitment.

Role conflict is a widely discussed concept in current literature. The primary consequence of role

---

Role Stress Problems

Role ambiguity

Unclear role expectations.

Role conflict

Incompatible, competing role expectations within a single role or multiple roles.

Role incongruity

Values are incompatible with role expectations.

Role overload or underload

Too much is expected in the time available, or the role is too complex (overload); minimal role expectations that do not use the abilities of the role incumbent (underload).

Role overqualification or underqualification

Nurse's abilities and motivation exceed those required (overqualification); nurse lacks necessary resources (underqualification).

---

conflict is role stress. If unreconciled, role stress and role strain lead to *burnout*, a syndrome of mental and physical exhaustion involving negative self-concept, negative job attitude, and loss of concern for clients.

Shead (1991, p. 737) discusses four major causes of role conflict for nurses. A widely discussed causative factor is professional-bureaucratic work conflict. Nurses who are prepared to provide independent practice and use professional judgment experience conflict in bureaucracies that are more concerned about getting routine tasks completed. The organization's reward systems may contribute to conflict between nurses, who identify with their profession, and supervisors, who identify with the organization. Disproportionate power also creates stress. Increased professionalism often means increased conflict and stress, unless the bureaucratic structure is flexible enough to deal with the professional modality.

A second cause of role conflict arises from different views concerning what nursing is and should be. Role value orientations vary considerably among practitioners; some nurses have a more traditional view of the nurse's role than new managers or new professionals. The role of the professional nurse continues to change; nurses are becoming increasingly involved in planning and organizing health care activities and are becoming more responsible for delivering total client care services. The nurse's role is becoming one of managing client care activities in general. In this new role, nurses have greater responsibility and accountability and may experience increased stress as a result.

A third cause of conflict is a discrepancy between the nursing and medical view of what the nurse's role should be. Physicians may view the caring ideology of nurses as secondary in importance to their own, idealize curing aspects of care, and view the nurse as a handmaiden. Nurses use behavioral science and communication skills to develop their professional relationship with clients; physicians have traditionally employed a clinical, biologic approach. This variance can create role strain if (a) the physician expects the nurse to handle the client as the physician does and (b) the physician does not listen to the nurse's concerns and suggestions about the client.

A fourth source of conflict arises from the public image of nursing. Personal expectations and self-image may conflict with perceived public expectations. The public may regard the ideal nurse as a dedicated angel of mercy, whereas the media often malign the image by portraying the nurse as a sex symbol or other negative stereotype.

CONSIDER...

- role conflicts in your professional experience. What are the sources of your role conflicts? Are there role conflicts that are unique to your practice setting? Do other nursing colleagues experience the same role conflicts? What attitudes or behaviors do you or your colleagues manifest as a result of role conflicts? How do these attitudes or behaviors affect client care?

MANAGING ROLE STRESS AND ROLE STRAIN

Nurses may use various methods to resolve role stress related to role conflict or ambiguity. Their strategies are influenced by the situation, such as the availability of resources, the nurse's position in the setting, and flexibility of the organization.

1. *Redefine the role.* Redefinition may be a formal process, such as the writing of a job description, or an informal negotiation process, which produces a more immediate solution. Written job descriptions need to be explicit in terms of performance expectations and goals and objectives that can be used to appraise performance. Informal negotia-

tion may involve reallocating workloads and clarifying role performance expectations.

2. *Modify the environment.* Modifications may include changes in the organization of nursing care delivery, in the physical environment, or the allocation of resources such as money, equipment, and personnel.

3. *Delegate some functions.* A nurse manager may need to delegate some responsibilities to an assistant. A nurse clinician with multiple family and professional roles may need to delegate some family responsibilities to a spouse or children. However, changing self-expectations in usual roles and relinquishing familiar tasks to others presents difficulties for some. Women often experience guilt when they leave their children in the care of others or do not perform usual tasks, such as cooking dinner every night. Two common strategies women use coping with multiple roles include (a) setting priorities and (b) dividing tasks within the family. The family sets priorities to determine which tasks are vital and which can

be omitted or delayed. To divide tasks, the nurse may need to relinquish certain household or parent tasks and allow flexibility in how they are completed.

Nurses can manage role strain by using stress reduction techniques commonly considered for client. In addition, Hamilton (1984), Scully (1980), and Wilson (1986) suggest the following:

• Plan a daily relaxation program with meaningful quiet times to reduce tension. For example, take a walk in the park, listen to music, or take a hot bath.
• Establish an activity program to direct energy outward.
• Become more assertive to overcome feelings of powerlessness in relationships with others. Learn to say no.
• Manage time better by delegating to others and combining tasks.
• Take a course in biofeedback, yoga, meditation, or some other advanced relaxation technique.
• Learn to accept failures and learn from them.

RESEARCH NOTE

How Do Nurses Balance Personal and Professional Caregiving Careers?

Traditionally, research has focused on work as separate and distinct from family; now there is increasing recognition of the spillover effects, both positive and negative, in balancing personal and professional careers. In one study, researchers sought to understand more fully the experiences of nurses whose personal and professional lives both center on the provision of care to others. The objectives were to investigate (a) the subjective dimensions of the care that nurses provide at home and at work, (b) the challenges and opportunities associated with such care, and (c) the outcomes of balancing two careers that center on the provision of care. Of particular interest to the researchers were the feelings associated with providing care to others and the perceived tensions and benefits that result from these combined roles.

Forty full-time nurses who were also responsible for providing care to individuals in their private lives volunteered for a qualitative study of combined caregiving careers. Each respondent kept a diary of caregiving activities during two representative 24-hour periods and was interviewed prior to and after diary recording. Findings revealed that most nurses experienced high levels of stress associated with caregiving in both their professional and private lives. In general, they were relatively satisfied with their lives in both spheres and felt a slightly greater sense of control in their work lives than in their home lives. Regarding the tensions and conflicts they alluded to, the following themes emerged: an ethic of high expectation, feeling torn between two worlds, a sense of working in isolation, and working in overdrive. The rewards and benefits included remuneration, recognition and self-esteem, opportunities for personal growth, and opportunities for family growth. Ways to enhance the quality of their lives were also identified.

Implications: Nurses who provide care in both their personal and professional lives do cope and, in many cases, manage well. However, nurses need to consider ways to enhance the quality of their lives, both at home and at work.

SOURCE: "Nurses' Work: Balancing Personal and Professional Caregiving Careers" by M. M. Ross, E. Rideout, and M. Carson, *Canadian Journal of Nursing Research*, 26, (4), pp. 43–59.

- Learn to ask for help, and share your feelings with colleagues.
- Learn to support your colleagues in times of need. Give them a chance to "ventilate" feelings and listen to their concerns.
- Learn to handle problems constructively instead of defensively.
- Accept what cannot be changed. There are certain limitations in every situation.
- If working in an intensive care unit (ICU), establish a structured emotional support group. Most observers of the intensive care setting recommend that ICU nurses participate in some type of emotional support group. These groups are identified by various names: ventilation groups, discussion forums, or regular staff meetings for the purpose of dealing with feelings and anxieties generated in the work setting.

CONSIDER...

- your own strategies for dealing with role stress. Which strategies have been effective? Which have not?
- how your practice setting supports nurses in dealing with role stress. Explore the availability of support groups or counselors for nurses or other employees who are experiencing stress. If none exist, how might you develop and implement a support system for employees experiencing personal or professional stress?

ENHANCING PROFESSIONAL SELF-CONCEPT AND ROLE IMAGE

Nurses who seek to maintain or improve both their personal and professional selves are more effective in caring for their clients. They are also more effective in communicating with other health professionals and in promoting a positive image of nursing in the community. Strasen (1992, p. 2) defines *professional self-concept* as the set of beliefs and images held to be true as a result of specific professional socialization. The development of professional self-concept is based on one's personal self-concept. An individual's personal self-concept and professional self-concept affect one another. The characteristics of a person who has a positive self-concept include the following (Strader & Decker, 1995, p. 88):

- Future orientation; ability to minimize past failures
- Ability to cope with life's problems and disappointments
- Ability to help and accept help from others
- Ability to see and value the uniqueness of all individuals
- Ability to feel all aspects of emotion but not allow the feelings to affect behavior negatively or affect interactions with people who are not responsible for the situation

Because a person's subconscious mind acts positively or negatively on the information it receives, nurses can change their self-concepts by controlling what goes into the subconscious mind. Nurses who perceive themselves as successful will use their energy and creativity to explore ways to become even more successful. Positive thoughts help them to succeed.

To develop a positive self-concept, Strader and Decker (1995, pp. 88–89) suggest the following steps:

- Accept your present self but have a better self in mind.
- Set goals that are high but attainable.
- Develop expertise in some area to increase your value to yourself and to your employing agency. This may involve continuing education or obtaining certification in a specialized area of practice.

CONSIDER...

- how a positive self-concept in individual nurses might improve the quality of client care and the profession of nursing.
- your own professional goals. What attitudinal changes will you need to make to reach your goals? What strategies would you implement to achieve your future goals? How will the achievement of your goals affect your personal and professional self-concepts? How can you help nursing colleagues define and achieve their professional goals?
- ways in which you can improve the image of nurses and nursing in the medical and general communities; for example, among physicians and other health professionals, the public, the media, politicians and legislators, and so on.

READINGS FOR ENRICHMENT

Benner, P. (1984). *From novice to expert: Excellence and power in clinical nursing practice.* Menlo Park, CA: Addison-Wesley Nursing.

This book is a major contribution to nursing. Dr. Benner takes observations reported by nurses in actual practice and analyzes them according to a model of skill acquisition that was developed by professors Hubert L. Dreyfus and Stuart E. Dreyfus. Dr. Benner's analysis provides a vivid description of nursing practice as rendered by expert nurses. The book discloses what expert nurses do in specific client care situations and how beginners and experts do it differently; how, as their clinical careers develop, nurses themselves change their intellectual orientation, integrate and sort out their knowledge, and refocus their decision making on a basis different from the process-oriented process they were taught. Benner's analysis has many profound implications for nurses in administration, education, and practice.

Christman, L. (1991, September). Perspectives on role socialization of nurses. *Nursing Outlook, 39;* 209–212.

This Dean Emeritus of Rush University College of Nursing provides insightful concepts about role socialization as it is applied to nurses. He includes the influence of Florence Nightingale, the way in which the emphasis on art and discipline obscured nursing's role, the feminist disdain for nursing, ethics of associate degree preparation, and different themes for the future.

Muscari, M. E., Archer, K. E., & Harrington, T. L. (1994, October). Developing your professional identity: How to feel more confident and get the respect you desire. *Nursing 94, 24;* 96–100.

This assistant professor and two senior nursing students outline ten important ways a nurse can develop a solid, professional identity. Continuing development enables nurses to see their work as more than a job.

SUMMARY

Nurses must understand the roles they and others play and societal expectations associated with those roles. Any role consists of three elements: the ideal role, the perceived role, and the performed role. Role performance is influenced by such factors as health status, values, and situational pressures. Five determinants form boundaries for nursing roles: conceptual frameworks, the nursing process, standards of practice, nurse practice acts, and a code of ethics.

Nurses function in a variety of roles that are not exclusive of one another; in reality, they often occur together and serve to clarify the nurse's activities. These roles include caregiver, teacher, counselor, client advocate, change agent, leader, manager, researcher, consultant, collaborator, case manager, and quality care evaluator.

Nurses are fulfilling expanded nursing roles, for example, those of the nurse generalist, the nurse clinician, clinical nurse specialist, nurse anesthetist, and advanced nurse practitioner.

Socialization is a lifelong process by which people become functioning participants of a society or a group. It is a reciprocal learning process that is brought about by interaction with other people and establishes boundaries of behavior. Socialization to professional nursing practice is the process whereby the values and norms of the nursing profession are internalized into the nurse's own behavior and self-concept. The nurse acquires the knowledge, skills, and attitudes characteristic of the profession.

Socialization for professional nursing requires the development of critical values, including a strong commitment to the service that nursing provides to the public, a belief in the dignity and worth of each person, a commitment to education, and autonomy.

Various models of the socialization process have been developed. Such models may serve as guidelines to establish the phase and extent of an individual's socialization.

Nurses are prone to role stress and strain for a variety of reasons unique to their role in the health care and social systems. Common problems are role conflict, role ambiguity, role overload, and role incongruity. Strategies to handle role stress differ from strategies to manage role strain. Nurses can positively influence their self-concepts and role images to improve work satisfaction and provide quality care.

SELECTED REFERENCES

American Nurses Association. (1991). *Standards of clinical nursing practice.* Kansas City, MO: ANA.

Benner, P. (1984). *From novice to expert: Excellence and power in clinical nursing practice.* Menlo Park, CA: Addison-Wesley Nursing.

Benner, P., & Wrubel, J. (1989). *The primacy of caring: Stress and coping in health and illness.* Menlo Park, CA: Addison-Wesley Nursing.

Brooten, D. A., Hayman, L., & Naylor, M. (1978). *Leadership for change: A guide for the frustrated nurse.* Philadelphia: Lippincott.

Dalton, G. W., Thompson, P. H., & Price, R. L. (1977, Summer). The four stages of professional careers—A new look at performance by professionals. *Organizational Dynamics,* 19–42.

Davis, F. (1966, September). Professional socialization as subjective experiences: The process of doctrinal conversion among student nurses. Paper. Evian, France: *Sixth World Congress of Sociology.*

DeYoung, L. (1985). *Dynamics of nursing* (5th ed.). St. Louis: Mosby.

Disparti, J. (1988). Nutrition and self care. In Caliandro, G., & Judkins, B. L. *Primary nursing practice.* Glenview, IL: Scott, Foresman.

Dreyfus, S. E., & Dreyfus, H. L. February 1980. A five-stage model of the mental activities involved in directed skill acquisition. Unpublished report supported by the Air Force Office of Scientific Research (AFSC), USAF (Contract F49620-79-C-0063), University of California at Berkeley.

Epstein, C. (1982). *The nurse leader: Philosophy and practice.* Reston, VA: Reston Publishing.

Fralic, M. F., Kowalski, P. M., & Llewellyn, F. A. (1991, April). The staff nurse as quality monitor. *American Journal of Nursing, 91,* 40–42.

Hamilton, J. M. (1984, July/August). Effective ways to relieve stress. *Nursing Life, 4,* 24–27.

Hardy, M. E., & Conway, M. E. (1988). *Role theory: Perspectives for healthy professionals* (2nd ed.). Norwalk, CT: Appleton & Lange.

Hardy, M. E., & Hardy, W. L. (1988). Role stress and strain. In Hardy, M. E. & Conway, M. E. *Role theory: Perspectives for health professionals* (2nd ed.) (pp. 159–239). Norwalk, CT: Appleton & Lange.

Hinshaw, A. S. (1977, November.) *Socialization and resocialization of nurses for professional nursing practice.* National League for Nursing Pub. No. 15-1659. New York: National League for Nursing.

Hinshaw, A. S. (1986). Socialization and resocialization of nurses for professional nursing practice. In Hein, E. C., & Nicholson, M. J. (Eds.). *Contemporary leadership behavior: Selected readings* (2nd ed.). Boston: Little, Brown.

Jenny, J. (1990, October). Self-esteem: A problem for nurses. *Canadian Nurse, 86*(10), 19–21.

Kane, D. (1993, October-December.) Invest in yourself. Coping with multiple roles: Mother/wife/nurse. *Nursing Forum, 28,* 17–21.

Kelman, H. (1961). Process of opinion changes. *Public Opinion Quarterly, 25*(1), 57.

Kemp, V. H. (1986). An overview of change and leadership. In Hein, E. C., & Nicholson, M. J. (Eds.). *Contemporary leadership behaviors: Selected readings* (2nd ed.). Boston: Little, Brown.

Kramer, M. (1974). *Reality shock: Why nurses leave nursing.* St. Louis: Mosby.

Lancaster, J., & Lancaster, W. (Eds.). (1982). *Concepts for advanced nursing practice: The nurse as a change agent.* St. Louis: Mosby.

Leddy, S., & Pepper, J. M. (1993). *Conceptual bases of professional nursing* (3rd ed.). Philadelphia: Lippincott.

Lippitt, R., & Lippitt, G. L. (1977). Consulting process in action. In Jones, J. E., & Pfeiffer, J. W. (Eds.). *The 1977 annual handbook for group facilitators.* La Jolla, CA: University Associates.

Merton, R. K. (1968). *Social theory and social structure.* Glencoe, IL: Free Press.

Pranulis, M. F., Renwanz-Boyle, A., Kontas, A. S., & Hodson, W. L. (1995). Identifying nurses vulnerable to role conflict. *International Nursing Review, 42,* 45–50.

Redman, B. K. (1993). *The process of patient education* (7th ed.). St. Louis: Mosby.

Scully, R. (1980, May). Stress in the nurse. *American Journal of Nursing, 80,* 912–914.

Shead, H. (1991, June). Role conflict in student nurses: Towards a positive approach for the 1990s. *Journal of Advanced Nursing, 16,* 736–740.

Simpson, I. H. (1967, Winter). Patterns of socialization into professions: The case of student nurses. *Sociological Inquiry, 37,* 47–54.

Starzomski, R. (1983, September). The place of research in nursing. *Canadian Nurse, 79,* 34–35.

Strader, M. K., & Decker, P. J. (1995). *Role transition to patient care management.* Norwalk, CT: Appleton & Lange.

Strasen, L. L. (1992). *The image of professional nursing: Strategies for action.* Philadelphia: Lippincott.

Styles, M. M. (1978, June). Why publish? *Image: Journal of Nursing Scholarship, 10,* 28–32.

Styles, M. M. (1982). *On nursing: Toward a new endowment.* St. Louis: Mosby.

Watson, I. (1981, Summer). Socialization of the nursing student in a professional nursing education program. *Nursing Papers, 13,* 19–24.

Watson, J. (1979). *Nursing—The philosophy and science of caring.* Boston: Little, Brown.

Wilson, H. S. (1985). *Research in nursing.* Menlo Park, CA: Addison-Wesley Nursing.

Wilson, L. K. (1986, May/June). High-gear nursing: How it can run you down and what you can do about it. *Nursing Life, 6,* 44–47.

Yura, H., Ozimek, D., & Walsh, M. B. (1981). *Nursing leadership: Theory and process.* New York: Appleton-Century-Croft.

Health Promoter

OBJECTIVES

- Differentiate health preventive or protective care and health promotion.

- Discuss essential components of health promotion.

- Identify various types and sites of health promotion programs.

- Compare three health promotion models: those of Pender, Kulbock, and Neuman.

- Discuss Prochaska and DiClemente's five-stage model of behavior change.

- Discuss the nurse's role in health promotion.

"I believe promotion of health is far more important than the care of the sick. I believe there is more to be gained by helping every man learn how to be healthy than by preparing the most skilled therapists for services to those in crises."
—Virginia Henderson

Health promotion is an important component of nursing practice. It is a way of thinking that revolves around a philosophy of wholeness, wellness, and well-being.

- In the past two decades, the public has become increasingly aware of and interested in health promotion. Many people are aware of the relationship between life-style and illness and are developing health-promoting habits, such as taking adequate exercise, rest, and relaxation; maintaining good nutrition; and controlling the use of tobacco, alcohol, and other drugs.
- The vision of health promotion was expressed nationally in Canada in 1974 with the publication of the Lalonde Report, "A New Perspective on the Health of Canadians" and in the United States in 1979 in the Surgeon General's report *Healthy People*. Both of these reports emphasize the role that individuals can play in modifying their life-styles and personal behaviors to improve their health status. These reports also consider, to a lesser extent, environmental factors influencing health.

- The Surgeon General's report was followed in 1980 by *Objectives for the Nation*, developed by the U.S. Public Health Service, in particular, the Office of Health Information and Promotion (OHIP) (U.S. Surgeon General, 1980). This report addressed more specifically the broad goals set forth in *Healthy People* by listing strategies to achieve each objective. These strategies included not only personal behavior changes but also the roles of institutions, legislation, and policy. The objectives cover 15 areas, 5 of which specifically address health promotion: exercise and fitness, smoking, stress control, nutrition, and alcohol and drugs.
- The World Health Organization (WHO) has viewed the initial emphasis on individual life-style behavior change as blaming the victim because this approach does not consider society's responsibility for promoting the public's health, in areas such as legislation, organizational change, and community development (WHO, 1986).
- In the mid 1980s, the Canadian government undertook a large restructuring of its approach to health care. This report, known as the Epp Report, emerged from a synthesis of the Lalonde Report and the World Health Organization document. Its framework emphasizes two approaches (Epp, 1986):
1. To reduce inequities between low- and high-income groups. This approach is structured in

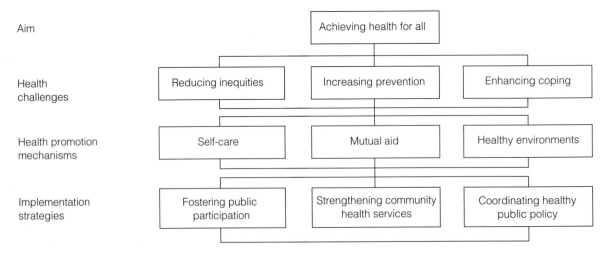

Figure 8–1 *A framework for health promotion.*

SOURCE: *Achieving Health for All: A Framework for Health Promotion: Report of the Minister of National Health and Welfare*, by J. Epp, November 1986, Ottawa, Canada: Government Printing Office.

terms of broad social responsibility rather than individual responsibility.

2. Three levels of concern—health challenges, health promotion mechanisms, and implementation strategies. In each of these levels, attention is given to the role of broad institutional or environmental change (Figure 8–1).

- In September 1990, *Healthy People 2000* was presented to the American public. This document encompasses 298 health-related objectives that provide a framework for a national health promotion, health protection, and preventive service strategy (United States Department of Health and Human Services [USDHHS], 1991, p. 89). Individual nurses and 24 national nursing organizations were involved in the development of *Healthy People 2000* (Brown, Mattson, Newman & Sirles, 1992, p. 204).

- Health promotion, then, includes programs that modify both the environment and the behavior of individuals. It involves education in individual life-styles, community development, organizational change, and—at the political level—legislation.

DEFINING HEALTH PROMOTION

Considerable differences appear in the literature regarding the use of the terms *health promotion*, *primary prevention*, *health protection*, and *illness prevention*. Leavell and Clark (1965, p. 21) define three levels of prevention: primary, secondary, and tertiary. There are five steps that describe these levels: **Primary prevention** focuses on (1) health promotion and (2) protection against specific health problems. **Secondary prevention** focuses on (1) early identification of health problems and (2) prompt intervention to alleviate health problems. **Tertiary prevention** focuses on restoration and rehabilitation to an optimal level of functioning.

In the model used by Leavell and Clark, primary prevention precedes any disease symptoms. The purpose of primary prevention is to encourage optimal health and to increase the person's resistance to illness. Examples of primary prevention include health education concerning the hazards of smoking and specific protection against a particular disease, such as the vaccine against poliomyelitis.

The second level, secondary prevention, presumes the presence of a disease or illness. Screening procedures, such as a blood sugar test for a client with diabetes mellitus, and the Denver Developmental Screening Tests to assess developmental delays, are facets of secondary prevention. Screening procedures facilitate early discovery and allow treatment to begin before the illness progresses. Disability limitation, another step in secondary prevention, is also more effective in the early stages of a disease.

Tertiary prevention relates to situations where a disability is already present. The goal of tertiary prevention is to restore individuals to their optimal level of functioning within the limitations imposed by their condition.

Pender (1987, p. 4) considers **health promotion** distinct from primary prevention. She defines health promotion as "activities directed toward increasing the level of well being," and primary prevention as "activities directed toward decreasing the probability of specific illnesses." In this instance, health promotion is considered to be an approach behavior, whereas primary prevention is considered avoidance behavior. Health promotion is not disease oriented; that is, no specific problem is being avoided. By contrast, primary prevention activities are geared toward avoiding specific problems (Pender, 1987, p. 5).

Stachtchenko and Jenicek (1990, p. 53) support Pender's conceptual differences between the terms health promotion and primary prevention (or health protection). They describe health promotion as broad in scope, involving not only life-style changes but also the process of granting individuals and communities more control over determinants of health. Health prevention programs focus on risk reduction and are targeted toward specific populations.

Healthy People 2000 is a document that describes specific objectives in health promotion and disease prevention for adults and children. The box on page 146 outlines the *Healthy People 2000* priority areas. *Healthy People 2000* differentiates health promotion, health protection, and preventive health services, outlining specific activities for each category:

- **Health promotion**—individual and community activities to promote healthful life-styles. Examples of health promotion activities include improving nutrition, preventing alcohol and drug misuse, restricting smoking, maintaining fitness, and exercising.

- **Health protection**—actions by government and industry to minimize environmental health threats. Health protection relates to activities such as maintaining occupational safety, controlling radiation and toxic agents, and preventing infectious diseases and accidents.

Healthy People 2000 Priority Areas

Health Promotion

1. Physical activity and fitness
2. Nutrition
3. Tobacco
4. Alcohol and other drugs
5. Family planning
6. Mental health and mental disorders
7. Violent and abusive behavior
8. Educational and community-based programs

Health Protection

9. Unintentional injuries
10. Occupational safety and health
11. Environmental health
12. Food and drug safety
13. Oral health

Preventive Services

14. Maternal and infant health
15. Heart disease and stroke
16. Cancer
17. Diabetes and chronic disabling conditions
18. HIV infection
19. Sexually transmitted diseases
20. Immunization and infectious diseases
21. Clinical preventive services

Surveillance and Data Systems

22. Surveillance and data systems

SOURCE: Adapted from *Healthy People 2000: National Health Promotion and Disease Prevention* by the United States Department of Health and Human Services, September 1990, DHHS Pub. No. (PHS) 91-50212, Washington, D.C.: U.S. Government Printing Office.

- **Preventive health services**—actions that health care providers take to prevent health problems. These services include control of high blood pressure, control of sexually transmitted diseases, immunization, family planning, and health care during pregnancy and infancy. See also the discussion of *Healthy People 2000* in Chapter 3.

The difficulty in separating the terms *health promotion*, *health prevention*, and *health protection* lies in the fact that an activity may be carried out for numerous reasons. For example, a 40-year-old male may begin a program of walking 3 miles each day. If the goal of his program is to "decrease the risk of heart disease," then the activity would be considered prevention. By contrast, if his walking regimen is instituted to "increase his overall health and feeling of well-being," then the activity would be considered health promotion behavior.

A chief scientist for nursing from WHO, Amelia Mangay Maglacas, uses the terms *positive health* and *positive health promotion* and presents them in a broader context. According to Maglacas, *positive health* for all does not mean the eradication of every disease or the healing of every body part. Rather, health should be considered in the context of its contribution to social and economic development, so that all people have the necessary social and economic support to lead satisfying lives (1988, p. 67). *Positive health promotion* is the process of enabling people to improve and to increase their control over their own health. The aim of positive health promotion is to improve health potential and maintain health balance. One attains this goal of positive health by caring for oneself and for others, by controlling life's circumstances with careful and conscientious decision making, and by ensuring that conditions in society allow people to attain health.

A summary of essential components of health promotion proposed by Schultz (1995, p. 32) are shown in the box on page 147. These points are incorporated into her definition of health promotion:

> Health promotion facilitates an individual or a community in a process of self-determining a present health status, in order to actively choose ways of altering personal or communal health habits for improvement, and to develop resources and skills to alter the environment so

Concepts of Health Promotion

- Health promotion maintains and enhances health.
- Health promotion develops the resources and skills of the person or community.
- Health promotion alters personal or communal habits and the environment.
- Health promotion defines health as a continuum.
- Health promotion is self-directed.

SOURCE: "What Is Health Promotion?" by A. Schultz, 1995, *Canadian Nurse, 91*(7), 31–34.

that health is being maintained or a self-determined higher level of health can be achieved.

CONSIDER . . .

- whether you agree with Pender's conceptual differences between the terms *health promotion* and *primary prevention.*
- whether health promotion can be offered to all clients regardless of their age, health and illness status.

HEALTH PROMOTION ACTIVITIES

Health promotion organizations, wellness centers, and traditional health care centers all offer a different approach to client care. Table 8–1 demonstrates these differences. Health promotion activities can be carried out on a governmental level (e.g., a national program to improve knowledge of nutrition) or on a personal level (e.g., an individual exercise program).

Health promotion programs on an individual level can be active or passive. With *passive* strategies, the client is a recipient of the health promotion effort. Many health professionals participate in national programs to define and institute these passive strategies. Examples of passive government strategies are maintaining the cleanliness of water and promoting a healthy environment by enforcing sewage regulations to decrease the spread of disease. *Active* strategies depend on individuals' commitment to and involvement in adopting a program directed toward their health promotion. Active strategies are important in that they encourage individuals to take control of their lives and assume the responsibility for their health. Examples of active strategies that

TABLE 8–1   Focus of Traditional Health Care Contrasted with Health Promotion and Wellness

	Traditional	Health Promotion	Wellness
Primary goal	Identify and correct problem	Disease prevention and risk reduction	Increased health
Dominant message	"Health care professionals will take care of you."	"You will live longer if you avoid illness."	"You are responsible, and your efforts to be well will be supported."
Change agent	Treatment	Information and behavior change	Positive experience and cultural influences
Target	The problem	Individuals, families, and communities	Clients within cultures
Duration of intervention	Ends when the problems clear up	Length of class or program	Ongoing

SOURCE: Adapted from *A Primer of Health Promotion: Creating Healthy Organizational Cultures* by J. P. Opatz, 1985, Washington, D.C.: Oryn Publications, p. 101.

involve changes in life-style are (1) a diet management program to improve nutrition, (2) a self-help program to reduce stress related to parenting, (3) an exercise program to improve muscle strength and endurance, or (4) a combination diet and exercise regimen for weight reduction or control. For optimal health and well-being, a combination of both active and passive strategies is suggested.

Types of Health Promotion Programs

A variety of programs can be used for the promotion of health, including (1) information dissemination, (2) health appraisal and wellness assessment, (3) lifestyle and behavior change, and (4) environmental control programs.

Information dissemination is the most basic type of health promotion program. This method makes use of a variety of media to offer information to the public about the risk of particular life-style choices and personal behavior, as well as the benefits of changing that behavior and improving the quality of life. Billboards, posters, brochures, newspaper features, books, and health fairs all offer opportunities for the dissemination of health promotion information. Alcohol and drug abuse, driving under the influence of alcohol, hypertension, and the need for immunizations are some of the topics frequently discussed. Recently, information about acquired immune deficiency syndrome (AIDS), including how it is transmitted, techniques for prevention, and the issue of sexual responsibility, has been distributed. The intent is to reduce unjustified fear, correct misinformation, and educate the public about this disease. Information dissemination is a useful strategy for raising the level of knowledge and awareness of individuals and groups about health habits.

Health risk appraisal/wellness assessment programs are used to apprise individuals of the risk factors that are inherent in their lives in order to motivate them to reduce specific risks and develop positive health habits. Wellness assessment programs are focused on more positive methods of enhancement, in contrast to the risk factor approach used in the health appraisal. A variety of tools are available to facilitate these assessments. Some of these tools are computer based and can therefore be offered to educational institutions and industries at a reasonable cost. For detailed information on assessment tools see Chapter 16.

Life-style and behavior change programs require the participation of the individual and are geared toward enhancing the quality of life and extending the life span. Individuals generally consider life-style changes after they have been informed of the need to change their health behavior and become aware of the potential benefits of the process. Many programs are available to the public, both on a group and individual basis, some of which address stress management, nutrition awareness, weight control, smoking cessation, and exercise.

Environmental control programs have been developed in response to the recent growth in the number of contaminants of human origin that have been introduced into our environment. The amount of contaminants that are already present in the air, food, and water will affect the health of our descendants for several generations. The most common concerns of community groups are toxic and nuclear wastes, nuclear power plants, air and water pollution, and herbicide and pesticide spraying.

Sites for Health Promotion Activities

Health promotion programs are found in many settings. Programs and activities may be offered to individuals and families in the home or in the community setting and at schools, hospitals, or worksites. Some individuals may feel more comfortable having the nurse, diet counselor, or fitness expert come to their home for teaching and follow-up on individual needs. This type of program, however, is not cost-effective for most individuals. Many people prefer the group approach, find it more motivating, and enjoy the socializing and group support. Most programs offered in the community are group oriented.

Community programs are frequently offered by cities and towns. The type of program depends on the current concerns and the expertise of the sponsoring department or group. Program offerings may include health promotion, specific protection, and screening for early detection of disease. The local health department may offer a townwide immunization program or blood pressure screening. The fire department may disseminate fire prevention information; the police may offer a bicycle safety program for children or a safe-driving campaign for young adults.

Hospitals began the emphasis on health promotion and prevention by focusing on the health of their employees. Because of the stress involved in caring for the sick and the various shifts that nurses and other health care workers must work, the life-styles and health habits of health care employees were given priority.

Programs offered by health care organizations initially began with the specific focus of prevention. Examples include infection control, fire prevention and fire drills, limiting exposure to X rays, and the prevention of back injuries. Gradually, issues related to the health and life-style of the employee were addressed with programs on topics such as smoking cessation, exercise and fitness, stress reduction, and time management. Increasingly, hospitals have offered a variety of these programs and others (e.g., women's health) to the community as well as to their employees. This community activity of the health care institution enhances the public image of the hospital, increases the health of the surrounding population, and generates some additional income.

School health promotion programs may serve as a foundation for children of all ages to learn basic knowledge about personal hygiene and issues in the health sciences. Because school is the focus of a child's life for so many years, the school provides a cost-effective and convenient setting for health-focused programs. The school nurse may teach programs about basic nutrition, dental care, activity and play, drug and alcohol abuse, domestic violence, child abuse, and issues related to sexuality and pregnancy. Classroom teachers may include health-related topics in their lesson plans, for example, the way the normal heart functions or the need for clean air and water in the environment.

Worksite programs for health promotion have developed out of the need for businesses to control the rising cost of health care and employee absenteeism. Many industries feel that both employers and employees can benefit from healthy life-style behavior. The convenience of the worksite setting makes these programs particularly attractive to many adults who would otherwise not be aware of them or motivated to attend them. Health promotion programs may be held in the company cafeteria so that employees can watch a film or have a discussion group during their lunch break. Worksite programs may include programs that address air quality standards for the office, classroom, or plant; programs aimed at specific populations, such as accident prevention for the machine worker or back-saver programs for the individual involved in heavy lifting; programs to screen for high blood pressure; or health enhancement programs, such as fitness infor-

mation and relaxation techniques. Benefits to the worker may include an increased feeling of well-being, fitness, weight control, and decreased stress. Benefits to the employer may include an increase in employee motivation and productivity, an increase in employee morale, a decrease in absenteeism, and a lower rate of employee turnover, all of which may decrease business and health care costs.

CONSIDER...

- the accessibility of preventive care services to people of all ages and economic status in your community.
- places where health information is made available to the public in your community.
- how you would improve your current worksite wellness program.
- the effectiveness of environmental control programs in your community.
- health promotion activities you would like to see implemented in your community if there were no limits in such resources as time, expertise, and money.
- health promotion activities you would plan for (a) elderly clients, (b) adolescents, and (c) school-age children.
- health promotion interventions that could be incorporated into a nursing care plan for a client with an existing health problem, such as chronic lung disease, diabetes mellitus, or cardiac disease.

HEALTH PROMOTION MODELS

The health belief model (HBM) discussed in Chapter 3 focuses on a person's susceptibility to disease. According to Pender (1987, p. 44), HBM is considered appropriate for explaining health-protecting or preventive behaviors, but it is not considered an appropriate model for health-promoting behaviors. Three health promotion models follow.

Pender's Health Promotion Model

Nola Pender's health promotion model (1987, p. 57–72) focuses on *health-promoting* behaviors rather than health-protecting or preventive behaviors (Figure 8–2). Its organization is similar to that of the health belief model. Determinants of health-

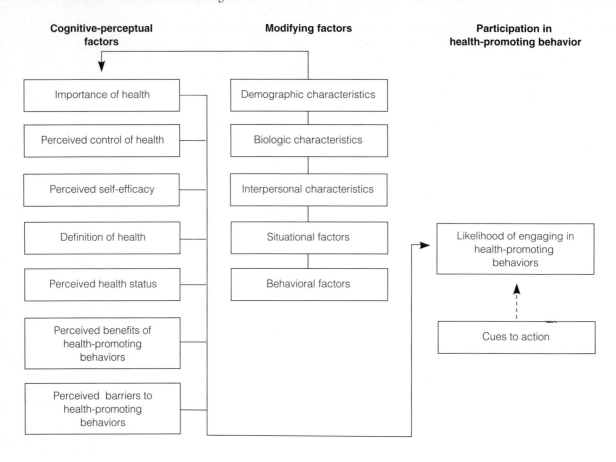

Figure 8–2 *Health promotion model.*

SOURCE: *Health Promotion in Nursing* (2nd ed.) by N. J. Pender, 1987, Norwalk, CT: Appleton & Lange, p. 58. Reprinted with permission.

promoting behaviors are categorized into (a) cognitive-perceptual factors, (b) modifying factors, and (c) cues to action.

Cognitive-Perceptual Factors

Cognitive-perceptual factors are considered to be the *primary motivational mechanisms* for acquiring and maintaining health promoting behaviors. They include the following:

- *The importance of health.* Placing a high value on health results in information-seeking behavior, such as reading health-related pamphlets.
- *Perceived control.* People who perceive that they have control over their own health are more likely to use preventive services than people who feel powerless. (See the section on "Locus of Control" in Chapter 3.) Control over health can relate

to such behaviors as not smoking and using seat belts in automobiles.

- *Perceived self-efficacy.* This concept refers to the conviction that a person can successfully carry out the behavior necessary to achieve a desired outcome, such as maintaining an exercise program to lose weight. Often people who have serious doubts about their capabilities decrease their efforts and give up, whereas those with a strong sense of efficacy exert greater effort to master problems or challenges.
- *Definition of health.* A person's definition of health may influence the extent to which the person engages in health-promoting behaviors.
- *Perceived health status.* Perceived health status may affect the frequency and intensity of health-promoting behaviors.

- *Perceived benefits of health-promoting behaviors.* Perceived benefits (e.g., physical fitness, psychologic well-being, and stress reduction) affect the person's level of participation in health-promoting behaviors and may facilitate continued practice. Repetition of such behavior itself can strengthen and reinforce beliefs about benefits.
- *Perceived barriers.* A person's perceptions about available time, access to facilities, and difficulty performing the activity may act as barriers to health-promoting behaviors. These barriers may be imagined or real.

Modifying Factors

Factors that modify the cognitive-perceptual factors include the following:

- *Demographic factors*, such as age, sex, race, ethnicity, education, and income
- *Biologic characteristics*, such as percentage of body fat and total body weight, which are related to exercise adherence
- *Interpersonal influences* such as expectations of significant others, family patterns of health care, and interactions with health professionals
- *Situational factors*, such as ease of access to health promotion alternatives and availability of environmental options (e.g., vending machines and restaurant menus that provide healthful options)
- *Behavioral factors*, such as previous experience, knowledge, and skill in health-promoting actions

Cues to Action

The likelihood that a person will take health-promoting action may depend on (a) cues of *internal origin*, such as personal awareness of the potential for growth or increased feelings of well-being; and (b) cues of *external origin*, such as conversations with others about their health behavior patterns and mass media information about personal and family health and environmental concerns.

Kulbok's Resource Model of Preventive Health Behavior

The Resource model of preventive health behavior developed by Kulbok (1985, pp. 67–81) proposes that people act in ways that maximize their "stock in health." It hypothesizes that the greater a person's social and health resources, the more frequently the person will perform preventive behaviors.

Social resources refer to education level and family income. *Health resources* refer to general psychologic well-being; perceptions about health, health status, and energy level; the capability to take care of one's own health; participation in social groups; and number and closeness of friends and relatives. *Preventive health behaviors* relate to physical activity, diet, sleeping, smoking, drinking alcoholic beverages, drinking caffeinated beverages, dental hygiene, use of seat belts, use of professional health

---

RESEARCH NOTE

What Determines a Health-Promoting Life-Style?

One researcher sought to create an integrative review and analysis of research literature on health promotion published between 1983 and 1991. The review focused on identifying the determinants of a health-promoting life-style. Pender's health promotion model (HPM) (Pender, 1987) provided the organizing framework for conducting the review. Twenty-three published research papers were reviewed; six concerned children and adolescents, and the remaining seventeen concerned adults.

Findings revealed that the strongest predictor of a health-promoting life-style was self-efficacy. This was followed by social support, perceived benefits, self-concept, perceived barriers, and health definition. The most frequently studied determinants, such as health locus of control and health value, were not found to be strong predictors.

Implications: Further research is needed to provide more varied data about the determinants of health promotion life-styles and practices of people of all ages. Most of the research tools currently in use have been tested on an adult population and may not be appropriate for children, adolescents, and older adults. In addition, Pender's health promotion model has been tested only on well individuals, not on ill individuals.

SOURCE: "Determinants of a Health-Promoting Lifestyle: An Integrative Review" by A. M. Gillis, March 1993, *Journal of Advanced Nursing, 18,* 345–353.

services for prevention of disease, and behavior to control high blood pressure.

Neuman's Systems Model

In her health promotion model, nurse theorist Betty Neuman (1995) includes levels of prevention (primary, secondary, and tertiary) and factors that strengthen a person's lines or barriers of defense. For additional information, see Chapter 2, and the book *The Neuman Systems Model* (1995).

CONSIDER . . .

- determinants (primary instructors) of health-promoting behaviors cited in Pender's and Kulbok's models that may influence your own health behavior.
- what barriers can deter positive health-promoting behaviors in adolescents and older adults.
- how demographic factors such as age, sex, race, ethnicity, education, and income may influence health-promoting behaviors.

STAGES OF HEALTH BEHAVIOR CHANGE

Health behavior change is a cyclic phenomenon in which people progress through several stages. In the first stage, the person does not think seriously about changing a behavior; by the time the person reaches the final stage, he or she is successfully maintaining the change in behavior. Several behavior change models have been proposed. The stage model proposed by Prochaska and DiClemente (1982, 1992) is discussed here. The stages are (a) precontemplation, (b) contemplation, (c) preparation, (d) action, and (e) maintenance. If the person does not succeed in changing behavior, relapse occurs.

In the *precontemplation stage*, the person does not think about changing behavior, nor is the person interested in information about the behavior. The negative aspects of making the change outweigh the benefits. Some people may believe the behavior is not under their control and may become defensive when confronted with information.

During the *contemplative stage*, the person seriously considers changing a specific behavior, actively gathers information, and verbalizes plans to change the behavior in the near future. Belief in the value of the change and self-confidence in the ability to change both increase in this phase. It is com-

mon for a person to feel some ambivalence when weighing the losses against the rewards of changing the behavior. Some people may stay in the contemplative stage for months or years.

The *preparation stage* occurs when the person undertakes cognitive and behavioral activities that prepare the person for change. At this stage, the person believes that the advantages of changing the behavior outweigh the disadvantages and makes specific plans to accomplish the change. Some people in this stage change small aspects of the behavior, such as cutting out sugar in their coffee.

The *action stage* occurs when the person actively implements behavioral and cognitive strategies to interrupt previous behavior patterns and adopt new ones. To prevent recurrences to previous behavior, the action stage needs to continue for several weeks or months.

During the *maintenance stage*, the person integrates newly adopted behavior patterns into his or her life-style. This stage lasts until the person no longer experiences temptation to return to previous unhealthy behaviors.

These five stages are cyclical; people generally move through one stage before progressing to the next. However, at any point in time a person may regress to any previous stage. Sudden or gradual relapses to previous behavior patterns may occur during the action or maintenance stages, for example. Individuals who relapse may return to the stage of precontemplation, contemplation, or preparation before their next attempt to change. To identify whether the client is in the precontemplative or contemplative stages, ask whether the client is thinking about changing a behavior in the next 6 months or a year. Those in precontemplation will answer no; those in contemplation or preparation will answer yes. Table 8–2 relates nursing strategies appropriate for each stage of health behavior change.

CONSIDER . . .

- a client under your care who is considering a health behavior change. At what stage of Prochaska and DiClemente's model is the client? What barriers exist in the client's experience that might interfere with the client's goal? What activities or interventions might you suggest or do to help the client successfully make the health behavior change?
- your own experience in changing an unhealthy behavior (e.g., quitting smoking, losing

TABLE 8-2   Examples of Nursing Strategies for Each Stage of Health Behavior Change

Stage	Nursing Strategies
Precontemplation	• Raise the client's awareness of healthy behaviors, such as exercising, altering the diet, quitting smoking, using sunscreen, and undergoing regular mammography screening. • Provide personalized information about the benefits of specific health behaviors; for example, relate the client's cough to smoking or excessive fat intake to heart disease. • Explore the client's beliefs and feelings related to the health behavior. • Identify previous successful changes (e.g., previous weight loss) to increase the client's self-confidence, and offer positive feedback.
Contemplation	• Continue to provide the interventions cited in the previous stage. In addition, provide adequate and accurate information about available alternatives to encourage clients to make appropriate choices and actively participate in decision making. • Encourage the client to express ambivalent feelings. Include spouses, if appropriate (e.g., for dietary alterations). • Help the client further clarify values in relation to the health behavior, and encourage the client to consider how it would feel, for example, to be at an appropriate weight or to be an ex-smoker. • Help the client identify social pressures that encourage positive health behaviors, such as exercise facilities or bans on smoking at work.
Preparation	• Assist the client to make specific plans to implement the change; for example, discuss self-help groups and other available support persons or groups. • Help the client identify stimuli that trigger unhealthy behavior and consider ways to remove or minimize these stimuli (e.g., altering the environment or removing oneself from a troublesome area). • Teach the client to substitute activities to counteract the unhealthy behavior, such as relaxation exercises, internal dialogues, or thought stopping (suddenly saying "stop" loudly). • Plan appropriate rewards (e.g., a movie, dining out) for clients to give themselves for having achieved their goals.
Action	• Review plans and instructions discussed in the preparation phase. • Help the client set realistic goals. • Encourage positive self-talk that supports the behavior change. • Provide positive feedback, support, and encouragement for partial or complete achievement of goals.
Maintenance	• Encourage continuing use of support networks and open discussion of problems related to maintaining healthy behavior. • Identify and encourage strategies that support healthy behavior.

SOURCES: "Toward a More Integrative Model of Change" by J. Prochaska and C. DiClemente, 1982, *Psychotherapy: Theory, Research, and Practice, 19,* 276–288; "Stages of Change in the Modification of Problem Behaviors" by J. Prochaska and C. DiClemente, 1992, *Progress in Behavior Modification, 28,* 183–218; "A Stage-Based Approach to Helping People Change Health Behaviors" by V. S. Conn, 1994, *Clinical Nurse Specialist, 8*(4), 187–193.

weight, maintaining proper nutrition, reducing stress). How did you progress through the stages of the Prochaska and DiClemente model? What barriers to health behavior change did you experience? How did you overcome the barriers and effect a successful health behavior change?

- what barriers exist in your community that interfere with individual and family health behavior changes. What supports exist in your community to assist individuals and families in making health behavior changes? How might you promote and support health behavior changes in your community?

THE NURSE'S ROLE IN HEALTH PROMOTION

Individuals and communities who seek to increase their responsibility for personal health and self-care require health education. The trend toward health promotion has created the opportunity for nurses to strengthen the profession's influence on health promotion, disseminate information that promotes an educated public, and assist individuals and communities to change long-standing health behaviors. Health promotion activities involve collaborative relationships with both clients and physicians. The role of the nurse is to work *with* people, not *for* them—that is, to act as a facilitator of the process of assessing, evaluating, and understanding health. The nurse may act as advocate, consultant, teacher, or coordinator of services. For examples of the nurse's role in health promotion, see the accompanying box.

In these roles, the nurse may work with individuals of all age groups and diverse family units or concentrate on a specific population, such as new parents, school-age children, or older adults. In any case, the nursing process is a basic tool for the nurse in a health promotion role. Although the process is the same, the nurse emphasizes teaching the client (who can be either an individual or a family unit) self-care responsibility. Adult clients decide the goals, determine the health promotion plans, and take the responsibility for the success of the plans.

For detailed information about nursing interventions that promote the health of individuals and families, see Chapter 16.

The Nurse's Role in Health Promotion

- Model healthy life-style behaviors and attitudes.
- Facilitate client involvement in the assessment, implementation, and evaluation of health goals.
- Teach clients self-care strategies to enhance fitness, improve nutrition, manage stress, and enhance relationships.
- Assist individuals, families, and communities to increase their levels of health.
- Educate clients to be effective health care consumers.
- Assist clients, families, and communities to develop and choose health-promoting options.
- Guide clients' development in effective problem solving and decision making.
- Reinforce clients' personal and family health-promoting behaviors.
- Advocate in the community for changes that promote a healthy environment.

CONSIDER . . .

- types of health promotion activities you have previously been involved in.
- any difficulties you have previously encountered in initiating or maintaining clients' health-promoting behaviors.
- what personal responsibility means in relation to health and how that affects the nurse's role in health promotion.

READINGS FOR ENRICHMENT

Ahijevych, K., & Bernhard, L. (1994, March/April). Health-promoting behaviors of African American women. *Nursing Research, 43,* 86–89.

Information about the health behaviors of African-American women is limited. This study describes the health-promoting life-style behaviors of 187 African-American women and compares the findings with those of other published reports on the Health Promoting Lifestyle Profile (HPLP) instrument. The profile included the following behaviors: self-actualization, health responsibility, exercise, nutrition, interpersonal support, and stress management.

Alford, D. M. & Futrell, M. (1992, September/October). Wellness and health promotion of the elderly. AAN working paper. *Nursing Outlook, 40,* 221–226.

In 1991, the United Nations Social Development Commission proposed a set of principles for older persons that outlines both the rights and the responsibilities of older adults to promote and protect their health (Nusberg, 1991). One of the tasks of the American Academy of Nursing (AAN) is to formulate health policy. The Expert Panel on Older Adults, one of the working groups of the AAN, requested interested members to formulate a policy paper on wellness and health promotion of older adults for presentation at the AAN meeting in Los Angeles in October 1991. This draft paper has been published and invites all readers to review and comment on these policy recommendations. The paper discusses recommendations for changes in curriculum, self-care, social policy, research, accessibility of care, and health/wellness care delivery to older persons. Ten additional recommendations conclude this working paper.

Hales, D. (1992). *An invitation to health* (5th ed.). Redwood City, CA: Benjamin/Cummings.

This 600-page book includes comprehensive coverage of key concepts in health, wellness, and health promotion, such as stress management, nutrition, weight management, physical fitness, responsible sexuality, avoidance of harmful habits, personal health risks, personal safety, and environmental health. Strategies for change, self-surveys, discussions of controversial topics, and personal narratives are provided throughout the book.

Kolcaba, K., & Wykle, M. (1994, September/October). Health promotion in long-term care facilities. *Geriatric Nursing, 15;* 255–269.

These authors surveyed 140 long-term care facilities and measured two domains of health promotion in long-term care: (a) screening procedures (early detection of disease) and (b) typical health-promoting activities, such as vaccinations, exercise classes, group work, and health education for residents. The major purpose of the study was to determine the extent to which health screening and health promotion were being practiced in these facilities.

Salsberry, P. J. (1993, September/October). Assuming responsibility for one's health: An analysis of a key assumption in nursing's agenda for health care reform. *Nursing Outlook, 41,* 212–216.

Nursing's proposal for health care reform includes an expanded role for the consumer of health care and an emphasis on personal responsibility for health. This author states that these tenets mark a significant philosophic shift in the underpinnings of the health care system and that they require explanation and analysis. The delivery system has shifted from a societal-focused responsibility to an individual-focused responsibility. Three fundamental questions regarding this shift are addressed in this article: (1) Why include such tenets now? (2) What does personal responsibility in the context of health mean? (Three interpretations are provided.) (3) What are the consequences of including personal responsibility in a health care reform package?

SUMMARY

The goal of health promotion is to raise the level of health of an individual, family, or community. Health promotion activities are directed toward developing client resources that maintain or enhance well-being. Health protection activities are geared toward preventing specific diseases, such as obtaining immunizations to prevent poliomyelitis.

Health promotion strategies may be active or passive. With active strategies, the client participates in making life-style changes. With passive strategies, the client is the recipient of a health promotion effort, such as maintaining an appropriate water supply. A variety of programs can be used for health promotion, including (a) information dissemination, (b) health appraisal and wellness assessment, (c) life-style and behavior change, and (d) environmental control programs. These programs are found in many settings— in the home, schools, community centers, hospitals, and worksites.

Three health promotion models are described. Pender's health promotion model categorizes determinants of health promoting behaviors as cognitive-perceptual factors, modifying factors, and variables affecting the likelihood of action. Cognitive-perceptual factors, the primary motivational factors, include the person's perception of the importance of health, perceived control, perceived self-efficacy, definition of health, perceived health status, perceived benefits of health-promoting behaviors, and perceived barriers. These factors may be modified by demographic factors, biologic characteristics, interpersonal influences, situational factors, and behavioral factors. Cues to action may be of either internal origin or external origin.

Kulbok's resource model of preventive health behavior hypothesizes that the greater the person's social and health resources, the more frequently the person will perform preventive behaviors. Neuman's systems model includes dimensions of health promotion designed to strengthen a person's lines of defense and addresses primary, secondary, and tertiary levels of prevention.

Prochaska and DiClemente propose a five-stage model for health behavior change. The stages are (a) precontemplation, (b) contemplation, (c) preparation, (d) action, and (e) maintenance. If the person is not successful in changing behavior, relapse may occur during the action or maintenance stages. However, at any point in these stages, people may move to any previous stage. An understanding of these stages enables the nurse to provide appropriate nursing interventions.

The nurse's role in health promotion is to act as a facilitator of the process of assessing, evaluating, and understanding health.

SELECTED REFERENCES

Barnes, D., Eribes, C., Juarbe, T., Nelson, M., Proctor, S., Sawyer, L., Shaul, M. & Meleis, A. I. (1995, January/February). Primary health care and primary care: A confusion of philosophies. *Nursing Outlook, 43*, 7–16.

Brown, K. C., Mattson, A. H., Newman, K. D., & Sirles, A. T. (1992, Winter). A community health nursing curriculum and Healthy People 2000. *Clinical Nurse Specialist, 6* (4), 203–208.

Conn, V. S. (1994, July). A stage-based approach to helping people change health behaviors. *Clinical Nurse Specialist, 8*, 187–193.

Edelman, C., & Mandle, C. L. (Eds.). (1990). *Health promotion through the life span.* St. Louis: Mosby.

Epp, J. (1986, November). *Achieving health for all: A framework for health promotion. Report of the Minister of National Health and Welfare.* Ottawa, Canada: Government Printing Office.

Gilbert, B. (1994, October). Employee assistance programs. *AAOHN Journal, 42*, 488–493.

Gillis, A. J. (1994, December). A change for the better. *Canadian Nurse, 90*, 27–30.

Green, L. Kreuter, M., Deeds, S., & Partridge, R. (1980). *Health education planning: A diagnostic approach.* Palo Alto, CA: Mayfield.

Hartweg, D. L. (1993, July/August). Self-care actions of healthy middle-aged women to promote well-being. *Nursing Research, 42*, 221–227.

Hawranik, P., & Walker, J. (1995, August). Targeting seniors. *Canadian Nurse, 91*, 35–39.

Kar, S. B., Smitz, M., & Dyer, D. A. (1983, March/April). A psychosocial model of health behaviors: Implications for nutrition education, research and policy. *Health Values, 7*, 29–37.

Kelly, M. P. (1992, November). Health promotion in primary care: Taking account of the patient's point of view. *Journal of Advanced Nursing, 17*, 1291–1296.

Kulbok, P. P. (1985, June). Social resources, health resources, and preventive behaviors: Patterns and predictions. *Public Health Nursing, 2*, 67–81.

Lalonde, M. (1974). *A new perspective on the health of Canadians.* Ottawa: Government of Canada.

Lauver, D. (1992, Winter). A theory of care-seeking behavior. *Image: Journal of Nursing Scholarship, 24*, 281–287.

Leavell, H. R., & Clark, E. G. (1965). *Preventive medicine for the doctor in the community* (3rd ed.). New York: McGraw-Hill.

Maglacas, A. M. (1988, March/April). Health for all: Nursing's role. *Nursing Outlook, 36*, 266–271.

Minkler, M. (1994, July/August). Association for work-site health promotion: Practitioner's forum. *American Journal of Health Promotion, 8*, 403–413.

Neuman, B. (1995). *The Neuman Systems Model* (3rd ed.). Norwalk, CT: Appleton & Lange.

Nusberg, C. (1991). UN takes action on principles for older persons. *Aging International, 18*(1), 3–6.

Pender, N. J. (1987). *Health promotion in nursing practice* (2nd ed.). Norwalk, CT: Appleton & Lange.

Prochaska, J., & DiClemente, C. (1982). Toward a more integrative model of change. *Psychotherapy: Theory, Research, and Practice, 19*, 276–288.

Prochaska, J., & DiClemente, C. (1992). Stages of change in the modification of problem behaviors. *Progress in Behavior Modification, 28*, 183–218.

Salsbury, P. J. (1993, September/October). Assuming responsibility for one's health: An analysis of a key assumption in nursing's agenda for health care reform. *Nursing Outlook, 41*, 212–216.

Schultz, A. (1995, August). What is health promotion? *Canadian Nurse, 91*, 31–34.

Smillie, C. (1992, July/August). Preparing health professionals for a collaborative health promotion role. *Canadian Journal of Public Health, 93*, 279–282.

Stachtchenko, S., & Jenicek, M. (1990, January-February). Conceptual differences between prevention and health promotion: Research implications for community health programs. *Canadian Journal of Public Health, 81*, 53–59.

Thorne, S. (1993, December). Health belief systems in perspective. *Journal of Advanced Nursing, 18*, 1931–1941.

Underwood, E. J., VanBerkel, C., Scott, F., Siracusa, L., & Gibson, B. (1993, December). The environmental connection. *Canadian Nurse, 89*, 33–35.

United States Department of Health and Human Services. (1990, September). *Healthy people 2000: National health promotion and disease prevention objectives.* DHHS Pub. No. (PHS) 91-50212. Washington, D.C.: U. S. Government Printing Office.

U. S. Surgeon General. (1979). *Healthy people: The Surgeon General's report on health promotion and disease prevention.* DHHS Pub. No. 79-55071. Washington, D.C.: Government Printing Office.

U. S. Surgeon General. (1980). *Health promotion/disease prevention: Objectives for the nation.* Washington, D.C.: Department of Health and Human Services.

World Health Organization. (1984). *Report of the working group on the concept and principles of health promotion.* Copenhagen: Author.

World Health Organization. (1986). *Framework for health promotion training.* Copenhagen: Author.

9

Learner and Teacher

OBJECTIVES

- Discuss the three main constructs of learning theory.

- Explain the three domains of learning.

- Identify guidelines for effective teaching and learning.

- Explain essential aspects of a teaching plan and of apply-

ing the nursing process for learning.

"Teaching is more difficult than learning because what teaching calls for is this: to let learn. The real teacher, in fact, lets nothing else be learned than—learning….The teacher is ahead of his apprentices in this alone, that he has still far more to learn than they—he has to let them learn."

—Martin Heidegger, 1968

Nurses have both learning and teaching responsibilities. They must continue to learn so that they can maintain their knowledge and skills amid the many changes in health care. They teach clients and their families, other health care professionals, and nursing assistants to whom they delegate care, and they share their expertise with other nurses and health professionals.

- There are many theories about learning. These are generally based on assumptions about people, the nature of knowledge, and how people learn. The *eclectic* approach presumes that no one theory is more correct than another.
- Learning is thought to be a complex process.
- There are also beliefs about how teaching can be most effective. These are commonly referred to as principles of teaching.
- Both learning and teaching are active processes.

LEARNING

People, including clients, have a variety of learning needs. A learning need is a need to change behavior or "a gap between the information an individual knows and the information necessary to perform a function or care for self" (Gessner, 1989, p. 593). **Learning** is a change in human disposition or capability that persists over a period of time and that cannot be solely accounted for by growth. Learning is represented by a change in behavior. See the accompanying box for attributes of learning.

An important aspect of learning is the individual's desire to learn and to act on the learning, referred to as **compliance.** In the health care context compliance is the extent to which a person's behavior coincides with medical or health advice. Compliance is best illustrated when the person recognizes and accepts the need to learn, willingly expends the energy required to learn, and then follows through with the appropriate behaviors that reflect the learning. For example, a person diagnosed as having diabetes willingly learns about the special diet needed, and then plans and follows the learned diet.

Attributes of Learning

Learning is:

- An experience that occurs inside the learner.
- The discovery of the personal meaning and relevance of ideas.
- A consequence of experience.
- A collaborative and cooperative process.
- An evolutionary process.
- A process that is both intellectual and emotional.

Andragogy is "the art and science of helping adults learn" (Knowles, 1980, p. 43) in contrast to **pedagogy,** the discipline concerned with helping children learn. Nurses can use the following andragogic concepts about learners as a guide for client teaching (Knowles, 1984):

- As people mature, they move from dependence to independence.
- An adult's previous experiences can be used as a resource for learning.
- An adult's readiness to learn is often related to a developmental task or social role.
- An adult is more oriented to learning when the material is immediately useful, not useful sometime in the future.

Theories of Learning

Theories about how and why people learn can be traced back to the 17th century. Three main theoretical constructs are behaviorism, cognitivism, and humanism.

Behaviorism

Behaviorism was originally advanced by Edward Thorndike, who believed that transfer of knowledge could occur if the new situation closely resembled the old situation. To Thorndike, the term *understanding* was used in the context of building connections. One of his major contributions applicable to teaching is that learning should be based on the learner's behavior. In addition to Thorndike, major behaviorist theorists include I. Pavlov, B. F. Skinner, and A. Bandura.

Behaviorists believe that the environment influences behavior and how a person controls it; moreover, they maintain that it is the essential factor determining human action. In the behaviorist school of thought, an act is called a *response* when it can be traced to the effects of a stimulus.

Skinner's Operant Conditioning Theory Skinner postulates two types of **conditioning** (behavioral responses to a stimulus) that cause the response or behavior. The first type of conditioning, termed *classical conditioning*, is illustrated by Pavlov's well-known experiments with dogs. Pavlov (1849–1936) conditioned dogs to salivate in response to the sound of a tuning fork, a sound they heard when they received food. Classical conditioning is a procedure in which conditioned responses are established by the association of a new stimulus that is known to cause an unconditioned response. The resulting response is the conditioned response to the *new* (unrelated) stimulus.

The second type of conditioning is what Skinner refers to as *operant conditioning*, a process by which the frequency of a response can be increased or decreased depending on when, how, and to what extent it is reinforced. Skinner believes that humans, like animals, will always repeat actions that bring pleasure. He considers the consequences of an action, what he terms **reinforcement,** to be all-important. Positive consequences foster repetition of the action; the absence of consequences causes the action to cease.

Extinction is the process in which a conditioned behavior is "unlearned" because the reinforcement has been removed. Greater effort, however, is required to extinguish a behavior than to condition it. The procedure involves removing the *unconditional stimulus* or the reward from the training situation. When the conditioning procedure is again instigated following complete extinction, it does not take the subject as long to show the conditioned response as it did in the original conditioning.

Studies of conditioning produced a number of laws of learning that were thought to be universal; that is, they were thought to apply to all ages, all cultures, and all types of behavior—motor, cognitive, emotional, and social. Examples follow:

- The more quickly reinforcement follows a response, the more effective the reinforcement.
- A response made in the presence of one stimulus generalizes to similar stimuli.
- Behavior that is reinforced only part of the time takes longer to extinguish than behavior that is reinforced continuously.

Bandura's Modeling Theory Social learning theorists such as Bandura agree with Skinner that the environment exerts a great deal of control over overt behavior; however, they believe that the entire learning process involves three highly interdependent factors:

1. Characteristics of the person
2. The person's behavior
3. The environment

These factors influence and control each other through a process that Bandura calls *reciprocal determinism.* The major contribution of Bandura's reciprocal determinism is the concept that the child's behavior affects or "creates" that child's environment. This differs from Skinner's belief that the environment, viewed as a set of stimuli, controls behavior.

Bandura claims that most learning comes from observational learning and instruction rather than from overt trial-by-error behavior. **Observational learning** is the acquisition of new skills or the alteration of old behaviors simply by watching other children and adults. It is especially important for acquiring behavior in situations where mistakes are life-threatening or costly, e.g., driving a car or performing brain surgery.

Bandura's research focuses on **imitation,** the process by which individuals copy or reproduce what they have observed, and **modeling,** the process by which a person learns by observing the behavior of others. Imitation is regarded as one of the most powerful socialization forces. Various imitative behaviors are reinforced by a process of operant conditioning. For example, a boy may be praised for being "just like his father." The child may even self-reinforce the imitations by repeating an adult's words of praise. According to Bandura, models influence others mainly by providing information rather than by eliciting matching behavior, so that learning can occur without even once performing the model's behavior.

In recent years, Bandura's theory has become more cognitive, and he now calls his theory a "social cognitive theory." Learning is defined as "knowledge acquisition through cognitive processing information" (1986, p. xii). For example, television's effects on children depend on both cognitive and imitative processes. Whether the child can comprehend the story affects the child's perceptions of the model and the tendency to imitate the model.

Cognitivism

Cognitivism depicts learning as a complex cognitive activity. Major cognitive theorists include J. Piaget, K. Lewin, R. Gagne, and B. Bloom. Cognitivists view learning as the development of understandings and appreciations that help the individual function in a larger context. Learning is based on a change of perception, which itself is influenced by the senses and both internal and external variables. In other words, learning is largely a mental or intellectual or thinking process. (See cognitive learning processes on page 164.) The learner structures and processes information. Perceptions are selectively chosen by the individual and personal characteristics have an impact on how a cue is perceived. Cognitivists also emphasize the importance of social, emotional, and physical contexts in which learning occurs such as the teacher-learner relationship and environment. Developmental readiness and individual readiness (expressed as motivation) are other key factors associated with cognitive approaches.

Piaget's Phases of Cognitive Development According to Piaget, cognitive development is an orderly, sequential process in which a variety of new experiences (stimuli) must exist before intellectual abilities can develop. Piaget's cognitive developmental process is divided into five major phases: sensorimotor, preconceptual, intuitive, concrete operations, and formal operations. A person develops through each of these phases, and each phase has unique characteristics.

The *sensorimotor* phase lasts from birth to 2 years of age. It includes reflexive actions, perceptions of events centered on the body, objects as an extension of self, mental acknowledgement of the external environment, and discovery of new goals and ways to attain these goals. The *preconceptual* phase occurs from 2 to 4 years of age and includes an egocentric approach to accommodate the demands of the environment. Everything is significant and relates to "me." In the *intuitive phase*, extending from 4 to 7 years old, the child is able to think of one idea at a time, can use words to express thoughts, and includes others in the environment. The *concrete operations* phase (7 to 11 years old) involves a beginning understanding of relationships such as size, right and left, different viewpoints, and the ability to solve concrete problems. In the *formal operations* phase, occurring at 11 to 15 years of age, the person is able to use rational thinking and reasoning that is deductive and futuristic.

In each phase, the person uses three primary abilities: assimilation, accommodation, and adaptation. *Assimilation* is the process through which humans encounter and react to new situations by using the mechanisms they already possess. In this way, people acquire new knowledge and skills as well as insights into the world around them. *Accommodation* is the process of change whereby cognitive processes mature sufficiently to allow the person to solve problems that were unsolvable before. This adjustment is possible chiefly because new knowledge has been assimilated. *Adaptation*, or coping behavior, is the ability to handle the demands made by the environment.

Nurses can employ Piaget's theory of cognitive development when developing teaching strategies. For example, a nurse can expect a toddler to be egocentric and literal; therefore, explanations to the toddler should focus on the needs of the toddler rather than on the needs of others. Further, a 13-year-old can be expected to use rational thinking and to reason; therefore, when explaining the need for a medication, a nurse can outline the consequences of taking and not taking the medication, enabling the adolescent to make a rational decision.

Lewin's Field Theory Lewin's field theory involves theories of motivation and perception, which were considered precursors of the more recent cognitive theories. Lewin believed that learning involved four different types of changes: change in cognitive structure, change in motivation, change in one's sense of belonging to the group, and gain in voluntary muscle control. His well known theory of change has three basic stages: unfreezing, moving, and refreezing. These stages are discussed in detail in Chapter 13.

Gagne's Information Processing Theory Gagne postulates eight levels of intellectual skills: (1) signal; (2) stimulus-response; (3) chaining, which involves at least two stimulus-response connections; (4) verbal association, which involves assembling verbal chains from previous learning; (5) multiple discrimination involving differentiated responses to variable stimuli; (6) concept formation, which involves identifying and responding to a class of objects that serve as stimuli; (7) principle formation, which involves applying a principle that is made up of at least one chain of two or more concepts; (8) problem solving, which involves processing at least two or more principles to produce a higher level principle.

Bloom's Domains of Learning Bloom (1956) has identified three domains, or areas of learning: cognitive, affective, and psychomotor. The *cognitive domain* includes six intellectual skills such as knowing, comprehending, and applying in order from simple to complex. The *affective domain* includes feelings, emotions, interests, attitudes, and appreciations. It involves five major categories. The *psychomotor domain* includes motor skills such as giving an injection. It includes seven categories from perception (lowest level) to origination (highest level). See Table 9–1. Nurses should include each of these three domains in client teaching plans. For example, teaching a client how to irrigate a colostomy is the psychomotor domain. An important part of such a teaching plan is to teach the client why a specific amount of fluid is used and when the irrigation should be carried out; this is the cognitive domain. Helping the client accept the colostomy and maintain self-esteem is in the affective domain.

Each of these domains has a developed hierarchical classification system; that is, the behaviors in each category are arranged from the simplest to the most complex.

Humanism

Humanistic learning theory focuses on both cognitive and affective (feelings and attitudes) areas of the learner. It focuses on the whole person and therefore is pertinent to a holistic philosophy of care. Prominent members of this school of thought include Abraham Maslow and Carl Rogers. According to humanistic theory, learning is believed to be self-motivated, self-initiated, and self-evaluated. Each individual is viewed as a unique composite of biologic, psychologic, social, cultural, and spiritual factors. Learning focuses on self-development and achieving full potential; it is best when it is relevant to the learner. Autonomy and self-determination are important; the learner identifies the learning needs and takes the initiative to meet these needs. The learner is thus an active participant and takes responsibility for meeting individual learning needs.

Maslow's hierarchy of needs suggests a way of prioritizing nursing interventions so that physiologic needs are met first, followed by safety and security needs, love and belonging needs, esteem and self-esteem needs, and ultimately, growth needs. Carl Rogers was particularly concerned with personalized approaches. He emphasized that independence, creativity, and self-reliance are all facilitated when self-criticism and self-evaluation are of primary importance; evaluation by others is of secondary importance.

Using Learning Theories

The major attributes of *behaviorist* theories include the careful identification of what is to be taught and the immediate identification of and reward for correct responses. However, the theory is not easily applied to complex learning situations and is limiting in terms of the learner's role in the teaching process. Nurses applying behavioristic theory will:

- Provide sufficient practice time and both immediate and repeat testing and redemonstration.
- Provide opportunities for learners to solve problems by trial and error.
- Select teaching strategies that avoid distracting information and evoke the desired response.
- Praise the learner for correct behavior and provide positive feedback at intervals throughout the learning experience.
- Provide role models of desired behavior.

The major attributes of *cognitive* theory are its recognition of developmental levels of learners, and acknowledgements of the learner's motivation and environment. However, some or many of the motivational and environmental factors may be beyond the teacher's control. Nurses applying cognitive theory will:

- Provide a social, emotional, and physical environment conducive to learning.
- Encourage a positive teacher-learner relationship.
- Select multisensory teaching strategies since perception is influenced by the senses.
- Recognize that personal characteristics have an impact on how cues are perceived and develop appropriate teaching approaches to target different learning styles.
- Assess a person's developmental and individual readiness to learn and adapt teaching strategies to the learner's developmental level.
- Select behavioral objectives and strategies that encompass the cognitive, affective, and psychomotor domains of learning.

The major attributes of *humanism* are its focus on the feeling and attitudes of learners, the importance of the individual in identifying learning needs, in taking responsibility for them, and on the

TABLE 9-1   Major Categories in Each Learning Domain

Category/Description	Client Learning Example
Cognitive Domain	
Knowledge Remembers previously learned material	A client learns the side effects of a medication and describes them two days later.
Comprehension Understands the meaning of learned material	A client describes how the side effects of a medication can be recognized and what to do about them.
Application Applies newly learned material in new concrete situations	A client learns to take the medication after meals to minimize side effects.
Analysis Breaks learned material into component parts and separates important from unimportant material	A client describes which side effects are serious and when the physician is to be notified.
Synthesis Takes parts of learned material and puts them together to form new material	A client learns to take steps to prevent side effects of a medication.
Evaluation Judges the value of the learned material	A client describes how the knowledge of new material can help prevent accidents at work.
Affective Domain	
Receiving Willingness to attend to particular stimuli	A female client is willing to listen to a nurse's description of the preparation for breast surgery.
Responding Actively participates by listening and responding	The female client asks questions about the preparation for the scheduled surgery.
Valuing Attaches a value or worth to a particular object, phenomenon, or behavior	The female client refuses to look at the incision following her breast removal.
Organization Develops a value system by bringing together different values and resolving conflicts	The client accepts changes brought about by the breast surgery.
Characterization Acts according to a value system	After surgery, the client returns to a life-style consistent with her value system.
Psychomotor Domain	
Perception Uses the senses to obtain cues to guide motor activity	A male client immediately calls a nurse when he sees another client fall from his bed.
Set Refers to readiness to take immediate action: includes mental, physical, and emotional sets	The client becomes ready to act when he sees the client who fell from his bed preparing to get out of his chair.
Guided Response Performs an act under the guidance of a nurse	A client moves himself from his bed to a wheelchair with a nurse's guidance.
Mechanism Performs a learned activity with confidence and proficiency	The client moves himself between his bed and a wheelchair quickly and competently.
Complex Overt Response Performs a motor skill competently, accurately, and smoothly	The client moves between the bed and the wheelchair at the same time adjusting his intravenous line and his catheter.
Adaptation Performs skills and adapts them to special circumstances	The client stops transferring to the wheelchair and adjusts his intravenous line when it stops dripping.
Origination Creates new movement patterns to suit a particular problem	The client transfers from his bed to the wheelchair in a different way to avoid pull on the intravenous line.

Sources: Adapted from *Stating Objectives for Classroom Instruction* (3rd ed.) by N. E. Gronlund, 1985, New York: Macmillan, pp. 34–40; and *Taxonomy of Educational Objectives. Vol. 1: Cognitive Domain,* ed. B. S. Bloom, 1956, New York: David McKay, pp. 18–24.

self-motivation of the learners to work toward self-reliance and independence. Nurses applying humanistic theory will:

- Encourage the learners to establish goals and promote self-directed learning.
- Encourage active learning by serving as a facilitator, mentor, or resource for the learner.
- Expose the learner to new relevant information and ask appropriate questions to encourage the learner to seek answers.

Cognitive Learning Processes

Learning involves three cognitive (mental) processes: acquiring information, processing the information, and using the information. These three processes can occur sequentially or simultaneously.

Acquiring Information

Acquiring information involves two processes: sensory reception and discrimination. Sensory reception is made possible by the neurosensory system. Stimuli in the environment signal the appropriate sense, such as sight, hearing, or smell. Impulses then travel by the nervous system to the brain. Sensory reception generally is continuous, but it is not always a conscious process.

The second aspect of acquiring information is discrimination. Discrimination is the ability to determine which stimuli are relevant in a particular situation. Stimuli can be objects, ideas, actions, or facts. They may be internal (i.e., inside the body) or external. Discrimination is the most difficult where there are multiple, complex stimuli.

Processing Information

Processing provides meaning to the information. Information is processed in three steps: association, generalization, and the formation of concepts. *Association* is the joining of two or many ideas. For example, a person may associate an object such as a needle with the word *needle* and/or with the experience of pain. *Generalization* is the perceiving of similarities among various stimuli, for example, the similarities between three different computers. *Concept formation* is the organization of stimuli that have some attributes in common. For example, a nurse who understands the concept of caring appreciates the characteristics associated with caring. The nurse can then help others to convey caring in the health care setting.

Using Information

Using information is the application of information in the cognitive, affective, and psychomotor areas. See "Bloom's Domains of Learning," earlier in this chapter. The ability to formulate and relate concepts is an essential critical thinking skill (see Chapter 12). In addition, relating concepts is essential for creative thinking and problem solving.

Factors Facilitating Learning

Motivation

Motivation to learn is the desire to learn. It greatly influences how quickly and how much a person learns. Motivation is generally greatest when a person recognizes a need and believes the need will be met through learning. It is not enough for the need to be identified and verbalized by the nurse; it must be experienced by the client. Often the nurse's task is to help the client personally work through the problem and identify the need. Sometimes clients or support persons need help identifying relevant situational elements before they can see a need. For instance, clients with heart disease may need to know the effects of smoking before they recognize the need to stop smoking. Or adolescents may need to know the consequences of an untreated sexually transmitted disease before they see the need for treatment.

Readiness

Readiness to learn is the behavior that reflects motivation at a specific time. Readiness reflects a client's willingness and ability to learn. The nurse's role is often to encourage the development of readiness.

Active Involvement

Active involvement in the process makes learning more meaningful. If the learner actively participates in planning and discussion, learning is faster and retention is better. Passive learning, such as listening to a lecture or watching a film, does not foster optimal learning.

Once learners have succeeded in accomplishing a task or understanding a concept, they gain self-confidence in their ability to learn. This reduces their anxiety about failure and can motivate greater learning. Successful learners have increased confidence with which to accept failure. People learn best when they believe they are accepted and will not be judged. The person who expects to be judged as a "poor" or "good" client will not learn as well as the person who feels no such threat.

Feedback

Feedback is information relating a person's performance to a desired goal. It has to be meaningful to the learner. Feedback that accompanies practice of psychomotor skills helps the person to learn those skills. Support of desired behavior through praise, positively worded corrections, and suggestions of alternative methods are ways of providing positive feedback. Negative feedback such as ridicule, anger, or sarcasm can lead people to withdraw from learning. Such feedback, viewed as a type of punishment, may cause the client to avoid the teacher in order to avoid punishment.

Simple to Complex

Learning is facilitated by material that is logically organized and proceeds from the *simple to the complex.* Such organization enables the learner to comprehend new information, assimilate it with previous learning, and form new understandings. Of course, simple and complex are relative terms, depending on the level at which the person is learning. What is simple for one person may be complex for another.

Repetition

Repetition of key concepts and facts facilitates retention of newly learned material. Practice of psychomotor skills, particularly with feedback from the nurse, improves performance of those skills and facilitates their transfer to another setting. Also when a person appreciates the relevance of specific material, learning is facilitated.

Timing

People retain information and psychomotor skills best when the *time between learning and use is short;* the longer the time interval, the more is forgotten. For example, a woman who is taught to administer her own insulin but is not permitted to do so until discharge from hospital is unlikely to remember much of what she learned. However, if she is allowed to give her own injections while in hospital, her learning will be enhanced.

Environment

An *optimal learning environment* facilitates learning by reducing distraction and providing physical and psychologic comfort. It has adequate lighting that is free from glare, a comfortable room temperature, and good ventilation. Most students know what it is like to try to learn in a hot, stuffy room; the subsequent drowsiness interferes with concentration. Noise can also distract the student and interfere with listening and thinking. To facilitate learning in a hospital setting, nurses should choose a time when there are no visitors present and interruptions are unlikely. Privacy is essential for some learning. For example, when a client is learning to irrigate a colostomy, the presence of others can be embarrassing and thus interfere with learning. When a client is particularly anxious, having support persons present often gives the client confidence.

Factors Inhibiting Learning

Many factors inhibit learning. Some of the most common are described below and in Table 9–2.

Emotions

A greatly *elevated anxiety* level can impede learning. Clients or families who are very worried may not hear spoken words or may retain only part of the communication. Extreme anxiety might be reduced by medications or by information that relieves uncertainty. By contrast, clients who appear disinterested and unconcerned may need to be cautioned about potential problems to enhance their motivation to learn.

Physiologic Events

Learning can be inhibited by *physiologic events* such as a critical illness, pain, or impaired hearing. Because the client cannot concentrate and apply energy to learning, the learning itself is impaired. The nurse should try to reduce the physiologic barriers to learning as much as possible before teaching. Providing analgesics and rest before teaching is often helpful.

Cultural Barriers

There are also *cultural barriers* to learning, such as language or values. Obviously the client who does not understand the nurse's language will learn little. Western medicine may conflict with cultural healing beliefs and practices. Nurses must deal directly with this conflict to be effective, otherwise the client may be partially or totally noncompliant with recommended treatments. Another impediment to

TABLE 9–2 Barriers to Learning

Barrier	Explanation	Nursing Implications
Acute illness	Client requires all resources and energy to cope with illness.	Defer teaching until client is less ill.
Pain	Pain decreases ability to concentrate.	Deal with pain before teaching.
Age	Vision, hearing, and motor control can be impaired in the elderly.	Consider sensory and motor defects in teaching plan.
Prognosis	Client can be preoccupied with illness and unable to concentrate on new information.	Defer teaching to a better time.
Biorhythms	Mental and physical performances have a circadian rhythm.	Adapt time of teaching to suit client.
Emotion (e.g., anxiety, denial, depression, grief)	Emotions require energy and distract from learning.	Deal with emotions first and possible misinformation.
Language and ethnic background	Client may not be fluent in the nurse's language.	Obtain services of an interpreter or nurse with appropriate language skills.
Iatrogenic barriers	The nurse may set up barriers by appearing condescending or hurried, ignoring client cues, or appearing incompetent or unsure.	Establish a helping relationship and be sensitive to the client's needs. Plan and prepare for teaching ahead of time with current information appropriate for the learner.

learning is *differing values* held by the client and the health team. For example, a client who comes from a culture that does not value slimness may have difficulty learning about a reducing diet.

NURSES AS LEARNERS

There are several ways in which the nurse may learn, including continued formal academic education, institution-based human resource development (HRD) programs, encouraged or legislatively mandated continuing education, or episodic individual selected educational pursuits.

Continued formal academic education includes postbaccalaureate study at the master's or doctoral degree levels. Education at the graduate level requires critical thinking and knowledge of the research process. Graduate study may be in nursing or in other disciplines that potentiate the nurses' practice. For example, nurses in administration may choose to pursue master's degrees in nursing administration, health care administration, or business administration. There are many factors the nurse

must consider in choosing a graduate program. Chapter 23 provides guidelines for preparing for graduate study and selecting and applying to a graduate program.

Institution-based human resource development programs are administered by the employer. Swansburg (1995, p. 2) defines human resource development as "the process by which corporate management stimulates the motivation of employees to perform productively. HRD provides the stimuli that motivate nursing personnel to provide nursing care services to clients at quality and quantity standards that keep the health care entity reputable and financially solvent, the nurses satisfied with their professional accomplishments and quality of work life, and the clients treated successfully." Human resource development programs are designed to upgrade the knowledge of skills of employees. For example, an employer might offer programs to orient new staff members, to inform nurses about a new institutional policy, to familiarize nurses with a new piece of equipment or a new technique, to prepare nurses for certification at specialty or advanced levels of practice, or to implement a nurse theorist's conceptual framework as the guideline for nursing practice within the institution. Some human resource development programs also offer nurses tuition benefits to enroll in work-related courses or to attend professional conferences. It is important for the nurse to remember that the primary intended benefit of human resource development programs is for the institution; however, nurses who take advantage of institution-based programs can also benefit their own professional practice.

The term *continuing education* refers to formalized experiences designed to enlarge the knowledge or skills of nurses. Continuing education programs tend to be more specific and shorter than formal advanced academic degree study. Continuing education is the responsibility of each practicing nurse. Constant updating and growth are essential for the nurse to keep abreast of scientific and technologic change and changes within the nursing profession. Continuing education can be part of an employer's human resource development program or may be offered by professional organizations or continuing education departments of colleges or universities. Continuing education may also be obtained through self-study programs offered through professional journals or through home study programs provided by private, public, and professional educational organizations.

Some states require nurses to obtain a certain number of continuing education (CE) credits to renew their professional licenses. In these states, required CE contact hours vary from 15 to 30 hours for every 2-year licensure period. Depending on the state, all, some, or none of these hours may be acquired though home study. Some states require specific content instruction as part of the legislated continuing education requirement, for example, current study in violence or AIDS. Nurses who hold licensure in several states must meet the continuing education requirements for each state.

Some professional organizations require continuing education to meet certification and recertification requirements for specialty practice. For example, to be certified as a pediatric nurse by the American Nurses Association, the nurse must have completed 30 contact hours of continuing education applicable to pediatric nursing within the previous 3 years (American Nurses Credentialing Center [ANCC], 1995, p. 7). This continuing education requirement is in addition to other requirements.

Episodic learning activities are determined by the individual nurse. Episodic learning activities are those activities that are distinct and separate from formal or planned education. Subscribing to and reading professional journals and newsletters or commercial newspapers are examples of nurses' episodic educational activities. The learning the nurse gains through these activities can be just as important as formal educational pursuits. Through reading about the contemporary understanding of health care in professional or commercial literature, the nurse gains an awareness of how nurses can influence the health care system. Nurses can also gain knowledge of personal benefit, such as liability and malpractice issues, advanced practice and licensure issues, and portable pension plans.

RESEARCH NOTE

How Do Nurses Learn Caring in Clinical Practice?

One nurse researcher conducted a study to discover, describe, and analyze how nursing students learn caring in the clinical area. Eighteen female baccalaureate students were interviewed, 17 of whom were European American and one African American. Each student described how she created caring with patients. The researcher created two constitutive patterns: creative caring and learning caring. Creative caring incorporated seven themes: connecting, sharing, taking a holistic view, touching, advocating, being competent, and feeling good. Learning methods of caring incorporated five themes: modeling, reversing, imagining, sensing, and construct-

ing. Students also expressed awareness of "noncaring" behaviors of staff members. The author pointed out that "caring breakdown" was a powerful way for the participants to learn about caring.

Implications: There appears to be a need to further explore ways for nurses to learn caring. It also points out the need for nursing curricula to emphasize theories, concepts, and principles of caring and how they are applied in clinical areas.

SOURCE: Koslowski, M. M. R. (1995, May). Clinical learning experiences and professional nurse caring: A critical phenomenological study of female baccalaureate nursing students. *Journal of Nursing Education, 34,* 235–242.

CONSIDER...

- the various learning activities you have participated in during the last year. How many were episodic activities? How many were part of the human resource development program of your employer? How many were done to meet continuing education requirements for relicensure or recertification? How many were done for personal satisfaction?
- your personal goals related to professional learning activities. Are your learning activities directed toward becoming certified? To achieving an academic degree? For personal satisfaction?
- how many professional journals do you subscribe to and read in a month? In a year? How often do you read the newspaper, news magazines, or other commercial media in order to learn about health care issues in society?

TEACHING

Teaching is a system of activities intended to produce learning. The teaching process is intentionally designed to produce specific learning.

The teaching/learning process involves dynamic interaction between teacher and learner. Each participant in the process communicates information, emotions, perceptions, and attitudes to the other.

The relationship between the teacher and the learner is essentially one of trust and respect. The learner trusts that the teacher has the knowledge and skill to teach, and the teacher respects the learner's ability to attain the recognized goals. Once a nurse starts to instruct a client and/or a co-worker, it is important that the teaching process continue until the participants reach the learning goals, change the goals, or decide that the goals cannot be met.

Nurses have a responsibility to keep their clinical knowledge current. The American Nurses Association (ANA) lists four standards of clinical nursing practice that relate directly to learning and teaching. See the accompanying box.

Teaching Guidelines

The following guidelines for effective learning/teaching may be helpful to nurses:

- Teaching activities should help a learner meet individual learning objectives. These objectives

---

American Nurses Association Standards of Clinical Nursing Practice Related to Teaching and Learning

- *Standard II. Performance Appraisal:* The nurse evaluates his/her own nursing practice in relation to professional practice standards and relevant statutes and regulations. This standard infers that the nurse should regularly engage in professional appraisal, evaluating strengths and areas for development. Also the nurse participates in peer reviews, seeks feedback from others, and takes action to achieve identified goals. Through such actions, the nurse can identify learning needs and devise a plan to meet them.

- *Standard III. Education:* The nurse acquires and maintains current knowledge in nursing practice. This standard requires the nurse to participate in educational activities related to clinical knowledge and professional issues. Also, the nurse seeks experience to maintain clinical skills and seeks knowledge and skills appropriate to the practice setting.

- *Standard IV. Collegiality:* The nurse contributes to the professional development of peers, colleagues, and others. This standard suggests that nurses share information with others and give constructive feedback to others regarding their performance. The nurse also contributes to an environment that is conducive to learning of nursing students.

- *Standard VII. Research:* The nurse uses research findings in practice. This standard suggests that the nurse participate in research according to individual educational level and practice environment and use research findings in practice.

SOURCE: Adapted from American Nurses Association *Standards of Clinical Nursing Practice*, 1991, Kansas City, MO.

---

should be determined by the client (learner) and the nurse (teacher). If certain activities do not assist the learner, these need to be reassessed; perhaps other activities can replace them. For example, explanation alone may not be able to teach a client to handle a syringe. Actually handling the syringe may be more effective.

- Rapport between teacher and learner is essential. A relationship that is both accepting and constructive will best assist learning. The nurse should take time to establish rapport before teaching.

- The teacher who uses the client's previous learning in the present situation encourages the client and facilitates learning new skills. For example, a

Characteristics of Effective Teaching

- Holds the learner's interest.
- Fosters a positive self-concept in the learner; learner believes learning is possible and probable.
- Supports the learner with positive reinforcement.
- Makes partners of the learner and the teacher.
- Is accurate and current.
- Is appropriate for the learner's age, condition, and abilities.
- Is optimistic, positive, and nonthreatening.
- Is directed at helping the learner meet learning objectives.
- Uses several methods of teaching to accommodate a variety of learning styles; provides learning opportunities through hearing, seeing, and doing.
- Is cost-effective (cost of nurse's time spent teaching is less than the cost of treating health problems occurring when clients do not follow recommended treatments, fail to take medications correctly, or do not adapt life-style to changing health needs).

person who already knows how to cook can use this knowledge when learning to prepare food for a special diet.

- The nurse-teacher must be able to communicate clearly and concisely. The words the nurse uses need to have the same meaning to the learner as to the teacher. For example, a client who is taught not to put water on an area of skin may think a wet washcloth is permissible for washing the area. In effect, the nurse needs to explain that no water or moisture should touch the area.
- A knowledge of the learners and the factors that affect their learning should be established before planning the teaching.
- When a person in involved in planning, learning is often enhanced.
- Teaching that involves a number of the learners' senses often enhances learning. For example, when learning about changing a surgical dressing, the nurse can tell the client about the procedure (hearing), show how to change the dressing (sight), and show how to manipulate the equipment (touch).
- The anticipated behavioral changes that indicate that learning has taken place must always be within the context of the client's life-style and

resources. For example, it would probably not be reasonable to expect a woman to soak in a tub of hot water four times a day if she did not have a bathtub and had to heat water on a stove.

See the accompanying box for the characteristics of effective teaching.

ASSESSING

A comprehensive assessment of learning needs incorporates data from the nursing history and physical assessment and addresses the client's support system. It also considers client characteristics that may influence the learning process: readiness to learn, motivation to learn, and reading and comprehension level, for example.

The nurse's own knowledge of common learning needs required by clients experiencing similar health problems is another source of information. Learning needs change as the client's health status changes, so nurses must constantly reassess them.

Nursing History

Several elements in the nursing history provide clues to learning needs. These elements include, (a) age, (b) the client's understanding and perceptions of the health problem, (c) health beliefs and practices, (d) cultural factors, (e) economic factors, (f) learning style, and (g) client's support system.

Age   Age provides information on the person's developmental status that may indicate distinctive health teaching content and teaching approaches. Simple questions to school-age children and adolescents will elicit information on what they know. Observing children in play provides information about their motor and intellectual development as well as relationships with other children. For the elderly person, conversation and questioning may reveal slow recall or limited psychomotor skills and learning difficulties.

Client's Understanding of Health Problem Clients' perceptions of their current health problems and concerns may indicate knowledge deficits and/or misinformation. In addition, the effects of the problem on the client's usual activities can alert the nurse to other areas requiring instruction. For example, persons who cannot arrange self-care at home often need information about community resources and services.

Health Beliefs and Practices A client's health beliefs and practices are important to consider in any teaching plan. The health belief model described in Chapter 3 provides a predictor of preventive health behavior. However, even if a nurse is convinced that a particular client's health beliefs should be changed, doing so may not be possible because so many factors are involved in a person's health beliefs.

Cultural Factors Many cultural groups have their own beliefs and practices, a number of them related to diet, health, illness, and life-style. It is therefore important to know how the practices and values held by clients impinge on their learning needs.

Folk beliefs of certain groups may also affect learning. Although the client may readily understand the health care information being taught, this learning may not be implemented in the home, where folk medical practices prevail. For additional information, see Chapter 18 and the section on transcultural teaching on page 178.

Economic Factors Economic factors can also affect a client's learning. For example, a client who cannot afford to obtain a new sterile syringe for each injection of insulin may find it difficult to learn to administer the insulin when the nurse teaches that a new syringe should be used each time.

Learning Style Considerable research has been done on people's learning styles. The best way to learn varies with the individual. Some people are visual learners and learn best by watching. Other people do not visualize an activity well; they learn best by actually manipulating equipment and discovering how it works. Other people can learn well from reading things presented in an orderly fashion. Still other people learn best in groups relating to other people. For some, stressing the thinking part of a skill and the logic of something will promote learning. For other people, stressing the feeling part or interpersonal aspect motivates and promotes learning.

The nurse seldom has the time or skills to assess each learner, identify the person's particular learning style, and then adapt teaching accordingly; what the nurse can do, however, is to ask clients how they have learned things best in the past or how they like to learn. Many people know what helps them learn, and the nurse can use this information in planning the teaching. Using a variety of teaching techniques and varying activities during teaching are good ways to match learners with learning styles. One technique will be most effective for some clients, whereas other techniques will be suited to clients with different learning styles.

Client Support System The nurse explores the client's support system to determine the extent to which others may enhance learning and offer support. Family members or a close friend may help the client perform required skills at home and maintain required life-style changes.

Physical Examination

The general survey part of the physical examination provides useful clues to the client's learning needs, such as mental status, energy level, and nutritional status. Other parts of the physical examination reveal data about the client's physical capacity to learn and to perform self-care activities. Visual ability, hearing ability, and muscle coordination affect the selection of content and approaches to teaching, for example.

Readiness to Learn

Clients who are ready to learn often behave differently from those who are not. A client who is ready may search out information, for instance, by asking questions, reading books or articles, talking to others, and generally showing interest. The person unready to learn is more likely to avoid the subject or situation. In addition, the unready client may change the subject when it is brought up by the nurse.

The nurse assesses for:

- *Physical readiness.* Is the client able to focus on things other than physical status, or are pain, fatigue, and immobility using up all of the client's time and energy?
- *Emotional readiness.* Is the client emotionally ready to learn self-care activities? Clients who are extremely anxious, depressed, or grieving over their health status are not ready.
- *Cognitive readiness.* Can the client think clearly at this point? Are the effects of anesthesia and analgesia altering the client's level of consciousness?

Nurses can promote readiness to learn by providing physical and emotional support during the critical stage of recovery. As the client stabilizes physically and emotionally, the nurse can provide opportunities to learn and encouragement.

Determining Readability Level of Written Materials Using the SMOG Index

To determine the reading level of learning materials for clients, choose 30 sentences in the reading. Pick 10 from the beginning, 10 from the middle, and 10 from the end of the reading. Count all the words with 3 or more syllables; total these. Find the number in the list below, and read across to find the reading grade level.

Number of Words with 3 or More Syllables	Reading Grade Level
0–2	4
3–6	5
7–12	6
13–20	7
21–30	8
31–42	9
43–56	10
57–72	11
73–90	12

To decrease the reading level of and simplify the client educational material,
- Use smaller words.
- Avoid words with several syllables.
- Write shorter sentences.
- Explain terms that must be used.
- Use easy, common words.

Sources: Adapted from "Patient Educational Materials: Are They Readable?" by S. T. Stephens, January/February 1992, *Oncology Nursing Forum, 19,* p. 84; and "Self-Care Instructions: Do Patients Understand Educational materials? by M. Wong, February 1992, *Focus on Critical Care, 19,* 47–49.

Motivation

As discussed earlier, motivation relates to whether the client wants to learn and is usually greatest when the client is ready, the learning need is recognized, and the information being offered is meaningful to the client.

Nurses can increase a client's motivation in several ways:

- By relating the learning to something the client values and helping the client see the relevance of the learning
- By helping the client make the learning situation pleasant and nonthreatening

- By encouraging self-direction and independence
- By demonstrating a positive attitude about the client's ability to learn
- By offering continuing support and encouragement as the client attempts to learn (i.e., positive reinforcement)
- By creating a learning situation where the client is likely to succeed (succeeding in small tasks motivates the client to continue learning)

Reading Level

The nurse should not assume that a client's reading level is equal to the highest grade or level of formal education the client has completed. An eighth-grade reading level or lower is recommended for health education material designed for the general client population (Estey, Musseau & Keehn, 1991). The nurse can use the SMOG index to assess the reading levels of client educational material and thereby determine its appropriateness for the population who will be reading it. See the accompanying box.

DIAGNOSING

Nursing diagnoses pertinent to a client's learning needs are all grouped under the diagnostic category of **Knowledge deficit**. This diagnosis can be written in a number of ways. In all situations, the nurse specifies which deficit the client has.

Examples using the NANDA label as the client response include the following:

- **Knowledge deficit: low-calorie diet** related to inexperience with newly ordered therapy
- **Knowledge deficit: diabetic diet** related to unfamiliarity with prescribed treatment
- **Knowledge deficit: home safety hazards** related to denial of declining health and lack of interest in learning

Another way to deal with identified learning needs of clients is to write the knowledge deficit as the etiology, or second part, of the diagnosis statement. Such nursing diagnoses are written in the following format:

Risk for (specify) related to knowledge deficit (or lack of skill)

Examples include the following:

- **Risk for altered parenting** related to knowledge deficit: skills in infant care and feeding

- **Risk for infection** related to knowledge deficit: sexually transmitted diseases and their prevention

Other nursing diagnoses in which **Knowledge deficit** can be the etiology follow:

- **Risk for injury**
- **Ineffective breast-feeding**
- **Impaired adjustment**
- **Ineffective individual coping**
- **Altered health maintenance**
- **Health-seeking behaviors**
- **Noncompliance**
- **Ineffective individual management of therapeutic regimens**

PLANNING

Developing a teaching plan (see a sample teaching plan for wound care on the facing page) is accomplished in a series of steps. Involving the client at this time promotes the formation of a meaningful plan and stimulates client motivation. The client who helps formulate the teaching plan is more likely to achieve the desired outcomes.

Determining Teaching Priorities

The client's learning needs must be ranked according to priority. The client and the nurse should do this together, with the client's priorities always being considered. Once a client's priorities have been addressed, the client is generally more motivated to concentrate on other identified learning needs. For example, a man who wants to know all about coronary artery disease may not be ready to learn how to change his life-style until he meets his own need to learn more about the disease. Nurses can also use theoretical frameworks, such as Maslow's hierarchy of needs, to establish priorities.

Setting Learning Objectives/Outcomes

Learning objectives can be considered the same as outcome criteria for other nursing diagnoses. They are written in the same way. Like client outcomes, learning objectives

- State the client (learner) behavior or performance, not nurse behavior. For example, "Will write his own diets as instructed" (client behavior), not "To teach the client about his diet" (nurse behavior).

Selected Verbs for Learning Objectives

Cognitive Domain	Affective Domain	Psychomotor Domain
compares	alters	adapts
contrasts	answers	arranges
defines	attends	assembles
describes	chooses	begins
draws	complies	calculates
differentiates	conforms	calibrates
explains	completes	changes
identifies	defends	constructs
labels	differentiates	creates
lists	discusses	demonstrates
matches	displays	dismantles
names	follows	manipulates
prepares	helps	measures
plans	initiates	moves
recites	joins	organizes
restates	justifies	proceeds
selects	modifies	rearranges
solves	participates	reacts
sorts	responds	shows
states	revises	starts
summarizes	shares	works
underlines	uses	
writes	verifies	

SOURCE: Adapted from *Stating Objectives for Classroom Instruction* (3rd ed.) by N. E. Gronlund, 1985, Toronto: Collier Macmillan, pp. 37–40.

- Reflect an observable, measurable activity. The performance may be visible (e.g., walking) or invisible (e.g., adding a column of figures). However, it is necessary to be able to deduce whether an unobservable activity has been mastered from some performance that represents the activity. Therefore, the performance of an objective might be written: "Writes the total for a column of figures in the indicated space" (observable), not "Adds a column of figures" (unobservable). Selected measurable verbs used for learning objectives are shown in the accompanying box. Avoid using words such as knows, understand, believes, and appreciates; there are neither observable nor measurable.

Teaching Plan: Wound Care

Assessment of Learner: A 24-year-old male college student suffered a 2.5 inch (7 cm) laceration on the left lower anterior leg during a hockey game. The laceration was cleansed, sutured, and bandaged. The client was given an appointment to return to the health clinic in ten days for suture removal. Client states that he lives in the college dormitory and is able to care for wound if given instructions. Client is able to understand and read English.

Nursing Diagnosis: **Knowledge deficit** related to care of sutured wound.

Long-term Goal: Client's wound will heal completely without infection, or other complication.

Intermediate Goal: At clinic appointment, client's wound will be healing without signs of infection, loss of function, or other complication.

Short-Term Goal: Client will respond to questions regarding wound care and perform return demonstration of wound cleansing and bandaging.

Behavioral Objectives	Content Outline	Teaching Methods
Upon completion of the instructional session, the client will		
1. Describe normal wound healing	I. Normal wound healing	Describe normal wound healing with the use of audiovisuals.
2. Describe signs and symptoms of wound infection	II. Infection Signs and symptoms include wound warm to touch, malalignment of wound edges, and purulent wound drainage. Signs of systemic infection include fever and malaise.	Discuss the mechanism of wound infection. Use audiovisuals to demonstrate infected wound appearance. Provide handout describing signs and symptoms of wound infection.
3. Identify equipment needed for wound care	III. Wound care equipment a. Cleansing solution as prescribed by physician (e.g., clear water, mild soap and water, antimicrobial solution, or hydrogen peroxide). b. Bandaging material: Telfa, gauze wrap, adhesive tape.	Demonstrate equipment needed for cleansing and bandaging wound. Provide handout listing equipment needed.
4. Demonstrate wound cleansing and bandaging	IV. Demonstration of wound cleansing and bandaging on the client's wound or a mannikin	Demonstrate wound cleansing and bandaging on the client's wound or a mannikin. Provide handout describing procedure for cleansing and bandaging wound.
5. Describe appropriate action if questions or complications arise	V. Resources available for client questions include health clinic, emergency department.	Discuss available resources. Provide handout listing available resources and follow-up treatment plan.
6. Identify date, time, and location of follow-up appointment for suture removal	VI. Follow-up treatment plan; where and when	Provide written instructions.

Evaluation: The client will
1. Respond to questions regarding self-care of wound
2. Return demonstration of wound cleansing and bandaging
3. State contact person and telephone number to obtain assistance
4. State date, time, and location of follow-up appointment

- May add conditions/modifiers as required to clarify what, where, when, or how the behavior will be performed. Examples are "Walks to the end of the hall and back *without crutches*" (condition), "Irrigates his colostomy *independently* (condition) as taught," or "States *three* (condition) factors that affect blood sugar level."
- Include criteria specifying the time by which learning should have occurred. For example, "The client will state three things that affect blood sugar level *by end of second diabetic class.*"

Choosing Content

The content, or what is to be taught, is determined by learning objectives. For instance, "Identify appropriate sites for insulin injection" means the nurse must include content about the body sites suitable for insulin injections. Nurses can select among many sources of information including books, nursing journals, and other nurses and physicians. Whatever sources the nurse chooses, content should be

- Accurate.
- Current.
- Based on learning objectives.
- Adjusted for the learner's age, culture, and ability
- Consistent with information the nurse is teaching.
- Selected with consideration for how much time and resources are available for teaching.

Selecting Teaching Strategies

The method of teaching the nurse chooses should be suited to the individual, to the material to be learned, and to the teacher. For example, the person who cannot read needs material presented in other ways; a discussion is usually not the best strategy for teaching to give an injection; and a teacher using group discussion for teaching should be a competent group leader. As stated earlier, some people are visually oriented and learn best through seeing; others learn best through hearing and having the skill explained. See Table 9–3 for selected teaching strategies.

Ordering Learning Experiences

To save nurses time in constructing their own teaching guides, some health agencies have developed teaching guides for teaching sessions that nurses commonly give. These guides standardize content and teaching methods and make it easier for the nurse to plan and implement client teaching. Whether the nurse is implementing a plan devised by another or developing an individualized teaching plan, some guidelines can help the nurse order the learning experience.

- Start with something the learner is concerned about; for example, before learning how to administer insulin to himself, an adolescent wants to know how he can adjust his life-style and still play football.
- Begin with what the learner knows, and proceed to the unknown. This gives the learner confidence. Sometimes you will not know the client's knowledge or skill base and will need to elicit this information, either by asking questions or by having the client fill out a form, such as a pretest.
- Address first any area that is causing the client anxiety. A high level of anxiety can impair concentration in other areas. For example, a woman highly anxious about turning her husband in bed might not be able to learn about bathing him until she has successfully learned to turn him.
- Teach the basics first, then proceed to the variations or adjustments. It is very confusing to learners to have to consider possible adjustments and variations before they master the basic concepts. For example, when teaching a female client how to insert a retention catheter, it is best to teach the basic procedure before teaching any adjustments that might be needed if the catheter stops draining after insertion.
- Schedule time for review of content and questions the learner(s) may have to clarify information.

IMPLEMENTING

The nurse needs to be flexible in implementing any teaching plan, because the plan may need revising. The client may tire sooner than anticipated, or be faced with too much information too quickly; the client's needs may change; or external factors may intervene. For instance, the nurse and the client, Mr. Brown, have planned to irrigate his colostomy at 10 A.M. but when the time comes, Mr. Brown wants additional information before actually doing it himself.

In this case, the nurse alters the teaching plan and discusses the desired information, provides written information, and defers teaching the psychomotor

TABLE 9-3 **Selected Teaching Strategies**

Strategy	Major Type of Learning	Characteristics
Explanation or description (e.g., lecture)	Cognitive	Teacher controls content and pace. Learner is passive; therefore retains less information than when a participant. Feedback is determined by teacher. May be given to individual or group.
One-to-one discussion	Affective, cognitive	Encourages participation by learner. Permits reinforcement and repetition at learner's level. Permits introduction of sensitive subjects.
Answering questions	Cognitive	Teacher controls most of content and pace. Teacher must understand question and what it means to learner. Learner may need to overcome cultural perception that asking questions is impolite and may embarrass the teacher. Can be used with individuals and groups. Teacher sometimes needs to confirm whether question has been answered by asking learner, for example, "Does that answer your question?"
Demonstration	Psychomotor	Often used with explanation. Can be used with individuals, small or large groups. Does not permit use of equipment by learners; learner is passive.
Discovery	Cognitive, affective	Teacher guides problem-solving situation. Learner is active participant; therefore retention of information is high.
Group discussions	Affective, cognitive	Learner can obtain assistance from supportive group. Group members learn from one another. Teacher needs to keep the discussion focused and prevent monopolization by one or two learners.
Practice	Psychomotor	Allows repetition and immediate feedback. Permits "hands-on" experience.
Printed and audiovisual materials	Cognitive	Forms include books, pamphlets, films, programmed instruction, and computer learning. Learners can proceed at their own speed. Nurse can act as resource person, need not be present during learning. Potentially ineffective if reading level is too high. Teacher needs to select language that meets learner needs if English is a second language.
Role playing	Affective, cognitive	Permits expression of attitudes, values, and emotions. Can assist in development of communication skills. Involves active participation by learner. Teacher must create supportive, safe environment for learners to minimize anxiety.
Modeling	Affective, psychomotor	Nurse sets example by attitude, psychomotor skill.
Computer-assisted learning programs	All types of learning	Learner is active. Learner controls pace. Provides immediate reinforcement and review. Use with individuals or groups.

skill until the next day. It is also important for nurses to use teaching techniques that enhance learning and reduce or eliminate any barriers to learning such as pain or fatigue.

Guidelines for Teaching

When implementing a teaching plan, the nurse may find the following eight guidelines helpful.

1. The optimal time for each session depends largely on the learner. Some people, for example, learn best at the beginning of the day, when they are most rested; others prefer late afternoon, when no other activities are scheduled. Whenever possible, ask the client for help to choose the best time.

2. The pace of each teaching session also affects learning. Nurses should be sensitive to any signs that the pace is too fast or too slow. A client who appears confused or does not comprehend material when questioned may be finding the pace too fast. When the client appears bored and loses interest, the pace may be too slow, the learning period may be too long, or the client may be tired.

3. An environment can detract from or assist learning; for example, noise or interruptions usually interfere with concentration, whereas a comfortable environment promotes learning.

4. Teaching aids can foster learning and help focus a learner's attention. To ensure the transfer of learning, the nurse should use the type of supplies or equipment the client will eventually use. Before the teaching session, the nurse needs to assemble all equipment and visual aids and ensure that all audiovisual equipment is functioning effectively.

5. Learning is more effective when the learners discover the content for themselves. Ways to increase learning include stimulating motivation and stimulating self-direction, for example, by providing specific, realistic, achievable objectives, giving feedback, and helping the learner derive satisfaction from learning. The nurse may also encourage self-directed independent learning by encouraging the client to explore sources of information required.

6. Repetition—for example, summarizing content, rephrasing (using other words), and approaching the material from another point of view—reinforces learning. For instance, after discussing the kinds of foods that can be included in a diet, the nurse describes the foods again, but in the context of the three meals eaten during one day.

7. It is helpful to employ "organizers" to introduce material to be learned. Advanced organizers provide a means of connecting unknown material to known material and generating logical relationships. For example: "You understand how urine flows down a catheter from the bladder. Now I will show you how to inject fluid so that it flows up the catheter into the bladder." The details that follow are then seen within its framework, and the details have added meaning.

8. Using a layperson's vocabulary enhances communication. Often nurses use terms and abbreviations that have meaning to other health professionals but make little sense to clients. Even words such as *urine* or *feces* may be unfamiliar to clients, and abbreviations such as "RR" (recovery room) or "PAR" (postanesthesia room) are often misunderstood.

Special Teaching Strategies

There are a number of special teaching strategies that nurses can use: client contracting, group teaching, computer-assisted instruction, discovery/problem solving, and behavior modification. Any strategy the nurse selects must be appropriate for the learner and the learning objectives.

Client Contracting

Client contracting involves establishing a contract with a client that specifies certain objectives and when they are to be met. The contract, drawn up and signed by the client and the nurse, specifies not only the learning objectives but also the responsibilities of the client and the nurse, and the teaching plan. The agreement allows for freedom, mutual respect, and mutual responsibility.

Group Teaching

Group instruction is economical, and it provides members with an opportunity to share with and learn from others. A small group allows for discussion in which everyone can participate. A large group often necessitates a lecture technique or use of films, videos, slides, or role-playing by teachers.

It is important that all members involved in group instruction have a need in common (e.g., prenatal health or preoperative instruction). It is also important that sociocultural factors be considered in the formation of a group. Whereas middle-class Americans may value sharing experiences with others, people from a culture such as Japan may consider it inappropriate to reveal their thoughts and feelings.

Computer-Assisted Instruction (CAI)

Computer-assisted instruction (CAI) is becoming more popular. Initially, cognitive learning of facts was the primary use of computer educational methods. Now, however, computers can also be used to teach the following:

- Complex problem-solving skills
- Application of information
- Psychomotor skills

Programs can be used for

- Individual health care professionals or clients using one computer.
- Families of small groups of three to five clients gathered around one computer taking turns running the program and answering questions together.
- Large groups, with the computer display screen projected onto an overhead screen and a teacher or one learner using the keyboard.

Individuals using a computer are able to set the pace that meets their learning needs. Small groups are less able to do this, and large groups progress through the program at a pace that may be too slow for some learners and too fast for others. It is therefore helpful to group learners of similar needs and abilities together. Whether using the computer alone or in large groups, learners read and view informational material, answer questions, and receive immediate feedback. The correct answer is usually indicated by the use of colors, flashing signs, or written praise. When the learner selects an incorrect answer, the computer responds with an explanation of why that was not the best answer and encouragement to try again. Many programs ask learners whether they want to review material on which the question and answer were based. Some computer programs feature simulated situations that allow learners to manipulate objects on the screen to learn psychomotor skills. When used to teach such skills, CAI must be followed up with practice on actual equipment supervised by the teacher.

Some clients may have a negative attitude about computers that could act as a barrier to learning. The nurse helps these clients by explaining the steps to start and run the program, to turn the computer on and off, and where and when to insert the computer disk so that the client can use the program when the nurse is not present. Most media catalogs, professional journals, and health care libraries contain information about computer programs available to the nurse for client education. The media specialist or librarian in a health care facility or college is an excellent resource to help the nurse locate appropriate compute programs. Computer educational material is also available for clients with different language needs, for clients with special visual needs, and for clients at different growth and development levels.

Discovery/Problem-Solving

In using the discovery/problem-solving technique, the nurse presents some initial information and then asks the learners a question or presents a situation related to the information. The learner applies the new information to the situation and decides what to do. Learners can work alone or in groups. This technique is well suited to family learning. The teacher guides the learners through the thinking process necessary to reach the best solution to the question or the best action to take in the situation. This may also be referred to as anticipatory problem solving. For example, the nurse-educator might present information on diabetes and blood glucose management. Then, the nurse might ask the learners how they think their insulin and/or diet should be adjusted if their morning glucose was too low. In this way, clients learn what critical components they need to consider to reach the best solution to the problem.

Behavior Modification

Behavior modification is an outgrowth of behavioral learning theory. Its basic assumptions include (a) human behaviors are learned and can be selectively strengthened, weakened, eliminated, or replaced and (b) a person's behavior is under conscious control. Under this system, desirable behavior is regarded and undesirable behavior is ignored. The client's response is the key to behavior change. For example, clients trying to quit smoking are not criticized when they smoke, but they are praised or rewarded when they go without a cigarette for a certain period of time. For some people a learning contract is combined with behavior modification, and includes the following pertinent features:

- Positive reinforcement (e.g., praise) is used.
- The client participates in the development of the learning plan.

- Undesirable behavior is ignored, not criticized.
- The expectation of the client and the nurse is that the task will be mastered (i.e., the behavior will change).
- Success is maximized through positive reinforcement; failure and the threat of failure are minimized.

CONSIDER...

- the teaching strategies you employ with clients in your clinical setting. Based on the strategies discussed on pages 176–177, which do you consider the most and least effective? Why?
- barriers that may influence the learning ability of older adults and children. What strategies would you employ to overcome these barriers? What teaching tools would you select for children?
- strategies you would use to teach a 15-year-old diabetic about insulin injections. Include strategies for the cognitive, affective, and psychomotor domains.

Transcultural Client Teaching

The nurse and clients of different cultural and ethnic backgrounds have additional barriers to overcome in the teaching-learning process. These barriers include language and communication problems, differing concepts of time, conflicting cultural healing practices, beliefs that may positively or negatively influence compliance with health teaching, and unique high-risk or high-frequency health problems needing health promotion instruction. See Chapter 18 for detailed information. Nurses should consider the following guidelines when teaching clients from various ethnic backgrounds:

- *Obtain teaching materials, pamphlets, and instructions in languages used by clients in the health care setting.* Nurses who are unable to read the foreign language material for themselves can have the translator read the material to them. The nurse can then evaluate the quality of the information and update it with the translator's help as needed.
- *Use visual aids, such as pictures, charts or diagrams, to communicate meaning.* Audiovisual material may be helpful if the English is spoken clearly and slowly. Even if understanding the verbal message is a problem for the client, seeing a skill or procedure may be helpful. In some instances, a translator can be asked to clarify the video.

Alternatively the video may be available in several languages, and the nurse can request the necessary version from the company.

- *Use concrete rather than abstract words.* Use simple language (short sentences, short words), and present only one idea at a time.
- *Allow time for questions.* This helps the client mentally separate one idea or skill from another.
- *Avoid the use of medical terminology or health care language,* such as "taking your vital signs" or "apical pulse." Rather, nurses should say they are going to take a blood pressure or listen to the client's heart.
- *If understanding another's pronunciation is a problem, validate brief information in writing.* For example, during assessments, write down numbers, words, or phrases, and have the client read them to verify accuracy.
- *Use humor very cautiously.* Meaning can change in the translation process.
- *Do not use slang words or colloquialisms.* These may be interpreted literally.
- *Do not assume that a client who nods, uses eye contact or smiles is indicating an understanding of what is being taught.* These responses may simply be the client's way of indicating respect. The client may feel that asking the nurse questions or stating a lack of understanding is inappropriate because it might embarrass the nurse or cause the nurse to "lose face."
- *Invite and encourage questions during teaching.* Let clients know they are urged to ask questions and be involved in making information more clear. When asking questions to evaluate client understanding, avoid asking negative questions. These can be interpreted differently by people for whom English is a second language. "Do you understand how far you can bend your hip after surgery?" is better than the negative question "You don't understand how far you can bend your hip after surgery, do you?" With particularly difficult information or skills teaching, the nurse might say, "Most people have some trouble with this. May I please help you go through this one more time?" In some cultures, expressing a need is not appropriate, and expressing confusion or asking to be shown something again is considered rude.
- *When explaining procedures, or functioning related to personal areas of the body, it may be appropriate to have a nurse of the same sex do the teaching.* Because

of modesty concerns in many cultures and beliefs about what is considered appropriate and inappropriate male-female interaction, it is wise to have a female nurse teach a female client about personal care, birth control, sexually transmitted diseases (STDs), and other potentially sensitive areas. If a translator is needed during explanation of procedures or teaching, the translator should also be female.

- *Include the family in planning and teaching.* This promotes trust and mutual respect. Identify the authoritative family member and incorporate that person into the planning and teaching to promote compliance and support of health teaching. In some cultures, the male head of household is the critical family member to include in health teaching; in other cultures, it is the eldest female member.

- *Consider the client's time orientation.* The client may be oriented to the past, present, future, or a combination of all three. The client may be more oriented to the present than the nurse is. Cultures with a predominant orientation to the present include Mexican Americans, Navajo Native Americans, Appalachians, Eskimos, and Filipino Americans. For such clients, preventing future problems may be less significant, and teaching them how to do so may be more difficult. For example, teaching a client why and when to take medications may be more difficult if the client is oriented to the present. In such instances, the nurse can emphasize preventing short-term problems rather than long-term problems. Failure to keep clinic appointments or to arrive on time is common in clients who have a present-time orientation. The nurse can help by arranging transportation and by accommodating these clients when they do come rather than rescheduling an appointment that they probably will not keep.

Schedules may be very flexible in present-oriented societies, with sleeping and eating patterns varying greatly. Teaching clients to take medications at bedtime or with a meal does not necessarily mean that these activities will occur at the same time each day. For this reason, the nurse should assess the client's daily routine before teaching the client to pair a treatment or medication with an event the nurse assumes occurs at the same time every day. When teaching a client when to take medication, the nurse should determine whether a clock or watch is available to the client and whether the client can tell time.

- *Identify cultural health practices and beliefs.* Noncompliance with health teaching may be related to conflict with folk medicine beliefs. Noncompliance may also be related to lack of understanding or a fatalism, a belief system in which life events are held to be predestined or fixed in advance and the individual is powerless to change them. To encourage compliance, the nurse may need to involve the client in learning about the causes and preventability of certain health problems.

The nurse should treat the client's cultural healing beliefs with respect and try to identify whether any are in agreement or in conflict with what is being taught. The nurse can then focus on the ones in agreement to promote the integration of new learning with familiar health practices. The client will need an explanation of why certain folk healing practices are harmful and must be stopped and how the recommended health practices will improve health.

The nurse might begin assessment by assuming that the client has already tried culturally accepted remedies for the health problem and that because these have not worked, the client is now seeking help from the health care system. The nurse should identify what folk remedies were tried and whether any are still being used. Some practices may put the client at risk. Self-medication is common in some cultures and should be assessed. These medications can include not only herbal remedies and over-the-counter drugs but also injectable drugs, such as antibiotics or vitamins, which in some countries can be obtained without a doctor's prescription.

EVALUATING

Evaluating Learning

Evaluating is both an ongoing and a final process in which the client, the nurse, and often, the support persons determine what has been learned. This process is the same as evaluating client achievement of goals and outcomes for other nursing diagnoses. Learning is measured against the predetermined learning objectives selected in the planning phase of the teaching process. Thus, the objectives serve not only to direct the teaching plan but also to provide outcome criteria for evaluation. For example, the objective "Selects foods that are low in carbohydrates" can be evaluated by asking the client to name such foods or to select low-carbohydrate foods from a list.

The best method for evaluating depends on the type of learning. In *cognitive learning*, the client demonstrates acquisition of knowledge. Examples of the evaluation tools for cognitive learning include the following:

- Direct observation of behavior (e.g., observing the client selecting the solution to a problem using the new knowledge).
- Written measurements (e.g., tests).
- Oral questioning (e.g., asking the client to restate information or correct verbal responses to questions).
- Self-reports and self-monitoring. These can be useful during follow-up phone calls and home visits. Evaluating individual self-paced learning, as might occur with computer-assisted instruction, often incorporates self-monitoring.

The acquisition of *psychomotor skills* is best evaluated by observing how well the client carries out a procedure such as changing a dressing or carrying out a urinary self-catheterization.

Affective learning is more difficult to evaluate. Whether attitudes or values have been learned may be inferred by listening to the client's responses to questions, noting how the client speaks about relevant subjects, and by observing client's behavior that expresses feelings and values. For example, have parents learned to value health sufficiently to have their children immunized? Do clients who state that they value health actually use condoms every time they have sex with a new partner?

Following evaluation, the nurse may find it necessary to modify or repeat the teaching plan if the objectives have not been met or have been met only partially. For the hospitalized client, follow-up teaching in the home or by phone may be needed.

Behavior change does not always take place immediately after learning. Often individuals accept change intellectually first and then change their behavior only periodically (for example, Mrs. Green, who knows that she must lose weight, diets and exercises off and on). If the new behavior is to replace the old behavior, it must emerge gradually; otherwise, the old behavior may prevail. The nurse can assist clients with behavior change by allowing for client vacillation and by providing encouragement.

Evaluating Teaching

It is important for nurses to evaluate their own teaching. This is the same as evaluating the effectiveness of nursing interventions for other nursing diagnoses. Evaluation should include a consideration of all factors—the timing, the teaching strategies, the amount of information, whether the teaching was helpful, and so on. The nurse may find, for example, that the client was overwhelmed with too much information, was bored, or was motivated to learn more.

Both the client and the nurse should evaluate the learning experience. The client may tell the nurse what was helpful, interesting, and so on. Feedback questionnaires and videotapes of the learning sessions can also be helpful.

The nurse should not feel ineffective as a teacher if the client forgets some of what is taught. Forgetting is normal and should be anticipated. Having the client write down information, repeating it during teaching, giving handouts on the information and having the client be active in the learning process all promote retention.

DOCUMENTING

Documentation of the teaching process is essential, because it provides a legal record that the teaching took place and communicates the teaching to other health professionals. If teaching is not documented, legally it did not occur. It is also important to document the responses of the client and support persons. What did the client or support person say or do to indicate that learning occurred? The nurse records this in the client's chart as evidence of learning. The parts of the teaching process that should be documented in the client's chart include the following:

- Diagnosed learning needs
- Learning objectives
- Topics taught
- Client outcomes
- Need for additional teaching
- Resources provided

The written teaching plan that the nurse uses as a resource to guide future teaching sessions might also include these elements:

- Actual information and skills taught
- Teaching strategies used
- Time framework and content for each class

CONSIDER...

- the learning needs of clients in your specific practice setting. Is the instruction given by different health care providers consistent in its content? What problems might occur if there is inconsistency in instruction? How might you go about correcting these inconsistencies?
- the specific health problems of your community (e.g., AIDS, teenage pregnancy, sexually transmitted disease, domestic violence). How might the nurse assist in solving community health problems through the teaching role?
- how the nurse might influence through education others' understanding of nurses' knowledge, skill, and roles. Do nurses speak in community education programs? In what way are nurses involved in the education of other health professionals? In what ways are nurses politically proactive regarding health care and nursing practice?

SUMMARY

Teaching clients, families, and other health professionals is a major nursing role. Learning is represented by a change in behavior.

Three main theories of learning are behaviorism, cognitivism, and humanism. Behaviorism *focuses on careful identification of what is to be taught and the immediate identification of a reward for correct responses.* Cognitivism, *which has a more holistic view of learning, emphasizes the importance of an integrated learning experience, one that develops understandings and appreciations that help the person function in a larger context. It also stresses the importance of social, emotions, and physical contexts in which learning occurs. The teacher-learner relationship is also an important factor in cognitive learning theory.* Humanism *focuses on the feelings and attitudes of the learner and stresses that individuals can become highly self-motivated learners. The learner identifies the learning needs and takes responsibility for meeting them.*

Bloom has identified three learning domains: cognitive, affective, and psychomotor. The cognitive *domain includes six intellectual skills: knowledge, comprehension, application, analysis, synthesis, and evaluation. The* affective *domain includes five categories: receiving, responding, valuing, organization, and characterization. The* psychomotor *domain includes seven categories: perception, set, guided, responses, mechanism, complex overt response, adaptation, and origination.*

READINGS FOR ENRICHMENT

Dobrzykowski, T. M. (1994, Dec.). Teaching strategies to promote critical thinking skills in nursing staff. *Journal of Continuing Education, 25,* 272–276.

In this article, the author describes strategies to help nurses attain and advance critical thinking skills. As a foundation to understanding these strategies, the author defines *critical thinking, inductive reasoning,* and *deductive reasoning* and also describes a critical thinking model developed by Dreyfus and Dreyfus. Benner's research is also described. Among the teaching strategies highlighted are an orientation program, mentoring, and individual and group activities.

Schoenly, L. (1994, Sept./Oct.). Teaching in the affective domain. *Journal of Continuing Education in Nursing, 25,* 209–212.

The author points out that in order to prepare caring nurses, teaching must also be targeted to the affective domain. The author describes five hierarchical categories of teaching in the affective domain: receiving, responding, valuing, organization, and value or value complex. This continuum of values development moves the learner toward self-actualization.

The writer further describes teaching strategies for learning in the affective domain, including questioning, case studies, role-playing, simulation gaming, values clarification, and values inquiry.

Weinrich, S. P., & Boyd, M. (1992, Jan.). Education in the elderly—adapting and evaluating teaching tools. *Journal of Gerontological Nursing, 18,* 15–20.

The population of older adults is increasing, and their multiple health problems, coupled with physical and psychosocial changes related to aging, make the educational needs of this population particularly complex. The article gives specific guidelines for selecting written and audiovisual material for educating the older client. A case example and clinical implications are included.

A number of factors facilitate learning, including motivation, readiness, active involvement, success at learning feedback, and moving from simple to complex. Factors such as extreme anxiety, certain physiologic processes, and cultural barriers impede learning.

Teaching is a system of activities intended to produce learning. Rapport between the teacher and the learner is essential for effective teaching. Teaching, like the nursing process, consists of five activities: assessing the learner, diagnosing learning needs, developing a teaching plan, implementing the plan, and evaluating learning out-comes and teaching effectiveness. Learning objectives guide the content of the teaching plan and are written in terms of client behavior. Teaching strategies should be suited to the client, the material to be learned, and the teacher. It should be adjusted to the client's developmental level and health status.

A teaching plan is a written plan consisting of learning objectives, content to teach, a time frame for teaching, and strategies to use in teaching the content. The plan must be revised when the client's needs change or the teaching strategies prove ineffective. Adaptations in teaching will facilitate learning for clients who are illiterate, elderly, or from non-Western cultural and ethnic backgrounds. Barriers to overcome transcultural teaching include language and communication problems, different concepts of time, and cultural beliefs and practices that conflict with those of Western medicine.

Evaluation of the teaching/learning process is both an ongoing and a final process. Documentation of client teaching is essential to communicate the teaching to other health professionals and to provide a record for legal purposes.

SELECTED REFERENCES

American Nurses Association. (1991). *Standards of clinical nursing practice.* Washington, D.C.: Author.

American Nurses Credentialing Center. (1995). *1995 Certification Catalog.* Washington, D.C.: Author.

Bandura, A. (1971). Analysis of modeling processes. In A. Bandura (Ed.), *Psychological modeling.* Chicago: Aldine.

Bloom, B. S. (Ed.). (1956). *Taxonomy of educational objectives.* Book 1, *Cognitive domain.* New York: Longman.

Chally, P. S. (1992, March). Empowerment through teaching. *Journal of Nursing Education, 31,* 117–120.

Dobrzykowski, J. M. (1994, Nov./Dec.). Teaching strategies to promote critical thinking skills in nursing staff. *Journal of Continuing Education in Nursing, 25,* 272–276.

Estey, A., Musseau, A., & Keehn, L. (1991, Oct.) Comprehensive levels of patients reading health information. *Patient Education and Counseling, 18,* 165–169.

Foulk, D., Lafferty, J., & Ryan, R. (1991, Sept./Oct.). Developing culturally sensitive materials for AIDS education specifically targeted to migrant farm workers. *Journal of Health Education, 22,* 283–286.

Gagne, R. M. (1974). *Essentials of learning of instruction.* Hinsdale, IL: Dryden Press.

Gessner, B. A. (1989, Sept.). Adult education: The cornerstone of patient teaching. *Nursing Clinics of North America, 24,* 589–595.

Giger, J. N., & Davidhizar, R. E. (1991). *Transcultural nursing.* St. Louis: Mosby.

Gronlund, N. E. (1985). *Stating objectives for classroom instruction* (3rd ed.). New York: Macmillan.

Kick, E. (1989, Sept.). Patient teaching for elders. *Nursing Clinics of North America, 24,* 681–686.

Knowles, M. S. (1980). *The modern practice of adult education: From pedagogy to andragogy.* Chicago: Follet.

Knowles, M. S. (1984). *Andragogy in action.* San Francisco: Jossey-Bass.

Lewin, K. (1948). *Resolving social conflicts.* G. W. Lewin, ed. New York: Harper and Brothers.

Lewin, K. (1951). *Field theory in social science.* New York: Harper and Row.

Logan, J., & Boss, M. (1993, March). Nurses' learning patterns. *Canadian Nurse, 89,* 18–22.

Maslow, A. H. (1970). *Motivation and personality.* New York: Harper and Row.

Miller, P. H. (1989). *Theories of developmental psychology* (2nd ed.) New York: Freeman.

North American Nursing Diagnosis Association. (1992). *NANDA nursing diagnoses: Definitions and classification 1994–1995.* Philadelphia: NANDA.

Pavlov, I. P. (1927). *Conditioned reflexes* (trans. G. V. Anrep). London: Oxford U. Press.

Piaget, J. (1966). *Origins of intelligence in children.* New York: Norton.

Redman, B. K. (1992). *The process of patient education* (7th ed.). St. Louis: Mosby.

Rogers, C. R. (1961). *On becoming a person.* Boston: Houghton-Mifflin.

Rogers, C. R. (1969). *Freedom to learn.* Columbus, Ohio: Chas. E. Merrill.

Schoenly, L. (1994, Sept./Oct.) Teaching in the affective domain. *Journal of Continuing Education in Nursing, 25,* 209–212.

Skinner, B. F. (1953). *Science and human behavior.* New York: Macmillan.

Swansburg, R. C. (1995). *Nursing staff development: A component of human resource development.* Boston: Jones and Bartlett.

Thorndike, E. L. (1913). *The psychology of learning.* New York: Teachers College.

Whitman, N. I., Graham, B. A., Gleit, C. J., & Boyd, M. D. (1992). *Teaching in nursing practice* (2nd ed.). Norwalk, CT: Appleton & Lange.

Wong, M. (1992, Feb.) Self-care instructions: Do patients understand educational materials? *Focus on Critical Care, 19,* 47–49.

Leader and Manager

by Diane Whitehead

OBJECTIVES

- Differentiate leadership from management

- Compare and contrast the following leadership styles: charismatic, authoritarian, democratic, laissez-faire, situational, and transformational.

- Describe the management concepts of authority, accountability, planning, organizing, leading, controlling, and power.

- Compare and contrast the following nursing delivery models: case method, functional method, team nursing, primary nursing, case management, managed care, differentiated practice, and shared governance.

- Discuss the impact of downsizing, restructuring, and health care reform on the role of the professional nurse.

> "Let whoever is in charge keep this simple question in her head (*not*, how can I always do this right thing myself, but) how can I provide for this right thing to be always done?"
>
> —Florence Nightingale

Today's professional nurses assume leadership and management responsibilities regardless of the activity in which they are involved.

- Although leadership and management roles are different, they are frequently intertwined. **Leadership** is defined as "the process of influencing others" (Tappen, 1995, p. xii). **Management** involves not only leadership but also planning, organizing, motivating, and controlling both human and material resources to achieve designated outcomes (Bleich, 1995, p. 5). Douglas (1992, p. 6) distinguishes managers from leaders in this way: "Managers are people who do things right and leaders are people who do the right things." See Table 10–1 for a comparison of leader and manager roles.
- The ability to advocate for the client is linked to the nurse's leadership ability (see Chapter 5).
- The nurse may be a leader or manager in the care of the individual client, the client's family, groups of clients, or the community. Regardless of the setting, the nurse must demonstrate leadership and management skills in interacting with nursing colleagues, nursing students, physicians, and other health professionals.

NURSING LEADERSHIP

The purposes of nursing leadership vary according to the context in which it is exhibited. These purposes may include (a) improving the health status of individual clients or families, (b) increasing the effectiveness and level of satisfaction among professional colleagues who provide care, and (c) improving the attitudes of citizens and legislators toward the nursing profession and their expectations of it (Leddy & Pepper, 1993, p. 383). Additionally, nurses as leaders promote the concept of caring by advocating for changes that promote physical, psychologic, and social well-being in the society as a whole.

On a wider scope, nurses must apply leadership skills as they apply nursing knowledge to personal concerns. Nurses can demonstrate these leadership skills in their involvement in such organizations as Mothers Against Drunk Drivers (MADD), the American Cancer Society, and the American Heart Association. Nurses demonstrate leadership activities as they advocate for the homeless, older adults, victims of acquired immune deficiency syndrome (AIDS), abused children, and environmental protec-

TABLE 10–1 Comparison of Leader and Manager Roles

Leaders	Managers
May or may not have official appointment to the position.	Are appointed officially to the position.
Have power and authority to enforce decisions only so long as followers are willing to be led.	Have power and authority to enforce decisions.
Influence others toward goal setting, either formally or informally.	Carry out predetermined policies, rules, and regulations.
Interested in risk taking and exploring new ideas.	Maintain an orderly, controlled, rational, and equitable structure.
Relate to people personally in an intuitive and empathetic manner.	Relate to people according to their roles.
Feel rewarded by personal achievements.	Feel rewarded when fulfilling organizational mission or goals.
May or may not be successful as managers.	Are managers as long as the appointment holds.

SOURCE: *The Effective Nurse: Leader and Manager* (4th ed.) by L. M. Douglass, 1992, St. Louis: Mosby-Year Book, p. 6. Used with permission.

tion programs. In recent years, professional nurses have demonstrated a wide range of leadership and management skills to politicians and legislators in all parts of the country in their efforts to advocate and plan for a system of affordable health care for all residents of the United States through Nursing's Agenda for Health Care Reform (American Nurses Association [ANA], 1991a).

Leadership occurs when someone influences others to act. Whereas managers are assigned their roles, leaders achieve their roles. One may be designated the leader and demonstrate no leadership skills, while another person may have no formal leadership title yet demonstrate excellent leadership skills.

Leadership Characteristics

What are the characteristics of successful leadership? Hellriegel and Slocum (1993, pp. 469–479) emphasize the following core leadership skills:

- *Empowerment.* Leaders who empower others share influence and control with group members in deciding how to achieve the organization's goals. Through empowerment, the leader gives others a sense of achievement, belonging, and self-esteem. One way in which the nursing leader can empower the staff is to discuss with them ideas about providing client care.
- *Intuition.* By using intuition, a leader can build trust with others, scan a situation, anticipate the need for change, and quickly move to institute appropriate change. Intuition involves having a "feel" for the environment and the needs and desires of others. Effective nurse leaders heighten their sense of intuition in order to keep abreast of the needs of clients and staff.
- *Self-understanding.* Self-understanding includes an ability to recognize one's strengths and weaknesses. Building on one's strengths and correcting or working on weaknesses are essential for effective leadership.
- *Vision.* Leaders with a vision imagine a different and better situation and identify ways of achieving it. Visionary leadership does not mean constantly imagining new and original goals; a vision may be as simple as incorporating caring and efficiency in meeting the needs of employees and clients.
- *Values congruence.* Values congruence is the ability to understand and accept the mission and objectives of the organization and the values of employees and to reconcile them. In this era of

health reform and cost containment, values congruence is an essential leadership characteristic.

Does the fact that effective leaders share certain characteristics imply that they all act the same? Not necessarily. Besides having the above characteristics, most effective leaders demonstrate the following: (a) achievement and ambition, (b) the ability to learn from adversity, (c) high dedication to the job, (d) sound analytic and problem-solving skills, (e) a high level of people skills, and (f) a high level of innovation.

Leadership Style

Leadership style refers to "the individual's pattern of relating to others or how the leader gets along with members of the work group" (Wywialowski, 1993, p. 127). Several leadership styles have been described: charismatic leadership; authoritarian, or directive leadership; democratic, or participative leadership; laissez-faire, or nondirectional, leadership; situational leadership; and transformational leadership.

Charismatic leadership is characterized by an emotional relationship between the leader and the group members in which the leader "inspires others by obtaining an emotional commitment from followers and by arousing strong feelings of loyalty and enthusiasm" (Marriner-Tomey, 1992, p. 261). A charismatic relationship exists when the leader can communicate a plan for change and the followers adhere to the plan because of their faith and belief in the leader's abilities (Marriner-Tomey, 1993, pp. 19–20). The followers of a charismatic leader may be able to overcome extreme hardship to achieve the goal because of their faith in the leader.

In *authoritarian leadership*, the leader makes the decisions for the group. This style of leadership has also been referred to as *directive* or *autocratic leadership*. Authoritarian leadership is likened to a dictatorship and presupposes that the group is incapable of making its own decisions. The leader determines policies, giving orders and directions to the group members. Authoritarian leadership generally has negative connotations and often makes group members dissatisfied. Because of the differences in status between the leader and group members, the degree of openness and trust between leader and group members is minimal or absent. Under this type of leadership, procedures are well defined, activities are predictable, and the group may feel secure. Although productivity is usually high, the group members' needs for creativity, autonomy, and self-motivation are not met (Tappen, 1995, pp. 80–81). Authoritarian leadership may, however, be most effective in situations requiring immediate decisions, such as cardiac arrest, fire on the unit, airplane crash, or other emergency, when one person must assume responsibility without being challenged by other team members. Similarly, when group members are unable or unwilling to participate in making a decision, the authoritarian style effects resolution of the problem and enables the individual or group to move on. This style can also be effective when a project must be completed quickly and efficiently.

In *democratic, or participative, leadership*, the leader acts as a catalyst or facilitator, actively guiding the group toward achieving the group goals. Providing constructive criticism, offering information, making suggestions, and asking questions become the focus of the participative leader. This type of leadership demands that the leader have faith in the group members to accomplish the goals. Democratic leadership is based on the following principles (Tappen, 1995, p. 82):

1. Every group member should participate in decision making.

2. Freedom of belief and action is allowed within reasonable bounds that are set by society and by the group.

3. Each individual is responsible for himself or herself and for the welfare of the group.

4. There should be concern and consideration for each group member as a unique individual.

Although democratic leadership has been shown to be less efficient and more cumbersome than authoritarian leadership, it allows for more self-motivation and more creativity among group members. Democratic leadership calls for a great deal of cooperation and coordination among group members. This style of leadership can be extremely effective in the health care setting (Tappen, 1995, p. 83).

The *laissez-faire, or nondirectional leader* is described as "inactive, passive, and permissive; offering few commands, questions, suggestions, or criticism" (Tappen, 1995, p. 83). Although there are various degrees of nondirectional leadership, leadership participation is, in general, minimal. The group's members may act independently of each other and suffer from a lack of cooperation or coordination. Apathy, chaos, and frustration may arise. The laissez-faire approach works best when group members have both personal and professional maturity, so that once the group has made a decision, the members become committed to it and have the required expertise to implement it. Individual group members then perform tasks in their area of expertise, with the leader acting as a resource person. Table 10–2 compares the authoritarian, democratic, and laissez-faire leadership styles.

In *situational leadership*, levels of direction and support vary according to the level of maturity of the employees or group. The leader assumes one of four styles (Hellriegel & Slocum, 1993, p. 484):

1. *Directive.* A leadership style characterized by the giving of clear instructions and specific direction to immature employees.

RESEARCH NOTE

What Management Styles Do Staff Nurses Find Most Desirable?

Increasing productivity without increasing costs continues to be a primary goal in today's health care environment. Employing a management style that promotes staff nurse satisfaction may be one method to meet this goal. Nakata and Saylor describe their nonexperimental study, which explores the perceived and desired management styles of nurse managers and the relationship between perceived management style and job satisfaction. The results indicate that staff nurses perceive that a benevolent-authoritative style of management prevails, but they desire a participative management style.

Implications: The use of a participative management style may provide a more positive, problem-solving, collaborative approach to decision making. The staff may be able to provide innovative ways of dealing with unit-specific problems and to understand how these decisions may affect the entire institution. The significant correlation between job satisfaction and management style and staff nurses' desire for a more participative style of management reinforces the need for nurse managers to be aware of the style of management they employ.

Source: Data from "Management Style and Staff Nurse Satisfaction in a Changing Environment" by J. A. Nakata and C. Saylor, 1994, *Nursing Administration Quarterly, 18*(3), pp. 51–57.

TABLE 10–2 Comparison of Authoritarian, Democratic, and Laissez-Faire Leadership Styles

	Authoritarian	Democratic	Laissez-Faire
Degree of freedom	Little freedom	Moderate freedom	Much freedom
Degree of control	High control	Moderate control	No control
Decision making	By the leader	Leader and group together	By the group or by no one
Leader activity level	High	High	Minimal
Assumption of responsibility	Primarily the leader	Shared	Abdicated
Output of the group	High quantity, good quality	Creative, high quality	Variable, may be of poor quality
Efficiency	Very efficient	Less efficient than authoritarian	Inefficient

SOURCE: *Nursing Leadership and Management: Concepts and Practice* (3rd ed.) by R. M. Tappen, 1995, Philadelphia: F. A. Davis, p. 82. Reprinted with permission.

2. *Coaching.* A leadership style characterized by expanding two-way communication and helping maturing employees build confidence and motivation.

3. *Supporting.* A leadership style characterized by active two-way communication and support of mature employees' efforts to use their talents.

4. *Delegating.* A hands-off leadership style in which the highly mature employees are given responsibilities for carrying out plans and making task decisions.

The situational leadership model poses some questions. First, can leaders actually choose one of these four leadership styles when faced with a new situation? Second, how do such factors as personality traits and the leaders' power base influence the leader's choice of style? Third, what should the leader choose for a group whose members are at different levels of maturity?

An important issue in situational leadership is the value placed on the accomplishment of tasks and on the interpersonal relationships between leader and group members and among group members. For example, the nurse manager encourages input from staff members when planning daily work assignments so that the needs of both staff and clients are met. The nurse manager may also solicit input from staff members when doing both short-range and long-range planning for the unit. However, when a new staff member is being oriented to the unit, the nurse manager may be more directive in making

assignments until the staff member develops experience and professional maturity. In emergency situations or situations in which the task needs to be completed quickly, the nurse manager may be more authoritative in directing the actions of all staff members.

Transformational leadership theory, which was developed in the 1980s, "reconsiders the characteristics of the leader-manager, reemphasizes the vision that the leader-manager shares with the group, and stresses the importance of preparing people for change (Tappen, 1995, p. 99). This model combines elements of earlier theories and recognizes the influence of the leader, workers, tasks, and environment. Transformational leadership is characterized by four primary factors (Tappen 1995, pp. 99–100):

1. *Charisma.* Charismatic leaders are highly respected and are viewed with reverence, dedication, and awe. They set high standards, challenging their staff to go beyond the expected level of effort.

2. *Inspirational motivation.* The leader shares visions with the staff that appeal to both their emotions and their ideals.

3. *Intellectual stimulation.* The leader stimulates followers to question the status quo: to question critically what they are doing and why.

4. *Contingent reward.* The leader recognizes mutually agreed-upon goals and rewards the employee's achievements.

It is expected that transformational leadership will become critically vital in the creation of a health care system that embodies community well-being, basic care for all, cost-effectiveness, and holistic nursing care. The transformational leader is a myth-maker and storyteller, painting vivid descriptions of an inspiring, uplifting future everyone will build together. A recent survey of 2500 health care leaders identified six factors in transformational leadership that will effect these changes as we move into the 21st century: (1) mastering change, (2) systems thinking, (3) shared vision, (4) continuous quality improvement, (5) an ability to redefine health care, and (6) a commitment to serving the public and community (Trofino, 1995, p. 45).

Caring leadership is a concept that is an extension of transformational leadership. The term *caring leadership* was introduced in 1991 by a Fortune 500 executive, who stated: "Good management is largely a matter of love. Or if you're uncomfortable with the word call it caring, because proper management involves caring for people, not manipulating them" (Brandt, 1994, p. 68). Caring leadership recognizes the importance of caring in the practice of nursing, combining concepts from both caring and leadership theories.

Effective leadership is a learned process requiring an understanding of the needs and goals that motivate people, the knowledge to apply the leadership skills, and the interpersonal skills to influence others. Much has been written about effective leadership and style; some descriptive statements about effective leaders are listed in the box at the left. Humanistic leadership can serve as a means of creating an environment "that is stimulating, motivating, and empowering to the professional nurse" (Glennon, 1992, p. 41). Strategies for humanistic and caring leadership are identified in the box below.

Characteristics of Effective Leaders

- Use a leadership style that is natural to them.
- Use a leadership style appropriate to the task and the members.
- Assess the effects of their behavior on others and the effects of others' behavior on themselves.
- Are sensitive to forces acting for and against change.
- Express an optimistic view about human nature.
- Are energetic.
- Are open and encourage openness, so that real issues are confronted.
- Facilitate personal relationships.
- Plan and organize activities of the group.
- Are consistent in behavior toward group members.
- Delegate tasks and responsibilities to develop members' abilities, not merely to get tasks performed.
- Involve members in all decisions.
- Value and use group members' contributions.
- Encourage creativity.
- Encourage feedback about their leadership style.

Strategies for Putting Humanistic and Caring Leadership into Action

- Praise or positively recognize staff and colleagues.
- Always think good thoughts about yourself and others.
- Work on discovering group members' unique personal and professional needs.
- Always give before you get—give colleagues and staff a reason for doing whatever it is that you are asking of them.
- Smile often—it generates enthusiasm and goodwill.
- Recognize the expertise of others.
- Remember the names of the people you work with.
- Think, act, and look successful.
- Always greet others with a positive, affirmative statement.
- Foster an atmosphere of collegiality and mutual trust.
- Write informal appreciation notes; this shows appreciation and reinforces positive performance.
- Get out of the nurse's station or office; make a point of circulating among those who work in your circle of influence.
- Foster creativity, independence, and professional growth.
- Talk less and listen more; encourage communication and the sharing of ideas and information.
- Don't condemn, criticize, or complain; instead, work on ways to improve the situation or solve the problem.
- Accept responsibility.

SOURCES: Adapted from "Empowering Nurses through Enlightened Leadership" by T. K. Glennon, Spring 1992, *Revolution: The Journal of Nurse Empowerment, 2,* pp. 40–44; and "Caring Leadership: Secret Path to Success" by M. A. Brandt, August 1994, *Nursing Management, 25,* pp. 68–72.

- nursing leaders you admire. What characteristics of leadership do they have that you admire? Are there characteristics that you don't like? What leadership style or styles do they employ to influence others? Do they emphasize one style or several styles? Are the nursing leaders you admire well liked by other colleagues and health professionals? Is it important to be liked when you are a leader?
- nursing heroes past and present. What qualities of leadership do they share? How important is risk taking to effective leadership?
- your own leadership activities. What characteristics of leadership do you have? What leadership style or styles are you most comfortable with? How might you improve your abilities as a leader?

NURSING MANAGEMENT

As a manager and provider of client care, the nurse coordinates various health care professionals and their services to help the client meet desired outcomes.

Theories of Management Style

Concern with management practices began in the latter part of the 19th century, as the United States began emerging as a leading industrial nation. Early management theory focused on how to get as much work as possible from each worker. The oldest and most widely accepted viewpoint on management is called the *traditional, or classical, viewpoint.*

The traditional style stresses the manager's role in a strict hierarchy and focuses on efficient and consistent job performance. Traditionalists are concerned with the formal relations among an organization's departments, tasks, and structural elements, and they stress the manager's role in a hierarchy. Superiors are assumed to have greater expertise and are therefore to be obeyed by subordinates. Time-and-motion studies, Gantt charts, and the development of early management principles were the work of the traditionalists. Characteristics of traditional management include adherence to routines and rules, impersonality, division of labor, hierarchy, financial motivation, and authority structure. The benefits of the traditional style include efficiency, consistency, clear structure, and an emphasis on productivity (Hell-

riegel & Slocum, 1993, pp. 41–44). Although most traditionalists today recognize the emotional and humanistic component of management, the focus on efficient and effective job performance remains overriding. Many managers and health care organizations still use the traditional management style today.

The expansion of labor unions in the 1930s, the Great Depression, and World War II heralded another era in management theory. Against the backdrop of change and reform, managers were forced to focus on the humanistic side of managing organizations. *Behavioral theory* moves beyond the traditionalists' mechanical view of the work world and stresses the importance of group dynamics and the leadership style of the manager. The behavioral viewpoint includes the following four basic assumptions (Hellriegel & Slocum, 1993, p. 56):

1. Workers are motivated by social needs and get a sense of identity through their associations with one another.
2. Workers are more responsive to the social forces exerted by their peers than to management's financial incentives and rules.
3. Workers respond to managers who can help them satisfy their needs.
4. Managers need to coordinate the work of their subordinates democratically in order to improve efficiency.

These assumptions really do not hold true for the workforce of the 1990s. Today's work world is more complex than the work world of the traditionalist and behaviorist. The post–World War II years brought a new management theory, *systems theory*. Just as the human body is a system consisting of organs, muscles, bones, and a circulatory system that links all the parts together, an organization is a system consisting of many departments that are linked by people working together. Systems theory approaches problems by looking at inputs, transformation processes, outputs, and feedback. Inputs are the physical, human, material, financial, and information resources that enter the system and leave as outputs. The technology used to convert the inputs are the transformation processes. Outputs are the original physical, human, material, financial, and information resources that are now in the form of goods and services. A vital part of systems theory is the feedback loops, which provide ongoing information about a system's status and performance. Another vital component of the systems theory is the interaction of the system with the environment. The manager within systems theory is responsible for planning, organizing, leading, and controlling in order to ease the transformation process (Hellriegel & Slocum, 1993, p. 57).

Contingency theory emerged in the mid 1960s in response to managers' unsuccessful attempts to apply traditional, behavioral, and systems concepts to managerial problems. Contingency theory is a blend of these concepts. Using contingency theory, the manager is expected to determine which method or combination of methods will be most effective in a given situation. To apply the contingency viewpoint effectively, the manager must be able to diagnose and understand a situation thoroughly, determine the most useful approach, and recognize the impact of the external environment, technology, and the people involved prior to acting (Hellriegel & Slocum, 1993, p. 61).

The contingency theory of management moves the manager away from the "one size fits all" approach. Managers are encouraged to analyze and understand the differences in each situation, selecting the solution that best suits the organization and individual in each situation.

Management Skills

Management skills fall into four categories: technical, interpersonal, conceptual, and communication (Hellriegel & Slocum, 1993, pp. 25–26).

1. *Technical skills.* Technical skills involve the ability to apply specific methods, procedures, and techniques in a specialized field. Nursing managers may use technical skills in varying degrees but are concerned more with identifying and developing the technical skills that others in the organization need.

2. *Interpersonal skills.* The abilities to lead, motivate, manage conflict, and work with others are a key part of every manager's job. Although we sometimes forget, the most important resource in an organization is the people, and a manager with strong interpersonal skills can be extremely effective.

3. *Conceptual skills.* Conceptual skills involve viewing the organization as a whole. Using thinking and planning abilities assists the manager to set priorities, recognize correlations and patterns, and scan the environment for trends.

4. *Communication skills.* Managers spend a great deal of time communicating with others. The impor-

tance of good written, oral, and nonverbal communication skills cannot be overly stressed. At a time when health care agencies expect managers to work in an ever-changing environment, competent communication skills are a must.

The relative importance and skill mix at each level of management change as one moves from first-line managers to middle and top management. Interpersonal and communication skills are of equal importance to all levels of management. The professional nurse may be promoted into a middle management position because of excellent technical nursing skills. These new managers often rely on their nursing expertise, unaware that they also need to develop other skills associated with business and finance. Duffield (1994, p. 64) explored the responsibilities of first-line managers. She found consensus that the first-line manager is required not only to maintain the technical skills associated with managing client care but also to master the technical skills of finance and business management, such as budget and finance, human resource management, and development of policies and procedures.

The higher a manager's position in the organization, the greater the need for conceptual and interpersonal skills. Many of the responsibilities of top nurse managers, such as allocating resources and developing overall strategies, require a broad outlook and ability to see the "big picture." The ability to provide visionary leadership will become an even more highly valued managerial skill in the coming years. This means creating a vision with which people can identify and to which they can commit (Hellriegel & Slocum, 1993, p. 29). Offering educational programs such as workshops, seminars, and mentor programs is one way the organization and profession can help the new nurse manager build on the knowledge founded on the nursing discipline (Duffield, 1994, p. 63).

Management Roles

Nurses function differently in various types of organizations. An autocratic organization confers primary knowledge and power to one person and places other persons in subordinate roles. Bureaucratic organizations exert control through policy, structured jobs, and compartmentalized actions. Other organizations decentralize control and emphasize self-direction and self-discipline of members. Still another type of organization is the component of a system that interacts interdependently with other components and adapts dynamically to change. This type of organization is particularly beneficial for the nurse who manages the care of individuals, families, and communities. On a larger scale, the nurse manager must work in the organizational framework of the employing agency.

Authority is defined as the official power given by the organization to direct the work of others (Marquis & Huston, 1994, p. 125). It is an integral component of managing. Authority is conveyed through leadership actions; it is determined largely by the situation, and it is always associated with responsibility and accountability.

Accountability is the ability and willingness to assume responsibility for one's actions and to accept the consequences of one's behavior. Accountability can be viewed within a hierarchic systems framework, starting at the individual level, through the institutional/professional level, and then to the societal level. At the individual or client level, accountability is reflected in the nurse's ethical integrity. At the institutional level, it is reflected in the statement of philosophy and objectives of the nursing department and nursing audits. At the professional level, accountability is reflected in standards of practice developed by national or provincial nursing associations. At the societal level, it is reflected in legislated nurse practice acts.

To be successful, the nurse manager must exert authority and assume accountability in implementing the managerial roles of planning, organizing, leading and delegating, and controlling.

Planning

Planning is often considered the first and most basic management function. Planning is a process that includes the following steps (Hellriegel & Slocum, 1993, p. 246):

- *Choosing an organization's mission and objectives.* The mission identifies the business in which the organization is engaged. The organization describes itself in terms of the goods or services it supplies, markets it serves or plans to serve, and the client needs it aims to satisfy. The objectives are the results to be achieved and should be stated in terms of both quality and quantity of results, and target dates should be established.

- *Devising departmental objectives.* The nursing unit should reflect the more global objectives of the nursing department and health care agency.

- *Selecting strategies to achieve objectives.* Strategies are the courses of action the unit staff will take in order to achieve the unit's objectives.
- *Deciding on the allocation of resources.* Distribution of money, personnel, equipment, and physical space is included in resource allocation.

Nurse managers must keep in mind that plans are the means, not the ends. Quick fixes may cause one to neglect the big picture. Planning can help the nurse manager (1) identify future opportunities, (2) anticipate and avoid future problems, and (3) develop strategies and courses of action.

Organizing

Organizing is the formal system of working relationships. The nurse manager is responsible for identifying particular tasks and assigning them to individuals or teams who have the training and expertise to carry them out. Along with organizing, the nurse manager is responsible for coordinating activities to meet the unit's objectives. Health care reform, downsizing, and restructuring have all impacted the management role of organizing.

Leading and Delegating

The beginning of this chapter discussed many of the elements of effective leadership. These elements, even when combined with the motivation to lead and basic leadership skills, will not necessarily make an effective leader; power is also an essential component of leading. **Power** is defined as "the ability to make things happen the way one wants it to happen" (Hellriegel & Slocum, 1993, p. 472). Frameworks for understanding power are discussed in Chapter 22.

Another component of leading is *delegating*. The delegation function in the health care field is often complex because of the number and diversity of caregivers, the amount of different knowledge and skills needed to provide care, and the intricacy of the relationships among staff, client, and environment (Tappen, 1995, p. 307).

Delegation is a major tool in making the most efficient use of time. Delegation is a high-level implementation skill. To delegate effectively, the nurse must be aware of the needs and goals of the client and family, the nursing activities that can help the client meet the goals, and the skills and knowledge of various nursing and support personnel.

In delegating, the nurse must also determine how many and what type of personnel are needed. This information may be indicated on the client's records.

Other sources of information are the client, the charge nurse, other nursing personnel, and the nurse's own judgment. Nurses may require assistance to give client care quickly in certain situations and to ensure the client's safety.

After establishing that assistance is required, the nurse must identify what type of help is needed, how long help will be required, when it will be required, and what assistance is available. Before beginning the nursing activity, the nurse must arrange for assistance, usually by asking the appropriate person on the unit. Delegation does not require that the nurse have the personal knowledge and expertise to perform a specific nursing activity, but it does require that the nurse know who does have the knowledge

and expertise. For example, the nurse may call the dietitian to assist a client in choosing foods from a menu or request a social worker to assist a client who needs financial assistance and homemaker services after discharge.

An important aspect of delegation is the development of the potential of nursing and support personnel. By knowing the background, experience, knowledge, skill, and strengths of each person, a nurse can delegate responsibilities that help develop each person's competence. Nursing personnel to whom aspects of care have been delegated need to be supervised and evaluated. The amount of supervision required is highly variable and depends on the knowledge and skills of each person. As the person who assigns the activity and observes the performance, the nurse contributes to the evaluation process. Because individual motivation varies, the nurse needs to realize that not all persons perform equally. Thus, the nurse must evaluate standards of performance against written job descriptions, rather than by comparing one person's performance to that of another. It is essential, too, for the nurse to realize that people require ongoing feedback about their performance and to give feedback, including both positive and negative input, in an objective manner.

Characteristics of effective nurse managers as described by Sullivan and Decker (1988, p. 576) are listed in the accompanying box.

Controlling

Controlling is a method to ensure that behaviors and performances are consistent with the planning process. Control is not something managers do *to* employees, but rather *with* them. Formal, structured, bureaucratic controls, such as tightly written job descriptions, extensive rules and procedures, and top-down authority, are familiar control mechanisms. Increasingly in health care agencies, more flexible controls such as continuous quality improvement (CQI), shared governance, and team building help make control an easier and integral part of the management process.

The discussion of management roles would be incomplete without a few words on "the games people play" within the world of work. A lack of understanding of the politics of work can cause even the most competent and committed nurse to feel helpless and frustrated.

Many nurses feel that being politically astute is a genetic trait, that they have neither the ability nor

---

Characteristics of Effective Nurse Managers

- Have a face; that is, they join committees and groups and "work the crowd."

- Prepare themselves by pursuing educational programs that are directed toward their goals.

- Present a positive image; that is, they know the unwritten dress code and follow it, and their carriage and energy proclaim confidence.

- Demonstrate an above-average grasp of written and oral communication skills, expressing themselves clearly, concisely, and with impact.

- Network effectively. They have a circle of people internally and externally from whom to draw information and support. They carry business cards so as to be ready to validate new liaisons.

- Have mentors and sponsors and a clear awareness of the responsibilities and obligations inherent in these types of relationships.

- Know their organization's values (i.e., where their organization is headed and why).

- Do not wound the lion or lioness; that is, they know the "hot buttons" and do not push them or publicly make moves that discredit themselves or others.

- Mobilize resources. Know who or what can be of help in given situations and how to mobilize these resources.

- Have a vision of what may or could be and assume leadership in moving toward those goals.

SOURCE: *Effective Management in Nursing* (2nd ed.) by E. J. Sullivan and P. J. Decker, 1988, Redwood City, CA: Addison-Wesley Nursing, pp. 576–577. Reprinted with permission.

desire to "get involved in that political mess." These nurses soon discover that power and politics are inevitable in today's workplace. First, there will always be those people who will do anything to obtain and hang on to power. Second, hard work is usually measured by the manager in charge, not by the rules and regulations on the top shelf. Menke and Ogborn (1993, pp. 35–37) describe the following behaviors that nurses should develop to negotiate the politics of the workplace.

1. *Read the environment.* Observe where the power lies in the organization. Historically, power has rested in those who bring in the money and those who supply the resources for those in power.

2. *Listen.* Listen to everyone, everywhere. Move slowly, and don't be anxious to exhibit everything you know.

3. *Read.* Read organizational charts, policies and procedure statements, and professional journals. Learn to identify what is "hot" and what is not.

4. *Detach.* Don't hook up with people who are on the losing side. Detach and stay independent until you know the political ropes.

5. *Analyze.* Identify your own potential weaknesses. For example, are you the only male, the only nurse with a baccalaureate degree, or the only newcomer? If so, you may have to work a little harder to achieve your goal.

6. *Create competence.* A firm handshake, offering your name, and politeness never go out of style. Summarizing your project status with your manager while sharing credit for success when due keeps your manager aware of what is going on.

7. *Never gossip about the manager.* Keep the manager from being blind-sided and embarrassed. Don't whine!

8. *Always roll with the punches.* Remain enthusiastic! The nurse may never like being in the political game, but being knowledgeable will make it easier to understand and survive it.

CONSIDER...

- the organizational structure of your practice setting. How many levels of management are there? How many of these levels are managed by nurses? Identify advantages and disadvantages to having nurses in mid-level and high management positions in health care organizations.

- the activities of nurse managers at the unit level of your practice setting. What management activities do they perform? What management activities do staff nurses perform? What management activities do you perform? How do the management responsibilities of the staff nurse differ from those of the nurse manager? What is the relationship between good unit management and effective client care?

- the experience and educational background of nurse managers at all levels of your organization. What are their clinical nursing experiences? What is their education? Do they have formal or informal education in management or business? Do the experience levels and educational backgrounds differ among nurse managers at different levels of organizational or unit management? How could you best prepare yourself for management responsibility?

NURSING DELIVERY MODELS

Common configurations for the delivery of nursing care include the case method, the functional method, team nursing, primary nursing, case management, managed care, differentiated practice, and shared governance.

Case Method

Case method nursing, also referred to as *total care*, is one of the earliest models of nursing care. This method was used by private-duty nurses in providing total care to the client (Wywialowski, 1993, pp. 40–41). This method is client centered: One nurse is assigned to and is responsible for the comprehensive care of a group of clients during an 8- or 12-hour shift. For each client, the nurse assesses needs, makes nursing plans, formulates diagnoses, implements care, and evaluates the effectiveness of care. In this method, a client has consistent contact with one nurse during a shift but may have different nurses on other shifts. The case method, considered the precursor of primary nursing, continues to be used in a variety of practice settings, such as intensive care nursing. With the shortage of nursing personnel during World War II, the case method could no longer be the chief mode of care for clients. To meet staff shortages, managers hired personnel with less educational preparation than the professional nurse and developed on-the-job training programs for auxiliary helpers. The case method became unfeasible in such situations, and the functional method was developed in response.

Functional Method

The **functional nursing method,** which evolved from concepts of scientific management used in the field of business administration, focuses on the jobs to be completed. In this task-oriented approach, personnel with less preparation than the professional nurse perform less complex care tasks. The functional method is based on a production and efficiency model that gives authority and responsibility to the person assigning the work, for example, the nurse manager. Clearly defined job descriptions, procedures, policies, and lines of communication are required. The functional approach to nursing is economical and efficient and permits centralized direction and control. Its disadvantages are fragmentation of care (the client receives care from several different categories of nursing personnel) and the possibility that nonquantifiable aspects of care, such as meeting the client's emotional needs, may be overlooked.

Team Nursing

In the early 1950s, Eleanor Lambertsen (1953) and her colleagues proposed a system of team nursing to overcome the fragmentation of care resulting from the task-oriented functional approach and to meet the increasing demands for professional nurses created by advances in technologic aspects of care. **Team nursing** is the delivery of individualized nursing care to clients by a nursing team lead by a professional nurse. A nursing team consists of registered nurses, licensed practical nurses, and, often, nursing assistants. This team is responsible for providing coordinated nursing care to a group of clients during an 8- or 12-hour shift. Compared to the functional system, team nursing emphasizes humanistic values and responds to the needs of both clients and employees. It emphasizes individualized client care on a personal level rather than task-oriented care on an impersonal level. The professional nurse leader motivates employees to learn and develop skills and instructs them, supervises them, and provides assignments that offer the potential for growth.

Primary Nursing

Primary nursing, a system in which one nurse is responsible for total care of a number of clients 24 hours a day, 7 days a week, was introduced at the Loeb Center for Nursing and Rehabilitation in the Bronx, New York. Primary nursing is a method of providing comprehensive, individualized, and consistent care.

Primary nursing uses the nurse's technical knowledge and management skills. The primary nurse assesses and prioritizes each client's needs, identifies nursing diagnoses, develops a plan of care with the client, and evaluates the effectiveness of care. Associates provide some care, but the primary nurse coordinates it and communicates information about the client's health to other nurses and health professionals. Primary nursing encompasses all aspects of the professional role, including teaching, advocacy, decision making, and continuity of care. The primary nurse is the first-line manager of the client's care, allocating resources and directly communicating with other care providers (Lyon, 1993, p. 166).

Case Management

Case management, a more recent model of nursing care delivery, was pioneered at the New England Medical Center in the 1980s. Initially, public health and psychiatric-mental health nurses served as case managers. Today, case management is used in insurance-based programs, employer-based health programs, workers' compensation programs, maternal-child health settings, mental health settings, and hospital-based nursing practice. Case management as defined in some hospitals may bear little resemblance to the community health models. Although the nurse in primary or team nursing models is often referred to as the case manager, the true purpose of the case management model is to assist the client through a complex, fragmented health care system across many settings, without undue costs, and with enhancement of the quality of life (Lyon, 1993, p. 164).

Although various case management models are in place throughout the United States, all share five common goals (Christensen & Bender, 1994, p. 67):

1. Outcomes that are based on standards of care

2. Well-coordinated continuity of care through collaborative practice patterns

3. Efficient use of resources to reduce wasted time, energy, and materials

4. Timely discharge within diagnostic-related group (DRG) length of stay parameters

5. Professional development and satisfaction

The activities of case management require the nurse to integrate a variety of disciplines and services in coordinating care throughout the client's span of illness (Allred, Arford, Michel, Veitch, Dring & Carter, 1995, p. 33). Collaboration, coordination, information processing and information exchange are imperative in this role. The case manager role differs from the traditional role of the nurse manager or staff nurse. A lack of understanding of this role in the midst of the changing health care environment can cause confusion for the case manager, nurse manager, and staff nurse.

According to Bower (1992, p. 25), the American Nurses Association (ANA) recommends that case managers have a minimum educational preparation of a baccalaureate in nursing and 3 years of clinical experience.

Shared Governance

Marelli (1993, p. 97) describes **shared governance** as "an organizational model that gives staff the authority for decisions, autonomy to make those decisions, and control over the implementation and outcomes of the decisions." The focus of this model is to encourage nurses to participate in decision making at all levels of the organization, either at their own request or as part of their job criteria. More commonly, nurses participate through serving in decision-making groups, such as committees and task forces. The decisions they make may address employment conditions, cost-effectiveness, long-range planning, productivity, and wages and benefits. The underlying principle of shared governance is that employees will be more committed to the organization's goals if they have had input into planning and decision making. In the past decade, over 1000 hospitals in the United States have implemented a shared governance design for nursing. During the next decade, whole-system shared governance, which moves into community-based care, will need to be explored (Porter-O'Grady, 1995, p. 187).

Porter-O'Grady (1994b, p. 187) sees shared governance as a tool that facilitates the maturing of the nursing professional: "It has facilitated the creation of a structure supportive of behaviors reflecting an adult, collaborative, and active decision-maker in any clinical partnership that will advance the integrative role of the nurse and the care of the patient."

Managed Care

Managed care is a method of organizing care delivery that emphasizes communication and coordination of care among health care team members. Managed care differs from case management in that it is unit based and designed to promote and support care at the client's bedside in the acute-care setting. Case management may be used as a cost-containment strategy in managed care. Managed care has gained popularity with the health care reform movement in the United States. "Managed care is viewed as a system that provides the generalized structure and focus when managing the use, cost, quality, and effectiveness of health care services" (Cohen & Cesta, 1993, p. 33).

Both case management and managed care use critical pathways to track the client's progress. **Critical pathways** are treatment plans that all health team members use to plan the sequence of client care based on medical diagnosis and projected length of stay (see Chapter 4). The current status and anticipated future of the health care system are pushing for efficiency and effectiveness, are emphasizing outcomes and decreased use of unnecessary resources, and are promoting client satisfaction (Capuano, 1995, p. 34). Often, critical pathways focus on high-cost, high-volume areas involving many physicians and specialties. Critical pathways become a tool necessary for the financial survival of a delivery system within a managed care environment. Providing high-quality care within a highly regulated environment requires the identification and elimination of excessive, inefficient systems and a high degree of collaboration. The involvement of physicians, clinical nurse specialists, and a multidisciplinary staff are key to developing and implementing successful critical pathways.

Differentiated Practice

Differentiated practice is a structure of providing care that allows nurses to carry out various roles and functions, according to their education, experience, and competence. Differentiated practice models recognize the broad domain of professional nursing, the multiple roles and responsibilities that nurses assume, and the contribution of all nursing personnel as valuable and unique. Differentiated practice can improve client care and contribute to client safety. Used effectively, differentiated practice models allow for the effective and efficient use of resources. Most important, if used properly, differentiated practice increases nurses' ability to provide safe, effective care based on their expertise and, in turn, increases their professional satisfaction (Koerner & Karpiuk 1994, p. 10).

As early as 1967, a Harvard Business School research project identified the role of differentiated practice in nursing. Not only are technical tasks involved but also such factors as time frame, space, personal development, ethical action, interpersonal effectiveness, critical thinking and commitment to lifelong learning. As the nursing paradigm changes, the areas of communication and critical thinking, rather than technical skills, expand. The American Hospital Association sees the need for differentiated practice in responding to change in the health care system, client acuity, payment systems, and reward systems (Allender, Egan & Newman, 1995, p. 42). Differentiated practice models include nurses prepared at all educational levels: bachelor's degree, master's degree, and doctorate, recognizing the diversity of these roles.

The newer models of case management, managed care, differentiated practice, and shared governance may be the keys to meeting the demands of the future by (1) increasing demand for quality and excellence in service across the continuum of care; (2) facilitating the use of appropriate, efficient skill mix and delivery of client-centered care; (3) reducing health care costs; and (4) rewarding performance based on measured team outcomes, including the value of interdependent contributions (Wenzel 1995, p. 62).

CONSIDER...

- your own experience with the various nursing delivery models. Which models do you prefer, and why? Which models promote the value of the professional nurse? Are there models that tend to devalue the abilities of the professional nurse?
- key factors in determining the appropriate-ness of a specific nursing delivery model for a specific practice setting. Are there models of nursing delivery that are more appropriate for some practice settings and less appropriate for others?
- how you might implement a different model of nursing delivery in your current practice setting.

MENTORS AND PRECEPTORS

Mentoring has been widely used as a strategy for career development in nursing during the last 20 years. Mentors are "competent, experienced professionals who develop a relationship with a novice for the purpose of providing advice, support, information, and feedback in order to encourage development of the individual" (Schutzenhofer, 1995, p. 487). Most nursing literature describes the nurse-mentor relationship as important for career development in nursing administration or nursing education. Through mentoring, the experienced nurse can also foster the professional growth of the new graduate, who may choose to mentor those who follow. Marriner-Tomey (1992, p. 210) describes three phases to the mentoring process:

1. *The invitational stage.* In this stage, the mentor must be willing to use time and energy to nurture an individual who is goal directed, willing to learn, and respectfully trusting of the mentor. The nurse-mentor invites the new nurse to share knowledge, skill, and personal experiences of professional growth.

2. *The questioning stage.* In this stage, the novice experiences self-doubt and fear of being unable to meet the goals. The mentor helps the protégé clarify goals and the strategies for achieving them, shares personal experiences, and serves as a sounding board and a source of support during times of doubt.

3. *The transitional stage.* In this stage, the mentor assists the protégé to become aware of the protégé's own strengths and uniqueness. The protégé now is able to mentor someone else.

In the clinical area, the term **preceptor** is used to describe mentoring relationships in which the experienced nurse assists the new nurse in improving clinical nursing skill and judgment. The preceptor also instills understanding of the routines, policies, and procedures of the institution and the unit.

Mentors provide support. Often, the mentor relationship is one of teacher-learner. The mentor instructs the protégé in the expected role, introduces the protégé to those who are important to the achievement of goals, listens to and helps the protégé evaluate ideas in light of institutional policy, and challenges the protégé to advance professional practice. Marriner-Tomey (1992, p. 210) describes a mentor as "a confidant who becomes a role model and a sounding board for decision making."

Nurses who wish to improve and advance their professional practice, whether in education, administration, or clinical practice, should seek mentors to assist them. Mentors usually are of the same sex, 8 to 14 years older, and have a position of authority in the organization. Most are knowledgeable individuals who are willing to share their knowledge and experience. Mentors often choose protégés because of their leadership or managerial qualities. Mentoring is a process that can promote the personal and professional growth of both mentor and protégé.

CONSIDER...

- your own mentoring experiences. Were you mentored or did you seek out a mentor as a new graduate or as a new employee in a new practice setting? What qualities would you seek in a mentor? If you were mentored, how did your mentor assist you in your socialization to your work setting, the organization, the nursing profession?
- whether there are or should be differences between mentors and preceptors? If there are differences, what are they?
- your own ability to mentor a new graduate or new employee. What knowledge, attitudes, and skills do you have that would make you an effective mentor? What knowledge, attitudes, and skills do you need to become an effective mentor? How will you develop the knowledge, attitudes, and skills?

NETWORKING

To function effectively in all nursing roles, but especially in leadership and management roles, the nurse needs to network with other professionals. Marriner-Tomey (1993, p. 175) describes **networking** as a process in which people communicate, share ideas and information, and offer support and direction to each other. Networking builds linkages with people throughout the profession, both within and outside the work environment. Getting to know people helps build a trust relationship that can facilitate the achievement of professional goals. It is easier to access people one knows than it is to access strangers.

Networking is a long-term, deliberate process, a powerful tool for building relationships. Networking requires time, commitment, and follow-through (Andrica, 1994, p. 284). Networking is an opportunity for nurses to develop their careers, share information, organize for political action, and effectively promote change (Strader & Decker, 1995, p. 481). Active membership in professional organizations may be the nurse's most important networking tool. Other networking opportunities include (1) continuing-education or university classes, (2) socializing with professional colleagues, and (3) keeping in touch with former professors and nursing associates. Strader and Decker (1995, p. 482) offer a few important tips in networking: Be discreet, deliver on your promises, and don't burn bridges.

CHANGING TIMES

Health Care Reform

"There is no question that health care is at the limit of its resources. The forces driving a newer profile for the health care system are many and varied, and rival anything previously conceived in both complexity and intensity" (Porter-O'Grady, 1994, p. 34).

The old paradigm of health care focused on the following (Porter-O'Grady, 1994, p. 35):

1. Rewarding sickness. Frequently, health care workers received payment only when someone became ill.

2. Lack of preventive services and personal accountability for health.

3. A design created primarily for and by physicians and based on a medical model of health.

4. A triad of payors, physicians, and hospitals, which did not respond well to change outside the established system.

5. High costs. Health care under the established system was the single largest budget item in the federal government.

The ANA has recognized the need for nursing to take action toward reform. Historically, nursing has been blocked from having any great power in health care decisions. Hospital-based nursing services usually have been reimbursed under billing codes for "daily room rate," a practice that deemphasizes and devalues the knowledge and skill that a nurse brings to the client's care. In the health care reform debate, male-dominated groups, such as health care insurers, hospital administrators, physicians, and the medical-industrial complex, appear to have minimized the importance of nursing in major decision-making directed toward an improved health care system. For the key components of Nursing's Agenda for Health Care Reform (ANA, 1991a) see Chapter 4.

In preparation for upcoming health care reform, health care agencies have instituted two measures: downsizing and restructuring of patient care delivery.

Downsizing

Downsizing is a polite term for layoffs: employer cuts in human resources in order to reduce expenses. Downsizing is not exclusive to health care: Virtually all industries, from manufacturing to service industries, have experienced some degree of downsizing in recent years. Russ (1994, pp. 66–67) offers the following strategies to help nurses prepare for potential downsizing:

1. *Network.* Reestablish your network by calling a colleague for career or personal advice. Participate in meetings of professional nursing organizations.

2. *Update your résumé.* Even if you have a secure job, an updated résumé reflecting your accomplishments and future goals is important. Occasionally "testing the waters" to brush up on your interview skills and seeing what positions are available in the market may also be advisable.

3. *Develop a portfolio.* Keep documentation of your previous work accomplishments. Reports, memos, completed projects, and published articles that reflect your achievements and potential should be neatly compiled for future employers.

4. *Compile a reference list.* Keep a list of people with whom you have worked and who will attest to your merits. Be sure to get permission to use a contact and always send written thanks.

5. *Remain active during the layoff period.* "Sleeping in" will not get you a new position. Rather, continue to attend professional meetings and social gatherings and to investigate employment agencies, want ads, and human resource departments.

6. *Fight depression, denial, and anger.* These are common responses to downsizing. Don't burn bridges and "bad mouth" your old employer. Remember to remain positive and keep your cup half full, not half empty!

Reengineering

Downsizing, reorganization, computerization, and decentralization of services may reshape business structure, but they do not necessarily reengineer how those services are delivered. Health care administrators view reengineering as a way to enter the 21st century with a flexible, lean, efficient corporation. The single largest reengineering program in the health care industry is called *patient-focused care.*

Health care consultants and analysts view the current model of service delivery as inefficient, fragmented, and expensive. Patient-focused care entails components that require reengineering of health care (Richardson, 1995, pp. 31–34):

1. *Hospital architecture.* Self-sufficient service units replace departments. The clients in these units have commonality of care, often reflecting DRG groupings.

2. *Teams.* Specialized self-governed teams responsible for delivery of services are organized. These self-directed work teams may be constructed or titled differently, but all focus on developing an intact work group responsible for the entire work process.

3. *Information technology.* To reduce the amount of time nurses spend writing, scheduling, and communicating, up-to-date technology is essential. Automated medication dispensers, bedside computers, voice messaging, pneumatic tubes, and fax machines are common in the reengineered environment.

4. *Multiskilling and cross-training.* In the most common from of multiskilling and cross-training, a staff member who is skilled in one discipline obtains the knowledge and skill of another discipline. The staff member goes through the process of obtaining licensure, if required. For example, many respiratory therapists are currently seeking licensure as registered nurses. A more cost-effective development is the creation of the generic health care worker. Depending on the needs of the agency, the multiskilled worker would receive prescribed training. Currently, many colleges and universities have introduced programs for certification in multiskilled health care practitioners.

Much controversy surrounds patient-focused care. Clearly, there is a financial benefit: Estimates of a 40% decrease in personnel costs are commonly quoted. Health care consultants and administrators also maintain that patient-focused care increases satisfaction among clients, staff, and physicians alike. Some consultants, however, state that patient-focused care reduces the number of staff having contact with a patient during a stay by 75% (Clouten & Weber, 1994, p. 35).

CONSIDER...

- the role of the professional nurse in a changing health care system. What new knowledge, attitudes, and skills are essential for the nurse to prepare for the changes in health care?
  How can the nurse best prepare for changes in health and nursing care delivery?
- the concept of the multiskilled worker and the historical work activities of nursing. Are there activities that other health care professionals or paraprofessionals currently do that previously were done by nurses? How might this merging of roles affect nursing? How might it affect the other health care professionals and paraprofessionals?

SUMMARY

Leadership and management are the responsibility of all professional nurses. Knowledge of the different, yet intertwined, roles of leader and manager are vital to nurses' ability to work within the health care system.

The ability of the professional nurse to advocate for clients is linked to leadership and management skills. As an individual, family, or community advocate, professional nurses may offer a wide variety of support and services.

Leadership styles include charismatic, authoritarian, democratic, laissez-faire, situational, and transformational. Effective leadership is a learned process involving understanding of the needs and goals that motivate others and interpersonal skills to influence others.

Management involves the basic functions of planning, organizing, leading, and delegating. The degree to which a nurse carries out these functions depends on the position the nurse holds in the organization. Regardless of degree, authority and accountability remain important to the process.

Nursing delivery models include the case method, the functional method, team nursing, primary nursing, case management, managed care, differentiated practice, and shared governance. Emphasis on efficiency, outcomes, cost-effectiveness, and client satisfaction have become buzzwords within the newer delivery models.

READINGS FOR ENRICHMENT

Covey, S. R. (1989). *The 7 habits of highly effective people: Powerful lessons in personal change.* New York: Simon and Schuster.

This national best-seller presents a paradigm of seven habits, starting with three self-mastery habits that move a person from dependence to independence (private victories), and followed by other habits that move a person toward effective interdependence (public victories). The seven habits become the basis of a person's character, "creating an empowering center of correct maps from which an individual can effectively solve problems, maximize opportunities, and continually learn and integrate other principles in an upward spiral of growth." (p.52). Covey inspires readers to integrate personal, family, and professional responsibilities into their lives. He emphasizes the need to restore the "character" ethic in our society. The character ethic is based on the idea that there are *principles* that govern human effectiveness.

Johnson, J. E., Costa, L. L., Marshall, S. B., Moran, M. J., & Henderson, C. S. (June 1994). Succession management: A model for developing nursing leaders. *Nursing Management, 25,* 50–55.

This article describes a management system that assists motivated individuals to enter and ascend the management hierarchy. Authors discuss key steps in developing the program, creating management options for nurses, and promoting the program's effectiveness.

Mentors and preceptorships should be encouraged. Mentoring and preceptorships can assist in the personal and professional growth of both the novice and professional nurse.

Personal integrity, honesty, and a concern for human dignity should guide all the nurse's leadership and management decisions.

SELECTED REFERENCES

Allender, C. D., Egan, E. C., and Newman, M. A. (1995). An instrument for measuring differentiated nursing practice. *Nursing Management, 26*(4), 42–45.

Allred, C. A., Arford, P. H. Michel, Y., Veitch, J. S., Dring, R., & Carter, V. (1995). Case management: The relationship between structure and environment. *Nursing Economics, 13*(1), 32–41.

American Nurses Association. (1991a). *Nursing's agenda for health care reform.* Washington, D.C.: ANA.

American Nurses Association. (1991b). *Standards of clinical nursing practice.* Washington, D.C.: ANA.

Andrica, D. C. (1994). Networking: To do or not to do and how to. *Nursing Economics, 12*(8), 284.

Bleich, M. R. (1995). Managing and leading. In P. S. Yoder-Wise (Ed.), *Leading and Managing in Nursing* (pp. 2–21). St. Louis: Mosby-Year Book.

Bower, K. A. (1992). *Case management by nurses.* Washington, D.C.: American Nurses Association.

Brandt, M. A. (1994). Caring leadership: Secret and path to success. *Nursing Management, 25*(8), 68–72.

Capuano, T. A. (1995). Clinical pathways. *Nursing Management, 26*(1), 34–37.

Christensen, P., & Bender, L. (1994). Models of nursing care in a changing environment: Current challenges and future directions. *Orthopaedic Nursing, 13*(2), 64–70.

Clark, C. M., Steinbinder, A., & Anderson, R. (1994). Implementing clinical paths in a managed care environment. *Nursing Economics, 12*(4), 230–234.

Clouten, K., & Weber, R. (1994). Patient-focused care: Playing to win. *Nursing Management, 25*(2), 34–36.

Cohen, E. L. & Cesta, T. G. (1993). *Nursing case management: From concepts to evaluation.* St. Louis: Mosby-Year Book.

Curtin, L. (1994). 25 years: A slightly irreverent retrospective. *Nursing Management, 25*(6), 9–32.

Douglass, L. M. 1992. *The effective nurse: Leader and manager.* St Louis: Mosby-Year Book.

Duffield, C. (1994). Nursing unit managers: Defining a role. *Nursing Management, 25*(4), 63–67.

French, J. R. & Raven, B. H. (1960). The bases of social power. In D. Cartwright & A. Zanders (Eds.). *Group dynamics: Research and theory* (2nd ed.). New York: Harper and Row.

Glennon, T. K. (1992, Spring). Empowering nurses through enlightened leadership. *Revolution: The Journal of Nurse Empowerment, 2,* 40–44.

Hellriegel, D., & Slocum, J. W. (1993). *Management* (6th ed.). Reading, MA: Addison-Wesley.

Koerner, J. G., & Karpiuk, K. L. (1994). *Implementing differentiated nursing practice.* Gaithersburg, MD: Aspen.

Lambertsen, Eleanor C. *Nursing Team—Organization and Functioning.* Published for the Division of Nursing Education by the Bureau of Publications, Teachers College, Columbia University, 1953.

Leddy, S., & Pepper, J. M. (1993). *Conceptual bases of professional nursing* (3rd ed.). Philadelphia: Lippincott.

Lyon, J. C. (1993). Models of nursing care delivery and case management: Clarification of terms. *Nursing Economics, 11*(3), 163–169.

Marelli, T. M. (1993). *The nurse manager's survival guide: Practical answers to everyday problems.* St. Louis: Mosby-Year Book.

Marriner-Tomey, A. (1992). *Guide to nursing management* (4th ed.) St. Louis: Mosby-Year Book.

Marriner-Tomey, A. (1993). *Transformational leadership in nursing.* St. Louis: Mosby-Year Book.

Marquis, B. L., & Huston, C. J. (1994). *Management decision making for nurses* (2nd ed.) Philadelphia: Lippincott.

Menke, K., & Ogborn, S. E. (1993). Politics and the nurse manager. *Nursing Management, 23*(12), 35–37.

Mundinger, M. (1994). Health care reform: Will nursing respond? *Nursing & Health Care, 15*(1), 28–33.

Nightingale, F. (1992). *Notes on nursing: What it is and what it is not.* Philadelphia: Lippincott. (Original work published 1859).

Pederson, A., & Easton, L. S. (1994). Teamwork: Bringing order out of chaos. *Nursing Management, 26*(6), 34–35.

Porter-O'Grady, T. (1994a). Building partnerships in health care: Creating whole systems change. *Nursing & Health Care, 15*(1), 34–38.

Porter-O'Grady, T. (1994b). Whole systems shared governance: Creating the seamless organization. *Nursing Economics, 12*(4), 187–195.

Richardson, T. (1995, Summer). Patient focused care. *Revolution: The Journal of Nursing Empowerment,* 31–34, 37–38.

Russ, A. (1994). Downsizing: A survival kit for employees. *Nursing Management, 25*(8), 66–67.

Schutzenhofer, K. K. (1995). Power, politics and influence. In P. S. Yoder-Wise, *Leading and managing in nursing.* St. Louis: Mosby-Year Book.

Stearley, H. (1995, Summer). Patient focused care: Is it the end of hospital nursing? *Revolution: The Journal of Nursing Empowerment,* 40–43.

Strader, M. K., & Decker, P. J. (1995). *Role transition to patient care management.* East Norwalk, CT: Appleton & Lange.

Sullivan, E. J., & Decker, P. J. (1988). *Effective management in nursing* (2nd ed.). Menlo Park, CA: Addison-Wesley Nursing.

Tappen, R. M. (1995). *Nursing leadership and management: Concepts and practice* (3rd ed.). Philadelphia: F. A. Davis.

Trofino, J. (1995). Transformational leadership in health care. *Nursing Management, 26*(8), 42–47.

Wenzel, K. (1995). Redesigning patient care delivery. *Nursing Management, 26*(8), 60–62.

Wywialowski, E. (1993). *Managing client care.* St. Louis: Mosby-Year Book.

Yoder-Wise, P. S. (1995). *Leading and managing in nursing.* St. Louis: Mosby-Year Book.

11

CHAPTER

Research Consumer

by Divina Grossman

OBJECTIVES

- Discuss the steps of the research process.

- Describe the nurse's role in protecting the rights of human subjects in research.

- Differentiate the qualitative from the quantitative approaches in nursing research.

- Identify the criteria for using research in nursing practice.

- Evaluate critically the dimensions of a research report.

"Nursing is essentially a special type of human caring. Some perceive human caring and science to be antithetical. Science, for some, conjures up images of test tubes, laboratories and increasing remoteness from the real world. This is not the whole story…. [Science] is a means of achieving the kind of caring that is not simple sentiment, but a kind of caring that includes deliberate, scientifically selected action. Science can be an effective tool of the humanist. It is not his enemy."

—Rosemary Ellis, 1970

A national newspaper health columnist (Brody, 1991) wrote, "The Florence Nightingales of the nation are busily adding a Louis Pasteur component to their profession." This statement reflects the growing public recognition of the role that nurses play in generating research to help deliver quality and cost-effective care and to help clients and families cope with illness.

- Nursing research is more than just scientific investigation conducted by a person educated and credentialed as a nurse. It refers instead to research directed toward building a body of nursing knowledge about "human responses to actual or potential health problems" (American Nurses Association [ANA], 1980, p. 9) and to the effects of nursing action on human responses. The human responses may be (a) reactions of individuals, groups, or families to actual health problems, such as the caregiving burden on the family of an older individual with Alzheimer's disease; and (b) concerns of individuals and groups about potential health problems, such as accident prevention or stress management in a factory or assembly plant.
- Nursing research also reflects the traditional nursing perspective. In this view, the client is seen as a whole person with physiologic, psychologic, spiritual, social, cultural, and economic aspects:

  For example, when a person has a head injury, the nurse needs to understand the body's processes for dealing with the increased pressure within the head and the changes this brings about in the patient's condition. At the same time, the nurse focuses on care that can maintain the person's cognitive, that is, thinking and feeling processes. A nurse would also examine the person's life patterns that could lead to other head injuries. (Roy, 1985, pp. 2–3)

- In addition to reflecting the concern for the whole person, a nursing perspective implies 24-hour responsibility. Thus, this viewpoint encompasses all of the factors in a client's environment, such as fatigue, noise, sensory deprivation, nutrition, and positioning, that may influence coping patterns. Diers (1979, pp. 13–15) identifies three distinguishing properties of nursing research:

1. The final focus of nursing research must be on a difference that matters for improving client care.
2. Nursing research has the potential for contributing to developing theory and the body of scientific knowledge.
3. A research problem becomes a nursing problem when nurses have access to and control over the phenomena being studied.

WHY NURSING RESEARCH IS FUNDAMENTAL

The information revolution that is transforming the present and shaping the future has made reading, understanding, and using nursing research as fundamental to professional practice as the knowledge of asepsis, application of the nursing process, and communication skills. Polit and Hungler (1995, pp. 3–4) cite four reasons why research is important in nursing:

1. As a profession, nursing needs research to evolve and expand a scientific body of knowledge that is unique and separate from other disciplines.
2. Research is important to maintain nursing's scientific accountability to clients, families, and the public in general.
3. The current concerns regarding the economics and efficacy of health care require nursing to document through research how its services contribute to health care delivery.
4. When multiple interventions are possible in a given client-care situation, nursing research is essential to the clinical decision-making process.

HISTORY OF NURSING RESEARCH

As early as 1854, Florence Nightingale demonstrated the importance of research in the delivery of nursing care. When Nightingale arrived in the

Crimea in November of 1854, she found the military hospital barracks overcrowded, filthy, rat- and flea-infested, and lacking in food, drugs, and essential medical supplies. As a result of these conditions, men died from starvation and such diseases as dysentery, cholera, and typhus (Woodham-Smith, 1950, pp. 151–167). By systematically collecting, organizing, and reporting data, Nightingale was able to institute sanitary reforms and significantly reduce mortality rates from contagious disease.

Although the Nightingale tradition influenced the establishment of American nursing schools in 1873, the research approach did not take hold until the beginning of the 20th century. Recognizing the need, nursing leader Isabel Stewart integrated research into the graduate nursing curriculum at Teachers College,

Columbia University and published the first research journal in nursing, the *Nursing Education Bulletin*, in the late 1920s. The journal *Nursing Research* was established in 1952 to serve as a vehicle to communicate nurses' research and scholarly productivity (Donahue, 1985, pp. 449–452). The publication of many other nursing research journals followed, some dedicated to research and others combining clinical and research publications. See the boxes at the left.

Today, nurses are actively generating, publishing, and applying research in practice to improve client care and enhance nursing's scientific knowledge base. The *Standards of Clinical Nursing Practice* published by the American Nurses Association (1991) include research as one of the standards of professional performance. The investigative functions of nurses at various educational levels was also previously addressed by the ANA's Commission on Nursing Research (1981). See the box at the right and on page 204.

Examples of Research Journals in Nursing

Nursing Research
Advances in Nursing Science
Image: The Journal of Nursing Scholarship
Research in Nursing and Health
Western Journal of Nursing Research
Applied Nursing Research
International Journal of Nursing Studies
Scholarly Inquiry for Nursing Practice

Examples of Clinical and Specialty Nursing Journals that Publish Research

Nursing Outlook
American Journal of Nursing
MedSurg Nursing
Journal of Gerontologic Nursing
Journal of Neuroscience Nursing
Heart and Lung
American Journal of Critical Care
Journal of Pediatric Nursing
Journal of Professional Nursing
Journal of Nursing Education
Journal of Nursing Administration
Nursing Administration Quarterly

American Nurses Association's Standard of Professional Performance Pertaining to Research

Standard VII: RESEARCH

The nurse uses research findings in practice.

Measurement Criteria:

1. The nurse uses interventions substantiated by research as appropriate to the individual's position, education, and practice environment.

2. The nurse participates in research activities as appropriate to the individual's position, education, and practice environment. Such activities may include:

  • Identification of clinical problems suitable for nursing research.

  • Participation in data collection.

  • Participation in a unit, organization, or community research committee or program.

  • Sharing of research activities with others.

  • Conducting research.

  • Critiquing research for application to practice.

  • Using research findings in the development of policies, procedures, and guidelines for client care.

SOURCE: *Standards of Clinical Nursing Practice* by the American Nurses Association, 1991, Washington, D.C.: Author.

Investigative Functions of Nurses at Various Educational Levels

Associate Degree in Nursing

- Demonstrates awareness of the value or relevance of research in nursing.

- Assists in identifying problem areas in nursing.

- Assists in collecting data within an established, structured format.

Baccalaureate Degree in Nursing

- Reads, interprets, and evaluates research for applicability to nursing practice.

- Identifies nursing problems that need to be investigated and participates in the implementation of scientific studies.

- Uses nursing practice as a means of gathering data to refine and extend practice.

- Applies established findings of nursing and other health-related research to nursing practice.

- Shares research findings with colleagues.

Master's Degree in Nursing

- Analyzes and reformulates nursing practice problems so that scientific knowledge and scientific methods can be used to find solutions.

- Enhances the quality and clinical relevance of nursing research by providing expertise in clinical problems and by providing knowledge about the way in which these clinical services are delivered.

- Facilitates investigations of problems in clinical settings through such activities as contributing to a climate supportive of investigative activities, collaborating with others in investigations, and enhancing nursing's access to clients and data.

- Conducts investigations for the purpose of monitoring the quality of the practice of nursing in a clinical setting.

- Assists others to apply scientific knowledge in nursing practice.

Doctoral Degree in Nursing or a Related Discipline

- Provides leadership for the integration of scientific knowledge with other sources of knowledge for the advancement of practice.

- Conducts investigations to evaluate the contribution of nursing activities to the well-being of clients.

- Develops methods to monitor the quality of the practice of nursing in a clinical setting and to evaluate contributions of nursing activities to the well-being of clients.

Graduate of a Research-Oriented Doctoral Program

- Develops theoretical explanations of phenomena relevant to nursing by empirical research and analytic processes.

- Uses analytic and empirical methods to discover ways to modify or extend existing scientific knowledge so that it is relevant to nursing.

- Develops methods for scientific inquiry of phenomena relevant to nursing.

SOURCE: *Guidelines for the Investigative Functions of Nurses* by the American Nurses Association, Commission on Nursing Research, 1981, Kansas City, MO: Author.

In 1985, the United States Congress passed a bill creating a Center for Nursing Research in the National Institutes of Health (NIH) to house the research activities conducted by the Division of Nursing at the Department of Health and Human Services (DHHS). In 1993, the Center for Nursing Research was promoted to the Institute for Nursing Research, gaining equal status with other institutes within the NIH. In 1993, nursing scientists recommended that research priorities for the years 1995 to 1999 include developing community-based nursing models, promoting behaviors that prevent AIDS in women, devising ways to remedy cognitive impairment, and helping clients cope with chronic illness (*American Journal of Nursing*, 1993, p. 70).

The American Nurses Association's Cabinet on Nursing Research formulated in 1985 a set of priority goals to advance nursing research in the 21st century. These goals, listed in the box at the right, include the development of a cadre of nurse scientists by the year 2000. Currently, there are 62 doctoral programs in nursing and some 75 nursing research centers in the United States (Sigma Theta Tau International, 1995). The breadth and diversity of nursing research is reflected in examples of nursing studies shown in the box at the right.

American Nurses Association's Priorities for Nursing Research in the 21st Century

1. To ensure an increased supply of nurse scientists by the year 2000.

2. To generate knowledge about well-being and optimum functioning of human beings, the effective delivery of nursing services, excellence in nursing education, and the impact of the profession on health policy.

3. To develop environments that support nursing inquiry, including opportunities to initiate and implement nursing investigations and access to subjects, personnel, research facilities, and equipment.

4. To disseminate the results of nursing research to clinicians, the scientific community, the general public, and health policy makers and to increase the use of the results.

SOURCE: *Directions for Nursing Research: Toward the Twenty-First Century* by the American Nurses Association, Cabinet of Nursing Research, 1985, Kansas City, MO: Author.

Examples of Nursing Studies

Cole and Slocumb (1995) explored factors influencing the practice of safer sex behaviors in heterosexual male adolescents and young adults.

Grossman, Jorda, and Farr (1994) compared blood pressure rhythms in school-age children of normotensive and hypertensive parents.

Libbus and Russell (1995) examined the congruence of decisions between patients and their potential surrogates about life-sustaining therapies.

McCarthy, Daun, and Hutson (1993) evaluated the effects of meperidine on the febrile response on Sprague-Dawley rats injected with bacterial endotoxin.

Good (1995) compared the effects of jaw relaxation and music, individually and combined, on sensory and affective pain in patients following abdominal surgery.

Stiles (1994) described the application of phenomenology in delineating the meaning of spiritual relationship between hospice nurses and families.

Kalisch and Kalisch (1995) examined the experiences of nurses who served in Bataan and Corregidor during World War II.

Brown and Grimes (1995) evaluated patient outcomes of nurse practitioners and nurse midwives as compared with those of physicians in primary care.

Coyne, Baier, Perra, and Sherer (1994) determined the effect of the elevation of the head of the bed after diagnostic coronary angiography on patient comfort and on the incidence and timing of postprocedural complications.

Zeimer, Cooper, & Pigeon (1996) evaluated the effectiveness of a polyethylene film dressing with a perimeter adhesive system in reducing nipple pain and improving nipple skin condition in breast-feeding women.

NURSING KNOWLEDGE

Every discipline has its own way of generating, organizing, and testing knowledge. In nursing, the decisions made and the actions taken are based on different types of knowledge. Carper (1978, pp. 13–23) discussed four types of nursing knowledge.

Empirical Knowledge

Otherwise known as science, **empirical knowledge** is systematically organized into theories and laws for the purpose of describing, explaining, and predicting phenomena. The science of nursing requires factual, objective, and verifiable evidence to explain relationships among phenomena.

A nurse who tells a client who is about to receive an intravenous dye injection prior to an intravenous pyelography (IVP), "Mr. Jones, you will feel warm and flushed immediately after receiving the injection," is providing sensory information. Research has established that such information reduces client anxiety and distress. This type of nursing intervention before a diagnostic test is based on empirical knowledge gained through research conducted by Johnson and colleagues (1972, 1974).

Esthetic Knowledge

Esthetic knowledge, referred to as the art of nursing, is gained by subjective acquaintance and direct feeling of experience. According to Orem (1971), the art of nursing is "expressed by the individual nurse through creativity and style in designing and providing nursing that is effective and satisfying" (p. 155).

A nurse who discerns pain and discomfort from nonverbal cues displayed by the client and who proceeds to smooth the bed linens, reposition the client, and offer a dose of pain medication is demonstrating the use of esthetic knowledge, or the art of nursing.

Personal Knowledge

Personal knowledge is a type of knowledge considered in nursing to be the most difficult to master and to teach. Personal knowledge involves the "therapeutic use of self," emphasizing the knowing, encountering, and actualizing of the client's individual self. Carper (1978, p. 16) states that personal knowledge is "concerned with the kind of knowing that promotes wholeness and integrity in the personal encounter, the achievement of engagement rather than detachment…."

As an example, a nurse who had been caring for a client over a period of a few days suddenly found that "something was wrong. I became afraid something would happen." Less than a half-hour after the nurse's observation, the client progressed into full-blown pulmonary edema and had to be moved to the critical care unit. The nurse in this situation drew on an intimate and personal knowledge of the client and applied it in the assessment and intervention.

Ethical Knowledge

Ethical knowledge derives from a moral code dictating that nurses are responsible for promoting health, relieving suffering, and preserving life. Ethics focuses on nurses' moral obligations: what is good, what is right, or what ought to be done in certain situations. When a nurse advocates on behalf of a critically ill client who expresses a wish not to be placed on a ventilator because, "I do not want to suffer anymore," the nurse exercises a nursing action that is motivated by ethical knowledge.

CONSIDER…

- how your own knowledge of nursing fits into Carper's four types of knowledge: empirical knowledge, esthetic knowledge, personal knowledge, and ethical knowledge. What are the sources of the different types of knowledge that you have (e.g., school, family, culture, religion)?

THE RESEARCH PROCESS

Kerlinger (1986) defines research as "a systematic, controlled, empirical, and critical investigation of natural phenomena guided by theory and hypotheses about presumed relations among such phenomena" (p. 10). Research is the application of the scientific approach to generate empirical knowledge. The steps in the research process are discussed below.

State a Research Question or Problem

The investigator's initial task is to narrow a broad area of interest to a circumscribed problem that specifies exactly the intent of the study. The ideas for research may arise from recurrent problems encountered in practice, questions that are difficult to resolve because of contradictions in the literature, or areas in which minimal or no research has been done.

Research Criteria

In formulating a research problem, Polit and Hungler (1995, pp. 47–49) suggest that three criteria be used: significance, researchability, and feasibility. A research problem has **significance** if it has the potential to contribute to nursing science by enhancing client care, testing or generating a theory, or resolving a day-to-day clinical problem. The question "So what?" must be answered adequately to determine if a research problem is significant.

Researchability means that the problem can be subjected to scientific investigation. Many significant problems that produce ambiguity and uncertainty in clinical situations may not be amenable to research. For instance, "Should nurses support voluntary euthanasia?" is a relevant, timely, and difficult question, but it cannot be answered through research.

Feasibility pertains to the availability of time as well as the material and human resources needed to investigate a research problem or question. Conducting a study involves the use of space, money, equipment, supplies, computers, subjects, research assistants, and consultants.

The following are sample research problems or questions derived from published research:

- What are the effects of biofeedback and progressive muscle relaxation on blood pressure in adults with essential hypertension?
- What are the effects of distraction on perceived pain and behavioral distress in children during an acute pain experience?
- What is the nature of coping and adaptation in clients with implanted cardioverter defibrillators?
- What are the factors associated with the progression of labor pain in primiparas and multiparas?
- What are clients' and nurses' perceptions of the use of physical restraints in the hospitalized elderly?

Dependent and Independent Variables

Research problems contain dependent and independent variables, except for descriptive research, which has no dependent variables. The **dependent variable** is the behavior, characteristic, or outcome that the researcher wishes to explain or predict. The **independent variable** is the presumed cause of or influence on the dependent variable. In the first example above, blood pressure is the dependent variable, whereas biofeedback and progressive muscle relaxation are the independent variables. In the second example, perceived pain and behavioral distress are the dependent variables, whereas distraction is the independent variable.

Define the Study's Purpose or Rationale

The statement of the study's purpose indicates what the researcher intends to do with the research problem identified. The study purpose includes *what* the researcher will do, *who* the subjects will be, and *where* the data will be collected. Depending on the level of research the study purpose may be a declarative statement, an interrogative statement, or a hypothesis (Brink & Wood, 1988, pp. 10–11).

In **Level I research,** the focus is on exploring or searching information because little or nothing is known about the phenomenon under investigation. The study purpose will be in the form of a declarative sentence and will describe what the researcher intends to do. The following is an example:

> The purpose of this study is to examine current nursing practices in the management of infectious or inflammatory fever among adult patients in postsurgical units in Queens Hospital.

In **Level II research,** the investigator asks a question that deals with relationships among concepts or among ideas within a concept. The purpose of the study is then stated in the form of an interrogative sentence or a question, as in this example:

> The purpose of this study is to answer the question, Is there a significant relationship between the circadian characteristics of blood pressure and parental history of essential hypertension in school-age children of normotensive and hypertensive parents examined at home? (Grossman, Jorda, & Farr, 1994, p. 232)

In **Level III research,** the investigator intends to predict the relationships among variables or concepts. The purpose of the study is stated in the form of one of more hypotheses. A **hypothesis** is a predictive statement or a relationship between two or more variables. In research, **variables** refer to attributes that take on different values—such as blood pressure, weight, temperature, and the like. Hypotheses are derived from a review of previous studies or from existing theory. An example of a hypothesis follows:

> The purpose of this study is to test the following hypothesis: Parents attending childbirth education classes at three private community hospitals who perceive greater confirmation of support expectations postnatally will have more positive outcomes, including relationship satisfaction, emotional affect, and attitudes toward the baby. (Coffman, Levitt, & Brown, 1994, p. 111)

Review the Related Literature

Before progressing with the development of the research design, the investigator determines what is known and what is not known about the problem. A thorough review of the literature provides the foundation on which to build new knowledge. Through a literature review, a researcher may also acquire information about available techniques, instruments, and methods of data analysis that have been used in prior research, as well as potential flaws or problems and how to avoid them.

Reviewing the literature enables the investigator to select or develop an appropriate theoretical framework for the research. A **theoretical framework** is a set of abstract and general concepts and propositions that provide a frame of reference for proposed study (Polit & Hungler, 1993, p. 109). Theoretical frameworks guide research "by providing an outline of the phenomena to be investigated, the methods to be used to investigate those phenomena, how theories about these phenomena are to be tested, and how data are to be collected" (Fawcett & Downs, 1992, p. 85). Thus, a nurse researcher who uses Orem's self-care model as a framework for studying educational needs of newly diagnosed type II diabetics will focus on individuals' identified self-care demands. If the same researcher uses King's open systems model, the researcher will view the process of teaching and learning as the interaction personal, interpersonal, and social systems.

Primary and Secondary Sources

In performing a literature review, the researcher focuses on primary rather than secondary sources. A **primary source** is a publication authored by the person who conducted the research investigation. Research articles from *Nursing Research* or *Research in Nursing and Health*, for example, are primary sources. A **secondary source** is a description of a study or studies prepared by someone other than the person who conducted the research. Review articles describing a number of studies on a particular topic are considered secondary sources. In conducting a literature search, a researcher may use secondary sources to identify references that may be pertinent primary sources for the proposed study.

Nursing Research Literature Indexes

The *Cumulative Index to Nursing and Allied Health Literature*, the *International Nursing Index*, and the *Cumulated Index Medicus* are excellent resources for locating published research on a topic or problem of interest. Other databases may also be useful in finding research abstracts: the *Annual Review of Nursing Research*, *Dissertation Abstracts International*, *Nursing Research Abstracts*, and *Psychological Abstracts*, to name a few.

Formulate Hypotheses and Define Variables

Some studies are intended to develop hypotheses, whereas others are intended to test hypotheses using statistical procedures. Hypothesis formulation requires not only sufficient knowledge about a topic to predict the outcome of the study but also **operational definitions,** definitions that specify the instruments or procedures by which concepts will be measured.

An operational definition contains two parts: the definition of the theoretical concept and the empirical indicators. **Empirical indicators** are the instruments or procedures used to measure the theoretical concept. The following are examples of operational definitions:

- *Blood pressure* is the force exerted by the circulating volume of blood on the walls of arteries, as measured by the oscillometric method with a Dinamap™ monitor.
- *Assertiveness* is a personality trait characterized by self-confidence, determination, and the ability to express oneself directly and honestly, as measured by the Rathus Assertiveness Inventory.

In the above examples, the first part of the operational definition describes the theoretical concept, and the second part indicates the instruments or methods used to measure the concept. Thus, the theoretical definition of blood pressure is "the force exerted by the circulating volume of blood on the walls of arteries" and the theoretical definition of assertiveness is "a personality trait characterized by self-confidence, determination, and the ability to express oneself directly and honestly." The empirical indicator for blood pressure is the Dinamap™ monitor, whereas the empirical indicator for assertiveness is the Rathus Assertiveness Inventory.

Select a Research Design to Test the Hypothesis

A research design is "the overall plan for obtaining answers to the research questions and for testing the research hypothesis" (Polit & Hungler, 1993, p. 129). The research design includes the study setting, the sample, the type of data to be collected, as well as strategies to control extraneous variables and reduce bias. There are three major types of research design:

- *Experimental design* is one in which the investigator manipulates the independent variable by administering an experimental treatment to some subjects while witholding it from others. Polit and Hungler (1995, pp. 158–160) describe the three elements of a true experiment:
  a. **Manipulation.** The investigator administers a treatment or intervention to some of the subjects in the study.
  b. **Control.** The investigator institutes some controls over the experimental situation, including the use of a control group.
  c. **Randomization.** The investigator assigns subjects randomly to the experimental or control groups.
- *Quasi-experimental design* is one in which there is manipulation of the independent variable but which lacks either the randomization or control that characterizes true experiments.
- *Nonexperimental design* is one in which there is *no* manipulation of the independent variable. Descriptive, retrospective, prospective, and correlational studies are examples of nonexperimental designs.

Select the Population, Sample, and Setting

At this stage, the researcher chooses the study population, selects a sample, and decides on the setting where the sample can be found. The **population** includes all possible members of the group who meet the criteria for the study. The **sample** is the segment of the population from whom the data will actually be collected.

Sampling is the process of selecting a portion of the population to represent the entire population (Polit & Hungler, 1995, p. 230). The researcher is truly interested in the occurrence of the phenomenon in the population, but because of time and resource constraints can study only a part of the population. Therefore, it is crucial that the sample obtained from the population be *representative*, or reflective of the predominant characteristics of the population.

The two main types of sampling are probability and nonprobability sampling. **Probability sampling** uses random selection to allow every member of the population an equal chance of being included in the sample. In this way, probability sampling reduces bias and ensures a sample that is more representative (Brink & Wood, 1988, p. 123). The most common type of a probability sample is a simple random sample. Here, a numbered list of all the members of the population is drawn and a simple random sample is then selected by means of a table of random numbers, or, in case of a telephone survey, by random digit dialing.

In **nonprobability sampling,** there is less likelihood of obtaining a sample that is representative because subjects are not selected at random. A convenience sample is a type of nonprobability sampling. A convenience sample contains subjects who happen to be available at the time of the data collection. For instance, a researcher who is surveying job satisfaction among staff nurses in downsized hospitals may simply visit different units in the hospital and distribute questionnaires to those nurses who happen to be present. The sampling bias is evident, and it would be difficult to ascertain how the results might be different if most or all of the nurses were present when the questionnaires were distributed.

Conduct a Pilot Study

A pilot study is a "dress rehearsal" before the actual study begins. A trial run of the research procedure is conducted in a few subjects for the following purposes (Polit & Hungler, 1995, p. 263):

- To examine the feasibility of the proposed study
- To test whether the subject recruitment plan is adequate
- To assess whether the instruments to be used are valid and reliable

By identifying any problems or flaws during the pilot study, the investigators can refine the proposed plan and strengthen the research methodology.

Collect the Data

The research process relies on **empirical data,** or information collected from the observable world. Conclusions and generalizations are derived from collected data. The most commonly used methods of collecting data in nursing are questionnaires, rating scales, interview, observation, and biophysical measures.

The validity and reliability of measurement tools need to be established prior to the start of data collection. **Validity** is the degree to which an instrument measures what it is supposed to measure. If a nurse measures anxiety, how would the nurse be sure that what is being measured is not fear or stress, which are related concepts? **Reliability** is the degree of consistency with which an instrument measures a concept or variable. If an instrument is reliable, repeated measurement of the same variable should yield similar or nearly similar results.

The selection of instruments should be dictated by the type of research question being asked, the type of population being studied, the availability of resources to acquire the instrument as well as the researcher's expertise and familiarity with the instrument. Rating scales are easy to administer, but investigators need to be cautious about the possibility of response biases or response sets in the data. A **response-set bias** is the measurement error introduced by the tendency of some people to respond to items in characteristic ways (e.g., always agreeing), independently of the item's content. Interviews tend to produce higher response rates than standardized questionnaires or rating scales, but the costs associated with interviews may be high. Interviewers may have to travel to certain geographic areas to locate the subjects, and each interview may be time consuming. A researcher must be aware of the strengths and weaknesses, advantages and disadvantages of different methods and instruments before making a choice.

Analyze the Data

In this step, the collected data are organized, coded, and analyzed for the purpose of answering the research question or testing the hypotheses. Even before data collection is initiated, there must be a systematic plan for analyzing the results. Data analysis may involve descriptive or inferential statistics. **Descriptive statistics**, procedures that summarize large volumes of data, are used to describe and synthesize data, showing patterns and trends. Descriptive statistics include measures of central tendency and measures of variability.

Measures of central tendency describe the center of a distribution of data, denoting where most of the subjects lie. These include the **mean, median,** and **mode. Measures of variability** indicate the degree of dispersion or spread of the data. These include the **range, variance,** and **standard deviation.** See the accompanying box for definitions of these measures. Typically in a research report, the mean (a measure of central tendency) and standard deviation (a measure of variability) are reported together to give the reader an idea of the nature of the data distribution.

The following is an example:

Systolic blood pressure
130 ± 30

The two statistics reported are the mean and the standard deviation. The number 130 indicates the mean systolic blood pressure, whereas 30 represents 1 standard deviation (SD) from the mean. Hence, 1 SD from the mean would include blood pressure from 100 mm Hg to 160 mm Hg (1 SD below to 1 SD above the mean).

Inferential statistics are those that permit researchers to infer whether relationships observed in a sample are likely to oooccur in a large population of concern. They may also be used in a study to draw conclusions about the population based on data collected from the sample. The type of data collected will determine the type of inferential statistical procedure that is used. By way of illustration, when two groups are being compared with respect to a numerical variable such as weight or blood pressure, a t-test may be used. A *t-test* is a statistical test used to determine whether two groups are significantly different from each other. When the relationship between two categorical variables is being examined, such as nurses' religion and their opinion regarding voluntary euthanasia (whether they agree

> ### Definitions of Measures of Central Tendency and Variability
>
> #### *Central Tendency*
>
> *mean* A measure of central tendency, computed by summing all scores and dividing by the number of subjects; commonly symbolized as $\overline{X}$ or M.
>
> *median* A measure of central tendency, representing the exact middle score or value in a distribution of scores; the median is the value above and below which 50% of the scores lie.
>
> *mode* The score or value that occurs most frequently in a distribution of scores.
>
> #### *Variability*
>
> *range* A measure of variability, consisting of the difference between the highest and lowest values in a distribution of scores.
>
> *variance* A measure of variability or dispersion, equal to the square of the standard deviation.
>
> *standard deviation* The most frequently used measure of variability, indicating the average to which scores deviate from the mean; commonly symbolized as SD or S.

with it or not), then the appropriate test will be a chi-square. A *chi-square* is a test of statistical significance used to assess whether a relationship exists between two variables. It is symbolized as X^2.

Statistical Significance

Nurse researchers attempt to determine after data have analyzed whether the results were **statistically significant.** Underlying this statement is the notion of probability. By convention, p (probability) less than 0.05 is considered the acceptable level of significance. A p value greater than 0.05 is considered statistically *in*significant. In research, the desire is to generalize beyond the sample, so there is a need to determine the probability that the results were due to chance or a "fluke" rather than a true occurrence in the population. Hence, a p value of 0.05 means that the probability of the findings being caused by chance alone is 5 in 100 (Munro, Visintainer & Page, 1983, p. 50).

Null Hypothesis and Statistical Significance

The **null hypothesis** is the basis for statistical significance testing. The null hypothesis states that there is no difference found in the study. To illustrate, the null hypothesis of a study may be, "There is no difference in client compliance between the clients followed by a physician (MD) and the clients followed by a nurse practitioner (NP)."

If the findings reveal a p value of .002, then the null hypothesis will be rejected, which is the same as stating that a statistically significant difference was found between the clients followed by the MD and the clients followed by the NP. If the results show a p value of .13, then the null hypothesis will be accepted, which means that *no* statistically significant difference was found between the two groups.

Communicate Conclusions and Implications

Implicit in conducting research is the requirement to share the knowledge generated with others, either through publication in professional journals or by reporting the results verbally at professional conferences. Interpreting the results, communicating the findings, and suggesting directions for further study conclude the research process.

APPROACHES TO NURSING RESEARCH

There are two major approaches to investigating diverse phenomena in nursing research. These approaches originate from different philosophical perspectives and use different methods for collection and analysis of data.

Quantitative Research

Quantitative research is defined as "the systematic collection of numerical information, often under conditions of considerable control, and the analysis of that information using statistical procedures" (Polit & Hungler, 1995, p. 24). The quantitative approach is most frequently associated with *logical positivism*, a philosophical doctrine that asserts that scientific knowledge is the only kind of factual knowledge. Quantitative research is often viewed as "hard" science and tends to emphasize deductive reasoning and the *measurable* attributes of human experience.

The following are examples of research questions that lend themselves to a quantitative approach:

- What are the differential effects of continuous versus intermittent application of negative pressure on tracheal tissue during endotracheal suctioning?
- Is the auscultatory method effective in validating the location of a feeding tube? (Metheny, McSweeney, Wehrle, & Wiersema, 1990)
- Are there differences in the occurrence and size of bruises resulting from low-dose heparin therapy when administered in the abdomen, thigh, and arm? (Stewart-Fahs & Kinney, 1991)

Qualitative Research

Qualitative research is defined as "the systematic collection and analysis of more subjective narrative materials, using procedures in which there tends to be a minimum of researcher-imposed control" (Polit & Hungler, 1995, p. 24). Data are usually collected using structured methods and procedures and are analyzed using a number of statistical procedures.

The qualitative approach allows for exploration of the subjective experiences of human beings, a more holistic view that places value on the perceptions of clients and nurses in the nursing context (Taylor, 1993, p. 171). In the qualitative approach, no formal instruments are used; instead, loosely structured, narrative data are collected (Polit & Hungler, 1995, p. 15). Using the inductive method, data are analyzed by identifying themes and patterns that emerge from the data. The qualitative approach would be appropriate for the following types of research questions:

- What is the nature of the bereavement process in spouses of clients with terminal cancer?
- What is the nature of coping and adjustment after a radical prostatectomy?
- What is the process of family caregiving for older family relatives with Alzheimer's dementia as experienced by the caregiver?

PROTECTING THE RIGHTS OF HUMAN SUBJECTS

Because nursing research usually focuses on humans, a major nursing responsibility is to be aware of and to advocate on behalf of clients' rights. All clients must be informed about the consequences of consenting to serve as research subjects. The client needs to be able to assess whether an appropriate balance exists between the risks of participating in a study and the potential benefits, either to the client or to the development of knowledge.

Research ethics not only protects the rights of human subjects but also encompasses a broader range of principles. Most of these principles are reflected in the ANA's *Human Rights Guidelines for Nurses in Clinical and Other Research* (1975). These guidelines are based on historic documents, such as the Nuremberg Code (1949) and the Declaration of Helsinki (adopted in 1964 by the World Medical Assembly and revised in 1975), and on United States federal regulations, all of which set standards governing the conduct of research involving human subjects. The notorious Tuskegee study in Alabama, begun in 1932 and ended in 1972, illustrates how subjects' human rights were violated for a period of 40 years while a research study was being conducted. See the accompanying box.

All nurses who practice in settings where research is being conducted with human subjects or who participate in such research as data collectors or collaborators play an important role in safeguarding the following rights.

Right Not to Be Harmed

The Department of Health and Human Services defines **risk of harm** to a research subject as exposure to the possibility of injury going beyond everyday situations. The risk can be physical, emotional, legal, financial, or social. For instance, witholding standard care from a client in labor for the purpose of studying the course of natural childbirth clearly poses a potential physical danger. Risks can be less overt and involve psychologic factors, such as exposure to stress or anxiety, or social factors, such as loss of confidentiality or loss of privacy.

Right to Full Disclosure

Even though it may be possible to collect data about a client as part of everyday care without the client's particular knowledge or consent, to do so is considered unethical. **Full disclosure** is a basic right. It means that deception, either by witholding information about a client's participation in a study or by giving the client false or misleading information about what participating in the study will involve, will not occur.

Right of Self-Determination

Many clients in dependent positions, such as people in nursing homes, feel pressured to participate in studies. They feel that they must please the doctors and nurses who are responsible for their treatment

Lessons from Tuskegee: When Subjects' Rights Are Violated

The Tuskegee study began in 1932 and ended in 1972. The supposed purpose of this study was to determine the natural history of *untreated* syphilis in a population of some 412 mostly poor and illiterate African-American men in Tuskegee, Alabama, an area that had the highest syphilis rate in the nation at the time. The subjects, all of whom were diagnosed with syphilis, were matched against uninfected control subjects. Even when it became known in the 1940s that penicillin was effective in treating syphilis, the drug was withheld from the subjects. Subjects were recruited without informed consent and were falsely promised special treatment, which in this case was a spinal tap performed to establish the neurologic effects of syphilis.

When the ethical violations came to light in 1972 through front-page stories in newspapers, people were outraged. The subsequent initiatives in Congress resulted in the creation of the National Commission for the Protection of Human Subjects in Biomedical and Behavioral Research. The Commission established the conduct for present-day ethical requirements governing the conduct of research on human subjects in the United States (Caplan, 1992, p. 29).

and care. The **right of self-determination** means that subjects should feel free from constraints, coercion, or any undue influence to participate in a study. Masked inducements, for instance, suggesting to potential participants that by taking part in the study they might become famous, make an important contribution to science, or receive special attention, must be strictly avoided. Nurses must be assertive in advocating for this essential right.

Right of Privacy and Confidentiality

Privacy enables a client to participate without worrying about later embarrassment. The anonymity of a study participant is ensured if even the investigator cannot link a specific subject to the information reported. **Confidentiality** means that any information a subject relates will not be made public or available to others without the subject's consent. Investigators must inform research subjects about the measures that provide for these rights. Such measures may include the use of pseudonyms or code numbers or reporting only aggregate or group data in published research.

Nurses who participate in scientific investigations that involve human subjects are in a key position to serve as advocates for research subjects.

RESEARCH UTILIZATION IN NURSING

Research utilization is the process in which study findings are used to initiate and support innovations in the delivery of nursing care. In the 1970s, the lag between publication of research and the transfer of findings into actual practice was recognized. This gap was demonstrated in Ketefian's study (1975, p. 91), in which she found that despite widely published research about the optimal placement time for oral glass thermometers (9 minutes), only 1 of 87 nurses surveyed was aware of the correct placement time.

The Western Interstate Commission for Higher Education (WICHEN) and the Conduct and Utilization of Research in Nursing (CURN) projects were developed to promote the dissemination and utilization of nursing research (Horsley, Crane & Bingle, 1978; Krueger, Nelson & Wolanin, 1978). As a result, research utilization training programs and research-based innovations were implemented.

Studies by Brett in 1987 and by Coyle and Sokop in 1990 revealed that the process of adoption of research-based innovations was consistent with the stages of Rogers' (1983) theory of diffusion innovation. According to this theory, a nurse passes through four stages before adopting research-based ideas or practices:

1. *Knowledge stage*—when a nurse learns about an innovation.

2. *Persuasion stage*—when a nurse develops a positive or negative attitude about the innovation.

3. *Decision stage*—when a nurse determines whether to adopt or reject the innovation.

4. *Implementation stage*—when the nurse uses the innovation regularly.

In Brett's (1987) as well as in Coyle and Sokop's (1990) studies, samples of 279 and 113 nurses, respectively, were asked about their awareness or use of 14 research-based innovations. The innovations were nursing practices that had previously been documented to be effective in prior research. Among the innovations were (1) internal rotation of the femur during injection into the dorsogluteal site, which results in decreased discomfort from the injection; (2) providing the client with sensory information about what the client will feel, see, hear, or taste during a diagnostic procedure, which reduces distress during the procedure; (3) a formally planned and structured preoperative education program before elective surgery, which improves client outcomes; and (4) the fact the clients' urine can be tested for glucose or acetone with equal accuracy using first- or second-voided specimens.

The average adoption scores of the nurses in Brett's (1987) and Coyle and Sokop's (1990) studies indicated that the nurses were in the stage of persuasion. Coyle and Sokop reported that more than half of the nurses in their sample were persuaded of the usefulness of 8 of the 14 research-based nursing practices. The researchers found that the majority of nurses became aware of the innovations through the professional nursing literature, followed by conferences and in-service programs, and observation of others who performed the practice. Further, no significant relationship was found among the adoption of an innovation and such characteristics as the nurse's level of education, years of experiences, professional membership, and time spent in continuing education.

Among clinical nurse specialists (CNS), Stetler and DiMaggio (1991, p. 154) found in field surveys that the most frequent level of research utilization (75%) was conceptual: Subjects used it to enhance their understanding or influence their thinking regarding issues. The remaining 21% indicated that they applied specific components of studies to their practice, mostly after making some modification. There were three categories of situations in which CNSs used research:

1. Complex client care situations through consultation or direct involvement

2. Development or revision of a program or exploration of new activities

3. Development of departmental documents, such as policies, procedures, and standards

Although the sample of the CNSs in Stetler and DiMaggio's (1991) study was small, nonrandom, and confined to one large medical center in New England, the results were congruent with those of studies of research use in non-nursing groups.

Inhibitors and Facilitators of Research Utilization

Factors that inhibit and facilitate the process of using research in clinical settings have been examined. In a survey of 59 nurses in a community hospital, Champion and Leach (1989, p. 705) reported that the availability of research findings and nurses' attitudes toward research were strongly correlated with research utilization. In a sample of 924 nurses, Funk, Champagne, Wiese, and Tornquist (1991, p. 92) found that the factors inhibiting the use of research in practice were the nurses' perceived lack of authority to change client care procedures; insufficient time to implement new ideas; lack of support and cooperation from physicians, administrators, and other staff; inadequate facilities for implementation; and lack of time to read research. In the same study, facilitators of research utilization were identified—enhancing administrative support and encouragement, improving accessibility of research reports, advancing the nurses' research knowledge base, and providing colleague support networks.

In a survey of 543 nurses, Pettengill, Gillies, and Clark (1994, p. 143) found that the factors facilitating research utilization were those that provided nurses with information about research developments. These factors included monthly research newsletters, research meetings, continuing education programs, computer networks, and research study guides. Factors inhibiting research utilization were lack of time, lack of interest among the nursing staff, lack of support from other health care disciplines, and prior negative experience in research activities.

To be able to integrate research as part of day-to-day practice, nurses must work to overcome the inhibitors and perpetuate the facilitators of research utilization. Key strategies for success follow:

- Nurses must develop a positive attitude toward research utilization, viewing it as a tool to attain clinical excellence.
- Nursing administrators need to provide time, facilities, equipment, and support personnel needed for research utilization activities.
- Administrators of hospitals and clinical agencies must create an environment that is conducive to research-based innovation.

Criteria for Research Utilization

If a nurse reads in a research journal that teaching guided imagery to clients was found to be effective in enabling clients to deal with postoperative pain, can the nurse utilize the intervention in his or her own clients? How would a nurse know that the research he or she reads is ready for use in practice?

Haller, Reynolds, and Horsley (1979) formulated criteria for utilization of research in nursing practice, based on the CURN project. These criteria are replication, scientific merit, risk, clinical merit, clinical control, feasibility, cost, and potential for clinical evaluation.

Replication

The criterion of replication requires that the results of a study be replicated a number of times before its findings are accepted as credible and applicable to practice. A change in current practice or procedure cannot be based solely on one study. Establishing a research base of three or more studies confirms that the findings are true and prevents nurses from committing a type I error. A **type I error** is the rejection of a null hypothesis that is true, that is, concluding that the intervention was effective when in reality it was not.

Scientific Merit

The scientific merit of a study is probably the single most important criterion in judging its readiness for application in practice. Scientific rigor is evident in all steps of the research project—the clarity of the research problem, adequacy of the literature review, and the appropriateness of the design, sampling, data collection procedures, and data analytic techniques. The validity and reliability of the instruments used must also be evaluated.

Internal validity and external validity are key concerns in this area. **Internal validity** is the degree to which the independent variable influences the dependent variable. A classic monograph by Campbell and Stanley (1963) discussed factors that threaten internal validity. An example is selection bias if subjects in a study are not randomly assigned to the experimental or control groups. If a statistically significant difference is found, it would be difficult to conclude whether the change in the dependent variable is truly attributable to the independent variable (the intervention) or whether it is related to some preexisting differences between the groups.

External validity pertains to the degree to which the findings of the study can be generalized to similar settings and populations. Even if statistically significant differences are demonstrated, findings can be generalized to other settings or populations only if these settings and populations are similar to those of the study.

Risk

The degree of risk involved in using the findings of a study is another criterion to be considered. Nursing interventions that have been found effective through research may be readily implemented if they carry little risk. According to Haller, Reynolds, and Horsley (1979), risk must be evaluated along with scientific merit. If a protocol entails serious risks, then the evaluation of scientific merit must be applied more stringently.

Clinical Merit

This criterion evaluates the degree to which research findings have the potential to solve an existing problem in the clinical setting. Nurses working in a neonatal nursery may be concerned about the pain that infants experience during blood drawing for laboratory tests or during surgical procedures. For nurses working in this unit, a published study by Campos (1994) that reported the effects of rocking and pacifiers on relieving heelstick pain in infants would be rated high for clinical merit.

Clinical Control

Clinical control refers to the degree to which nurses are in control of the circumstances related to the implementation and evaluation of the research-based innovation. Nurses may not be able to exert clinical control if a research-based protocol requires collaboration or decision making by a team of health professionals. There may also be instruments or methods documented to be effective in research but unavailable to nurses in certain settings.

Feasibility

This is defined as the degree to which resources—time, personnel, expertise, equipment—are available to implement the innovation. For instance, the introduction of a new intervention may require the ordering and purchasing of equipment or supplies and inservice training for nursing staff.

Cost

In this era of downsizing and restructuring, cost is always a vital consideration. Cost is closely related to feasibility. A cost-benefit analysis would be important in order to weigh the costs against the benefits of implementing a new intervention. Benefits may include improved client outcomes or improved staff satisfaction.

Potential for Clinical Evaluation

Potential for clinical evaluation pertains to the degree to which the department variables in the original research base can be evaluated by nurses in the clinical setting. Specifically, this criterion requires that nurses have control over the variables in the protocol and that they possess the knowledge and skills needed to measure the outcome of the innovation.

Clinical Example of Research Utilization

Jane Monroe, RN, is concerned about the use of heparin solution to flush clients' peripheral heparin locks because of the incompatibility between heparin and several drugs administered through the heparin locks (the antibiotics gentamicin and vancomycin, for example). Ms. Monroe hears that other hospitals have changed their flushing procedure by substituting saline for heparin solution. She decides to investigate the issue further by conducting a literature search in the hospital library.

Ms. Monroe not only retrieves several research articles comparing the effects of saline versus heparin solution for flushing heparin locks; she also finds a meta-analysis published by Goode and associates in *Nursing Research* in 1991. A **meta-analysis** is a technique for quantitatively combining and thus integrating the results of multiple studies on a given topic. For Ms. Monroe, the meta-analysis she found compiled the results of 15 studies that compared the effects of saline versus heparin solution on the patency of the peripheral heparin lock, the incidence of phlebitis, and the duration of the catheter.

The findings of the meta-analysis demonstrated no statistically significant differences in the occurrence of clotting (patency), the incidence of phlebitis, and the duration of the catheter when either saline or heparin solution was used for flushing purposes. However, because saline is cheaper than heparin solution, the hospitals in the meta-analysis saved from $19,000 to $40,000 from the change in procedure. Another strong argument for the change is the reported thrombocytopenia, thrombosis, hemorrhage, and drug incompatibility documented in some clients receiving routine doses of heparin solution for flushes.

In this example, all eight criteria for research utilization (listed above) are met. Replication is evident: There are 15 studies in adult medical-surgical or critical care clients that constitute the research base for the innovation. The research base is scientifically sound, with random double-blind designs, and adequate, with large samples used in six studies. The risks to the clients are minimal, whereas the risks associated with continuing heparin flush are potentially serious. The criterion of cost is also met: A vial of saline solution is cheaper than a vial of heparin flush solution.

After carefully evaluating the research articles she has read, Jane Monroe concludes that the research base is ripe for implementation. She presents a report of her findings to the policy and procedure committee at the hospital, which votes to switch from saline to heparin solution in flushing peripheral heparin locks.

Mechanisms for Research Utilization

Research utilization in the clinical setting may occur through a number of mechanisms. There are situations in which research utilization takes place through individual action by nurses. In other cases, research-based protocols are developed by groups of nurses for a unit or hospital and may require changes in existing hospital or agency procedure.

Individual Action

According to the ANA Standards of Clinical Nursing Practice, nurses are expected to use interventions that are based on research. Low-risk, low-cost interventions that have potential to improve client outcomes may be readily implemented by individual nurses. One example is an innovation listed in the Coyle and Sokop (1990, p. 177) study—internal rotation of the femur during dorsogluteal intramuscular injection to reduce client discomfort.

Research-Based Protocols and Procedures

Many hospitals and clinical agencies follow a compendium of policies, procedures, and protocols in specific client care situations. For example, there are procedures to be followed when irrigating a Foley catheter, administering nasogastric tube feeding, or performing wound care. Current research literature must be the basis for developing or revising these procedures or protocols.

Clinical Practice Guidelines

The implementation of research-based clinical practice guidelines from the Agency for Health Care Policy and Research (AHCPR) is another mechanism to use research in the management of specific clinical conditions. The AHCPR guidelines were developed by multidisciplinary panels of experts to assist practitioners and clients in making decisions regarding the efficacy and appropriateness of health care. The guidelines were based on an exhaustive search and analysis of published research and, in areas where research is lacking, used expert opinion and consensus.

Key nursing researchers and clinicians have been members and sometimes chairpersons of these panels. For example, Nancy Bergstrom of the University of Nebraska Medical Center School of Nursing chaired the expert panel that drafted the AHCPR guideline on the prevention of pressure ulcers. The box on the following page shows some recently published AHCPR clinical practice guidelines.

These and other guidelines are available free of cost from AHCPR (1-800-358-9525, or at the Center for Research Dissemination and Liaison, AHCPR Clearinghouse, P.O. Box 8547, Silver Spring, MD 20907).

Product Evaluation

The systematic application of research findings may also be helpful in the evaluation of new products before they are adopted for use in a clinical setting. Janken, Rudisill, and Benfield (1992, p. 188) described how the research utilization strategy was used in their institution to examine a new closed-system catheter for use in the endotracheal suctioning of mechanically ventilated patients. A group of staff nurses, clinical nurse specialists, the director of nursing, and the nurse researcher reviewed recent research literature on endotracheal suctioning. The research findings noted that decreased oxygen saturation was a significant adverse effect for clients who are being suctioned. Thus, the effect of the new closed-system catheter on oxygen saturation was one of the main outcomes that needed to be evaluated.

Selected AHCPR Clinical Practice Guidelines Publications

- *Pressure Ulcers in Adults: Prediction and Prevention*
- *Acute Pain Management: Operative or Medical Procedures and Trauma*
- *Early HIV Infection: Evaluation and Management*
- *Urinary Incontinence in Adults*
- *Acute Low Back Problems in Adults: Assessment and Treatment*
- *Cataract in Adults: Management of Functional Impairment*
- *Depression in Primary Care: Detection, Diagnosis, and Treatment*
- *Sickle Cell Disease: Screening, Diagnosis, Management, and Counseling*
- *Benign Prostatic Hyperplasia: Diagnosis and Treatment*
- *Management of Cancer Pain*
- *Unstable Angina: Diagnosis and Management*
- *Heart Failure: Evaluation and Care of Patients with Left-Ventricular Systolic Dysfunction*
- *Otitis Media with Effusion in Young Children*

Triggers

Factors called triggers, arising from various sources, may serve as a strong stimulus for change in clinical practice. Titler and colleagues (1995, p. 307) reported that triggers are used in the Iowa Model of Research in Practice for infusing research into practice to improve the quality of care.

Triggers may be *problem focused* or *knowledge focused*. Problem-focused triggers are clinical problems that are repeatedly encountered in practice, risk management, and quality improvement (QI) data, and total quality management (TQM) programs. By contrast, knowledge-focused triggers proceed from new or freshly recognized information from credible sources such as standards and practice guidelines from national agencies and organizations, philosophies of care, recent research publications, and nurse experts within the organization.

Research Utilization Groups

The formation of research utilization groups—composed of researchers and nurses—is another mecha-nism that may be used to promote research utilization. Beckstrand and McBride (1990, p. 170) reported how novice researchers (staff nurses) and experienced researchers (nursing faculty) working together successfully addressed the problem of estimating the insertion length of nasogastric tubes (NGT) in children through a review of the research literature and, later, through completed research projects. Research utilization groups may be organized to address specific clinical problems or conditions encountered in the practice setting.

CRITIQUING RESEARCH REPORTS

If professional nurses are to use research, they must first learn to conduct a critical appraisal of research reports published in the literature. A research critique enables the nurse as a research consumer to evaluate the scientific merit of the study and decide how the results may be useful in practice. Critiquing involves intensive scrutiny of a study, including its strengths and weaknesses, statistical and clinical significance, as well as the generalizability of the results.

Polit and Hungler (1993, pp. 383–387) proposed that the following elements be considered in conducting a research critique: substantive and theoretical dimensions, methodologic dimensions, ethical dimensions, interpretive dimensions, and presentation and stylistic dimensions.

- *Substantive and theoretical dimensions.* For these dimensions, the nurse needs to evaluate the significance of the research problem, the appropriateness of the conceptualizations and the theoretical framework of the study, and the congruence between the research question and the methods used to address it.
- *Methodologic dimensions.* The methodologic dimensions pertain to the appropriateness of the research design, the size and representativeness of the study sample as well as the sampling design, validity and reliability of the instruments, adequacy of the research procedures, and the appropriateness of data analytic techniques used in the study.
- *Ethical dimensions.* The nurse must determine whether the rights of human subjects were protected during the course of the study and whether any ethical problems compromised the

scientific merit of the study or the well-being of the subjects.

- *Interpretive dimensions.* For these dimensions, the nurse needs to ascertain the accuracy of the discussion, conclusions, and implications of the study results. The findings must be related back to the original hypotheses and the conceptual framework of the study. The implications and limitations of the study should be reviewed, together with the potential for replication or generalizability of the findings to similar populations.
- *Presentation and stylistic dimensions.* The manner in which the research plan and results are communicated refers to the presentation and stylistic dimensions. The research report must be detailed, logically organized, concise, and well written.

CONSIDER . . .

- problems in your practice setting that might be solved by nursing research. Are the problems you have identified researchable problems?
- resources (libraries, colleges and universities, schools of nursing and so on) that are available in your practice setting and in your community to assist you in researching nursing practice problems.

SUMMARY

Nursing research refers to research directed toward building a body of nursing knowledge about "human responses to actual or potential health problems." Research is important in nursing to expand the scientific body of knowledge, to maintain scientific accountability to the public, to document nursing's contribution to health care delivery, and to provide the bases for sound clinical decision making in client care.

The information revolution that is transforming the present and shaping the future has made reading, understanding, and using nursing research as fundamental to professional practice as are knowledge of asepsis, application of the nursing process, and communication skills. There are four types of nursing knowledge: empirical, esthetic, personal, and ethical knowledge. Empirical knowledge, or scientific knowledge, is generated by the research process. A good nursing research problem meets the criteria of significance, researchability, and feasibility. The Cumulative Index to Nursing and Allied Health Literature, *the* International Nursing Index, *and the* Cumulated Medical

READINGS FOR ENRICHMENT

Laurence, L., & Weinhouse, B. (1994). *Outrageous practices.* New York: Fawcett Columbine.

This book focuses on the lack of research studies related to women's health issues, such as hormone replacement therapy, breast cancer, heart disease in women, menopause, premenstrual syndrome (PMS), and other disease processes that have a higher incidence in women than in men. In many cases, research has been done on exclusively male populations, and women have been purposely excluded because of female-specific hormone changes, physiologic differences, and the potential for pregnancy during the study. The authors also discuss how women are treated differently from men in the health care system. These differences in treatment are grounded in assumptions by both researchers and physicians about women—assumptions based on studies that have been done exclusively in men.

Mateo, M. A., & Kirchoff, K. T. (1991). *Conducting and using nursing research in the clinical setting.* Baltimore: Williams & Wilkins.

This book provides a practical approach to the conduct and use of research for nurses in clinical practice settings. The text addresses issues relevant to practicing nurses who are beginning their involvement in nursing research, especially focusing on research in clinical settings, using research in practice, conducting research and disseminating research findings.

Moore, T. J. (1995). *Deadly medicine.* New York: Simon & Schuster.

This book chronicles the history of multiple studies over approximately 10 years in the effectiveness of cardiac arrhythmia suppressant therapy (CAST) in the treatment of clients diagnosed with cardiac dysrhythmias. It points out how inaccurate assumptions and errors in study design can cause errors in conclusions that can have fatal results in client populations.

Index *are excellent resources for locating published research on a phenomenon of interest.*

The quantitative and qualitative approaches are both valid approaches to investigations of nursing phenomena, although they proceed from different philosophic perspectives and use different methods of data collection and analysis.

The research process is conceptualized as a series of steps or phases that are dynamic and flexible. The steps of the research process provide the tools with which nurse scientists achieve their major aims or goals. These basic aims are to develop explanations of phenomena, called theories, and to find solutions to practical problems.

If nursing is to develop as a research-based practice, the clinical nurse must know the process and language of research, be sensitive to protecting the rights of human subjects, participate in identifying significant researchable problems, and be a discriminating consumer of research findings.

All nurses who practice in settings where research is conducted with human subjects or who participate in research as data collectors or collaborators play an important role in safeguarding the rights of human subjects.

SELECTED REFERENCES

American Journal of Nursing. (1993). Nursing research center is reborn as an institute. *American Journal of Nursing 93*(8), 69–70.

American Nurses Association. (1975). *Human rights guidelines for nurses in clinical and other research.* Kansas City, MO: Author.

American Nurses Association. (1980). *Nursing: A social policy statement.* Kansas City, MO: Author.

American Nurses Association, Commission on Nursing Research. (1981). *ANA guidelines for investigative functions of nurses.* Kansas City, MO: Author.

American Nurses Association, Cabinet on Nursing Research. (1985). *Directions for nursing research: Toward the twenty-first century.* Kansas City, MO: Author.

American Nurses Association. (1991). *Standards of clinical nursing practice.* Kansas City, MO: Author.

Beck, C. T. (1992). The lived experience of postpartum depression: A phenomenological study. *Nursing Research, 41* (3), 166–170.

Beckstrand, J., & McBride, A. B. (1990). How to form a research interest group. *Nursing Outlook, 38* (4), 168–171.

Brett, J. L. L. (1987). Use of nursing practice research findings. *Nursing Research, 36* (6), 344–349.

Brink, P. J., & Wood, M. J. (1988). *Basic steps in planning nursing research* (3rd ed.). Boston: Jones and Bartlett.

Brody, J. E. (1991, August 13). Beyond tender loving care, nurses are a force in research. *New York Times,* p. C3.

Brown, S. A., & Grimes, D. E. (1995). A meta-analysis of nurse practitioners and nurse midwives in primary care. *Nursing Research, 44* (6), 332–339.

Campbell, D. T., & Stanley, J. C. (1963). *Experimental and quasi-experimental designs for research.* Boston: Houghton Miflin.

Campos, R. G. (1994). Rocking and pacifiers: Two comforting interventions for heelstick pain. *Research in Nursing and Health, 17* (5), 321–331.

Caplan, A. L. (1992). When evil intrudes. *Hastings Center Report, 22* (6), 29–32.

Carper, B. A. (1978). Fundamental patterns of knowing in nursing. *Advances in Nursing Science, 1* (1), 13–23.

Caruso, C. C., Hadley, B. J., Shukla, R., Frame, P., & Khoury, J. (1992). Cooling effects and comfort of four cooling blanket temperatures in humans with fever. *Nursing Research, 41* (2) 68–72.

Champion, V. L., & Leach, A. (1989). Variables related to research utilization in nursing: An empirical investigation. *Journal of Advanced Nursing, 14* (9), 705–710.

Coffman, S., Levitt, M. J., & Brown, L. (1994). Effects of clarification of support expectations in prenatal couples. *Nursing Research, 43* (2), 111–116.

Cohen, I. B. (1984). Florence Nightingale. *Scientific American, 250* (3), 128–137.

Cole, F. L., & Slocumb, E. M. (1995). Factors influencing safer sexual behaviors in heterosexual late adolescent and young adult collegiate males. *Image: Journal of Nursing Scholarship, 27* (3), 217–223.

Coyle, L. A., & Sokop, A. G. (1990). Innovation adoption behavior among nurses. *Nursing Research, 39* (3), 176–180.

Coyne, C., Baier, W., Perra, B., & Sherer, B. K. (1994). Controlled trial of backrest elevation after coronary angiography. *American Journal of Critical Care, 3* (4), 282–288.

Czarnik, R. E., Stone, K. S., Everhart, C. C., & Preusser, B. A. (1991). Differential effects of continuous versus intermittent suction on tracheal tissue. *Heart and Lung, 20* (2), 144–151.

Diers, D. (1979). *Research in nursing practice.* Philadelphia: Lippincott.

Donahue, M. P. (1985). *Nursing: The finest art.* St. Louis: Mosby.

Ellis, R. (1970). Values and vicissitudes of the scientist nurse. *Nursing Research, 19* (5), 440–445.

Fawcett, J., & Downs, F. (1992). *The relationship of theory and research.* Norwalk, CT: Appleton-Century-Crofts.

Funk, S. G., Champagne, M. T., Wiese, R. A., & Tornquist, E. (1991). Barriers: The barriers to research utilization scale. *Applied Nursing Research, 4* (1), 39–45.

Good, M. (1995) A comparison of the effects of jaw relaxation and music on postoperative pain. *Nursing Research, 44* (1), 52–57.

Goode, C. J., Titler, M., Rakel, B., Ones, D. Z., Kleiber, C., Small, S., & Triolo, P. K. (1991). A meta-analysis of the effects of heparin flush and saline flush: Quality and cost implications. *Nursing Research, 40* (6), 324–330.

Grossman, D. G. S., Jorda, M. L., & Farr, L. A. (1994). Blood pressure rhythms in early school-age children of normotensive and hypertensive parents: A replication study. *Nursing Research, 43* (4), 232–237.

Haller, K. B., Reynolds, M. A., & Horsley, J. A. (1979). Developing research-based innovation protocols: Process, criteria, and issues. *Research in Nursing and Health, 2* (2), 45–51.

Horsley, J. A., Crane, J., & Bingle, J. D. (1978). Research utilization as an organizational process. *Journal of Nursing Administration, 8* (7), 4–6.

Janken, J. K., Rudisill, P., & Benfield, L. (1992). Product evaluation as a research utilization strategy. *Applied Nursing Research, 5* (4), 188–193.

Johnson, J. E. (1972). Effects of structuring patients' expectations on their reactions to threatening events. *Nursing Research, 21* (6), 499–504.

Johnson, J. E., & Rice, V. H. (1974). Sensory and distress components of pain. Implications for the study of pain. *Nursing Research, 23* (3), 203–209.

Kalisch, P. A., & Kalisch, B. J. (1995). Nurses under fire: The World War II experiences of nurses on Bataan and Corregidor. *Nursing Research, 44* (5), 260–271.

Kerlinger, F. N. (1986). *Foundations of behavioral research* (3rd ed.) New York: Holt, Rinehart, & Winston.

Ketefian, S. (1975). Application of selected nursing research findings into nursing practice. *Nursing Research, 24* (2), 89–92.

Krueger, J. C., Nelson, A. H., & Wolanin, M. O. (1978). *Nursing research: Development, collaboration, and utilization.* Germantown, MD: Aspen Systems.

Libbus, M. K., & Russell, C. (1995). Congruence of decisions between patients and their potential surrogates about life-sustaining therapies. *Image: Journal of Nursing Scholarship, 27* (2), 135–140.

McCarthy, D. O., Daun, J. M., & Hutson, P. R. (1993). Meperidine attenuates the febrile response to endotoxin and interleukin-1 alpha in rats. *Nursing Research, 42* (6), 363–367.

Metheny, N., McSweeney, M., Wehrle, M. A., & Wiersema, L. (1990). Effectiveness of the auscultatory method in predicting feeding tube location. *Nursing Research, 39* (5), 262–267,

Metheny, N., Reed, L., Berglund, B., & Wehrle (1994). Visual characteristics of aspirates from feeding tubes as a method for predicting tube location. *Nursing Research, 43* (5), 282–287.

Munro, B. H., Visintainer, M. A., & Page, E. B. (1986). *Statistical methods for health care research.* Philadelphia: Lippincott.

Orem, D. E. (1971). *Nursing: Concepts of practice.* New York: McGraw-Hill.

Pettengill, M. M., Gillies, D. A., & Clark, C. C. (1994). Factors encouraging and discouraging the use of nursing research findings. *Image: Journal of Nursing Scholarship, 26* (2), 143–147.

Polit, D. F., & Hungler, B. P. (1993). *Essentials of nursing research: Methods, appraisal, and utilization.* Philadelphia: Lippincott.

Polit, D. F., & Hungler, B. P. (1995). *Nursing research: Principles and methods* (5th ed.). Philadelphia: Lippincott.

Rogers, E. (1983). *Diffusion of innovations* (3rd ed.). New York: Free Press.

Roy, C. (1985). Nursing research makes a difference. *Nurses' Educational Funds Newsletter, 4* (1), 2–3.

Sigma Theta Tau International. (1995). Listing of Doctoral Programs in the United States. *Reflections, 21* (3), 18–19, 22–23.

Stetler, C. B., & DiMaggio, G. (1991). Research utilization among clinical nurse specialists. *Clinical Nurse Specialist, 5* (3), 151–155.

Stewart-Fahs, P. S., & Kinney, M. R. (1991). The abdomen, thigh, and arm as sites for subcutaneous heparin injections. *Nursing Research, 40* (4), 204–207.

Stiles, M. K. (1994). The shining stranger: Application of the phenomenological method in the investigation of the nurse-family spiritual relationship. *Cancer Nursing, 17* (1), 18–26.

Taylor, B. (1993). Phenomenology: One way to understand nursing practice. *International Journal of Nursing Studies, 30* (2), 171–179.

Titler, M. G., Kleiber, C., Steelman, V., Goode, C., Rakel, B., Barry-Walker, J., Small, S., & Buckwalter, K. (1995). Infusing research into practice to promote quality care. *Nursing Research, 43* (5), 307–313.

Woodham-Smith, C. (1950). *Florence Nightingale.* London: Constable & Co.

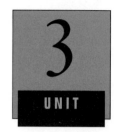

3

UNIT

Processes Guiding Professional Practice

12
CHAPTER

Critical Thinking and Decision Making

by Ruth Pease

OBJECTIVES

- Discuss characteristics, skills, and attitudes of critical thinking.

- Identify the elements of critical thinking according to Paul.

- Discuss the relationship between the nursing process, critical thinking, the problem-solving process, and the decision-making process.

- Explore ways of evaluating critical thinking.

> "Good thinking is hard work. That explains why so few people do it."
>
> — Henry Ford

Nurses must be critical thinkers because of the nature of the discipline and the nature of their work.

- Nurses are expected to solve client problems by performing critical analysis of the factors associated with the problems. This critical analysis, or *critical thinking*, allows the nurse to make better decisions.
- Creativity in thinking, problem solving, and decision making can enhance the effectiveness of the solutions or decisions made. Thus critical thinking, problem solving, and decision making are interrelated processes, with creativity enhancing the result.
- Critical thinking is not limited to problem solving or decision making; professional nurses use critical thinking to make reliable observations, draw sound conclusions, create new information and ideas, evaluate lines of reasoning, and improve their self-knowledge.
- Critical thinking is considered so important to nursing that the National League for Nursing (NLN) has added it as a mandatory criterion for the accreditation of schools of nursing (NLN, 1992).

CRITICAL THINKING

The thinking process that guides nursing practice must be organized, purposeful, and disciplined rather than random or undirected. This type of thinking is called critical thinking. Paul (1988, pp. 2–3) describes critical thinking as "the art of thinking about thinking." It is purposeful thinking in which the thinker systematically and habitually imposes criteria and intellectual standards on the thinking. The thinker is aware of and takes charge of the thinking process, guiding it according to the standards (Paul, 1995). Critical, in this context, does not mean "eager to find fault" but instead "capable of judging carefully and accurately."

Critical thinking is essential to safe, competent, skillful nursing practice (Kataoka-Yahiro & Saylor, 1994). The huge store of knowledge that nurses must use and the continuing rapid growth of this knowledge prevents nurses from being effective practitioners if they attempt to function only on the information acquired in school or outlined in books (Schank, 1990). Reilly and Oermann (1992, p. 217) state that "one cannot think critically about nursing without a basic knowledge of its concepts, theories, and content." As they plan and deliver care, nurses are expected to solve client problems by performing critical analysis of the factors associated with the problems. This critical analysis, or critical thinking, allows the nurse to make better decisions. Decisions that nurses must make about client care and about the distribution of limited resources force nurses to think and act in areas where there are no clear answers or no standardized procedures and where conflicting forces make decisions very complex. Nurses therefore need to embrace the attitudes that promote critical thinking and master critical thinking skills in order to process and evaluate both previously learned and new information.

Nurses use their critical-thinking skills in a variety of ways:

- *Nurses use knowledge from other subjects and fields.* Using insight from one subject to shed light on another subject requires critical thinking skills. Because nurses deal holistically with human responses, they must draw meaningful information from other subject areas (i.e., make interdisciplinary connections) in order to understand the meaning of the client data and plan effective interventions. Nursing students are required to take courses in the biologic and social sciences and in the humanities so that they can acquire a strong foundation on which to build their nursing knowledge and skill. For example, the nurse might use knowledge from nutrition, physiology, and physics to promote wound healing and prevent further injury to a client with a pressure ulcer.
- *Nurses deal with change in stressful environments.* Nurses work in rapidly changing situations. Treatments, medications, and technology change constantly, and a client's condition may change from minute to minute. Routine behaviors may therefore not be adequate to deal with the situation at hand. Familiarity with the routine for giving medications, for example, does not help the nurse deal with a client who is frightened of injections or with one who does not wish to take a medication. When unexpected situations arise, critical thinking enables the nurse to recognize important cues, respond quickly, and adapt interventions to meet specific client needs.

- *Nurses make important decisions.* During the course of a workday, nurses make vital decisions of many kinds. These decisions often determine the well-being of clients and even their very survival, so it is important that the decisions be sound. Nurses use critical thinking skills to collect and interpret the information needed to make decisions. Nurses must, for example, use good judgment to decide which observations must be reported to the physician immediately and which can be noted in the client record for the physician to address later, during the routine visit with the client.

See Table 12–1 describes the characteristics of critical thinking.

TABLE 12–1 Characteristics of Critical Thinking

Characteristic	Explanation	Example
Is rational and reflective.	It is based on reasons and evidence rather than on preference or self-interest. Critical thinkers do not "jump to conclusions." They take the time to collect data, weigh the facts, and think the matter through.	Sarah decided to become a nurse after watching a film in which nurses were shown as attractive and heroic. Michelle, who thinks more critically, asked a counselor about the job opportunities available for nurses. She also talked to several nurses. After gathering and weighing her facts, Michelle decided to go to nursing school.
Involves healthy, constructive skepticism.	Critical thinkers do not accept or reject ideas unless they understand them. They do not mindlessly follow rules but seek to understand the rationale behind them, following those that make sense and working to improve those that do not.	When a salesperson insisted that a new intravenous tubing was better than that being used on Nurse Mackey's unit, Nurse Mackey asked, "What do you mean by 'better'? What information do you have to show that this is so?"
Is autonomous.	Critical thinkers are not easily manipulated. They think for themselves, rather than being led by their peer group or passively accept the beliefs of others.	No one in Lin's family had ever gone beyond high school. Although her sisters did not understand why she wanted to work hard, Lin said, "I've thought it out, and this is what I want to do. I believe it will be worth the effort."
Includes creative thinking.	Critical thinkers create original ideas by finding connections among thoughts and concepts.	Nurse Wilson remembered a song his mother used to sing to him, and sang it to help comfort a frightened child in the hospital.
Is fair thinking.	Critical thinking is not biased or one-sided. Critical thinkers recognize the bias and prejudice of others' thinking. Seeks information from all points of view before taking a stand or action.	Nurse Maria Valdez, the unit manager, needed to make the schedule for the Christmas and New Year's holidays. Before responding to a nurse's request to be off for Christmas, she asked all staff members to submit their preference. Once she was able to determine that staffing was adequate for both holidays, she responded to the nurse's request.
Focuses on what to believe and do.	Critical thinking is used to decide on a course of action; make reliable observations; draw sound conclusions; solve problems; and evaluate policies, claims, and actions.	In the previous examples, Lin, Sarah, and Nurse Valdez decided what to do. Nurse Wilson creatively solved a problem. Nurse Mackey evaluated the salesperson's claim to decide what to believe and, ultimately, what to do.

Creativity, or original thinking, is a major component of critical thinking. When nurses incorporate creativity into their thinking, they are able to find unique solutions to unique problems. **Creative thinking** is thinking that results in the development of new ideas and products (Reilly & Oermann, 1992, p. 217). Creativity in problem solving and decision making is the ability to develop and implement new and better solutions (Strader, 1992, p. 243).

Strader (1992) describes four stages in the creative process: preparation, incubation, insight, and verification. During the *preparation stage*, the creative thinker gathers information related to the problem or concern. During the *incubation phase*, the creative thinker unconsciously considers and works on possible solutions or decisions. All possibilities, both old and new, are considered during this phase. Old possibilities that are considered may include a creative application of an effective solution used in a previous situation that was similar in nature to the present situation. During the *insight stage*, appropriate solutions emerge and are developed, and the solution believed to be most appropriate is implemented. Finally, during the *verification stage*, the implemented solution is evaluated for its effectiveness.

During the first three stages, unconscious, intuitive, and creative thinking occurs that can result in a unique solution to the problem at hand. Creative thinking is required when the nurse encounters a new situation or a client situation where traditional interventions are not effective. For example, Nurse Ned Rodriguez, a pediatric home health nurse, is caring for 9-year-old Pauline, who has ineffective respirations following abdominal surgery. The physician has ordered incentive spirometry (a treatment device that promotes alveolar expansion). Pauline is frightened by the equipment and tires quickly during the treatments. Ned offers Pauline a bottle of blow bubbles and a blowing wand. Pauline is delighted with blowing bubbles. Ned knows that the respiratory effort in blowing bubbles will promote alveolar expansion and suggests that Pauline blow bubbles between incentive spirometry treatments.

Creative thinkers must have knowledge of the problem. They must have assessed the present problem and be knowledgeable about the underlying facts and principles that apply. For example, in the previous situation, Ned knows the anatomy and physiology of respiratory function and is aware of the purpose of incentive spirometry. He also understands pediatric growth and development. In trying to assist Pauline, he builds on his knowledge and comes up with a creative solution. Strader (1992, p. 244) describes creative thinkers as

- Able to generate ideas rapidly.
- Flexible and spontaneous; that is, they are able to discard one viewpoint for another or change directions in thinking rapidly and easily.
- Able to provide original solutions to problems.
- Preferring complex thought processes to simple and easily understood ones.
- Independent and self-confident, even when under pressure.
- Exhibiting distinct individualism.

CONSIDER...

- a recent typical day in your nursing practice. Identify specific times when you had to make complicated choices. Why were they complicated? What kind of thinking helped you to make the decisions?
- a complicated choice you made recently in your personal life or a complex issue you read about. Was your thinking process similar or different from the thinking you use on the job? In what ways?

COGNITIVE CRITICAL THINKING SKILLS

Complex thinking processes such as critical analysis, problem solving, and decision making require the use of cognitive critical thinking skills. For example, when solving problems, nurses make inferences, differentiate facts from opinions, evaluate the credibility of information sources, and use a variety of other cognitive skills (see the box on page 226).

Critical analysis is a set of questions one can apply to a particular situation or idea to determine essential information and ideas and discard superfluous information and ideas. The questions are not sequential steps; rather, they are a set of criteria for judging an idea. Not all questions will need to be applied to every situation, but one should be aware of all the questions in order to choose those questions appropriate to a given situation. Socrates (born about 470 BC) was a Greek philosopher who developed the Socratic method of question and answer. The righthand box on page 226 lists Socratic questions to use in critical analysis. **Socratic questioning** is a technique one can use to look beneath the

Examples of Critical-Thinking Cognitive Skills

- Critical analysis
- Reasoning inductively
- Reasoning deductively
- Making valid inferences
- Differentiating fact from opinion
- Evaluating the credibility of information sources
- Clarifying concepts
- Recognizing assumptions

SOURCE: Adapted from *Critical Thinking* by R. Paul, 1993, Santa Rosa, CA: Foundation for Critical Thinking and Moral Critique, Sonoma State University, pp. 129–130.

Socratic Questions

Questions about the question (or problem)

- Is this question clear, understandable, and correctly identified?
- Is this question important?
- Could this question be broken down into smaller parts?
- How might _____ state this question?

Questions about assumptions

- You seem to be assuming _____; is that so?
- What could you assume instead? Why?
- Does this assumption always hold true?

Questions about point of view

- You seem to be using the perspective of _____. Why?
- What would someone who disagrees with your perspective say?
- Can you see this any other way?

Questions about evidence and reasons

- What evidence do you have for that?
- Is there any reason to doubt that evidence?
- How do you know?
- What would change your mind?

Questions about implications and consequences

- What effect would that have?
- What is the probability that will actually happen?
- What are the alternatives?
- What are the implications of that?

surface, recognize and examine assumptions, search for inconsistencies, examine multiple points of view, and differentiate what one knows from what one merely believes.

Nurses should employ Socratic questioning when listening to an end-of-shift report, reviewing a history or progress notes, planning care, or discussing a client's care with colleagues. When a nurse manager analyzes future trends, plans a change, determines whom to hire or fire, or simply reflects on ideas in print or other media, he or she should also engage in internal dialogue through use of Socratic questions. For example, the nurse asks such questions as: Have I gathered enough evidence to come to a conclusion about this idea? Have I considered a sufficient number of alternatives to come to a reliable nursing diagnosis? Have I considered all the consequences of this potential intervention?

Two other cognitive thinking skills which are used in complex thinking are inductive and deductive reasoning. When using **inductive reasoning,** generalizations are formed from a set of facts or observations. When viewed together, certain bits of information suggest a particular interpretation. For example, the nurse who observes that a client has dry skin, poor turgor, sunken eyes, and dark amber urine may make the generalization that the client is dehydrated. **Deductive reasoning,** by contrast, is reasoning from the general to the specific. The nurse starts with a conceptual framework—for example, Maslow's hierarchy of needs or a self-care framework—and makes descriptive interpretations

of the client's condition in relation to that framework. For example, the nurse who uses the needs framework might categorize data and define the client's problem in terms of elimination, nutrition, or protection needs. In a more simplistic example, inductive reasoning is like looking at the piece of a jigsaw puzzle and attempting to describe the whole (without seeing a picture of the completed puzzle). As the puzzler puts more and more pieces together, the whole picture becomes clearer. In deductive reasoning, the puzzler sees the whole picture (from the box cover) and puts the puzzle together by organiz-

TABLE 12–2 **Differentiating Types of Statements**

Statement	Description	Example
Facts	Can be verified through investigation.	Blood pressure is affected by blood volume.
Inferences	Conclusions drawn from the facts. Go beyond facts to make a statement about something not currently known.	If blood volume is decreased (e.g., in hemorrhagic shock), the blood pressure will drop.
Judgments	Evaluation of facts or information that reflect values or other criteria. A type of opinion.	It is harmful to the client's health if the blood pressure drops too low.
Opinions	Beliefs. Formed over time. Include judgments that may fit facts or be in error.	Nursing intervention can assist in maintaining the client's blood pressure within normal limits.

ing the pieces into border pieces, or colors, or some other grouping.

By using critical thinking, the nurse also differentiates facts, inferences, judgments, and opinions (Table 12–2).

ATTITUDES THAT FOSTER CRITICAL THINKING

Certain attitudes are crucial to critical thinking. These affective dimensions are based on the assumption that a rational person is motivated to develop, learn, and grow. A critical thinker, according to Paul (1995, p. 129) works to develop the following attitudes: independence of thought, fair-mindedness, insight into egocentricity and sociocentricity, intellectual humility and suspension of judgment, intellectual courage, integrity, perseverance, confidence in reason, interest in exploring thoughts underlying feeling and feelings underlying thoughts, and curiosity.

Independence of Thought

Critical thinking requires that individuals think for themselves. People acquire many beliefs as children, not because there are rational reasons for believing, but because there may have been rewards for believing or because they do not question authorities promoting the beliefs. As they mature and acquire knowledge and experience, critical thinkers examine their beliefs in the light of new evidence.

Being an independent thinker does not mean ignoring what others think and acting on one's own; rather, following the ideas of others makes one dependent only if one accepts those ideas without

question. Therefore, critical thinkers consider seriously a wide range of ideas, learn from them, and then make their own judgments about them. Nurses must be willing to challenge orders, activities, and rituals that have no rational support, such as the nursing traditions of wearing caps or white stockings, insisting all clients be bathed every day, assuming that all clients are motivated to change, and assuming that Western systems of medical care are the only valid methods of healing. Critical thinkers avoid succumbing to peer pressure and insist on seeing evidence for themselves. Further, critical thinkers admit when they do not know something and acknowledge acting in a certain way out of tradition or habit, rather than for a logical reason.

Fair-Mindedness

Critical thinkers are fair-minded, assessing all viewpoints with the same standards and not basing their judgments on personal or group bias or prejudice. Fair-mindedness helps one to consider opposing points of view and try to understand new ideas fully before rejecting or accepting them. Early educational reformer Carl Rogers (1969) proposed that one is not truly communicating with another person unless one allows the possibility that the other person may change one's own mind. The same applies to evidence: Critical thinkers strive to be open to the possibility that new evidence could change their mind.

Insight Into Egocentricity and Sociocentricity

Critical thinkers are open to the possibility that their personal biases or social pressures and customs could unduly affect their thinking. They actively try to examine their own biases and bring them to awareness each time they think or make a decision. For example, a nurse spends extensive time trying to teach a client how to prevent a future recurrence of some problem but is mystified when the client appears uninterested and does not follow the nurse's advice. The nurse's egocentric tendency to assume that all clients are motivated and interested in preventive care (just because the nurse is) resulted in inaccurate assessment of the client's desire to learn; both the nurse's and the client's time was wasted. Had the nurse assessed the client's cultural background and beliefs about what caused the disease (that is, had the nurse collected sufficient evidence), the nurse might have identified a more relevant problem and developed a better care plan.

Intellectual Humility and Suspension of Judgment

Intellectual humility means having an awareness of the limits of one's own knowledge. Critical thinkers are willing to admit what they don't know; they are willing to seek new information and to rethink their conclusions in light of new knowledge. They never assume that what everybody knows to be right will always be right, because new evidence may emerge. This particularly applies to what appears to be confirmed "knowledge."

In the 1960s, for example, it was accepted belief that a client recovering from a myocardial infarction should stay on absolute bed rest and use the bedpan for the first 2 to 3 days. Physicians consistently prescribed this practice, and nurses, too, believed it was best. This practice, however, was based on custom, and the unconfirmed assumptions that using the bedpan was less stressful than using a bedside commode.

Thus critical thinkers must remember that all knowledge is tentative and that they should hold principles and practices as tentative and follow them only as long as available evidence supports them. Critical thinkers should assume that new evidence may be discovered that will change current knowledge. This is a mark of humility in a thinker.

Intellectual Courage

With an attitude of courage, one is willing to consider and examine fairly one's own ideas or views, especially those to which one may have a strongly negative reaction. This type of courage comes from recognizing that beliefs are sometimes false or misleading. Values and beliefs are not always acquired "rationally." (Values are discussed in Chapter 5). Rational beliefs are those which have been examined and found to be supported by solid reasons and data. After such examination, it is inevitable that some ideas previously held to be true are found to contain questionable elements and that some truth will emerge from ideas considered dangerous or false. Courage is needed to be true to new thinking in such cases, especially if social penalties for nonconformity are severe.

For example, Evelyn is a nurse in a community where there is a negative attitude toward homosexuality and acquired immune deficiency syndrome (AIDS). Her friends believe that the homosexual lifestyle is unacceptable and that AIDS is a punishment. In caring for clients with AIDS, Evelyn learns to view them as individuals rather than labeling and condemning them. Because some of her friends have difficulty accepting her view, Evelyn risks losing them. It requires courage for Evelyn to stand up for what she knows to be right.

Lack of courage can cause people to become resistant to change. Old beliefs can provide a sense of security. People may be resistant to new ideas because they produce discomfort. Chapter 13 describes strategies for planning change.

Integrity

Intellectual integrity requires that individuals apply the same rigorous standards of proof to their own knowledge and beliefs as they apply to the knowledge and beliefs of others. Critical thinkers will question their own knowledge and beliefs as quickly and as thoroughly as they will challenge those of another. They are readily able to admit and evaluate inconsistencies within their own beliefs and between their own beliefs and those of another.

Perseverance

Nurses who are critical thinkers show perseverance in finding effective solutions to client and nursing problems. This determination enables them to clarify concepts and sort out related issues, in spite of difficulties and frustrations. Confusion and frustration are uncomfortable, but critical thinkers resist the temptation to find a quick and easy answer. Important questions tend to be complex and confusing and therefore often require a great deal of thought and research.

An example is the temptation for a committee to come to a hasty conclusion on a complex issue. The committee may be facing a challenging problem that has no simple answer, but external pressures may influence the members to come to a decision too quickly or to come to a conclusion without considering some relevant factors. A strongly opinionated leader or member may sway opinions, or general impatience and frustration with the task may discourage members. Critical thinkers, however, can temper these tendencies, promote thoughtful consideration of all aspects of the assignment, and avoid superficial "quick fixes."

Confidence in Reason

Critical thinkers believe that well-reasoned thinking will lead to trustworthy conclusions. Therefore, they will cultivate an attitude of confidence in the reasoning process and examine emotion-laden arguments using the standards for evaluating thought, by asking questions such as, "Is that argument fair? Is it based on sufficient evidence? Have opposing viewpoints been considered?" and so on. The critical thinker will develop skill in both inductive reasoning (forming generalizations from a set of facts or observations) and deductive reasoning (starting with a generalization and moving to specifics). As a critical thinker gains greater awareness of the thinking process, and more experience in improving such thinking, confidence in the thinking process will grow. This confident thinker will not be afraid of disagreement and, indeed, will be concerned when all agree too quickly. Such an individual can serve as a role model to colleagues, inspiring and encouraging them to think critically as well.

Interest in Exploring Thoughts Underlying Feelings and Feelings Underlying Thoughts

A critical thinker knows that emotions can influence thinking and that often feelings underlie thoughts. The rational, critical thinker adopts the attitude that feelings are real and need to be acknowledged. However, feelings need to be explored to determine whether they are based on reality or childhood interpretations, memories, or fears. Nurses need to identify, examine, and control, or modify feelings that are interfering with clear critical thinking. To deal with strong, negative emotion the nurse can take these steps:

1. Limit action for a while to avoid hasty conclusions and impulsive decisions.
2. Discuss negative feelings with a confidant.
3. Expend some of the energy generated by the emotion by, for example, walking or exercising.
4. Reflect on the situation and determine whether the emotional response was appropriate. After the strong emotion is dissipated, the nurse can then objectively move toward needed conclusions or make required decisions.

Curiosity

The internal conversation going on within the mind of a critical thinker is filled with questions: Why do we believe this? What causes that? Does it have to be this way? Could something else work? What would happen if we did it another way? Who says that is so? The curious individual may value tradition but is not afraid to examine traditions to be sure they are still valid.

Unexamined traditions are often called "sacred cows," in reference to the uncritical acquiescence of their advocates. Often, those who challenge traditional beliefs are viewed as dangerous and are rejected. When Copernicus questioned the idea that the earth was the center of the universe, for example, he was ridiculed by his colleagues and excommunicated from his church. Questioners tend to challenge the status quo, and remove the comfort of habit. But far more dangerous are individuals or disciplines that refuse to examine their beliefs and practices and fear new evidence that may influence change. Mitchell (1995) encourages nurses not to be afraid to continually reflect on traditional beliefs and values, to examine whether these beliefs withstand the tests of critical thinking, and to support others who engage in this process.

ELEMENTS AND STANDARDS OF CRITICAL THINKING

The critical thinker considers the elements of reasoning shown in Figure 12–1 (Paul, 1994b). These elements may be considered in any order and therefore are presented in a circular scheme. The relationship of Paul's elements of reasoning to the nursing process is shown in Table 12–3.

How can one know whether one's thinking is critical thinking? Paul (1995) proposes that thinkers

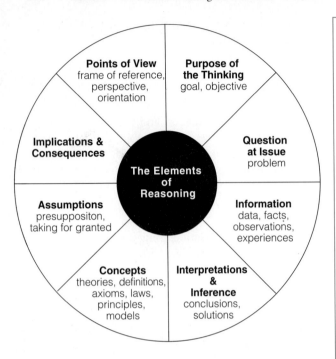

FIGURE 12–1 *The elements of reasoning.*

SOURCE: Critical Thinking Workshops, by R. Paul, 1994, Santa Rosa, CA: Foudnation for Critical Thinking, p. 111. Reprinted with permission.

Standards for Critical Thinkers

- Explore thinking that underlies emotions and feelings.
- Suspend judgment when there is insufficient data.
- Develop criteria for evaluation and apply them fairly and accurately.
- Evaluate the credibility of sources used to justify beliefs.
- Make interdisciplinary connections and use insights from one subject or experience to illuminate and correct other subjects.
- Differentiate facts from opinions.
- Examine assumptions that underlie thoughts and behavior.
- Distinguish relevant from irrelevant data and important from trivial data.
- Make plausible inferences and distinguish conclusions from the reasoning that supports them.

SOURCE: Adapted from "What, Then, is Critical Thinking?" by R. Paul, 1988, from the Eighth Annual and Sixth International Conference on Critical Thinking and Educational Reform, Rohnert Park, CA: Center for Critical Thinking and Moral Critique, Sonoma State University.

TABLE 12–3 **Relationship of Paul's Elements of Reasoning to the Nursing Process**

Paul's Elements of Reasoning	Parallels to the Nursing Process	Clinical Application
Information	Assessing	*Data:* A 45-year-old male Latino complains of severe headache; 20 lb overweight; blood pressure 180/95 mm Hg. States has been taking high blood pressure pills only when he has a headache. Is self-employed as gardener; lives with wife, mother-in-law, and four children.
		Given the above data, a critical thinker is aware that more data must be obtained about the client's cultural health values and reasons for stated behavior. Failure to think critically and to obtain additional data leads to inaccurate goals, diagnosis, and interventions.
Purpose of thinking	Goal setting	*Goal:* To increase compliance with medication regimen in order to relieve headaches and prevent a cerebrovascular accident (CVA). A critical thinking nurse will in addition try to determine the client's goals and to agree to mutual goals.
Question at issue	Diagnosing	A critical thinker will defer identifying the client's diagnosis until more data are obtained and the client's priorities are known. This prevents a premature diagnosis based on insufficient data.

TABLE 12–3 *continued*

Paul's Elements of Reasoning	Parallels to the Nursing Process	Clinical Application
Points of view		As a critical thinker, the nurse is aware that the client's point of view may differ from the nurse's. Although the nurse may support the Western medical belief system that puts high priority on preventing disease, the critical thinker is also aware that the client may hold other views of health/illness, therapy, and preventive measures.
Interpretation and inference (conclusions and recommendations)	Diagnosing	The critical thinker recognizes that the client's erratic use of the prescribed medication may have multiple causes (e.g., troublesome side effects, belief that illness is due to God's will and is not preventable) and will not infer a diagnosis with etiology until more data are obtained. Failure to think critically can lead to interpretations that are irrelevant, inadequate, and superficial (e.g., an erroneous interpretation that the client's problem is lack of sufficient knowledge).
Assumptions (presuppositions)		The critical thinker makes assumptions in accordance with a broad, unbiased database and mutually set client goals. The critical thinker avoids making unverified assumptions, such as that an increase in knowledge will increase this client's compliance, or that this client is motivated to prevent a CVA.
Concepts (theories, laws, principles, models)	Diagnosing Planning	The critical thinker uses concepts about motivation, change theory, and multicultural nursing to understand the client's behavior and motivation to change. Failure to think critically can lead to the exclusive reliance on a simplistic concept, such as "knowledge creates change."
Implications and consequences	Planning Implementing	The critical thinker considers the implications and consequences of selected nursing strategies before implementing plans of care. Plans of care, including outcomes, are based on ongoing assessment of the client's cultural values, beliefs, and needs. Failure to think critically may lead to ineffective interventions, such as client teaching that focuses *only* on resolving a knowledge deficit about the prescribed medication. The critical thinker recognizes that knowledge deficit may or may not be one of several problems.
Interpretation and inference	Evaluating	The critical thinker bases evaluation of client outcomes and the effectiveness of nursing interventions on well-developed, measurable criteria and considers rationally whether outcomes have been validated. Failure to think critically may lead to client noncompliance and an inference that the client did not learn effectively and that the client needs further instruction.

can use universal intellectual standards to assess reasoning. These standards are shown in the accompanying box. Such standards are more useful if they are made explicit. Making standards explicit promotes both the reliability and validity of the thinking and consequently strengthens the appropriateness of any actions that may result.

APPLICATIONS OF CRITICAL THINKING

Nurses function effectively some part of every day without thinking critically. Many small decisions are made based primarily on habit, with minimal thinking involved; examples include selecting what clothes to wear, choosing which route to take to work, and deciding what to eat for lunch. Psychomotor skills in nursing often involve minimal thinking, such as operating a familiar piece of equipment. But higher-order critical thinking skills are put into play as soon as a new idea is encountered or a less-than-routine decision must be made. When setting priorities for the day, a nurse employs critical thinking. When assessing a client, identifying potential and actual problems, and moving through the nursing process, the nurse involves critical thinking at each stage of the process. When analyzing a situation and planning strategies for conflict resolution or change, the nurse manager needs thinking attitudes and skills.

The nurse clinician and nurse manager seek to be aware of their thinking while they are thinking, as they apply standards for thinking, and as their thinking progresses.

Problem Solving

Nurses use critical thinking to rationally resolve problems related to direct client care. Nurse managers use critical thinking to resolve problems related to overall client care, unit administration, and staff interpersonal issues (see Chapter 10). Strader (1992, p. 228) defines **problem solving** as "the process used when a gap is perceived between an existing state (what *is* occurring) and a desired state (what *should be* occurring)." In problem solving, the nurse obtains information that clarifies the nature of the problem and suggests possible solutions. The nurse then carefully evaluates the possible solutions and chooses the best to implement. The situation is then carefully monitored over time to ensure its initial and continued effectiveness. The

---

RESEARCH NOTE

How Do Nurses Make Clinical Decisions?

Nurses use the clinical decision-making process to gather information, evaluate it, and make a judgment that results in the provision of client care. In one study, researchers sought to increase understanding of the clinical decision making of nurse practitioners. The sample consisted of 27 nurse practitioners, 6 of whom were obstetric/gynecologic nurse practitioners, 11 experienced family practitioners, and 10 inexperienced family nurse practitioners. All subjects cared for the same computer-simulated client whose case history, physical examination, and laboratory findings were based on an actual client with a vaginal discharge and genital rash. The computer ran interactively with videotape, making some client's responses, physical examination findings, and laboratory findings visible. Because the simulation allowed for natural language entry, the nurse practitioners were able to interview the client by typing in questions in their own words. Objective data were requested by the same process.

Findings indicated that all three groups used a process of clinical decision making in which diagnostic hypotheses helped them decide what data to collect. However, the nurse groups differed in their final diagnoses and in subsequent care decisions. The OB/GYN nurse practitioners tended to develop lists of diagnostic hypotheses

reflecting the client's chief complaint. In contrast, the experienced and inexperienced family nurse practitioners tended to acquire subjective and objective data that did not appear to be hypothesis driven. This clinical decision-making process was also more likely to result in correct diagnoses and more appropriate care decisions when used by the OB/GYN nurse practitioners. The authors believe that these findings confirm the idea that the two processes—namely, deciding what information to acquire and then deciding on the intervention—probably rely on different bodies of knowledge. Data acquisition (the approach favored by the family nurse practitioners) is process related, whereas diagnosis and management (the approach favored by the OB/GYN nurse practitioners) are content related.

Implications: These findings suggest that expertise in an area chiefly reflects an understanding of the significance of the data acquired thus making the correct diagnosis.

SOURCE: J. E. White, D. G. Nativio, S. N. Kobert, and S. J. Engberg, Summer, 1992, "Content and Process in Clinical Decision-Making by Nurse Practitioners." *Image: Journal of Nursing Scholarship, 24*(2), 153–158.

nurse does not discard the other solutions but holds them in reserve in the event that the first solution is not effective. The nurse may also encounter a similar problem in a different client situation where an alternative solution is determined to be the most effective. Therefore, problem solving for one situation contributes to the nurse's body of knowledge for problem solving in future similar situations.

There are various approaches to problem solving. Five of the most commonly used are trial and error, intuition, the nursing process, the scientific method/research process, and the modified scientific method.

Trial and Error

One way to solve problems is trial and error, in which a number of approaches are tried until a solution is found. However, without considering alternatives systematically, one cannot know why the solution works. Trial-and-error methods in nursing care can be dangerous because the client might suffer harm if an approach is inappropriate.

Intuition

Intuition as a problem-solving method has not been considered either sound or legitimate. Rather, it has been viewed as a form of guessing and, as such, an inappropriate basis for nursing decisions. However, according to Benner and Tanner (1987), intuition appears to be an essential and legitimate aspect of clinical judgment acquired through knowledge and experience. Intuitive judgment in nursing is developed through clinical experience with similar types of situations. In other words, nurses develop expertise in a specialty area, such as cardiovascular nursing, through continuous and meaningful exposure to clients who have experienced cardiovascular problems.

Intuition is based on experience and knowledge. The nurse must first have the knowledge base necessary to practice in the clinical area then use that knowledge in clinical practice. Clinical experience allows the nurse to recognize cues and patterns and begin to make correct decisions.

Experience is important in improving this skill of intuition because the rapidity of the judgment depends on the nurse having seen similar client situations many times before. Sometimes nurses use the words "I had a feeling" to describe a leap (or a condensing) in the critical thinking element of considering evidence. These nurses are able to judge

quickly which evidence is most important and to act upon that limited evidence. Thus, intuition might be said to be thinking that does not progress systematically in the linear fashion proposed by Paul, but that moves in a circular or other pattern less easy to identify or describe (Hezekiah, 1993). Using this kind of thinking, the nurse may process or prioritize data more rapidly than usual.

Paul (1995) urges thinkers to be cautious in acting on "intuitions." He defines intuition much as Benner and Tanner do, but suggests a problem: Sometimes, the inner sense that a nurse may believe to be true is true, but sometimes it is not. Paul proposes that a critical thinker does not blindly accept that which he or she thinks or believes but cannot account for; a critical thinker realizes how easy it is to confuse intuitions and prejudices. Critical thinkers may follow their "inner sense that something is so," but only with a healthy sense of intellectual humility.

The intuitive method of problem solving is gaining recognition as part of nursing practice. It is not a valid method of decision making for novices or students, however, because they usually lack the knowledge base and clinical experience on which to make a valid judgment.

CONSIDER...

- a time when you experienced an intuition. Recall the circumstances. Reflect on your thinking processes at the time. How did you determine whether the intuition you experienced was accurate?
- the pros and cons of encouraging more intuitive thinking among nurses.

Nursing Process

The nursing process is the systematic method of planning, providing, and evaluating nursing care. It is the method used by nurses to solve clients' problems. See Chapter 14.

Scientific Method/Research Process

The research process is a formalized, logical, systematic approach to solving problems. The classic scientific method is most useful when the researcher is working in a controlled situation. Health professionals require a modified approach of the scientific method for solving problems. This modified scientific problem solving method is used in the nursing

TABLE 12–4 Comparison Between the Research Process and the Modified Scientific Method

Research Process (Scientific Method)	Modified Scientific Method
State a research question or problem.	Define the problem.
Define the purpose of or the rationale for the study.	
Review related literature.	Gather information.
Formulate hypotheses and defining variables.	Analyze the information.
Select method to test hypotheses.	Develop solutions.
Select population, sample, and setting.	
Conduct pilot study.	Make a decision.
Collect the data.	Implement the decision.
Analyze the data.	Evaluate the decision.
Communicate conclusions and implications.	

process as well as the medical process. The research process is discussed in Chapter 11.

Table 12–4 compares the research process or scientific method with the modified scientific method. Critical thinking is important in all problem-solving processes as the nurse evaluates all potential solutions to a given problem and makes a decision to select the most appropriate solution for that situation.

Decision Making

Tschikota (1993, p. 389) states that "effective clinical decision making is critical to the future of professional nursing practice." Nurses make decisions in the course of solving problems, for example, in each step of the nursing process. Decision making, however, is also used in situations that do not involve problem solving. Nurses make value decisions (e.g., to keep client information confidential); time management decisions (e.g., taking clean linens to the client's room at the same time as the medication in order to save steps); scheduling decisions (e.g., to bathe the client before visiting hours); and priority decisions (e.g., which interventions are most urgent and which can be delegated).

Decision making is a critical-thinking process for choosing the best actions to meet a desired goal. **Decision making** is defined by Strader (1992, p. 233) as "the process of establishing criteria by which alternative courses of action are developed and selected." Decisions must be made whenever there are several mutually exclusive choices. For example, the individual who wishes to become a nurse in the United States has several possible courses of action: a diploma program, an associate degree program, or a baccalaureate program. Prospective students must choose. Therefore, they must evaluate the different types of programs, as well as personal circumstances, to make a decision appropriate to their situation.

Nurses must make decisions and assist clients to make decisions. When faced with several client needs at the same time, the nurse must decide which client to assist first. When a client is trying to make a decision about what course of treatment to follow, the nurse may need to provide the client with information or resources to assist the client in making a decision. Nurses must make decisions in their own personal and professional lives. For example, the nurse must decide whether to work in a hospital or community setting, whether to join a professional association, and whether to carry professional liability insurance.

According to Schaefer (1974, p. 1852) three conditions must prevail in decision making: freedom, rationality, and voluntary. *Freedom* means that the individual makes the decision without pressure from others and has the authority to make the decision. *Rationality* means that the best or optimal decision is made and that it is consistent with the decision maker's values and preferences. Rationality involves both deliberation and judgment. *Voluntarity* is making a choice voluntarily.

Tschikota (1993) states that clinical decision making is composed of six elements: cue, hypothesis, knowledge base, nursing intervention, search, and assumption (Table 12–5). Nurses use various combinations of these decision-making elements as part of their mental processing in making decisions.

Strader (1992) describes a seven-step decision making process:

1. *Identify the purpose.* In this step, the nurse identifies why a decision is needed and what needs to be determined.

TABLE 12–5 Elements of Decision Making

Element	Definition	Example
Cue	A piece of information or data	Vital signs, laboratory values, client history, signs and/or symptoms
Hypothesis	A projected or proposed possibility; may concern what is wrong with the client, what the nurse/doctor/client might do, think, or feel, or what possible doctor's orders or hospital policies might be used; often introduced by subjects with such words as *probably, might, if, could be, maybe, perhaps, sounds like,* or *looks like*	"Possible infection." "Possible allergic reaction." "Probable myocardial infarction." "If we change the intravenous flow rate, the blood pressure might change."
Knowledge base	Information, correct or incorrect, that is used as rationale or support for any statements made by the subject	"*Because the client has a fever,* he probably has an infection." "*When we increase the intravenous flow rate, we add to circulating volume;* therefore, the blood pressure should change."
Nursing intervention	Any proposed nursing action	"Increase the intravenous flow rate." "Administer prn acetominophen for fever."
Search	Indication of a desire for additional or supplmentary information about the situation	"I think we need to know what the client's hemoglobin and hematocrit are." "Do we know what the client was doing prior to experiencing the pain?"
Assumption	A conclusion for which there is insufficient information; may lead to a search	"I believe the client is experiencing depression." (This could be based on observation of behavior without an adequate history to support the statement.)

SOURCE: Adapted from "The Clinical Decision-Making Processes of Student Nurses" by S. Tschikota, November 1993, *Journal of Nursing Education, 32,* p. 393. Used with permission.

2. *Set the criteria.* When the nurse sets the criteria for decision making, three questions must be answered: what needs to be achieved, what needs to be preserved, and what needs to be avoided. For example, for a client with pain, the criteria would be as follows:
   a. What needs to be achieved? Relief of pain.
   b. What needs to be preserved? Physical functioning, cognitive functioning, psychologic functioning, client comfort.
   c. What needs to be avoided? Central nervous system depression, respiratory depression, nausea.

3. *Weight the criteria.* In this step, the decision maker sets priorities or ranks activities or services in order of importance from least important to most important as they relate to the specific situation. Because the weighting is specific to the situation, an activity may be ranked as most important in one situation and of less importance in another situation.

4. *Seek alternatives.* After establishing and weighting the criteria in the previous steps, the decision maker identifies all possible ways to meet the criterion. In clinical situations, the alternatives may be selected from a range of nursing interventions or client care strategies.

5. *Test alternatives.* The nurse analyzes the alternatives to ensure that there is an objective rationale

TABLE 12–6 Comparison Between the Nursing Process and the Decision-Making Process

Nursing Process	Decision-Making Process*
Assess	Identify the purpose
Diagnose	
Plan	Set the criteria
	Weight the criteria
	Seek alternatives
Implement	Test alternatives
	Troubleshoot
Evaluate	Evaluate the action

* The decision-making process parallels the nursing process but also is used during each step of the process.

in relation to the established criteria for choosing one strategy over another.

6. *Troubleshoot.* In troubleshooting, the nurse tries to determine what might go wrong as a result of a decision and develops plans to prevent, minimize, or overcome any problems.

7. *Evaluate the action.* In evaluating the strategies used, the nurse determines how effective they were and whether they achieved the initial purpose.

The decision-making process and the nursing process share similarities. The nurse uses decision making in all of the steps of the nursing process. Table 12–6 compares the steps of these processes.

DEVELOPING CRITICAL THINKING ATTITUDES AND SKILLS

After gaining an idea of what it means to think critically, solve problems, and make decisions, nurses need to become aware of their own thinking style and abilities. Acquiring critical thinking skills and a critical attitude then becomes a matter of practice. Critical thinking is not an "either-or" phenomenon; it exists on a continuum, along which people develop and use it more or less effectively. Some people make better evaluations than others; some people believe information from nearly any source; and still others

seldom believe anything without carefully evaluating the credibility of the information. Critical thinking is not easy. Solving problems and making decisions is risky. Sometimes the outcome is not what was desired. With effort, however, everyone can achieve some level of critical thinking to become effective problem solvers and decision makers.

Self-Assessment

The nurse should reflect on some of the attitudes discussed earlier that facilitate critical thinking, attitudes such as curiosity, fair-mindedness, humility, courage, and perseverance. A nurse might benefit first from a rigorous personal assessment to determine which attitudes he or she already possesses and which need to be cultivated. This could also be done with a partner or as a group. The nurse should determine which attitudes are held strongly and from a base for thinking and which are held minimally or not at all. The nurse should also reflect on situations where he or she made decisions that were later regretted and should analyze thinking processes and attitudes or ask a trusted colleague to assess them. Identifying weak or vulnerable skills and attitudes is also important.

Tolerating Dissonance and Ambiguity

The nurse should take deliberate efforts to cultivate critical thinking attitudes. For example, to develop fair-mindedness, the nurse could deliberately seek out information that is in opposition to her or his own views; this can help the nurse practice understanding opposing viewpoints and learn to be open to other viewpoints. It is a human tendency to seek out information that corresponds to one's previously held beliefs and to ignore evidence that may contradict cherished ideas. These phenomena are explained by the theory of **cognitive dissonance,** which holds that the mind rejects ideas that are not congruent with previously held concepts, resulting in "dissonance" (Festinger, 1957). Ideas that challenge rigidly held beliefs could cause cognitive dissonance and be rejected before receiving fair consideration. Nurses should increase their tolerance for ideas that contradict previously held beliefs, and they should practice suspending judgment. Suspending judgment means tolerating ambiguity for a time. If an issue is complex, it may not be resolved quickly or neatly, and judgment should be postponed. For a while, the nurse will need to say, "I don't know," and be comfortable with that answer until more is known. The thinker who can live with such ambiguity and cognitive dissonance will be at an advantage, and will not fall prey to quick fixes. Such a thinker will also be able to resist charismatic leaders who promise easy answers to problems. Although postponing judgment may not be feasible in emergency situations where fast action is required, it can usually be feasible in other situations.

Seeking Situations Where Good Thinking Is Practiced

Nurses should attend conferences in clinical or educational settings that support open examination of all sides of issues and respect opposing viewpoints. Nurses should always be suspicious of anyone who presents something as "proven fact" unless it is supported by sufficient and convincing evidence. Cultivating a questioning attitude, using either Socratic questioning or another technique, is critical. Nurses need to review the standards for evaluating thinking and apply them to their own thinking. If nurses are aware of their own thinking—while they are doing the thinking (metacognition)—they should detect thinking errors.

Creating Environments That Support Critical Thinking

A nurse cannot develop or maintain critical thinking attitudes in a vacuum. Nurses in leadership positions must be particularly aware of the climate for thinking that they establish, and they must actively create a stimulating environment that encourages differences of opinion and fair examination of ideas and options. As leaders, nurses should encourage colleagues to examine evidence carefully before they come to conclusions, and to avoid "group think," the tendency to defer unthinkingly to the will of the group.

Practicing and Enjoying

The more nurses practice applying standards to their own thinking, the easier they will find it to think better. Good thinking can also be fun. Sloane and MacHale (1995) present thinkers with short, sometimes humorous puzzles that help them break away from conventional assumptions and approach thinking from a new angle, which they call lateral thinking. Von Oech (1990) also presents activities that stimulate creative thinking and discourage rigid mind-sets. To practice critical thinking, nurses can try humor, brainstorming, questioning, and other strategies suggested earlier. Finally, it is important

not to give up when others resist good thinking to be a positive role model, to maintain high personal standards, and to support others. It will be worth the struggle because, as Socrates said, "The unexamined life is not worth living."

CONSIDER...

- what kind of thinker says, "My mind is made up; don't confuse me with facts."
- your first response when someone suggests a new way to do something, or a new idea. If you tend to reject new ideas too quickly, what critical thinking attitude do you need to develop? If you tend to adopt a new idea too quickly, what critical thinking attitude do you need to develop?

READINGS FOR ENRICHMENT

Bandman, E. L., & Bandman, B. (1995). *Critical thinking in nursing* (2nd ed.). Norwalk, CT: Appleton & Lange.

This 306-page book addresses critical thinking and applies it to nursing. Three major sections address practical reasoning in nursing, deductive reasoning in nursing, and inductive reasoning in nursing.

Wilkinson, J. (1996). *Nursing process: A critical thinking approach* (2nd ed.). Redwood City, CA: Addison-Wesley Nursing.

This interactive text provides exercises to develop the reader's critical thinking skills in applying the nursing process to both simulated and real client situations.

SUMMARY

Nurses need critical thinking skills and attitudes to be safe, competent, skillful practitioners. Critical thinking is a purposeful mental activity in which ideas are produced and evaluated and judgments made. It is thinking that is reasonable, rational, reflective, autonomous, creative, and fair and inspires an attitude of inquiry that focuses on deciding what to believe or do. Critical thinkers have certain attitudes: independence of thought, humility, courage, integrity, perseverance, empathy, and fair-mindedness. Nurses use critical thinking as they apply knowledge from other subjects and fields to nursing practice, deal with change in stressful environments, and make important decisions related to client care. A major component of critical thinking is creativity. When nurses incorporate creativity into their thinking, they are able to find unique solutions to unique problems.

Elements of reasoning, according to Paul, include purpose of thinking, question at issue, information, interpretation and inference, concepts, assumptions, implications and consequences, and points of view. Critical thinkers consider these elements when problem solving and making decisions.

Critical thinking consists of high-level cognitive processes that include problem solving and decision making. There are several problem solving methods: trial and error, intuition, the nursing process, the scientific method, and the modified scientific method. Nurses use the scientific method or research process when they participate in nursing and health research.

The nursing process and critical thinking are interrelated and interdependent, but they are not identical. Both involve problem solving, decision making, and creativity. Decisions must be made whenever there are several mutually exclusive choices. Nurses must make decisions in both their personal and professional lives. The steps of the decision-making process include identifying the purpose of the decision, setting the criteria, weighting the criteria, seeking alternatives, testing alternatives, troubleshooting, and evaluating the action. Everyone has at least some level of critical thinking skill, and that skill can be developed with practice. Some guidelines to enhance critical thinking skills and attitudes include performing a self-assessment, tolerating dissonance and ambiguity, seeking situations where good thinking is productive, creating environments that support critical thinking, and practicing and applying standards to one's thinking.

SELECTED REFERENCES

Bandman, E. L., & Bandman, B. (1995). *Critical thinking in nursing* (2nd ed.). Norwalk, CT: Appleton & Lange.

Benner, P., & Tanner, C. (1987, Jan.). How expert nurses use intuition. *American Journal of Nursing, 87,* 23–31.

Ennis, R. H. (1985). A logical basis for measuring critical thinking skills. *Educational Leadership, 43* (10), 44–48.

Facione, P. A. (1984). Toward a theory of critical thinking. *Liberal Education, 70,* (2), 253–261.

Kataoka-Yahiro, M. K., & Saylor, C. (1994). A critical thinking model for nursing judgment. *Journal of Nursing Education, 33* (8), 351–355.

McAllister, M. & Ryan, M. (1995). Feminist pedagogy: Developing creative approaches for teaching students of nursing. *Journal of Nursing Education, 34* (5), 243–245.

Miller, M. A. & Babcock, D. E. (1996). *Critical thinking applied to nursing.* St. Louis: Mosby.

Miller, M. S. & Malcolm, N. S. (1990). Critical thinking in the nursing curriculum. *Nursing and Health Care, 11,* (2) 67–73.

Mitchell, G. J. (1995). Reflection: The key to breaking with tradition. *Nursing Science Quarterly, 8,* 2:57.

National League for Nursing. (1992). *Criteria for the evaluation of baccalaureate and higher degree programs in nursing* (5th ed.). New York: Author.

Paul, R. W. (1985, May). Bloom's taxonomy and critical thinking instruction. *Educational Leadership,* 36–39.

Paul, R. (1988). What, then, is critical thinking? From the Eighth Annual and Sixth International Conference on Critical Thinking and Educational Reform. Rohnert Park, CA: Center for Critical Thinking and Moral Critique, Sonoma State University.

Paul, R. W. (1990). *Critical thinking.* Rohnert Park, CA: Sonoma State University.

Paul, R. W. (1994a). Overcoming the addiction to coverage. *Educational Vision, 2*(1), 11.

Paul, R. W. (1994b). *Critical thinking workshops* (manual). Rohnert Park, CA: Center for Critical Thinking and Moral Critique, Sonoma State University.

Paul, R. W. (1995). *Critical thinking: How to prepare students for a rapidly changing world.* Santa Rosa, CA: Foundation for Critical Thinking.

Reilly, D. E., & Oermann, M. H. (1992). Cognitive learning in the clinical setting. In *Clinical teaching in nursing education* (2nd ed.) (pp. 207–246). New York: National League for Nursing.

Rogers, C. R. (1969). *Freedom to learn.* Columbus: Charles E. Merrill.

Rubenfeld, M. G., & Scheffer, B. K. (1995). *Critical thinking in nursing: An interactive approach.* Philadelphia: Lippincott.

Schaefer, J. (1974, Oct.). The interrelatedness of decision making and the nursing process. *American Journal of Nursing, 74,* 1852–1855.

Schank, M. J. (1990). Wanted: Nurses with critical thinking skills. *Journal of Continuing Education in Nursing, 21*(2), 86–89.

Sloane, P., & MacHale, D. (1995). *Improve your lateral thinking.* New York: Sterling.

Strader, M. (1992). Critical thinking. In E. J. Sullivan & P. J. Decker (pp. 225–248). *Effective management in nursing* (3rd ed.). Redwood City, CA: Addison-Wesley Nursing.

Tschikota, S. (1993, Nov.). The clinical decision-making processes of student nurses. *Journal of Nursing Education, 32,* 389–398.

von Oech, R. (1990). *A whack on the side of the head: How you can be more creative.* New York: Warner.

West, T. G. (1979). *Plato's apology of Socrates: An interpretation, with a new translation.* Ithaca, NY: Cornell University Press.

13 CHAPTER

Change Process

OUTLINE

**Meanings and Types
of Change**

Change Theory
*Approaches to Planned Change
Frameworks*

Change Agent

Coping with Change
*Accepting Change
Resisting Change*

OBJECTIVES

- Differentiate spontaneous, developmental, and planned change.

- Explain the empirical-rational, normative-reeducative, and power-coercive approaches to change.

- Compare the change process models of Lewin, Lippitt, Havelock, and Rogers.

- Discuss types and characteristics of change agents.

- Identify essential aspects of Perlman and Takacs's ten stages of psychologic responses to change.

- Identify ways the change agent can facilitate change by enhancing motivating forces and decreasing resistive forces.

- Identify steps in the change process.

You see things; and you say, "Why?" But I dream things that never were; and I say, "Why not?"
—George Bernard Shaw,
Back to Methuselah, 1921

To be effective and influential in today's world, nurses need to understand change theory and apply its precepts in the workplace, in government and professional organizations, and in the community.

- Change is a dynamic process and a normal part of people's lives.
- Change is the means by which people grow, develop, and adapt. It can be positive or negative, planned or unplanned.
- The process of change is an integral part of many areas of nursing, such as teaching, client care, and health promotion.
- Change can involve individual clients, families, communities, organizations, nursing as a profession, and the entire health care delivery system.
- Change can involve gaining new knowledge, obtaining new skills, or adapting current knowledge in the light of new information.
- Change can be especially difficult when it presents challenges to one's values and beliefs, ways of thinking, or ways of relating.

MEANINGS AND TYPES OF CHANGE

Brooten, Hayman, and Naylor (1978) define *change* as "the process which leads to alteration in individual or institutional patterns of behavior." Mauksch and Miller define change as "the process by which alterations occur in the function and structure of society" (1981, p. 9).

The noun and verb forms of the word *change* have different meanings. The noun form denotes substitution of one thing for another, an alteration in the state or quality of a thing, or permutations constituting varied arrangements of a set or series of things. Used as a verb, *change* means to make a thing other than it was (outward directed change) or to become different, to undergo alterations, or to vary (inward directed change). Synonyms for the verb *change* include *alter, transform, convert,* and *vary*. All these terms suggest that a fundamental difference or substitution is the outcome of change.

Change is not always the result of rational decision making. It generally occurs in response to three different activities: (a) spontaneous reactions, (b) developmental activities, and (c) consciously planned activities. Both individuals and organizations can undergo change.

Spontaneous Change

Spontaneous change is also referred to as reactive or unplanned change because it is not fully anticipated, it cannot be avoided, and there is little or no time to plan response strategies. Examples of spontaneous change affecting an individual include an acute viral infection, a spinal cord injury, and the unsolicited offer of a new position.

On a larger scale, spontaneous change can be either short term or long term. Examples of short-term spontaneous change include an earthquake or other natural disaster, a major airplane crash that is near a small hospital, or a wildcat strike that closes a tertiary health care facility. The impact of human immunodeficiency virus (HIV) on the policies and practices of health care facilities is an example of change with long-term consequences.

Responses to spontaneous change can be either positive or negative. For example, the "cold" virus may create only minor inconveniences for one person but may lead to life-threatening illness in another. Likewise, an organization may respond successfully to the injuries resulting from a natural event if a well-developed disaster plan is in place; conversely, without such a plan the organization may experience disorganization, confusion, and major difficulties. The result of spontaneous change can be unpredictable. To ensure a successful response, spontaneous change demands flexibility and cohesiveness.

Developmental Change

Developmental change refers to physiopsychologic changes that occur during an individual's lifecycle or to the growth of an organization as it becomes more complex. Examples of developmental change of individuals include the increasing size and complexity of a human embryo and fetus and the decreasing physical capability of an older person. These changes are not consciously planned; they just happen. However, the individual may make plans for dealing with the changes. For example, an older person may make plans for dealing with the physical changes, such as moving to a smaller, one-floor residence which is easier to care for and in which it is easier to move around.

Organizations often grow and develop in unpredictable ways. A once-successful small health organization may no longer meet the increasing demands and needs of a community. As the organization evolves into a larger, more complex entity, it may undergo such unwanted change as overwork, task changes, less personalized service, and more formalized staff communication patterns. Such unavoidable changes necessitate development of organizational charts, revised job descriptions, and, often, formal staff meetings to meet the defined needs.

Planned Change

According to Lippitt (1973), **planned change** is an intended, purposive attempt by an individual, group, organization, or larger social system to influence the status quo of itself, another organism, or a situation. Problem-solving skills, decision-making skills, and interpersonal skills are important factors in planned change. An example of planned change is an individual who decides to improve his or her health status by attending a smoking cessation program or carrying out an exercise program. Organizations are continually involved in planned changes. In health care agencies changes are made in policies, in methods of care delivery, in staffing, and so on. Bringing about planned change is a major part of any nurse manager's role. The remainder of this chapter discusses change models, strategies, and ways to bring about successful change. The stages of health behavior change to promote health are discussed further in Chapter 8.

From a personal perspective, Alfaro-LeFevre (1995, p. 1) addresses four ways people change. See the accompanying box.

CONSIDER...

- your own responses toward change.
- spontaneous changes that have occurred in your personal and professional life. How did those changes affect you or your organization? What personal or professional strategies helped you or your organization adjust to the spontaneous changes? In what ways may positive (in your opinion) spontaneous changes be easier to deal with than negative spontaneous changes?
- developmental changes that might be identified in the clients seen in your practice setting. Do the policies, procedures, and plans

of care accommodate the identified developmental changes that are routinely occurring in your clients?
- developmental changes that are occurring in your organization. What are the staff reactions to these changes? How might the professional nurse cope with or assist colleagues to cope with organizational change?
- planned changes that have occurred in your personal or professional life during the last year. Do planned professional changes result in planned personal changes? Is it possible that planned professional changes might result in spontaneous personal changes?

Four Ways We Change

1. Pendulum change:	"I was wrong before, but now I'm right."
2. Change by exception:	"I'm right, except for ..."
3. Incremental change:	"I was *almost* right before, but now I'm right."
4. Paradigm change:	"What I knew before was *partially* right. What I know now is more right, but only part of what I'll know tomorrow."

Paradigm change is transformational

Paradigm change combines what's useful about *old* ways with what's useful about *new* ways and keeps us open to looking for *even better* ways.

We realize

- Our previous views were only part of the picture.
- What we now know is only part of what we'll know later.
- Change is no longer threatening: It enlarges and enriches.
- The unknown can then be friendly and interesting.
- Each insight smoothes the road, making the change process easier.

SOURCES: *Aquarian Conspiracy: Personal and Social Transformation in Our Time* by M. Ferguson, 1980, New York: Putnam; *Critical Thinking in Nursing: A Practical Approach* by R. Alfaro-LeFevre, 1995, Philadelphia: W. B. Saunders, p. 1. Reprinted with permission.

CHANGE THEORY

Approaches to Planned Change

Three broad strategies or approaches to planned change have been identified: empirical-rational, normative-reeducative, and power-coercive.

Empirical-Rational

The empirical-rational approach is based on two beliefs: that people are rational and that they will change if it is in their self-interests. Therefore, change will be adopted if the change can be rationally justified and shown to be advantageous to the people involved (Bennis, Benne & Chin, 1985, p. 23).

Normative-Reeducative

This approach is based on the assumption that human motivation depends on the sociocultural norms and the individual's commitment to these norms. The sociocultural norms are supported by the attitudes and value systems of the individuals. In this instance, change occurs if the people involved develop new attitudes and values and acquire new information. In this approach, knowledge is the power for change.

Power-Coercive

With the power-coercive approach, power lies with one or more persons of influence. The influence may come through political power, wealth, status, or ability. This approach does not deny the intelligence or rationality of people or the importance of their attitudes or values, but it recognizes the need to use power to attain change.

Hagerman and Tiffany (1994) in their research wrote that the rational-empirical and power-coercive approaches are less appropriate for nursing than the normative-reeducative approach. The latter is most compatible with contemporary life and to the advancement of scientific and democratic values (Bennis et al. 1985, p. 33).

Frameworks

Frameworks such as those of Lewin, Lippitt, and Havelock follow the normative-reeducative approach. See Table 13–1.

Lewin

Kurt Lewin (1948) originated change theory. He saw change as having three basic stages: unfreezing, moving, and refreezing. See Table 13–2. During the *unfreezing* stage, the motivation to establish some

TABLE 13–1　**Change Approaches**

Approach	Characteristics
Power-coercive	• Based on the application of power from a legitimate source. • Power is often economic or is political. • Minimal participation by target members. • Resistance may occur and morale may decrease. • Feelings and values of opposing forces are not a factor. • Model is nonparticipative and undemocratic.
Empirical-rational	• Knowledge is power. • Influence moves from those with knowledge to those without. • Once members of the target group have knowledge, they will accept or reject the idea. • Is a noncoercive model. • Appropriate for new technology. • Works well when the target group is discontented. • Fully participative and democratic.
Normative-reeducative	• Recognizes that change must deal with feelings, values, and needs. • Recognizes that not all responses of people to change are rational. • Information and rational arguments are often insufficient to bring about change. • Model is partially participative and democratic.

TABLE 13–2 **Comparison of Change Models**

Lewin	Lippitt	Havelock	Rogers
1. Unfreezing	1. Diagnose problem 2. Assess motivation 3. Assess change agent's motivations and resources	1. Building a relationship 2. Diagnosing the problem 3. Acquiring resources	1. Knowledge 2. Persuasion 3. Decision
2. Moving	4. Select progressive change objects 5. Choose change agent role	4. Choosing the solution 5. Gaining acceptance	4. Implementation
3. Refreezing	6. Maintain change 7. Terminate helping relationship	6. Stabilization	5. Confirmation

sort of change occurs. The individual becomes aware of the need for change. This stage is a cognitive process in which the person becomes aware of a problem or of a better method of accomplishing a task and hence of the need for change. Having identified this need, the individual must also identify restraining and driving forces. For example, a nurse who is instructing an adolescent client and his mother in dietary management of type I (juvenile-onset) diabetes may see the client's mother as a driving force, and the client's father and siblings, who don't want to change their sugar-loaded diet, as restraining forces.

In the second stage, *moving*, the actual change is planned in detail and then started. Information is gathered from one or several sources. At this stage, it is important that the people involved agree that the status quo is undesirable. In the above example, the nurse needs to help the family understand the importance of dietary management for diabetics and to enlist their support for the client. The nurse could ask the dietitian to meet with the client and his family to demonstrate how a diabetic diet can be nutritious and tasty. The nurse might also provide printed food exchange lists, sample menus, and recipes, as well as resources for diabetic information. As change agent, the nurse should work with the family to create an environment that is conducive to the change, including, perhaps, rewards to reinforce desired behaviors. An environment that fosters change should be supportive, nonthreatening, and educational (Olson, 1979, p. 327).

In the third stage, *refreezing*, the changes are integrated and stabilized. According to Welch (1979,

p. 309), those involved in the change integrate the idea into their own value system. Thus, in the example, the client and his family would come to value the importance of family involvement in dietary management of their diabetic son and sibling. The family may develop their own strategies for assisting their loved one to comply with the plan.

These three stages are described in Lewin's *force field theory*. Lewin recommended that before a change is begun, the forces operating for and against the change be analyzed. The forces for change are the *driving forces* and the forces against change are *restraining forces*. When the driving forces predominate, change occurs; when restraining forces predominate, change does not occur. It then becomes the responsibility of the change agent to use strategies to reduce the restraining forces and increase the driving forces. Reducing restraining forces usually is more effective than increasing the driving forces. This *unfreezing* is directed at the target system, that is, the individual, family, or group.

Lippitt

Gordon Lippitt described planned change as having seven phases (Lippitt et al., 1958). See Table 13–2. For a detailed discussion of each of these seven stages, see Welch (1979).

Havelock

Ronald Havelock (1973) modified Lewin's theory regarding planned change. See Table 13–2. His theory emphasizes planning the change process, which he believed takes the most time and involves the most significant changes (Welch, 1979, p. 313).

Rogers

Everett Rogers (1983) developed a *diffusion-innovation theory* rather than a planned change theory. He defines *diffusion* as the process by which an innovation is communicated through certain channels over time among the members of a social system. Diffusion that involves innovation becomes *social change* when the diffusion of new ideas results in widespread consequences. His framework, diffusion of innovation, emphasizes the reversible nature of change. Participants may initially adopt a proposal and later discontinue it, or they may initially reject it and adopt it at a later time. Rogers thus introduced the idea that an adopted change is not necessarily permanent. Rogers' three phases in the diffusion of innovation follow (Rogers & Shoemaker, 1971):

1. *Invention.* Collecting information about the proposed change. Data are collected and analyzed.

2. *Diffusion.* Communicating information or the idea to others. It includes disseminating information and estimating the case or difficulty of diffusing the new idea or information.

3. *Consequences.* The dissemination of information may result in the adoption or rejection of the change.

Rogers wrote that the factors associated with successful planned change are relativity, advantage, compatibility, complexity, divisibility, and communicability. His five steps to the diffusion of innovations, referred to as the *innovation-decision process*, follow:

1. *Knowledge.* The individual, called the decision-making unit, is introduced to change and begins to comprehend it.

2. *Persuasion.* The individual develops a favorable or unfavorable attitude toward the change.

3. *Decision.* The person makes a choice to adopt or not to adopt the change.

4. *Implementation.* The person acts on the choice. At this time, alterations may take place.

5. *Confirmation.* The individual looks for confirmation that the choice was right. If the person encounters mixed messages, the choice may be changed.

Rogers emphasized that for change to succeed, the people involved must be interested in the change and committed to implementing it. His theory is particularly useful for individuals who wish to track the adoption of technologic innovations (Hagerman & Tiffany, 1994, p. 60).

CONSIDER...

- how your own experiences with change relate to the different change theories described in this section.
- how the theories of change listed in Table 13–2 relate to the nursing process (see Chapter 14). What types of change might nurses attempt to influence in client care situations?
- how theories of change described in this section relate to theories of nursing as described in Chapter 2.

CHANGE AGENT

A **change agent** is a professional who relies on a systematic body of theoretical knowledge to guide the change process (Brooten et al., 1978). The change agent is the person or group who initiates, motivates, and implements the change. Change agents are leaders. The nurse uses critical thinking (see Chapter 12) and knowledge of change theory to act as an effective change agent in a variety of health care settings.

An effective change agent must be highly skilled. As the nurse moves through the process of change with clients, families, groups, communities, or institutions, the nurse assumes a variety of roles, depending on the type of change and the needs of the individuals involved in the change. Some of these roles may include "investigator, collaborator, consultant, facilitator, evaluator, teacher, observer, organizer, and manager" (Kaplan, 1991, p. 422). It is also important for the change agent to be accessible to all people involved in the change process. The change agent should be honest and straightforward about goals and problems. The accompanying box describes characteristics of effective change agents.

A key element in the change process is trust. The change agent must trust the participants in the change, and they in turn must trust the change agent. One of the greatest risks of change is that it can disrupt the system or even render it nonfunctional. For example, changing the method of nurse assignments could result in gaps and missed care for some clients. To avoid this problem, the change agent must closely observe the situation during the change process.

Change Agent Skills

- The ability to combine ideas from unconnected sources

- The ability to energize others by keeping the interest level up and demonstrating a high personal energy level

- Skill in human relations; well-developed interpersonal communication, group management, and problem-solving skills

- Integrative thinking; the ability to retain a "big picture" focus while dealing with each part of the system

- Sufficient flexibility to modify ideas when modifications will improve the change, but persistent enough to resist nonproductive tampering with the planned change

- Confidence and the tendency not to be easily discouraged

- Realistic thinking

- Trustworthiness; a track record of integrity and success with other changes

- Ability to articulate a "vision" through insights and versatile thinking

- Ability to handle resistance

SOURCE: *Effective Management in Nursing (3rd ed.)* by E. J. Sullivan and P. J. Decker, 1992, Redwood City, CA: Addison-Wesley Nursing, pp. 442–443. Reprinted with permission.

A change agent may be formally or informally designated. A *formally designated change agent* is one who has the role and responsibility for change, such as a clinical nurse-specialist expected to make changes beneficial to specified clients. This person has the authority to plan and implement change. An *informally designated change agent* does not have the authority to make change by virtue of a position but does have the leadership skills and respect of others and therefore can serve an important function in the change process. A change agent who has formal status carries authority, whereas an informal change agent can operate only through persuasion (Ehrenfeld, Bergman & Ziv, 1992, p. 23).

Change agents may also be internal or external. An *internal change agent* is a person who is part of the situation or system, for example, a charge nurse on a hospital unit or a public health nurse providing school health services to a specific school or within a school system. Internal change agents are familiar with the situation and the organization. However, they may have vested interests in the present system as well as biases. An *external change agent* comes to the situation from the "outside," for example, a nursing administrator from another hospital, a nurse-specialist from another health care facility, or a nurse-educator from a local college. External change agents are able to view the problem and the situation objectively and usually have no biases; they are often viewed as experts and are called consultants. However, they may not have personal knowledge of the situation and the problems. They may not be viewed as openly as an "insider"; therefore, they must develop a cooperative working relationship with the people involved in the change. A third option is to pair the external agent with the internal person to serve together as change agents. If this course is taken, it is critical that the two have similar philosophies about change and agree on the goals and process of the change (Kaplan, 1991, p. 420). There are advantages and disadvantages to each of these options, and it is important for any change agent to be aware of both in each situation.

The American Nurses Association (ANA), in *Standards of Clinical Nursing Practice* (1991, p. 13), identifies measurement criteria for the nurse's role in change: Nurses use "the results of quality of care activities to initiate changes in practice" and "to initiate changes throughout the health care delivery system."

CONSIDER . . .

- the formal and informal change agents in your practice setting. How do they effect change? Compare the characteristics of the individuals you have identified as formal and informal change agents.

- your experience with internal and external change agents. What specific characteristics are important in selecting internal change agents? In selecting external change agents?

- your own experience as a change agent. What are the feelings and experiences associated with acting as a change agent?

COPING WITH CHANGE

Although change is inevitable and necessary for growth, it is not always welcome and often produces anxiety. Even when change is well planned, it can be threatening because the process renders something different from the status quo. Change evokes emotional reactions, consumes considerable internal resources and energy, and often is associated with feelings of loss, grief, and pain. Various models have been used to explain the psychologic problems associated with change. A ten-step model proposed by Perlman and Takacs (1990, pp. 33–38) is discussed here. This model is based on the Kübler-Ross model of death and dying. The ten steps follow:

1. *Equilibrium*—Feelings of comfort and contentment with the status quo.

2. *Denial*—Holding onto familiar patterns and manifesting some active resistance to change because of a sense of uneasiness, lack of direction, and insecurity.

3. *Anger*—Blaming others for the predicament and expecting someone other than themselves to make things right.

4. *Bargaining*—Negotiating with others to prevent the inevitable from happening and to maintain the status quo.

5. *Chaos*—Feelings of confusion about the organization's identity and direction.

6. *Depression*—Feelings of sorrow and depletion of resources to cope. Fear of loss creates a *reactive depression; preparatory depression* facilitates eventual acceptance of the changes.

7. *Resignation*—Unhappily accepting the reality of the change and no longer resisting it.

8. *Openness*—Expending energies on what others recommend and being ready to learn about the change.

9. *Readiness*—Experiencing a "letting go" of the past and exploring new events.

10. *Reemergence*—Becoming fully operational as an employee and proactive in the work environment.

Characteristics of and interventions for each of these steps are shown in Table 13–3. Emotional reactions to change can increase resistance to change. It is important for change agents and recipients to deal effectively with these emotional dimensions.

Accepting Change

Accepting change often takes time, particularly when it does not fit into a person's attitudinal frame of reference; in such a case, change may not occur at all. For example, to stop smoking may not be accepted as a desirable behavior change by a person who values smoking and does not believe it is harmful. Optimally, this belief changes before the person tries to change the behavior. Stages in the acceptance of change are shown in the accompanying box. Some characteristics and beliefs that can help people survive the stress of change include the following (Brown, 1990, pp. 586–587):

- *Hardiness*—the ability to endure and grow in spite of difficult conditions
- *Positive outlook*—the ability to view change as an opportunity
- *Commitment*—the belief in the value of the change and the desire to work actively to promote the change
- *Control*—the sense that one can influence events; a sense of empowerment
- *Social support*—the feeling of support from and assistance of others involved in the change; the feeling that one is not alone
- *Stress management*—the ability to use stress management strategies to cope effectively with stressors associated with the change process
- *Timing*—the ability to determine the appropriate time to introduce change, to provide time for everyone to participate in all steps of the

---

Stages in the Acceptance of Change

The individual

1. Becomes aware of the new idea, system, or practice.

2. Seeks more information about the change.

3. Evaluates the information and relates it to the present situation.

4. Mentally tries out the proposed change.

5. Actually tries out the change, on a small scale if possible.

6. Adopts and integrates the change into the present system.

When a change is introduced, the nearer the people involved in the change are to the process, the easier the implementation of the change. These stages of acceptance can then naturally evolve.

SOURCE: "Effecting Change" by B. Stevens, February 1975, *Journal of Nursing Administration*, 5, p. 25. Used with permission.

TABLE 13-3   Growing with Change: The Emotional Voyage of the Change Process

Phase	Characteristics/Symptoms	Change Agent Interventions
1. Equilibrium	High energy level. State of emotional and intellectual balance. Sense of inner peace with personal and professional goals in sync.	Make employees aware of changes in the environment which will have impact on the status quo.
2. Denial	Energy is drained by the defense mechanism of rationalizing a denial of the reality of the change. Employees experience negative changes in physical health, emotional balance, logical thinking patterns, and normal behavior patterns.	Employ active listening skills; e.g., be empathetic, nonjudgmental, use reflective listening techniques. Nurturing behavior, avoiding isolation, and offering stress management workshops also will help.
3. Anger	Energy is used to ward off and actively resist the change by blaming others. Frustration, anger, rage, envy and resentment become visible.	Recognize the symptoms, legitimize employees' feelings and verbal expressions of anger, rage, envy and resentment. Active listening, assertiveness, and problem-solving skills needed by managers. Employees need to probe within for the source of their anger.
4. Bargaining	Energy is used in an attempt to eliminate the change. Talk is about "if only." Others try to solve the problem. "Bargains" are unrealistic and designed to compromise the change out of existence.	Search for real needs/problems and bring them into the open. Explore ways of achieving desired changes through conflict management skills and win-win negotiation skills.
5. Chaos	Diffused energy, feeling of powerlessness, insecurity, sense of disorientation. Loss of identity and direction. No sense of grounding or meaning. Breakdown of value system and belief. Defense mechanisms begin to lose usefulness and meaning.	Quiet time for reflection. Listening skills. Inner search for both employee and organization identity and meaning. Approval for being in state of flux.
6. Depression	No energy left to produce results. Former defense mechanisms no longer operable. Self-pity, remembering past, expressions of sorrow, feeling nothingness and emptiness.	Provide necessary information in a timely fashion. Allow sorrow and pain to be expressed openly. Long-term patience, take one step at a time as employees learn to let go.
7. Resignation	Energy expended in passively accepting change. Lack of enthusiasm.	Expect employees to be accountable for reactions to behavior. Allow them to move at their own pace.
8. Openness	Availability to renewed energy. Willingness to expend energy on what has been assigned to individual.	Patiently explain again, in detail, the desired change.
9. Readiness	Willingness to expend energy in exploring new events. Reunification of intellect and emotions begins.	Assume a directive management style: assign tasks, monitor tasks and results so as to provide direction and guidelines.
10. Reemergence	Rechanneled energy produces feelings of empowerment and employees become more proactive. Rebirth of growth and commitment. Employee initiates projects and ideas. Career questions answered.	Mutual answering of questions. Redefinition of career, mission and culture. Mutual understanding of role and identity. Employees will take action based on own decisions.

Source: "The Ten Stages of Change" by D. Perlman and G. J. Takacs, April 1990, *Nursing Management, 21*, p. 34. Used with permission of Springhouse Corporation®.

Guidelines for Experiencing Change

- In the initial stages, expect some confusion, uncertainty about expectations, and difficulty making decisions. Ask for more direction and clarification of expectations.

- Minimize the impact of the change by being honest about losses and gains associated with the change.

- Face one day or one step at a time.

- Accept help from others, or, if you are unable to do that, respond in ways that will encourage their support at a later time.

- Expect to feel some anger, discouragement, and resentment. Allow expression of these feelings, preferably with someone who can listen nonjudgmentally.

- Relinquish the past. Recount good memories, and then plan a "letting go" ritual, such as a burial or a graduation party.

- Accept some feelings of longing and sadness for the way things used to be.

- Seek out colleagues who are experiencing the same change or loss, particularly those who are supportive and encouraging.

- Visualize new skills and approaches required by the change, and consider ways to learn them.

- Seek new experiences, celebrate small successes, and share the experience with others.

- Look back periodically to realize the extent and effectiveness of the change.

SOURCE: Adapted from "Understanding the Seven Stages of Change," by J. Manion, April 1995, *American Journal of Nursing*, *95*, pp. 41–43.

change process, and to pace the implementation of change so as not to overwhelm those affected by it

Managing change requires adaptibility, flexibility, and resilience. Guidelines for coping with this transition are shown in the accompanying box.

Resisting Change

Resistance to change is not merely lack of acceptance but rather behavior intended to maintain the status quo—that is, to prevent the change. The change agent should anticipate some resistance to change, no matter how beneficial the change may seem. Resistance to change is often greatest when the idea is not concurrent with existing trends, such as trying to change from primary nursing to functional nursing when primary nursing is currently popular. Resistance is also usually great when the proposed change would alter a situation with which people are comfortable.

Robinson (1991, p. 823) suggests that some degree of resistance to change is a natural response and should not be viewed negatively. Resistance may help people adapt to the proposed change as they try to understand the meaning on a personal level, establish a thread of continuity, and then accept and grow with the change. See the box on page 250 for common reasons for resistance to change (restraining forces).

Watson (1973, pp. 118–119) proposed five stages in resistance, which lead eventually to successful change:

1. Resistance is undifferentiated.

2. The forces for and against change develop their arguments.

3. Resistance is mobilized to defeat the proposal. The resistance is either overcome or reduced.

4. Support for the change is strengthened.

5. Few opponents for the change are left, and they are isolated from the group.

To manage resistance, the leader (change agent) can analyze the field forces operating in the change (see the discussion of Lewin's theory, earlier in this chapter). After the analysis, three kinds of tactics can be used to "unfreeze" the system: (1) create discomfort, (2) induce guilt or anxiety, (3) provide psychologic safety (Tappen, 1995, p. 332). To create discomfort, the change agent can confront the target system with conflicting evidence that challenges the status quo. Often, the change agent meets with defensive responses that attempt to protect the individuals. By inducing guilt—for example, by pointing out that accepted goals are not being met—the change agent often upsets the balance of the driving and restraining forces. Then, by providing psychologic safety, the change agent can help the target system feel more comfortable and less threatened about the change. See the accompanying box.

Examples to Unfreeze a Target System

Producing discomfort
- Meet with small groups of nurses (target system) to discuss the inadequacies of the system of concern (e.g., staffing).

Inducing guilt and anxiety
- Demonstrate how the system is not meeting clients' needs for care.
- Explain that the administration wants the new system.
- Provide examples of how the old system has endangered client safety.

Providing psychologic safety
- Assure nurses (target system) that adequate numbers of nurses will be provided.
- Point out that sufficient time will be provided to implement the new system.
- Express confidence in the nurses' abilities to implement the change.
- Assure the nurses that there will be regular meetings to discuss progress.

Overcoming Resistance to Change

McKay (1993, p. 6) presents five realistic strategies for change agents to overcome resistance to change: Participation, communication, force field analysis, education, and avoidance of pitfalls.

Participation Through involving affected individuals in the decision-making process, the change agent decreases resistance to change by (a) decreasing potential feelings of alienation of the change targets, (b) socializing involved individuals into the change agent's ways of thinking, and (c) giving individuals a vested interest in the success of change, thus enhancing their commitment. Eliciting participation is a time-consuming process. Steps for increasing participation during the introduction of planned change follow:

1. Ask for input using questionnaires, surveys, brainstorming, and other group techniques.

2. Carefully consider the input, and objectively evaluate it. Convey a genuine desire and respect for input and value the suggestions provided.

3. Use those ideas that have merit.

4. Reject those ideas that are not practical.

5. Give credit to individuals whose ideas are being used.

6. Assure those whose ideas were rejected that their ideas were considered. Explain why the ideas were not used.

Communication Effective communication is vital to the success of planned change. Inadequate communication results in inaccurate perceptions and threatened self-interests that encourage resistive behaviors. Elements of successful communication are similar to those nurses use with clients: openness, attentive listening, providing a climate of trust, honesty, respect, empathy, and so on. All those who are potentially affected by the change need to list and receive direct information about the proposed change. The change agent should communicate in the early stages with other administrators who hold formal power so that the nurse can obtain managerial commitment to the change and with leaders at the change level who hold informal power. Written communication alone is inappropriate; face-to-face personalized oral communication is preferred. If information is complex, written and oral communications can be combined.

Force-Field Analysis Lewin's classical model of change theory (Lewin, 1948) can be used to consider the driving forces and the restraining forces. The change agent needs to consider strategies that will decrease restraining forces, increase the driving forces, or both. Common driving and restraining forces are shown in the box on page 250.

Education Obviously, education is required for overcoming resistance, but its effectiveness relies on a good relationship between the change agents and change targets. Education is essential (a) when the change involves a marked departure from past practices, because many new skills will need to be learned; (b) when resistance develops because of inaccurate or incomplete information; and (c) when an involved individual does not recognize the need for change.

Avoidance of Pitfalls Four common pitfalls are (a) rapid introduction of change (even when the plan is

Common Driving and Restraining Forces

Motivating Forces

- Perception that the change is challenging
- Economic gain
- Perception that the change will improve the situation
- Visualization of the future impact of change
- Potential for self-growth, recognition, achievement, and improved relationships.

Restraining Forces

- Fear that something of personal value will be lost (e.g., threat to job security or self-esteem)
- Misunderstanding of the change and its implications
- Low tolerance for change related to intellectual or emotional insecurity
- Perception that the change will not achieve goals; failure to see the big picture
- Lack of time or energy

Managing Resistance

1. Communicate with those who oppose the change. Get to the root of their reasons for opposition.
2. Clarify information and provide accurate feedback.
3. Be open to revisions but clear about what must remain.
4. Present the negative consequences of resistance (threats to organizational survival, compromised client care, and so on).
5. Emphasize the positive consequences of the change and how the individual or group will benefit. However, do not spend too much energy on rational analysis of why the change is good and why the arguments against it do not hold up. People's resistance frequently flows from feelings that are not rational.
6. Keep resisters involved in face-to-face contact with supporters. Encourage proponents to empathize with opponents, recognize valid objections, and relieve unnecessary fears.
7. Maintain a climate of trust, support, and confidence.
8. Divert attention by creating a different "disturbance." Energy can shift to a "more important" problem inside the system, thereby redirecting resistance. Alternatively attention can be brought to an external threat to create a "bully phenomenon." When members perceive a greater environmental threat (such as competition or restrictive governmental policies), they tend to unify internally.
9. Follow the "politics of change."

SOURCE: *Effective Management in Nursing (3rd ed.)* by E. J. Sullivan and P. J. Decker, 1992, Redwood City, CA: Addison-Wesley Nursing, pp. 444–445. Reprinted with permission.

clear and well thought out), (b) choosing strategies that differ vastly from traditional, long-standing practices, and (c) ignoring the "social aspect" of a change. Guidelines to manage resistance are shown in the box at the right.

Examples of Change

It is exciting to realize how effective nurses can be when they determine the need for change and plan strategies to bring it about. The following examples outline changes initiated by nurses who have identified a need to "do something" in each of four spheres of influence: the workplace, organizations, government, and the community.

The Workplace   At each of three shift meetings Nurse Hawkins, Head Nurse, listened to nurses complain about problems with getting clients' laboratory work done and reported to the unit in a timely manner. She conferred with other head nurses and with the attending and resident physicians on her unit. It appeared that similar complaints were widespread.

At the next meeting of head nurses, Nurse Hawkins described the problem. The group appointed a task force, with Nurse Hawkins as Chair, and asked it to present a plan to solve the problem at the next meeting. After gathering more data, the task force invited representatives from the attending and resident staff and the laboratory director to meet with them to review the data, consider alternative solutions, and select a plan to solve the problem.

By the next meeting of head nurses, a preliminary plan to alter the system of laboratory reporting had been devised, and all concerned were working cooperatively to implement the plan.

The Professional Organization Nurses on the Education Committee of a district nurses' association recognized the need to make a public policy statement concerning the care of clients with AIDS. Since the board of directors had recently expressed interest in promulgating such policy statements, the committee sensed the timing was right and that the board would welcome its draft despite the controversial subject matter.

Members of the committee researched and drafted a statement. The full committee offered a critique and selected an articulate spokesperson to present the statement to the association president and seek support before asking to have the statement presented to the board. Once the president had approved the statement, it was placed on the agenda for the next board meeting.

After making minor additions, the board approved it for distribution to the lay and nursing press and asked the Education Committee to suggest a nurse to present the statement at a local hearing of the City Council Health Committee.

The Government While the pressure to contain health care costs escalated through the first half of the 1980s, a coalition representing the shared interests of the ANA, the National League for Nursing (NLN), and the American Association of Colleges of Nursing (AACN) mounted a campaign to convince Congress of the cost-effectiveness of a center for nursing research within the National Institutes of Health (NIH). Despite incredible odds, including a presidential veto and opposition from the American Medical Association, the American Association of Medical Colleges, and the NIH administrations, the proposal was passed by Congress in the fall of 1985. The success of this effort demonstrates the effectiveness of carefully planned change including the collaboration of nursing organizations. It also illustrates the clout organized nurses can wield on any level and in any sphere.

The Community Every nurse plays several roles besides that of registered nurse. Each resides in a community, and many are parents. Some serve on school boards, belong to the League of Women Voters, or participate in religious, club, or scouting activities. There are numerous opportunities for nurses to contribute to the health and welfare of the communities in which they live. A group of nursing

students recognized a health problem within their community and developed a plan to intervene. Many of the students were parents of children in local elementary schools where a high percentage of children were being sent home daily with head lice. Because of previously enacted budget cuts, the district's school nurses were each responsible for between three and five schools. The students volunteered to work with the district nurses to provide screening and health teaching at each of the elementary schools, thereby helping to resolve the community's problem.

All nurses are affected by change; nobody can avoid it. Knowledgeable nurses make rational plans to deal with both opportunities to initiate and guide needed change as well as to respond to change that affects them in the workplace, government, organizations, and the community. To recognize these opportunities for change and respond to the factors that influence nursing from without, it is helpful to consider the history of nursing, current trends in nursing, and present political, social, technologic, and economic issues.

CONSIDER...

- what changes are needed in your professional skills and abilities to help you to become a more effective change agent. How will you approach these changes?
- a change that is needed in your practice setting. What are the different driving and restraining forces involved in the proposed change? What strategies might you implement to reduce the restraining forces? What strategies might you implement to enhance the driving forces? How might you obtain the assistance of formal and informal change agents in your practice setting to facilitate the change?
- the insistent call for health care reform that has been sounded in the United States since the mid 1980s. In countries with national medical systems (Canada, Australia, Great Britain), there has been concern about high taxes and insufficient funds to meet the health care needs of all citizens. How might nurses become active change agents in improving the health care system of their nation or state/province?

READINGS FOR ENRICHMENT

Bhola, H. S. (1994, May). The CLER model: Thinking through change. *Nursing Management, 25,* 59–63.

The CLER model, which is based on systems thinking, is a model for nurses to plan and implement change in interpersonal, institutional, and cultural settings. The acronym CLER stands for *C*onfigurations, *L*inkages, *E*nvironment(s), and *R*esources. This article discusses the concepts behind CLER and six characteristics of the model. Strategizing with CLER involves acceptance of three interactive components: the planner system (P), the change objective (O), and the adopter system (A).

Lane, A. J. (1992, September). Using Havelock's model to plan unit-based change. *Nursing Management, 23,* 58–60.

Lane states that the ability to change is critical to survival in today's complex health care arena. Nurse managers must understand the dynamics of change. This article details how to approach unit-level care using Havelock's six-phase approach.

Stelling, J., & Milne-Smith, J. (1994, Spring). Break-points and continuities: A case study of reactive change. *Nursing Administration Quarterly, 18*(3), 43–50.

This article discusses the radical changes nursing administrators effected on a pediatric psychiatry ward in response to major organizational changes. The changes were reactive; that is, they were adaptive changes to new surrounding circumstances. The authors present a case history of change on the ward to convey how the changes were accomplished. The changes included the following: A bachelor's degree in nursing science became mandatory for nursing staff, family systems nursing was introduced, and postdischarge nursing follow-up was instituted. The authors suggest that there were many driving forces, including a strong vision of nursing, sufficient pain or discomfort to motivate change, the ability to recognize and seize opportunities, and the linking of change to existing institutional practices, policies, and values.

SUMMARY

To be effective and influential in current and future health care delivery systems, nurses need to understand and apply change theory. Change generally occurs in response to three different activities: spontaneous reactions or events, developmental activities, and consciously planned activities. These three types of change can occur on an individual or organizational level.

The three most commonly used approaches to change are the empirical-rational approach, the power-coercive approach, and the normative-reeducative approach. In reality, all three of these approaches may operate in a situation of change simultaneously.

Lewin's theory of change has three stages: unfreezing, moving, and refreezing. His force-field analysis is a means of examining the driving forces for change and the restraining forces that would limit change. The analysis of the opposing forces is done in the unfreezing stage. Reducing restraining forces is usually more effective in accomplishing change than is increasing the driving forces.

Lippitt proposed a seven-stage process beginning with diagnosing the problem and ending with terminating the helping relationship. Havelock modified Lewin's theory to emphasize the planning stage of the change process. His six-stage theory begins with building a relationship and ends with stabilization and generating self-renewal. Rogers introduced the idea that adopted

change is not necessarily permanent. He developed a five-step diffusion innovation process.

A change agent seeks to facilitate the processes of change. An effective change agent uses an understanding of the change process to plan and implement any change. To be effective change agents, nurses require excellent skills of communication, problem solving, decision making, and teaching and must be able to project expertise, know how to use available resources, be able to inspire trust in themselves and others, and have a good sense of timing. A change agent may be formally or informally designated, internal or external. Nurses frequently act as formal or informal change agents in relation to clients, families, work settings, and communities. The change agent works to alter the driving and restraining forces and facilitates the acceptance of change by encouraging the participation of all involved in the change process. Effective communication is vital to the success of planned change.

Change is stressful, and the individuals experiencing change need to be supported and empowered. The stress is often associated with emotional reactions of denial, anger, feelings of loss, grief, and pain. An understanding of these responses enables both change agents and those experiencing the change to minimize the trauma associated with it. Managing change requires adaptability, flexibility, and resilience.

SELECTED REFERENCES

Alfaro-Lefevre, R. (1995). *Critical thinking in nursing: A practical approach*. Philadelphia: W. B. Saunders.

American Nurses Association. (1991). *Standards of clinical nursing practice*. Washington, DC: Author.

Bennis, W. G., Benne, K. D., & Chin, R., (Eds.). (1985). *The planning of change* (4th ed.). New York: Holt, Rinehart & Winston.

Brooten, D. A. (1984). *Managerial leadership in nursing*. Philadelphia: Lippincott.

Brooten, D. A., Hayman I., & Naylor, M. (1978). *Leadership for change: A guide for the frustrated nurse*. Philadelphia: Lippincott.

Brown, K. (1990, December). Managing Change. *AAOHN Journal, 38*, 586–587.

Carnall, C. A. (1990). *Managing change in organizations*. New York: Prentice Hall.

Ehrenfeld, M., Bergman, R., & Ziv, L. (1992, Jan./Feb.). Academia—a stimulus for change. *International Nursing Review, 39*, 23–26.

Hagerman, Z. J., & Tiffany, C. R. (1994, April). Evaluation of two planned change theories. *Nursing Management, 25*, 57–62.

Havelock, R. (1973). *The change agent's guide to innovations in education*. Englewood Cliffs, NJ: Educational Technology Publications.

Johnson Lutjens, L. R., & Tiffany, C. R. (1994, March). Evaluating planned change theories. *Nursing Management, 25*, 54–57.

Kaplan, S. M. (1991, Dec.). The nurse as change agent. *Dermatology Nursing, 3*, 419–422.

Kirkpatrick, D. L. (1985). *How to manage change effectively*. San Francisco: Jossey-Bass.

Lewin, K. (1948). *Resolving social conflicts*. New York: Harper and Brothers.

Lewin, K. (1951). *Field theory in social science*. New York: Harper and Row.

Lippitt, G. L. (1973). *Visualizing change: Model building and the change process*. La Jolla, CA: University Associates.

Lippitt, R., Watson, J., & Westley, B. (1958). *The dynamics of planned change*. New York: Harcourt Brace.

Manion, J. (1995, April). Understanding the seven stages of change. *American Journal of Nursing, 95*, 41–43.

Marriner-Tomey, A. (1992). *Guide to nursing management*. (4th ed.). St. Louis: Mosby-Year Book.

Mauksch, I. G., & Miller, M. H. (1981). *Implementing change in nursing*. St. Louis: Mosby.

McKay, L. (1993, March/April). Overcoming resistance to change. *Canadian Journal of Nursing Administration, 6*(1):6–9.

Olson, E. M. (1979, June). Strategies and techniques for the nurse change agent. *Nursing Clinics of North America, 14*, 323–336.

Perlman, D., & Takacs, G. J. (1990, April). The 10 stages of change. *Nursing Management, 21*, 33–38.

Robinson, J. (1991, July). Project 2000: The role of resistance in the process of professional growth. *Journal of Advanced Nursing, 16*, 820–824.

Rogers, E. (1983). *Diffusion of innovations* (3rd ed.). New York: Free Press.

Rogers, E., & Shoemaker, F. (1971). *Communication of innovations: A crosscultural approach*. New York: The Free Press of Glencoe.

Skinner, M. D. (1994, Spring). Getting to X. *Nursing Administration Quarterly, 18*, 58–63.

Spencer, S. A., & Adams, J. D. (1990). *Life changes: Growing through personal transitions*. San Luis Obispo, CA: Impact Publishers.

Spradley, B. W. (1980). Making change creatively. *Journal of Nursing Administration, 10*, 32–37.

Strader, M. K., & Decker, P. J. (1995). *Role transition to patient care management*. Norwalk, CT: Appleton & Lange.

Sullivan, E. J., & Decker, P. J. (1992). *Effective management in nursing* (3rd ed.). Redwood City, CA: Addison-Wesley Nursing.

Tappen, R. M. (1995). *Nursing leadership and management: Concepts and practice* (3rd ed.). Philadelphia: F. A. Davis.

Tiffany, C. R. (1994, Feb.) Analysis of planned change theories. *Nursing Management, 25*, 60–62.

Watson, G. (1973). Resistance to change. In G. Zaltman (Ed.) *Processes and phenomena of social change*. New York: Wiley.

Welch, L. B. (1979, June). Planned change in nursing: The theory. *Nursing Clinics of North America, 14*, 307–321.

CHAPTER

Nursing Process

OBJECTIVES

- Describe the components of the nursing process.

- Identify essential characteristics of the nursing process.

- Discuss the relationship among multidisciplinary assessments.

- Identify various types, components, and formats of nursing diagnoses.

- Discuss essential aspects of nursing prognosis.

- Identify essential guidelines for writing goals, expected outcomes, and nursing care plans.

- Describe the basic steps in the assessment, diagnostic, planning, implementation, and evaluation processes.

- Discuss three approaches to quality evaluation.

"The nursing process is the core and essence of nursing; it is central to all nursing actions; it is applicable in any setting and within any theoretical/conceptual reference. It is flexible and adaptable, adjustable to a number of variables, yet sufficiently structured so as to provide a base from which all systematic nursing actions can proceed."
—Yura and Walsh, 1983

The **nursing process** is a systematic, rational method of planning and providing individualized nursing care.

- The purpose of the nursing process is to identify a client's health status, actual or potential health care problems or needs; to establish plans to meet the identified needs; and to deliver specific nursing interventions to meet those needs.

- The nursing process is cyclic; that is, the components of the nursing process follow a logical sequence, but more than one component may be involved at any one time.

- The nursing process consists of a series of five components or phases: assessing, diagnosing, planning, implementing, and evaluating (Figure 14–1).

- The five phases of the nursing process are not discrete entities but overlapping, continuing subprocesses. Each phase of the nursing process affects the others; all phases are closely interrelated.

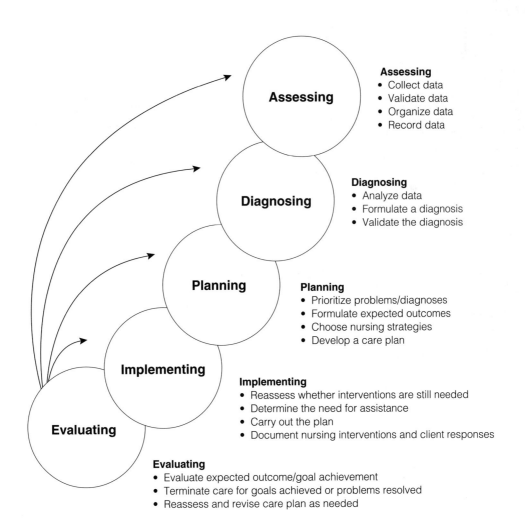

Assessing
- Collect data
- Validate data
- Organize data
- Record data

Diagnosing
- Analyze data
- Formulate a diagnosis
- Validate the diagnosis

Planning
- Prioritize problems/diagnoses
- Formulate expected outcomes
- Choose nursing strategies
- Develop a care plan

Implementing
- Reassess whether interventions are still needed
- Determine the need for assistance
- Carry out the plan
- Document nursing interventions and client responses

Evaluating
- Evaluate expected outcome/goal achievement
- Terminate care for goals achieved or problems resolved
- Reassess and revise care plan as needed

FIGURE 14–1 *The nursing process.*

Characteristics of the Nursing Process

- The system is open and flexible to meet the unique needs of client, family, group, or community.

- It is cyclic and dynamic. Because all phases are inter-related, there is no absolute beginning or end.

- It is client centered; it individualizes the approach to each client's particular needs.

- It is interpersonal and collaborative. It requires the nurse to communicate directly and consistently with clients to meet their needs.

- It is planned.

- It is goal directed.

- It permits creativity for the nurse and client in devising ways to solve the stated health problem.

- It emphasizes feedback, which leads either to reassessment of the problem or to revision of the care plan.

- It is universally applicable. The nursing process is used as a framework for nursing care in all types of health care settings, with clients of all age groups.

ANA Standards

Standard I: *Assessment*
The nurse collects client health data.

Measurement Criteria
1. The priority of data collection is determined by the client's immediate condition or needs.

2. Pertinent data are collected using appropriate assessment techniques.

3. Data collection involves the client, significant others, and health care providers when appropriate.

4. The data collection process is systematic and ongoing.

5. Relevant data are documented in a retrievable form.

SOURCE: Abstracted from *Standards of Clinical Nursing Practice*, by the American Nurses Association, 1991, Kansas City, MO: Author, p. 9. Used with permission.

CHARACTERISTICS OF THE NURSING PROCESS

The nursing process "provides the framework in which nurses use their knowledge and skills to express human caring" and to help clients meet their health needs (Wilkinson, 1996, p. 4). The nursing process is characterized by unique properties that enable it to respond to the changing health status of the client. See the accompanying box. Hence, the nursing process is *cyclic and dynamic* rather than static.

Decision making is involved in every component of the nursing process (Yura & Walsh, 1988, p. 108). Nurses can be highly creative when using the nursing process. They are not bound by standard responses and may apply their repertoire of knowledge and skills to assist clients.

THE ASSESSMENT PHASE

Assessment, the first phase of the nursing process, involves collecting, organizing, validating, and recording data. It must take place before a nursing diagnosis can be made. The ANA's *Standards of*

Clinical Nursing Practice (1991, p. 9) outlines nurses' accountability for collecting client data. See the accompanying box.

In effect, assessing is a continuous process carried out during all phases of the nursing process. For example, in the evaluation phase, assessment is done to determine the outcomes of the nursing strategies and to evaluate goal achievement. All phases of the nursing process depend on the accurate and complete collection of **data** (information).

The assessment process involves four closely related activities:

- Collecting data
- Organizing data
- Validating data
- Recording data

Collecting Data

Data collection is the process of gathering information about a client's health status. It must be both systematic and continuous to prevent the omission of significant data and reflect the changes in the client's health status.

A **database** (baseline data) is all the information about a client; it includes the nursing health history and physical assessment, the physician's history and physical examination, results of laboratory and diagnostic tests, and information contributed by other

TABLE 14–1   Factors That May Impede Client Data Collection

Client Factor	Effect	Nursing Action
Language difficulty (e.g., not fluent in English)	Unable to clearly communicate vital information.	Use simple, clear language with client. Obtain an interpreter.
High anxiety	Rapid, incoherent speech; distortion of information.	Attempt to reduce anxiety by speaking slowly and quietly; emphasize importance of providing accurate information to get appropriate help.
Fear that illness is incapacitating or life-threatening	May deny certain symptoms or deliberately give misleading facts.	Explore discrepancies between client statements and physical findings or data from other sources.
Acute illness and/or pain	Short responses; primary concern is intervention to alleviate the problem.	Provide required intervention before obtaining data. Ask closed questions to obtain essential data.
Limited mental capacity	Possibility of inaccurate, unreliable information.	Encourage client to provide as much information as able; then, use secondary sources.
Previous negative experience with health care professionals	Resists providing data; believes "it won't help me anyway. It didn't do any good before."	Acknowledge previous experience and the imperfection of health professionals. Request another chance to help. Convey competence. Respect client's thoughts and feelings.

health professionals, such as reports from consulting physicians, evaluations by physical and occupational therapists, and assessments by social workers.

Client data should include past history as well as information about current concerns and health promotion activities. The nurse should obtain such important past health history data as allergies, previous surgeries, hospitalizations or injuries, childhood illnesses, and chronic health problems. The nurse also obtains current data regarding present concerns or symptoms, such as pain, nausea, or dizziness; and personal health promotion practices, which may include nutritional patterns, rest and activity patterns, folk or cultural healing practices, and religious practices. To collect data accurately, both the client and nurse must actively participate. It is important that the nurse be aware of factors that may impede data collection and institute appropriate interventions. See Table 14–1.

The primary methods nurses use to assess clients are observation, interviewing, and examination. Nurses carry out observation whenever they come into contact with the client or support persons. The primary interviewing process is taking the client's health history. In obtaining the client's health history, the nurse may (1) obtain data on which the nurse will plan future nursing care, (2) develop rapport with the client that fosters greater cooperation and collaboration and allows the nurse to plan individualized care, and (3) provide the client with greater insight into the client's own health and illness behaviors. Examination is the major method used in the physical health assessment. During the physical assessment, the nurse further explores and validates information obtained during the history interview and uncovers additional health concerns.

In practice, the nurse uses all three methods simultaneously when assessing clients. For example, during the client interview, the nurse observes, listens, asks questions, and mentally retains information to explore in the physical assessment.

Organizing Data

To obtain data systematically, the nurse uses an organized assessment framework, often referred to as a *nursing health history* or *nursing assessment*. Data collected during the nursing health history are largely subjective. There are many frameworks available for the systematic collection and documentation of assessment data. The framework may be modified according to the client's physical status.

Nursing Conceptual Models

Most nursing education and health care agencies have developed their own structured assessment tools. Many of these are based on selected nursing theories (see Chapter 2). One example is Gordon's functional health pattern framework, a framework of 11 functional health patterns. Gordon uses the word *pattern* to signify a sequence of behavior. The nurse collects data about dysfunctional as well as functional behavior. Thus, by using Gordon's framework to organize data, nurses are able to discern emerging patterns (see the accompanying box).

Gordon's Typology of 11 Functional Health Patterns

- *Health-perception–health-management pattern.* Describes client's perceived pattern of health and well-being and how health is managed.

- *Nutritional-metabolic pattern.* Describes pattern of food and fluid consumption relative to metabolic need and pattern indicators of local nutrient supply.

- *Elimination pattern.* Describes patterns of excretory function (bowel, bladder, and skin).

- *Activity-exercise pattern.* Describes pattern of exercise, activity, leisure, and recreation.

- *Cognitive-perceptual pattern.* Describes sensory-perceptual and cognitive pattern.

- *Sleep-rest pattern.* Describes patterns of sleep, rest, and relaxation.

- *Self-perception–self-concept pattern.* Describes self-concept pattern and perceptions of self (e.g., body comfort, body image, feeling state).

- *Role-relationship pattern.* Describes pattern of role-engagements and relationships.

- *Sexuality-reproductive pattern.* Describes client's patterns of satisfaction and dissatisfaction with sexuality; describes reproductive patterns.

- *Coping–stress tolerance pattern.* Describes general coping pattern and effectiveness of the pattern in terms of stress tolerance.

- *Value-belief pattern.* Describes patterns of values, beliefs (including spiritual), or goals that guide choices or decisions.

SOURCE: *Nursing Diagnosis: Process and Application* (3rd ed.), by M. Gordon, St. Louis: Mosby, 1994, p. 93.

Wellness Models

Nurses use wellness models to assist clients to identify health risks and to explore life-style habits and health behaviors, beliefs, values, and attitudes that influence levels of wellness. Such models generally include the following (see Chapter 16 for details):

- Health history
- Physical fitness evaluation
- Nutritional assessment
- Life-stress analysis
- Life-style and health habits
- Health beliefs
- Sexual health
- Spiritual health
- Relationships
- Health risk appraisal

Nonnursing Models

Frameworks and models from other disciplines may also be helpful for organizing data. These frameworks are often narrower than the model required in nursing; therefore, the nurse usually needs to combine these with other approaches to obtain a complete history. Examples are (a) the body systems model of physicians, (b) Maslow's hierarchy of needs, and (c) developmental theories such as Havighurst's age periods and developmental tasks, Freud's five stages of development, Erikson's eight stages of development, Piaget's phases of cognitive development, and Kohlberg's stages of moral development.

Validating Data

If the nursing process is to be a successful framework for nursing care, the information gathered during the assessment phase must be complete, factual, and accurate. **Validation** is the act of "double-checking" or verifying data (cues) to confirm that they are accurate and factual. Validating data helps the nurse

- Ensure that assessment information is complete.
- Ensure that objective and related subjective data agree.
- Obtain additional information that may have been overlooked.
- Differentiate cues from inferences.
- Avoid jumping to conclusions and focusing in the wrong direction to identify problems.

Not all data require validation. For example, data such as height, weight, birth data, and most

TABLE 14–2 Validating Assessment Data

Guidelines	Example
Compare subjective and objective data to verify the client's statements with your observations.	Client's perceptions of "feeling hot" need to be compared with measurement of the body temperature.
Clarify any ambiguous or vague statements.	*Client:* "I've felt sick on and off for 6 weeks."
	Nurse: "Describe what your sickness is like. Tell me what you mean by 'on and off.'"
Be sure that your data consists of cues and not inferences.	*Observation:* Dry skin and reduced tissue turgor.
	Inference: Dehydration.
	Action: Collect additional data that are needed to make the inference in the diagnosing phase. For example, determine the client's fluid intake, amount and appearance of urine, and blood pressure.
Double-check data that are extremely abnormal.	*Observation:* A resting pulse of 40 beats per minute or a blood pressure of 180/95 mm Hg.
	Action: Use another piece of equipment as needed to confirm abnormalities, or ask someone else to collect the same data.
Determine the presence of factors that may interfere with accurate measurement.	A crying infant will have an abnormal respiratory rate and will need quieting before accurate assessment can be made.
Use references (textbooks, journals, research reports) to explain phenomena.	A nurse considers tiny purple or bluish-black swollen areas under the tongue of an elderly client to be abnormal until reading about physical changes of aging. Such varicosities are not uncommon.

laboratory studies that can be measured with an accurate scale of measurement can be accepted as factual. As a rule, the nurse validates data when there are discrepancies between data obtained in the nursing interview (subjective data) and the physical examination (objective data), or when the client's statements differ at different times in the assessment. Guidelines for validating data are shown in Table 14–2.

Cues are subjective or objective data that can be directly observed by the nurse; that is, cues include what the client says or what the nurse can see, hear, feel, smell, or measure. **Inferences** are the nurse's conclusions or interpretation of the cues; for example, if a nurse observes the cues that an incision is red, hot, and swollen, the nurse makes the inference that the incision is infected.

To collect data accurately, nurses need to be aware of their own biases, values, and beliefs and to separate fact from inference, interpretation, and assumption. For example, a nurse seeing a man clutching his chest might assume that he has a cardiac condition, when in fact he has severe indigestion. The acceptance of assumptions as fact is called **premature closure.** To build an accurate database and avoid premature closure, nurses must validate assumptions regarding the client's physical or emotional behavior. In the previous example, the nurse should ask the client why he is clutching his chest and should expeditiously obtain a pain history. The client's response may validate the nurse's assumptions or prompt further questioning. Failure to validate assumptions can lead to an inaccurate or incomplete nursing assessment.

Recording Data

To complete the assessment phase, the nurse records data. Accurate documentation is essential and should include all data collected about the client's health status. Data are recorded in a factual manner and not interpreted by the nurse.

CONSIDER . . .

- the various assessment instruments used by different health professionals in your agency. What are the similarities and differences between them? If there is overlapping information, what are the advantages or disadvantages to this redundancy? Are there areas of assessment not included? How might these deficiencies affect client care?
- what you would do if your assessment data differs from that of another health professional.
- whether nurses in your institution serve on committees that develop policies, procedures, and instruments related to client assessment. Why is nurse representation on these committees important? If nurses are not currently represented on these committees, how might you change this situation?

THE DIAGNOSTIC PHASE

In the diagnostic phase, nurses use critical thinking skills to interpret assessment data and identify client strengths and problems. Diagnosing is a pivotal step in the nursing process. All activities preceding this phase are directed toward formulating the nursing diagnoses; all the care-planning activities following this phase are based on the nursing diagnoses.

For clarity, this chapter uses the terms adapted from Carpenito (1995). The term **diagnosis** refers to the reasoning process (diagnostic reasoning); the standardized North American Nursing Diagnosis Association (NANDA) terms (see the box on the facing page) are called **diagnosis labels;** and the product (problem statement) is called a **nursing diagnosis.**

Taxonomy of Nursing Diagnosis

The first taxonomy of nursing diagnoses was alphabetical. The nonhierarchic alphabetical ordering (see page 261) was considered unscientific by some, and a hierarchic structure was sought. In 1982,

---

Human Response Patterns

1. Exchanging: mutual giving and receiving
2. Communicating: sending messages
3. Relating: establishing bonds
4. Valuing: assigning relative worth
5. Choosing: selection of alternatives
6. Moving: activity
7. Perceiving: reception of information
8. Knowing: meaning associated with information
9. Feeling: subjective awareness of information

NANDA accepted the "nine patterns of unitary man" as an organizing principle. In 1984, NANDA renamed the "patterns of unitary man" as "human response patterns" (Kim, McFarland & McLane, 1984, p. 49). See the box above.

Having undergone refinements, revisions, and acceptance of new diagnoses, the taxonomy is now called *Taxonomy I, Revised* (NANDA, 1990). All accepted nursing diagnoses now become subcategories of these nine human response patterns.

In 1990, the North American Nursing Diagnosis Association (NANDA) adopted an official working definition of *nursing diagnosis*, shown in the box on page 262, as well as a definition of **wellness diagnosis.** These definitions imply the following statements:

- *Professional nurses (registered nurses) are responsible for making nursing diagnoses*, even though other nursing personnel may contribute data to the process of diagnosing and may implement specified nursing care. The American Nurses Association (ANA) *Standards Clinical Nursing Practice* (1991, p. 9) reinforces that nurses are accountable for this phase of the nursing process (see the box on page 262). The Joint Commission for Accreditation of Healthcare Organizations (JCAHO) now requires evidence of nursing diagnosis in client's medical records as well (JCAHO, 1992, p. 2).
- *Nursing diagnoses describe a continuum of health states:* (a) **actual health problems** (deviations from health), (b) **potential health problems** (presence of risk factors that predispose persons

Approved Nursing Diagnosis Labels
North American Nursing Diagnosis Association

Activity intolerance
Activity intolerance, risk for
Adjustment, impaired
Airway clearance, ineffective
Anxiety
Aspiration, risk for
Body image disturbance
Body temperature, risk for
    altered
Breastfeeding, effective
    (potential for enhanced)
Breastfeeding, ineffective
Breastfeeding, interrupted
Breathing pattern, ineffective
Cardiac output, decreased
Caregiver role strain
Caregiver role strain, risk for
Communication, impaired verbal
Constipation
Constipation, colonic
Constipation, perceived
Coping, defensive
Coping (family), ineffective:
    Compromised
Coping (family), ineffective:
    Disabling
Coping (family), potential for
    growth
Coping (individual), ineffective
Decisional conflict (specify)
Denial, ineffective
Diarrhea
Disuse syndrome, risk for
Diversional activity deficit
Dysreflexia
Family processes, altered
Fatigue
Fear
Fluid volume deficit
Fluid volume deficit, risk for
Fluid volume excess
Gas exchange, impaired
Grieving, anticipatory
Grieving, dysfunctional
Growth and development, altered
Health maintenance, altered

Health-seeking behaviors (specify)
Home maintenance management,
    impaired
Hopelessness
Hyperthermia
Hypothermia
Incontinence, bowel
Incontinence, functional (urinary)
Incontinence, reflex (urinary)
Incontinence, stress (urinary)
Incontinence, total (urinary)
Incontinence, urge (urinary)
Infant feeding pattern, ineffective
Infection, risk for
Injury, risk for
Knowledge deficit (specify)
Management of therapeutic
    regimen, ineffective
Mobility, impaired physical
Noncompliance (specify)
Nutrition, altered: less than
    body requirements
Nutrition, altered: more than
    body requirements
Nutrition, altered: potential for
    more than body requirements
Oral mucous membrane, altered
Pain
Pain, chronic
Parental role conflict
Parenting, altered
Parenting, risk for altered
Peripheral neurovascular
    dysfunction, risk for
Personal identity disturbance
Poisoning, risk for
Post-trauma response
Powerlessness
Protection, altered
Rape-trauma syndrome
Rape-trauma syndrome:
    compound reaction
Rape-trauma syndrome:
    silent reaction
Relocation stress syndrome
Role performance, altered

Self-care deficit, bathing/hygiene
    (specify level)
Self-care deficit, dressing/grooming
    (specify level)
Self-care deficit, feeding
    (specify level)
Self-care deficit, toileting
    (specify level)
Self-esteem, chronic low
Self-esteem disturbance
Self-esteem, situational low
Self-mutilation, risk for
Sensory/perceptual alterations
    (specify): auditory, kinesthetic,
    gustatory, tactile, olfactory,
    visual
Sexual dysfunction
Sexuality patterns, altered
Skin integrity, impaired
Skin integrity, risk for impaired
Sleep-pattern disturbance
Social interaction, impaired
Social isolation
Spiritual distress (distress of the
    human spirit)
Suffocation, risk for
Swallowing, impaired
Therapeutic regimen (individuals),
    ineffective management of
Thermoregulation, ineffective
Thought processes, altered
Tissue integrity, impaired
Tissue perfusion, altered (specify
    type): cerebral, cardiopulmonary,
    gastrointestinal, peripheral,
    renal
Trauma, risk for
Unilateral neglect
Urinary elimination, altered
Urinary retention
Ventilation, inability to sustain
    spontaneous
Ventilatory weaning response
    (dysfunctional)
Violence, risk for: self-directed or
    directed at others

SOURCE: North American Nursing Diagnosis Association, *Nursing Diagnoses: Definitions and Classification, 1995–1996.* Philadelphia: NANDA. Used by permission.

NANDA Definitions

Nursing Diagnosis

"Nursing diagnosis is a clinical judgment about individual, family, or community responses to actual and potential health problems/life processes. Nursing diagnoses provide the basis for selection of nursing interventions to achieve outcomes for which the nurse is accountable."

Wellness Diagnosis

"A wellness diagnosis is a clinical judgment about an individual, family, or community in transition from a specific level of wellness to a higher level of wellness" (1990). It describes "human responses to levels of wellness in an individual, family, or community that have a potential for enhancement to a higher state" (1994).

SOURCE: *Taxonomy I, Revised*—1990, by the North American Nursing Diagnosis Association, 1990, St. Louis: Author, pp. 114, 117; and *NANDA Nursing Diagnoses: Definitions and Classifications—1995-1996* by the North American Nursing Diagnosis Association, 1994, St. Louis: Author.

---

and families to health problems), and (c) healthy responses (areas of enriched personal growth).

- *The domain of nursing diagnosis includes only those health states that nurses are able and licensed to treat.* For example, nurses are not educated to diagnose or treat diseases such as diabetes mellitus; this task is defined legally as within the practice of medicine. Yet they can diagnose and treat **Knowledge deficit, Ineffective individual coping,** or **Altered nutrition,** all of which may accompany diabetes mellitus.
- *A nursing diagnosis is a judgment made only after thorough, systematic data collection.*

Nursing diagnoses relate to **independent nursing functions,** that is, the areas of health care that are unique to nursing and separate and distinct from medical management. With regard to medical diagnoses, nurses are obligated to carry out physician-prescribed therapies and treatments, that is, **dependent nursing functions.**

Nurses may not prescribe *all* the care for a nursing diagnosis, but if the problem is a nursing diagnosis, the nurse can prescribe *most* of the interventions needed for prevention or resolution. For example, most clients with a nursing diagnosis of **Pain** have medical orders for analgesics, but there

are also many independent nursing interventions for alleviating pain.

Types of Nursing Diagnoses

There are various types of nursing diagnoses: actual, potential (at risk), possible, and wellness.

1. An *actual diagnosis* is a judgment about a client's response to a health problem that is present at the time of the nursing assessment. An actual nursing diagnosis is based on the presence of associated signs and symptoms. Examples are **Ineffective breathing pattern** and **Anxiety.**

2. A *potential* or *risk nursing diagnosis,* as defined by NANDA, is a clinical judgment that a client is more vulnerable to develop the problem than others in the same or similar situation. For example, the nurse lists a diagnosis of **Risk for infection** for the oncology client receiving radiation therapy who is admitted to the hospital because of gastrointestinal bleeding.

3. A *possible nursing diagnosis* is one in which evidence about a health problem is unclear or the causative factors are unknown. A possible diagnosis requires more data either to support or to refute it. For example, the nurse chooses the nursing diagnosis **Possible social isolation** for the client who is admitted with a diagnosis of AIDS-related *Pneumocystis carinii* pneumonia (PCP) and who has no visitors or phone calls.

ANA Standards

Standard II: Diagnosis

The nurse analyzes the assessment data in determining diagnoses.

Measurement Criteria

1. Diagnoses are derived from the assessment data.

2. Diagnoses are validated with the client, significant others, and health care providers, when possible.

3. Diagnoses are documented in a manner that facilitates the determination of expected outcomes and plan of care.

SOURCE: Abstracted from *Standards of Clinical Nursing Practice* by the American Nurses Association, 1991, Washington, DC: Author, p. 10. Used with permission.

TABLE 14–3   **Comparison of Nursing Diagnoses, Collaborative Problems, and Medical Diagnoses**

Nursing Diagnoses	Collaborative Problems	Medical Diagnoses
Example: **Activity intolerance** related to decreased cardiac output	*Example:* **Potential complication of myocardial infarction:** congestive heart failure	*Example:* **Myocardial infarction**
Describes human responses to disease process or health problem	Involve human responses—mainly physiologic complications of disease, tests, or treatments	Describes disease and pathology; does not consider other human responses
Oriented to individual	Oriented to pathophysiology	Oriented to pathology
Nurses responsible for diagnosing	Nurses responsible for diagnosing	Physician responsible for diagnosing; diagnosis not within the scope of nursing practice
Nurse orders most interventions to prevent and treat	Nurse collaborates with physician and other health care professionals to prevent and treat (requires at least some medical orders)	Physician orders primary interventions to prevent and treat
Nursing focus: treat and prevent	Nursing focus: prevent and monitor for onset or status of condition	Nursing focus: implement medical orders for treatment and monitor status of condition
Independent nursing actions	Some independent actions, but primarily for monitoring and preventing	Dependent nursing actions, primarily
Can change frequently	Present when disease or situation is present	Remains the same while disease is present
Has no universally accepted classification system; such systems are in the process of development	Has no universally accepted classification system	Has a well-developed classification system accepted by the medical profession
Consists of a one-, two- or three-part statement, usually including problem and etiology	Consists of a two-part statement of situation/pathophysiology and the potential complication	Consists usually of not more than three words

4. A *wellness diagnosis* is one indicating a healthy response of a client who desires a higher level of wellness. An example is **Potential for enhanced parenting.**

Collaborative Problems

Like "at risk" nursing diagnoses, **collaborative problems** are a type of potential problem. However, independent nursing interventions for collaborative problems focus mainly on monitoring the client's condition and preventing development of potential complications. Definitive treatment of the condition requires *both* medical and nursing interventions.

Because the number of physiologic complications for a given disease is limited, collaborative problems tend to be present any time a particular disease or treatment is present; that is, each disease or treatment has specific complications that are always associated with it. For examples, a statement of collaborative problems is "Potential complication of pneumonia: atelectasis, respiratory failure, pleural effusion, pericarditis, and meningitis."

Nursing diagnoses, by contrast, involve human responses, which vary greatly from one person to the next. Therefore, the same set of nursing diagnoses cannot be expected to occur with a particular disease or condition; moreover, a single nursing diagnosis may occur as a response to any number of diseases. For example, all postpartum clients have similar collaborative problems (potential complications), such as "Potential complication of childbearing: postpartum hemorrhage" or "Potential complication of childbearing: thrombophlebitis." But not all new mothers have the same nursing diagnoses. Some might experience **Altered parenting (delayed bonding),** but most will not; some might have a **Knowledge deficit** problem, whereas others will not. Table 14–3 compares nursing diagnoses, collaborative problems, and medical problems.

Components of a Nursing Diagnosis

A nursing diagnosis has three components: (1) the problem statement, (2) the etiology, and (3) the defining characteristics. Each components serves a specific purpose.

Problem Statement (Diagnostic Label)

The problem statement, or diagnostic label, describes the client's health problem or response for which nursing therapy is given. It describes the client's health status clearly and concisely in a few words. See the box on page 261 for a list of nursing diagnostic labels approved by NANDA. The purpose of the diagnostic label is to *direct the formation of client goals and outcome criteria.* It may also suggest some nursing interventions.

To be clinically useful, diagnostic labels need to be specific; when the word *specify* follows a label on this list, the nurse states the area in which the problem occurs, for example, **Knowledge deficit (medications)** or **Knowledge deficit (dietary adjustments).**

Qualifiers are words that have been added to some NANDA labels to give additional meaning to the diagnostic statement:

- *Altered* (a change from baseline)
- *Impaired* (made worse, weakened, damaged, reduced, deteriorated)
- *Decreased* (smaller in size, amount, or degree)
- *Ineffective* (not producing the desired effect)

TABLE 14–4 Components of a Nursing Diagnostic Label

Diagnosis	Definition	Etiology/Related Factors	Defining Characteristics
Activity intolerance	A state in which an individual has insufficient physiologic or psychologic energy to endure or complete required or desired daily activities	Sedentary life-style Generalized weakness Prolonged bedrest or immobility Sensory deficits Impaired motor function Fatigue Alterations in oxygen transport system Lack of motivation Obesity Acute or chronic pain	*Major (Must Be Present)* Altered response to activity (e.g., dyspnea, shortness of breath, tachypnea, rapid shallow respirations) Weak, thready pulse, tachycardia, irregular pulse, failure to return to resting after 3 minutes, EKG changes during activity Failure of blood pressure to increase with activity, hypotension, increased diastolic pressure of 15 mm Hg Weakness and fatigue *Minor (May Be Present)* Pallor, cyanosis, vertigo, diaphoresis, confusion

SOURCES: *Pocket Guide to Nursing Diagnosis* (6th ed.) by M. J. Kim, G. K. McFarland, and A. M. McLane (Eds.), 1995, St. Louis: Mosby, p. 2; *Nursing Diagnosis: Applications to Clinical Practice* (6th ed.) by L. J. Carpenito, 1995, Philadelphia: Lippincott, p. 105; and *Nursing Diagnosis and Intervention Pocket Guide* by J. M. Wilkinson, 1995, Menlo Park CA: Addison-Wesley Nursing, pp. 2–5.

TABLE 14-5 **Examples of Nursing Interventions to Address Different Etiologies**

Diagnostic Label (Problem)	Client	Etiology	Examples of Nursing Interventions
Ineffective breastfeeding	Ariel Dees	Breast engorgement	Teach Ms. Dees to massage her breasts before feeding.
			Use hot packs or hot shower before nursing infant.
	June Biden	Inexperience and lack of knowledge	Teach to feed infant on demand.
			Show Ms. Biden how to be sure infant is sucking and swallowing.
			Demonstrate different holding positions for feedings.

- *Acute* (severe or of short duration)
- *Chronic* (lasting a long time, recurring, or constant)

Each diagnostic label approved by NANDA carries a definition that clarifies the characteristics of the human response under consideration. For example, the definition of the label **Activity intolerance** is shown in Table 14–4.

Etiology (Related Factors and Risk Factors)

The etiology component of the diagnosis *identifies one or more probable causes of the health problem, gives direction to the required nursing therapy, and enables the nurse to individualize the client's care.* Etiology may include client behaviors, environmental factors, or interactions of the two. As shown in Table 14–4, the probable causes of **Activity intolerance** include sedentary life-style, generalized weakness, prolonged inactivity, and so on. Differentiating among possible causes in the nursing diagnosis is essential, because each may require different nursing interventions. Refer to Table 14–5 for an example of a health problem that has different etiologies and therefore requires different interventions.

NANDA uses the term *related factor* to describe the etiology or likely cause of actual nursing diagnoses. The term *risk factor* describes the etiology of *at risk* (potential) nursing diagnoses, because there are no subjective and objective signs present. Table 14–6 compares related and risk factors.

Defining Characteristics

Defining characteristics are the cluster of signs and symptoms that indicate the presence of a particular diagnostic label. For *actual* nursing diagnoses, the defining characteristics are the client's signs and symptoms. For *risk* nursing diagnoses, the defining characteristics are the same as the etiology: the risk factors that cause the client to be more than "normally" vulnerable to the problem.

Nursing diagnosis labels are similar to medical diagnoses in that they are associated with a standard set of defining characteristics that are universally accepted. *Major* defining characteristics are those that *must* be present for the diagnosis to be valid.

TABLE 14-6 **Comparison of Related Factors and Risk Factors**

	Related Factors	Risk Factors
Definition	Factor that is causing or contributing to an actual problem	Factors present that place client at risk for developing a problem that has not yet occurred
Use as etiology of:	Actual problems	Risk (potential) problems
Use when signs and symptoms of problem are:	Present	Not present

Minor characteristics may or may not be present. For example, for a nurse to make a diagnosis of **Activity intolerance,** the client would need to exhibit the defining characteristic of "altered response to activity," which might manifest as dyspnea, shortness of breath, tachypnea, or one of the other major symptoms listed in Table 14–4. For most nursing diagnoses, the list of defining characteristics is still being developed and refined. Partial listings have been published to assist nurses in developing and validating nursing diagnoses. Defining characteristics suggest criteria or client outcomes and may also suggest required nursing interventions.

The Diagnostic Process

In diagnosing, the nurse uses the critical-thinking skills of analysis and synthesis. *Analysis* is the separation into components, that is, breaking down the whole into its parts. *Synthesis* is the opposite, that is, putting together the parts into the whole.

The diagnostic process is used continuously by most nurses. An experienced nurse may enter a client's room and immediately observe significant data about the client. The nurse is able to do this as a result of attaining knowledge, skill, and expertise in the practice setting.

The diagnostic process has three steps:
* Analyzing data
* Identifying health problems, risks, and strengths
* Formulating diagnostic statements

Analyzing Data

In the diagnostic process, analyzing involves the following steps:

1. Compare data against standards (identify significant cues).
2. Cluster data (generate tentative hypotheses).
3. Identify gaps and inconsistencies.

These activities occur simultaneously rather than sequentially.

Comparing Data against Standards   The nurse compares the client's data to a wide range of stan-

---

RESEARCH NOTE

Three Nursing Diagnoses with Cultural Etiologies: Are They Adequate or Inadequate?

In one study, researchers examined the adequacy of three nursing diagnoses with cultural etiologies: **Impaired verbal communication** related to cultural differences, **Impaired social interaction** related to sociocultural dissonance, and **Noncompliance** related to patient value system.

For each of these three diagnoses the researchers determined (1) which of the current NANDA defining characteristics identified the culturally relevant behaviors and (2) what additions in the diagnostic definition, defining characteristics, and related factors were needed to identify clients' culturally relevant problems and needs.

The sample was derived from the membership lists of the International Transcultural Nursing Society and the American Nurses Association Council on Cultural Diversity in Nursing Practice. The majority of respondents (46.1%) of 580 potential subjects were educators and practitioners. Responses were received from 43 states, the District of Columbia, and seven foreign countries (Canada, Philippines, Sweden, Pakistan, Saudi Arabia, Israel, and Malawi). The subjects were also asked to write and rank other defining characteristics they used to make the diagnosis in clinical practice.

The findings revealed that no defining characteristic met the NANDA criteria for a major or minor defining characteristic. According to NANDA policy, a defining characteristic is major if it is present 80% to 100% of the time and minor if it is present 50% to 79% of the time under a given diagnosis. When categories were broken down, however, seven characteristics emerged as minor defining characteristics. In the second part of the study, 113 new defining characteristics were written by respondents. Based on these respondents' suggestions, the definitions for each diagnosis were reworked and new cultural-related factors were added.

Implications: The NANDA diagnostic classification system needs to be reevaluated and refocused into transculturally meaningful and useful perspectives. The suggestions offered by transcultural experts form a database for future research to expand the now-limited number of culturally relevant defining characteristics and related factors. Problems with the new suggestions in this study need to be resolved before they are used in clinical practice with culturally diverse clients.

Source: Geissler, E. M. (1992, Sept./Oct.). Nursing diagnoses: A study of cultural relevance. *Journal of Professional Nursing, 8*(5), 301–307.

TABLE 14-7 Comparing Client Cues to Standards and Norms

Type of Cue	Client Cues	Standard/Norm
Deviation from population norms	Height is 158 cm (5 ft, 2 in) tall. Woman with small frame. Weighs 109 kg (240 lb).	Height and weight tables indicate that the "ideal" weight for a woman 158 cm (5 ft, 2 in) tall with a small frame is 49–53 kg (108–121 lb).
Developmental delay	Child is 18 months old. Parents state child has not yet attempted to speak. Child laughs aloud and makes cooing sounds.	Children usually speak their first word by 10 months to 1 year of age.
Changes in client's usual health status	States, "I'm just not hungry these days." Ate only 15% of food on breakfast tray. Has lost 13 kg (30 lb) in past 3 months.	Client usually eats three balanced meals per day. Adults typically maintain stable weight.
Dysfunctional behavior	Amy's mother reports that Amy has not left her room for 2 days. Amy is 16. Amy has stopped attending school and has withdrawn from social contact.	Adolescents usually like to be with their peers; social group very important. Functional behavior includes school attendance.
Changes in client's usual behavior	Mrs. Stuart reports that lately her husband angers easily. "Yesterday he even yelled at the dog." "He just seems so tense."	Mr. Stuart is usually relaxed and easygoing. He is friendly and kind to animals.

dards, such as normal health patterns, normal vital signs, laboratory values, basic food groups, growth, and development. The nurse also uses personal knowledge—for example, of physiology, psychology, and sociology—as well as past experience when comparing the data.

Standards must be both relevant and reliable. The nurse compares the client data against standards and norms to identify significant or relevant cues. Refer to Table 14–7 for specific examples of client cues and norms to which they may be compared. A cue is considered significant if it (a) deviates from population norms, (b) indicates a developmental delay, (c) points to a change in the client's health status, (d) indicates dysfunctional behavior, or (e) indicates a change in the client's usual behavior.

Clustering Data Clustering or grouping data is a process of determining the relatedness of facts and finding patterns in the facts. This is the beginning of synthesis. The nurse examines data to determine whether any patterns are present, whether the data represent isolated incidents, and whether the data are significant.

The nurse may cluster data **inductively** by combining data from different assessment areas to form a pattern, or the nurse may begin with a framework, such as Gordon's functional health patterns, and cluster the subjective and objective data into the appropriate categories. The latter is a **deductive** approach to data clustering, or pattern formation.

Gordon (1994) states that clustering information involves a search in the nurse's memory stores for previously learned meaningful groups of clinical cues that are associated with a diagnostic category. Gordon believes that clustering occurs in conjunction with data collection and interpretation, as evidenced in remarks or thoughts such as, "I'm getting a picture of" or "This cue doesn't fit the picture."

Data clustering involves making inferences about the data. During data clustering, the nurse interprets the possible meaning of the cues and labels the cue clusters with tentative diagnostic hypotheses.

Identifying Gaps and Inconsistencies in Data
Skillful assessment minimizes gaps and inconsistencies in data. However, data analysis should include a final check to ensure that data are complete and

correct. *Gaps* are missing pieces of information needed to determine a data pattern. For example, information about a 15-month-old child's mobility may not specify whether the child crawls or walks. This information is essential for establishing the child's developmental stage.

Inconsistencies are conflicting data. Possible sources of conflicting data include measurement error, expectations, and conflicting or unreliable reports (Gordon 1994). For example, if the client reports a history of high blood pressure but the nurse obtains a low reading, the nurse should check the equipment and procedure for possible error.

Identifying Health Problems, Risks, and Strengths

After data are analyzed, the nurse and client can together identify strengths and problems. This is primarily a decision-making process. During data analysis, the nurse groups the data and labels the clusters with tentative diagnoses. However, for health problems to have a successful outcome, the client must acknowledge that the problem exists. The nurse, by contrast, determines whether the client needs help dealing with the problem.

When any kind of problem exists, the nurse must determine what type of problem it is. See Figure 14–2 for a decision tree to help differentiate nursing diagnoses, medical diagnoses, and collaborative problems. Also refer to Table 14–3 on page 263.

After verifying problems with the client and determining the type of problem (i.e., nursing diagnosis, medical diagnosis, or collaborative problem), the nurse examines the causal relationships between the problems and their related or risk factors. These are the problem *etiologies*—the physiologic, psychologic, sociologic, spiritual, or environmental factors believed to cause or contribute to the problem. The etiology gives direction to required nursing interventions. Therefore, if interventions are to be effective, the nurse must accurately identify the etiologies. When possible, the nurse should focus on etiologies that can be influenced by independent nursing actions.

At this stage, the nurse and client also establish the client's strengths, resources, and abilities to cope. Generally, people have a clearer perception of their problems or weaknesses than of their strengths and assets, which they often take for granted. By taking an inventory of strengths, the client can

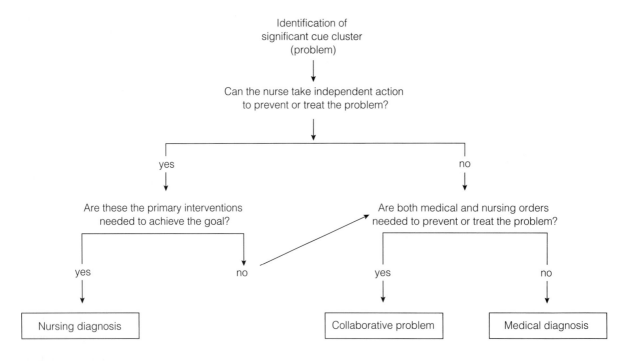

FIGURE 14–2 *Decision tree for differentiating among nursing diagnoses, collaborative problems, and medical diagnoses.*

develop a more balanced self-concept and self-image. Strengths can be an aid to mobilizing health and regenerative processes.

A client's strengths might be weight that is within the normal range for age and height, thus enabling the client to cope better with surgery. In another instance, a client's strengths might be absence of allergies and being a nonsmoker.

A client's strengths can be found in the nursing assessment record (health, home life, education, recreation, exercise, work, family and friends, religious beliefs, and sense of humor, for example), the health examination, and the client's records.

Formulating Diagnostic Statements

The basic format for a diagnostic statement is "Problem related to Etiology." However, nurses must be able to write one-, two-, three-, and four-part diagnostic statements, as well as some variations of each.

Basic Two-Part Statements   The basic two-part statement is used for actual, potential or risk, and possible nursing diagnoses. It includes the following:

1. Problem (P)—Statement of the client's response
2. Etiology (E)—Factors contributing to or probable causes of the responses

The two parts are joined by the words *related to* or *associated with* rather than *due to*. The phrase *due to* implies a cause-and-effect relationship; one clause causes or is responsible for the other clause. By contrast, the phrases *related to* and *associated with* merely imply a relationship. The phrase *related to* is most commonly used. If one part of the diagnostic statement changes, the other part may change as well. Examples of two-part nursing diagnoses are:

> **Colonic constipation** (problem) related to prolonged laxative use (etiology)

> **Ineffective breast feeding** (problem) related to breast engorgement (etiology)

Some NANDA labels contain the word *specify*. For these, the nurse must add words to indicate the problem more specifically. The format is still a two-part statement, for example,

> **Noncompliance** (specify)

> **Noncompliance (diabetic diet)** related to denial of having disease

For ease in alphabetizing, many NANDA lists are arranged with qualifying words after the main word (e.g., **Infection, risk for**). Avoid writing diagnostic statements in that manner; instead, write them as they would be stated in normal conversation (e.g., **Risk for infection**).

Basic Three-Part Statements   The basic three-part nursing diagnosis statement is called the **PES format** and includes

1. Problem (P)—Statement of the client's response
2. Etiology (E)—Factors contributing to or probable causes of the response
3. Signs and symptoms (S)—Defining characteristics manifested by the client

Actual nursing diagnoses can be documented by using the three-part statement (using *related to* and *as manifested by*, or *as evidenced by*), because the signs and symptoms have been identified. This format cannot be used for *risk* diagnoses, because the client does not have signs and symptoms of the diagnosis.

The PES format is especially recommended for beginning diagnosticians, because the signs and symptoms validate why the diagnosis was chosen and make the problem statement more descriptive. An example of the PES format is:

> **Self-esteem disturbance** related to rejection by husband (etiology) *as manifested by* hypersensitivity to criticism; states, "I don't know if I can manage by myself," and rejects positive feedback (signs and symptoms).

The disadvantage of this method is that it can create very long problem statements, thereby obscuring the problem and etiology. However, because the signs and symptoms can be helpful in planning nursing interventions, they should be easily accessible. To promote access without long problem statements, the nurse can record the signs and symptoms in the nursing progress notes instead of on the care plan. Another possibility, recommended for students, is to list the signs and symptoms on the care plan *below* the nursing diagnosis, grouping the subjective and objective data. The signs and symptoms are easily accessible, and the problem and etiology stand out clearly. For example:

> **Noncompliance (diabetic diet)** related to unresolved anger about diagnosis
>
> S— "I forget to take my pills."
>   "I can't live without sugar in my food."
> O— Weight 98 kg (215 lbs) (gain of 4.5 kg [10 lb])
>   Blood pressure 190/100 mm Hg

One-Part Statements Some diagnostic statements, such as wellness diagnoses and syndrome nursing diagnoses, consist of a NANDA label only. As the diagnostic labels are refined, they tend to become more specific, so that nursing interventions can be derived from the label itself. Therefore, an etiology is not needed. For example, adding an etiology to the labels **Rape-trauma syndrome, Post-trauma response,** and **Defensive coping** does not make the label any more descriptive or useful.

For some nursing diagnoses, it is difficult to write an etiology other than a medical diagnosis, or writing the etiology is somewhat redundant. **Reflex incontinence,** for instance, is fully described by its NANDA definition ("The state in which an individual experiences an involuntary loss of urine, occurring at somewhat predictable intervals when a specific bladder volume is reached"). The etiology of **Reflex incontinence** is "neurologic impairment" (e.g., spinal cord lesion that interferes with conduction of cerebral messages above the level of the reflex arc). This etiology does not suggest nursing actions, nor does it really add to the understanding of the problem label. Similarly, the nursing interventions for **Post-trauma response** would be much the same regardless of whether the etiology is "related to war experiences" or "related to earthquake."

There are currently four one-part NANDA labels reflecting healthy functioning: **Health-seeking behaviors, Family coping, Potential for growth, Effective breastfeeding,** and **Anticipatory grieving.** NANDA has specified that any new wellness diagnosis will be developed as a one-part statement beginning with the words "Potential for enhanced" followed by the desired higher-level wellness (for example, **Potential for enhanced parenting**).

Variations of Basic Formats Variations of the basic one-, two-, and three-part statements include the following:

1. Writing *unknown etiology* when the defining characteristics are present but the nurse does not know the cause of contributing factors. One example is **Noncompliance (medication regimen)** related to unknown etiology.

2. Using the phrase *complex factors* when there are too many etiologic factors or when they are too complex to state in a brief phrase. The actual causes of **Decisional conflict** and **Chronic low self-esteem,** for instance, may be long-term and complex, as in the following nursing diagnoses: **Decisional conflict** and **Chronic low self-esteem** related to complex factors.

3. Using the word *possible* to describe either the problem or the etiology. When the nurse believes more data is needed about the client's response (problem) or the etiology, the word *possible* is inserted. Examples are **Possible low self-esteem** related to loss of job and rejection by family; **Altered thought processes possibly** related to unfamiliar surroundings; and **Possible low self-esteem** related to unknown etiology.

4. Using *secondary to* to divide the etiology into two parts, thereby making the statement more descriptive and useful. The part following *secondary to* is often a pathophysiologic or disease process, as in **Risk for impaired skin integrity** related to decreased peripheral circulation secondary to diabetes.

5. Adding a second part to the general response or NANDA label to make it more precise. For example, the diagnosis **Impaired physical mobility** does not include the degree of mobility impairment. To make this label more specific, the nurse can add a colon and a descriptor, as follows:

   Impaired physical mobility (problem): inability to walk (descriptor) related to knee joint stiffness and pain secondary to muscle atrophy (etiology)

   Pain (problem): severe headache (descriptor) related to fear of addiction to narcotics (etiology)

6. Four-part statements are combinations of basic statements and variations 4 and 5, discussed above. For example, the nurse creates a four-part statement by using both variations 4 and 5 with a basic two-part statement, as in: (1) **Risk for impaired skin integrity:** (2) pressure sores related to (3) immobility (4) secondary to presence of casts and traction. A four-part statement is also created by using the basic three-part (PES) format and adding either variation 4 or 5; for example, (1) **Impaired skin integrity:** (2) pressure sore on left heel related to (3) immobility (4) as manifested by 2 cm × 2 cm red, excoriated area on the left heel and inability to move about in bed.

Collaborative Problems

Carpenito (1995) suggests that all collaborative problems begin with the diagnostic label "Potential Complication" ("PC"). Nurses should include in the diagnostic statement both the possible complication they are monitoring and the disease or treatment that is present to produce it. For example

>Potential complication of head injury: increased intracranial pressure

When monitoring for a group of complications associated with a disease or pathology, the nurse states the disease and follows it with a list of the complications:

>Potential complication of pregnancy-induced hypertension: seizures, fetal distress, pulmonary edema, hepatic/renal failure, premature labor, CNS hemorrhage

The PES format is not used for collaborative problems because they are potential problems. Therefore, the client has no signs or symptoms for the nurse to list.

There are some situations in which an etiology might be helpful in suggesting interventions, that is, when the complication is caused by something more specific than a disease process. Students should write the etiology, as in the following examples: (1) when it clarifies the problems statement, (2) when it can be concisely stated, and (3) when it helps to suggest nursing actions. Examples are:

>**Potential complication of childbirth** (disease/situation): **hemorrhage** (complication) related to: (1) uterine atony, (2) retained placental fragments, (3) bladder distention (etiologies)

>**Potential complication of diuretic therapy** (disease/situation): **dysrhythmias** (complication) related to low serum potassium (etiology)

Evaluating the Quality of the Diagnostic Statement

In addition to using the correct format, nurses must consider the content of their diagnostic statements. The statements should, for example, be accurate, concise, descriptive, and specific. The nurse must always validate the diagnostic statements with the client and compare the client's signs and symptoms to the NANDA defining characteristics. For high-risk problems, the nurse compares the client's risk factors to NANDA risk factors.

CONSIDER...

- the differences in nursing actions that arise from nursing diagnoses, medical diagnoses, and collaborative problems.

- in what situations the NANDA diagnosis **Pain** and other diagnoses are more useful as an etiology than as a diagnostic label. Why?
- which NANDA diagnoses may be applicable for any client throughout the perioperative period.
- how the family or significant others can affect the client's response.
- what additional nursing diagnosis labels related to your area of practice may need to be evaluated for inclusion on the NANDA list.

Nursing Prognosis

Carnevali and Thomas (1993, p. 9) modify the traditional five-phase nursing process by adding a new step between the diagnostic phase and the planning phase. This step, referred to as a *nursing prognosis*, involves the collection of prognostic data and making prognostic judgments. Carnevali and Thomas believe that both diagnostic and prognostic judgments serve as a foundation for planning nursing interventions. They influence goals, nursing interventions, and evaluations.

A prognosis is a forecast of the probable course and outcome of a problem or situation. A **nursing prognosis** is "a prediction of the possible or probable course of events and outcomes associated with a particular health status or situation under various treatment options or lack of treatment" (Carnevali & Thomas, 1993, p. 80).

Nurses are familiar with the concept of prognosis as it pertains to the medical domain. In that domain, prognostic data is related to human responses to pathology, pathophysiology, and psychopathology. Medical treatment decisions are made on the basis of both a medical diagnosis and a prognosis. In other words, prognostic judgments precede decisions about treatment. Pathologic processes that can be prevented or cured are treated in one way; those that cannot be cured or do not respond to treatment are treated another way.

By contrast, the nursing prognosis is similar in that it precedes treatment decisions, but it differs in that prognostic data relate to the client's functioning capacities and other data (see prognostic variables below). Nursing prognoses deal with the likelihood that the client and family or other support persons will be able to respond to the health problem in such a way that (Carnevali & Thomas, 1993, p. 87):

- Health, well-being, and effective functioning are promoted.

- Daily living is as effectively managed as capacities, external resources, and daily living permit.
- The resultant quality of life is satisfying.

Elements of Nursing Prognosis

The three components of prognosis are prognostic variables (indicators), outcomes, and trajectory. *Prognostic variables* are factors that the nurse considers to determine what the outcome and trajectory will be.

The nurse obtains information about prognostic variables by considering the following client data: (a) age, (b) past and current general health, (c) the effects of the health problem and its treatment, (d) the client's functional capacities for daily living, (e) demands of living placed on the functioning capacities of the client and family or other support persons (e.g., roles, functions, patterns of living), (f) availability of health care resources, and so on. The nurse may ask the following questions to determine prognostic variables related to nursing diagnoses:

- Has the client's illness altered mental, physical, and emotional capacities, and what are the implications for future functioning? For example, has the illness altered the client's vision, muscular capacity to manipulate equipment, intellectual capacity to learn, problem-solving skills to cope with change?
- What health risk factors are present, and how will these affect the client's outcomes?
- Is the client willing to adopt needed changes in life-style?
- What are the client's expectations of recovery?
- Are the family and home environment supportive? For example, are support persons available? If so, are they willing to learn necessary health care activities and seek help to assist the client?
- Does the client have adequate funds (or insurance coverage) for supplies, equipment, and food?
- Are appropriate ongoing health care resources available? For example, does the client have access to a diabetic clinic, self-help or support group, instructional classes, clearly written health care information, and appropriate health care specialists (e.g., dietitian)?

The second component of a nursing prognosis is the *prognostic outcome*. There are several types of outcomes (Carnevali & Thomas, 1993, p. 82):

1. Prevention or avoidance of a problem

2. Delay or minimization of the problem or dysfunction
3. Resolution of the diagnosed problem
4. Improvement or remission
5. Stabilization of a problem that will continue
6. Deterioration requiring palliative interventions

For all of these outcomes, the nurse may predict success, failure, or some degree of improvement.

Trajectory, the third component of a nursing prognosis, deals with the course of events as well as the outcomes. The nurse considers what is expected to happen, the direction of change, and the pattern or rate of change. Trajectories associated with different outcomes vary considerably. For example, the trajectory for resolution or deterioration of a problem may be rapid or slow; the onset of a problem may be delayed for a long or short time; the pattern of change may be continuous or characterized by fluctuations and plateaus; and some changes may be so subtle that they go unrecognized by the client. Nurses need to consider the client's anticipated course of events as a basis for setting realistic goals and evaluating the client's response to nursing interventions.

Stating the Prognosis

Just as medical prognosis is linked to medical diagnosis, the nursing prognosis is linked to each specific nursing diagnosis. Prognostic terms may include *resolution, stabilization, progression, continuation, good, poor,* and so on. Generally, a time span is included with the prognosis. Examples are shown in Table 14–8.

Most nursing prognoses are not absolute; they are conditional on a variety of uncertain variables. Carnevali and Thomas (1993, p. 86) refer to these types of prognoses as *contingent prognoses*. When this is the case, the qualifiers *if* and *then* are used to state the prognosis. For example, *if* this occurs, *then* the prognosis should be good, or *if* something fails to occur, *then* the prognosis will be poor.

Following the statement of prognosis, the nurse plans interventions that will influence the course of events and may prescribe interventions that attempt to

- Retain wellness.
- Prevent, delay, or minimize health problems at risk.
- Interfere with the normal dynamics and progress

TABLE 14–8   Relationship of Nursing Prognosis to Nursing Diagnosis

Nursing Diagnosis	Prognostic Variables	Nursing Prognosis
Chronic pain related to ineffective rest/activity patterns and excess weight secondary to rheumatoid arthritis	83-year old widower lives alone; children not available for help; cooks mostly fried foods for self and for cats. Weight is 25% above norm for height. Functional capacities for activities of daily living (ADLs) satisfactory. States pain increases with activity (e.g., walking to store for groceries and working in garden for a day). States willing to lose weight. Arthritic pain will continue episodically. Has good neighbors who will help with shopping and meals.	Decreased pain *if* • Alters diet to lose weight. • Accepts help from neighbor. • Schedules shorter activity periods in the garden.

of the health problem so as to shorten it, reduce its intensity, or remove it.

- Prevent complications and additional treatment-related (iatrogenic) problems.
- Minimize the negative effects of chronic problems and those that cause growing dysfunction and threat to life.

CONSIDER...

- two clients who have the same nursing diagnosis (etiology included). What factors influenced both the direction and rate of outcome in each situation?
- a client situation in which the medical prognosis is negative but the nursing prognosis is positive. Also consider the reverse situation—a positive medical diagnosis and a negative nursing diagnosis. What factors influenced these prognoses?

THE PLANNING PHASE

Planning is a deliberative, systematic phase of the nursing process that involves decision making and problem solving. In planning, the nurse refers to the client's assessment data and diagnostic statements for direction in formulating client goals and design-

ing the nursing strategies required to prevent, reduce, or eliminate the client's health problems. The product of the planning phase is a client care plan. The accompanying box describes the nurses' professional responsibilities for planning.

ANA Standards

Standard IV: Planning

The nurse develops a plan of care that prescribes interventions to attain expected outcomes.

Measurement Criteria

1. The plan is individualized to the client's condition or needs.

2. The plan is developed with the client, significant others, and health care providers, when appropriate.

3. The plan reflects current nursing practice.

4. The plan is documented.

5. The plan provides for continuity of care.

SOURCE: Abstracted from *Standards of Clinical Nursing Practice* by American Nurses Association, 1991, Washington, DC: Author, pp. 11, 12. Used with permission.

Steps in the Consulting Process

1. *Identify the problem.* Have the problem clearly in mind, including the circumstances surrounding it.

2. *Collect all pertinent data.* When consulting another health professional who is unfamiliar with the client, collect all the data relevant to the problem.

3. *Select the consultant.* Consult a recognized health professional who has the skills or knowledge required.

4. *Communicate the problem and pertinent information.* The information often varies with each client and each problem. It is important to include information about the client's strengths and problems. Convey the information clearly and objectively, and make sure the data are factual and not interpretive.

5. *Discuss the recommendations with the consultant.* The consultant may provide recommendations at the time the nurse describes the problem, or a later meeting may be necessary. For example, an oncology nursing consultant may give immediate recommendations regarding activity, positioning, timing of medication, or the consultant might prefer to obtain further data before making recommendations.

6. *Include the recommendations in the client's nursing care plan.* The recommendations become part of the client's record. After implementing the recommendations, the nurse evaluates and records their effectiveness.

Although planning is basically the nurse's responsibility, input from the client and support persons is essential if a plan is to be effective. Consulting with other health professionals is also part of planning. See the accompanying box for steps in the consulting process. Nurses do not plan *for* the client, but encourage the client to participate actively to the extent possible. In a home setting, the client's support persons and/or caregivers are the ones who implement the plan of care; thus, its effectiveness depends largely on them. They can also provide information about problems the nurse might not otherwise discover.

The planning process includes the following activities:

- Setting priorities
- Establishing client goals/expected outcomes
- Selecting nursing strategies
- Developing nursing care plans

Figure 14–3 provides an overview of the relationship between the nursing diagnoses and the written plan of care. The arrows between the columns indicate the specific relationships between each diagnosis and respective goals and nursing interventions.

Setting Priorities

Priority setting is the process of establishing a preferential order for nursing strategies. The nurse and client begin planning by deciding which nursing diagnosis requires attention first, which second, and so on. Instead of rank-ordering diagnoses, nurses can group them as having high, medium, or low priority. Life-threatening problems, such as loss of respiratory or cardiac functioning, are designated as *high priority*. Health-threatening problems, such as acute illness and decreased coping ability, may result in delayed development or cause destructive physical or emotional changes; thus, they are usually assigned *medium priority*. A *low-priority* problem is one that arises from normal developmental needs or that requires only minimal nursing support.

Using a framework makes priority setting easier. Although it is not, strictly speaking, a nursing framework, nurses frequently use Maslow's hierarchy of needs when setting priorities.

Priority setting does not require that all the high-priority diagnoses be resolved before the nurse addresses any others. The nurse may partially address a high-priority diagnosis and then deal with a diagnosis of lesser priority. Furthermore, because clients usually have several problems, the nurse often addresses more than one diagnosis at a time.

The priorities assigned to problems do not remain fixed; rather, they change as the client's responses, problems, and therapies change. The nurse assigns priorities on the basis of nursing judgment and, insofar as possible, client preference. The nurse must consider a variety of factors, for example, the client's values, beliefs, and priorities; the available resources; urgency of the problem; and medical treatment plan.

Establishing Client Goals/Expected Outcomes

The terms *goal* and *expected outcome* are sometimes used interchangeably. Some sources also use the terms *outcome criterion*, *objective*, and *predicted outcome*. The American Nurses Association (ANA) specifies outcome identification in *Standards of Clinical Nursing Practice*. See the box on page 275.

Care Planning

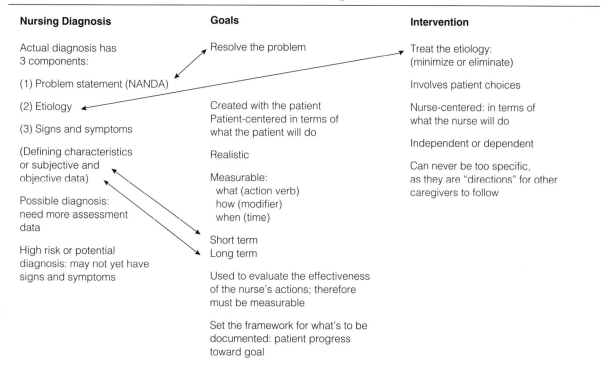

Nursing Diagnosis	Goals	Intervention
Actual diagnosis has 3 components:	Resolve the problem	Treat the etiology: (minimize or eliminate)
(1) Problem statement (NANDA)		Involves patient choices
(2) Etiology	Created with the patient Patient-centered in terms of what the patient will do	Nurse-centered: in terms of what the nurse will do
(3) Signs and symptoms		Independent or dependent
(Defining characteristics or subjective and objective data)	Realistic	Can never be too specific, as they are "directions" for other caregivers to follow
	Measurable: what (action verb) how (modifier) when (time)	
Possible diagnosis: need more assessment data		
High risk or potential diagnosis: may not yet have signs and symptoms	Short term Long term	
	Used to evaluate the effectiveness of the nurse's actions; therefore must be measurable	
	Set the framework for what's to be documented: patient progress toward goal	

FIGURE 14-3 *Relationship between the nursing diagnosis and a written plan of care.*

Source: A Guide for Care Planning by Patricia L. Newland, September/October 1994, *Nurse Educator, 19,* (5) p. 9. Used with permission.

Some nursing literature differentiates by defining *goals* as broad statements about the effects of nursing interventions and *expected outcomes* as the more specific, measurable criteria used to evaluate whether the goal has been met. For example:

Goal (broad): Nutritional status will improve.

Expected outcome (specific): Will gain 5 lb by April 25.

When goals are defined broadly, as in the above example, the client's care plan must include *both* goals and expected outcomes. In fact, they are sometimes combined into one statement linked by the words "as evidenced by," as follows:

Nutritional status will improve, as evidenced by weight gain of 5 lb by April 25.

Writing the broad goal first may help students to think of the specific outcomes that are needed. But even though broad goals can be a starting point for

ANA Standards

Standard III: Outcome Identification

The nurse identifies expected outcomes individualized to the client.

Measurement Criteria

1. Outcomes are derived from the diagnoses.

2. Outcomes are documented as measurable goals.

3. Outcomes are mutually formulated with the client and health care providers, when possible.

4. Outcomes are realistic in relation to the client's present and potential capabilities.

5. Outcomes are attainable in relation to resources available to the client.

6. Outcomes include a time estimate for attainment.

7. Outcomes provide direction for continuity of care.

Source: Abstracted from *Standards of Clinical Nursing Practice* by the American Nurses Association, 1991, Washington, DC: Author, pp. 11, 12. Used with permission.

planning, it is the specific, measurable outcomes that *must* be written on the care plan.

Goals may be short term or long term. A short-term goal might be "Client will raise right arm to shoulder height by Friday." In the same context, a long-term goal might be "Client will regain full use of right arm in 6 weeks." In an acute care setting, much of the nurse's time is spent on the client's immediate needs, so most goals are short term. Short-term goals also enable the nurse to evaluate client progress more accurately. Long-term goals are often used for clients who live at home and have chronic health problems and for clients in nursing homes, extended care facilities, and rehabilitation centers.

Goals/expected outcomes are derived from and relate to the client's nursing diagnoses—primarily from the first clause (problem). The problem clause contains the unhealthy response; it states what should change. Therefore, the *essential* client goals are derived from the problem clause. For example, if the nursing diagnosis is **Risk for fluid volume deficit** related to diarrhea and inadequate intake secondary to nausea, the *essential* goal statement might be "Client's fluid balance will be maintained, as evidenced by urinary and stool output in balance with fluid intake, normal skin turgor, and moist mucous membranes."

Goal/expected outcome statements generally have the following four components:

1. *Subject.* The subject, a noun, is the client, any part of the client, or some attribute of the client, such as the client's pulse or urinary output. Often, the subject is omitted in nursing care plan goals; it is assumed that the subject is the client unless indicated otherwise.

2. *Verb.* The verb denotes an action the client is to perform, for example, what the client is to do, learn, or experience. Verbs that denote directly observable behaviors, such as *administer, demonstrate, show, walk,* and so on, are used.

3. *Conditions or modifiers.* Conditions or modifiers may be added to the verb to explain the circumstances under which the behavior is to be performed. They explain what, where, when, or how. For example:

    Walks *with the help of a walker* (how).

    After *attending* two group diabetes classes, lists signs and symptoms of diabetes (when).

At home, maintains weight at existing level (where).

Discusses *four food groups and recommended daily servings* (what).

Conditions need not be included if the criterion of performance clearly indicates what is expected.

4. *Criterion of desired performance.* The criterion indicates the standard by which a performance is evaluated or the level at which the client will perform the specified behavior. These criteria may specify time or speed, accuracy, distance, and quality. To establish a time achievement criterion, the nurse needs to ask, "How long?" To establish an accuracy criterion, the nurse asks, "How well?" Similarly, the nurse asks, "How far?" and "What is the expected standard?" to establish distance and quality criteria, respectively. Examples are:

    Weighs 75 kg *by April* (time).

    Lists *five out of six* signs of diabetes (accuracy).

    Walks *one block per day* (time and distance).

    Administers insulin *using aseptic technique* (quality).

Table 14–9 illustrates the format that should be used to write outcomes, and the accompanying box provides a summary of the characteristics of well-stated outcomes.

Selecting Nursing Strategies

Nursing strategies chosen should focus on eliminating or reducing the etiology (cause) of the nursing diagnosis, which is the second clause of the diagnostic statement. Strategies for *potential* nursing diagnoses should focus on measures to reduce the client's risk factors and/or signs and symptoms, which are also found in the second clause.

Correct identification of the etiology during the diagnosing phase provides the framework for choosing successful nursing interventions. For example, **Activity intolerance** may have several etiologies—pain, weakness, sedentary life-style, anxiety, or cardiac dysrhythmias, for example. The interventions will vary according to the cause of the problem.

Often, the nurse and the client can establish a number of nursing strategies for each problem statement. Too many alternatives can be confusing. Usually three to five alternative nursing strategies for each health problem are satisfactory.

TABLE 14—9 Components of Goals/Expected Outcomes

Subject	Verb	Conditions/Modifiers	Criterion of Desired Performance
Client	drinks	2500 mL of fluid	daily (time)
Client	administers	correct insulin dose	using aseptic technique (quality standard)
Client	lists	three hazards of smoking (after reading literature)	(accuracy indicated by number of hazards)
Client	recalls	five symptoms of diabetes before discharge	(accuracy indicated by number of symptoms)
Client's ankle	measures	less than 10 inches in circumference	in 48 hours (time)

A recent development is a set of 433 standardized nursing interventions called the Nursing Interventions Classification (NIC). These interventions consist of 6 domains and 27 classes. See Table 14–10 on page 278. (McCloskey & Bulechek, 1996). The NIC interventions have yet to be reviewed by national nursing groups but have been put forth for clinical use and testing. Each broad intervention label includes a definition and a list of all the specific activities nurses perform to carry out the intervention. Not all the activities would be needed for every client, so the nurse chooses from the list those activities appropriate for the client, and individualizes them to fit the supplies, equipment, and so forth, available in the agency. See the box below for an example of one intervention label, definition, and a few of its specific activities. The NIC provides many benefits to nurse practitioners, nurse educators, nurse administrators, and the nursing profession as a whole (see the box on page 279).

Characteristics of Well-Stated Goals/Expected Outcomes

- Expected outcomes are derived primarily from the first clause of the nursing diagnosis, including the defining characteristics or subjective and objective data. The achievement of the outcomes demonstrates problem resolution or prevention.

- The expected outcome is possible to achieve.

- The expected outcome is stated in terms of client responses rather than nursing activities.

- Each expected outcome is a statement of *one* specific client response or behavior.

- Each expected outcome is specific and concrete, to facilitate measurement.

- Each expected outcome is appraisable or measurable, that is, the outcome can be seen, heard, felt, or measured by another person.

- The expected outcome is valued by the client and family.

- The expected outcome is compatible with the therapies of other professionals.

Example of a Standardized Nursing Intervention Label

Respiratory Monitoring

Definition: Collection and analysis of client data to ensure airway patency and adequate gas exchange.

Activities (5 examples are given from a list of 26).

Monitor rate, rhythm, depth, and effort of respirations

Monitor for noisy respirations such as crowing or snoring

Percuss anterior and posterior thorax from apices to bases bilaterally

Monitor for increased restlessness, anxiety, and air hunger

Monitor patient's ability to cough effectively

SOURCE: *Nursing Interventions Classification (NIC)* (2nd ed.) by J. C. McCloskey and G. M. Bulechek (Eds.), Iowa Intervention Project, 1996, St. Louis: Mosby-Year Book, p. 473. Used with permission.

TABLE 14–10 NIC Taxonomy

Level 1: Domains	Level 2: Classes (lettered for cross-referencing)
Domain 1 *Physiological: Basic* Care that supports physical functioning	A. Activity and Exercise Management: Interventions to organize or assist with physical activity and energy conservation and expenditure B. Elimination Management: Interventions to establish and maintain regular bowel and urinary elimination patterns and manage complications due to altered patterns C. Immobility Management: Interventions to manage restricted body movement and the sequelae D. Nutrition Support: Interventions to modify or maintain nutritional status E. Physical Comfort Promotion: Interventions to promote comfort using physical techniques F. Self-Care Facilitation: Interventions to provide or assist with routine activities of daily living
Domain 2 *Physiological: Complex* Care that supports homeostatic regulation	G. Electrolyte and Acid-Base Management: Interventions to regulate electrolyte/acid base balance and prevent complications H. Drug Management: Interventions to facilitate desired effects of pharmacological agents I. Neurologic Management: Interventions to optimize neurologic functions J. Perioperative Care: Interventions to provide care before, during, and immediately after surgery K. Respiratory Management: Interventions to promote airway patency and gas exchange L. Skin/Wound Management: Interventions to maintain or restore tissue integrity M. Thermoregulation: Interventions to maintain body temperature within a normal range N. Tissue Perfusion Management: Interventions to optimize circulation of blood and fluids to the tissue
Domain 3 *Behavioral* Care that supports psychosocial functioning and facilitates life-style changes	O. Behavior Therapy: Interventions to reinforce or promote desirable behaviors or alter undesirable behaviors P. Cognitive Therapy: Interventions to reinforce or promote desirable cognitive functioning or alter undesirable cognitive functioning Q. Communication Enhancement: Interventions to facilitate delivering and receiving verbal and nonverbal messages R. Coping Assistance: Interventions to assist another to build on own strengths, to adapt to a change in function, or to achieve a higher level of function S. Patient Education: Interventions to facilitate learning T. Psychological Comfort: Interventions to promote comforts using psychological techniques
Domain 4 *Safety* Care that supports protection against harm	U. Crisis Management: Interventions to provide immediate short-term help in both psychological and physiological crises V. Risk Management: Interventions to initiate risk-reduction activities and continue monitoring risks over time

TABLE 14–10 *continued*

Level 1: Domains	Level 2: Classes (lettered for cross-referencing)
Domain 5 *Family* Care that supports the family unit	W. Childbearing Care: Interventions to assist in understanding and coping with the psychological and physiological changes during the childbearing period
	X. Lifespan Care: Interventions to facilitate family unit functioning and promote the health and welfare of family members throughout the lifespan
Domain 6 *Health System* Care that supports effective use of the health care delivery system	Y. Health System Mediation: Interventions to facilitate the interface between patient/family and the health care system
	a. Health System Management: Interventions to provide and enhance support services for the delivery of care
	b. Information Management: Interventions to facilitate communication among health care providers

SOURCE: *Nursing Interventions Classification (NIC)* (2nd ed.) by J. C. McCloskey and G. M. Bulechek, Iowa Intervention Project, 1996, St. Louis: Mosby-Year Book, pp. 56–57. Used with permission.

Nursing strategies (or interventions) are identified and written during the planning step of the nursing process; however, they are actually performed during the implementing step. Nursing interventions are "any treatments, based upon clinical judgment and knowledge, that a nurse performs to enhance client outcomes; they include both direct and indirect care; nurse-initiated, physician-initiated, and other provider-initiated treatments" (McCloskey & Bulechek, 1996, p. xvii). Interventions can be categorized as independent, dependent, or collaborative.

Independent interventions are those activities that nurses are licensed to initiate on the basis of their knowledge and skills. They include physical care, ongoing assessment, emotional support and comfort, teaching, counseling, environmental management, and making referrals to other health care professionals. **Dependent interventions** are those activities carried out under the physician's orders or supervision, or according to specified routines. **Collaborative interventions** are actions the nurse carries out in collaboration with other health team members, such as physical therapists, social workers, dietitians, and physicians. Collaborative nursing activities reflect the overlapping responsibilities of, and collegial relationships between, health personnel.

Benefits of the Nursing Interventions Classification (NIC)

- Helps demonstrate the impact that nurses have on the health care delivery system.

- Standardizes and defines the knowledge base for nursing curricula and practice.

- Facilitates the appropriate selection of a nursing intervention.

- Facilitates communication of nursing treatments to other nurses and other providers.

- Enables researchers to examine the effectiveness and cost of nursing care.

- Assists educators to develop curricula that better articulate with clinical practice.

- Facilitates the teaching of clinical decision making to novice nurses.

- Assists administrators in planning more effectively for staff and equipment needs.

- Promotes the development of a reimbursement system for nursing services.

- Facilitates the development and use of nursing information systems.

- Communicates the nature of nursing to the public.

SOURCE: *Nursing Interventions Classification (NIC)* (2nd ed.) by J. C. McCloskey and G. M. Bulechek (Eds.), Iowa Intervention Project, 1996, St. Louis: Mosby-Year Book, p. x. Used with permission.

The amount of time the nurse spends in an independent versus a collaborative or dependent role varies according to the clinical area, type of institution, and specific position of the nurse. Guzzetta (1987, p. 634) estimates that a critical care nurse spends only about 10% of the day functioning in the independent nursing role. In other settings, such as home health care, nurses may function independently 50% of the time. Clinical nurse specialists may work independently 100% of the time.

The following criteria can help the nurse choose the best nursing strategy. The planned action must be

1. Safe and appropriate for the individual's age, health, and so on.
2. Achievable with the resources available.
3. Congruent with the client's values and beliefs.
4. Congruent with other therapies.
5. Based on nursing knowledge and experience or knowledge from relevant sciences (i.e., based on a rationale).
6. Within established standards of care as determined by state laws, professional associations (American Nurses Association, Canadian Nurses Association), and the policies of the institution.

Each state has nurse practice acts that govern the scope of nursing practice. What nurses can do varies somewhat from state to state. Nurses should know the laws of the state where they practice and remain aware of current changes.

Many agencies have policies to guide nursing activities and the activities of other health professionals. Policies are usually intended to safeguard clients. Rules for visiting hours and procedures to follow when a client has cardiac arrest are examples. If a policy does not benefit clients, nurses have a responsibility to bring this to the attention of the appropriate people.

After choosing the appropriate nursing interventions, the nurse writes them on the care plan as nursing orders. Components of nursing orders include the date, action verb, content area, time element, and signature as follows:

4/14/97   Pad (action verb) side rails (content area) during periods of restlessness and confusion (time element). J. Jonas RN.

Developing Nursing Care Plans

The nurse starts the care plan as soon as the client is admitted to the health care agency and constantly updates it throughout the client's stay, in response to changes in the client's condition and evaluations of goal achievement. A nursing care plan may be preplanned and preprinted, or it may be completely handwritten. Many agencies have devised preprinted, standardized guides for providing essential nursing care to specified groups of clients who have certain needs in common (e.g., all clients with pneumonia, all clients with a nursing diagnosis of **Ineffective breastfeeding,** or all clients undergoing cardiac catheterization). Standardized care plans, standards of care, protocols, policies, and procedures are developed and accepted by the nursing staff in order to

1. Ensure that the minimally acceptable standards of care are provided.
2. Promote efficient use of nurses' time by making it unnecessary to hand-write common activities that are done over and over for all (or most) clients on a nursing unit.

The use of standardized care plans is supported by the Joint Commission for the Accreditation of Healthcare Organization standards for nursing care (JCAHO, 1992), which no longer require a handwritten care plan for every client. Regardless of whether nursing orders are handwritten or chosen from a preprinted plan, nursing care must be individualized to fit the unique needs of each client. In practice, a care plan usually consists of both preprinted and handwritten sections.

Computerized care plans are increasingly being used to create and store nursing care plans. The computer can generate both standardized and individualized care plans. For an individualized plan, the nurse chooses the appropriate diagnoses from a menu suggested by the computer. The computer then lists possible goals and nursing interventions for those diagnoses; the nurse chooses those appropriate for the client and types in any additional goals and interventions not listed on the menu. The nurse can read the plan on the computer screen or print out an updated working copy each day.

A case management plan (sometimes called a collaborative care plan) is a multidisciplinary care plan that sequences the care that needs to be given each day during the projected length of stay for a specific type of case (Zander, 1992, p. 127). Like the traditional nursing care plan, a case management plan specifies goals and nursing orders to address client problems (including nursing diagnoses).

However, it includes medical and other treatments as well. For further information, see Chapter 4.

THE IMPLEMENTATION PHASE

Broadly defined, implementing consists of doing, delegating, and recording. The nurse performs or delegates the nursing orders that were developed in the planning step and then concludes the implementing step by recording nursing activities and the resulting client responses. See the accompanying box for professional standards describing nurses' accountability for implementing. Although the nurse may act on the client's behalf (e.g., referring the client to a community health nurse for home care), professional standards support client and family participation, as in all phases of the nursing process.

The process of implementing normally includes

- Reassessing the client
- Determining the need for nursing assistance
- Implementing the nursing strategies
- Communicating the nursing actions

Reassessing the Client

Assessing is carried out throughout the nursing process, whenever the nurse has contact with the client. Just before implementing, the nurse must reassess whether the intervention is still needed. Even though an order is written on the care plan, the situation or the client's condition may have changed. New data may, in the nurse's judgment, indicate a need to change the priorities of care or the nursing strategies.

Determining the Need for Nursing Assistance

When implementing some nursing strategies, the nurse may require assistance for one of the following reasons:

1. The nurse is unable to implement the nursing strategies safely alone (e.g., turning an obese client in bed).

2. It would reduce stress on the client (e.g., turning a person who experiences acute pain when moved).

3. The nurse lacks the knowledge or skills to implement a particular nursing activity (e.g., a nurse who is not familiar with a particular model of

---

ANA Standards

Standard V: Implementation
The nurse implements the interventions identified in the plan of care.

Measurement Criteria
1. Interventions are consistent with the established plan of care.
2. Interventions are implemented in a safe and appropriate manner.
3. Interventions are documented.

SOURCE: Abstracted from *Standards of Clinical Nursing Practice* by the American Nurses Association, 1991, Washington, DC: Author, p. 13. Used with permission.

---

intravenous infusion controller needs assistance the first time it is used).

Implementing Nursing Strategies

After reassessing the client and determining the need for assistance, the nurse implements the planned strategies. Nursing activities generally include caring, communicating, helping, teaching, counseling, acting as a client advocate and change agent, leading, and managing. In addition to performing nursing activities, nurses (a) assign and delegate care to other nursing personnel and (b) supervise and evaluate the nursing activities of others.

Communicating Nursing Actions

After carrying out the nursing orders, the nurse completes the implementing phase by recording the interventions, along with the client responses. Nursing actions must not be recorded in advance, because the nurse may determine on reassessing the client that the action should not or cannot be implemented.

In some instances, it is important to record a nursing action immediately after it is implemented. This is particularly true of the administration of medications and treatments because recorded data about a client must be up to date, accurate, and available to other nurses and health care professionals. Immediate recording helps safeguard the client, for example, from receiving a second dose of medication.

Nursing actions are communicated verbally as well as in writing. When a client's health is changing rapidly, the charge nurse and/or the physician may want to be kept up to date with verbal reports. Verbal reports are given to other nurses and other health professionals. Nurses also give verbal reports at a change of shift and on a client's discharge to another unit or health agency.

CONSIDER...

• reading the "Report on the NIC Project Nursing Interventions Used in Practice" by G. M. Bulechek, J. C. McCloskey, M. G. Titler, and J. A. Denehy, in the October 1994 issue of *American Journal of Nursing*, *94*, pp. 59–64. How does your daily practice correspond with the research findings on what interventions nurses use and how often they use them?
• which factors would support delegating a specific nursing strategy. What responsibility does the nurse have after delegating a task?

THE EVALUATION PHASE

Evaluation may be ongoing, intermittent, or terminal. *Ongoing evaluation* is done while or immediately after implementing a nursing order; it enables the nurse to make on-the-spot modifications in an intervention. *Intermittent evaluation*, performed at specified intervals (e.g., once a week), shows the extent of progress toward goal achievement and enables the nurse to correct any deficiencies and modify the care plan as needed. Evaluation continues (either ongoing or intermittently) until the client achieves the health goals and/or is discharged from nursing care. *Terminal evaluation* indicates the client's condition at the time of discharge. It includes the status of goal achievement and an evaluation of the client's self-care abilities with regard to follow-up care. Most agencies have a special discharge record for the terminal evaluation.

Through evaluating, nurses accept responsibility for their actions, indicate interest in the results of the nursing actions, and demonstrate a desire not to perpetuate ineffective actions but to adopt more effective ones. See the accompanying box for professional standards describing the nurse's responsibility for evaluating.

The evaluating and assessing phases overlap. As previously stated, assessment (data collection) is ongoing and continuous at every client contact. However, data are collected for different purposes at

---

ANA Standards

Standard VI: Evaluation

The nurse evaluates the client's progress toward attainment of outcomes.

Measurement Criteria

1. Evaluation is systematic and ongoing.
2. Client's responses to interventions are documented.
3. The effectiveness of interventions is evaluated in relation to outcomes.
4. Ongoing assessment data are used to revise diagnoses, outcomes, and the plan of care, as needed.
5. Revisions in diagnoses, outcomes, and the plan of care are documented.
6. The client, significant others, and health care providers are involved in the evaluation process, when appropriate.

SOURCE: Abstracted from *Standards of Clinical Nursing Practice* by the American Nurses Association, 1991, Washington, DC: Author, p. 14. Used with permission.

---

different points in the nursing process. During the assessing phase, the nurse collects data for the purpose of making diagnoses. During the evaluating step, the nurse collects data for the purpose of comparing it to preselected goals and judging the effectiveness of the nursing care. The *act* of assessing (data collection) is the same; the differences lie in (1) when the data are collected and (2) how the data are used.

The evaluation process has six components:

• Identifying the expected outcomes that the nurse will use to measure client goal achievement (this is done in the planning step)
• Collecting data related to the expected outcomes
• Comparing the data with the expected outcomes
• Judging whether the goals have been achieved
• Relating nursing actions to client outcomes
• Drawing conclusions about problem status
• Reviewing and modifying the nursing care plan

Identifying Expected Outcomes

The expected outcomes formulated in the planning step are the criteria used to evaluate the client's response to nursing care. Expected outcomes serve two purposes: They (1) establish the kind of evaluative data that need to be collected and (2) provide a standard against which the data are judged. For example, given the following expected outcomes, any nurse caring for the client should know what data to collect:

- Daily fluid intake will not be less than 2500 mL.
- Urinary output will balance with fluid intake.

Collecting Data

Using the clearly stated, precise, and measurable expected outcomes as a guide, the nurse collects data so that conclusions can be drawn about whether goals have been met. It is usually necessary to collect both objective and subjective data.

Some data may require interpretation. Examples of objective data requiring interpretation are the degree of tissue turgor of a dehydrated client or the degree of restlessness of a client with pain. When objective data need interpretation, the nurse may obtain the views of other nurses to substantiate changes. Examples of subjective data needing interpretation include complaints of nausea or pain by the client. When interpreting subjective data, the nurse must rely upon either (a) the client's statements (e.g., "My pain is worse now than it was after breakfast") or (b) objective indicators of the subjective data, even though these indicators may require further interpretation (e.g., decreased restlessness, decreased pulse and respiratory rates, and relaxed facial muscles as indicators of pain relief). Data must be recorded concisely and accurately to facilitate the third part of the evaluating process.

Judging Goal Achievement

If the first two parts of the evaluation process have been carried out effectively, it is relatively simple to determine whether a goal has been met. Both the nurse and client play an active role in comparing the client's actual response with the expected outcomes. Did the client drink 3000 mL of fluid in 24 hours? When determining whether a goal has been achieved, the nurse can draw one of three possible conclusions:

1. The goal was met; that is, the client response is the same as the expected outcome.

2. The goal was partially met; that is, either a short-term goal was achieved, but the long-term goal was not, or the expected outcome was only partially attained.

3. The goal was not met.

After determining whether a goal has been met, the nurse writes an evaluative statement (either on the care plan or in the nurse's notes). An evaluation statement consists of two parts: a conclusion and supporting data. The conclusion is a statement that the goal/expected outcome was met, partially met, or not met. The supporting data are the list of client responses that support the conclusion, for example:

> Goal met: Oral intake 300 mL more than output; skin turgor good; mucous membranes moist.

Relating Nursing Actions to Client Outcomes

The fourth aspect of the evaluating process is determining whether the nursing actions had any relation to the outcomes. It should never be assumed that a nursing action was the cause of or the only factor in meeting, partially meeting, or not meeting a goal.

Drawing Conclusions about Problem Status

The nurse uses the judgments about goal achievement (see preceding phase) to determine whether the care plan was effective in resolving, reducing, or preventing client problems. When goals have been met, the nurse can draw one of the following conclusions about the status of the client's problem:

- The actual problem stated in the nursing diagnosis has been resolved; or the potential problem is being prevented, and the risk factors no longer exist. In these instances, the nurse documents that the goals have been met and discontinues the care for the problem.
- The potential problem stated in the nursing diagnosis is being prevented, but the risk factors are still present. In this case, the nurse keeps the problem on the care plan.
- The actual problem still exists even though some goals are being met. Therefore, the nursing interventions must be continued even though this one goal was met.

When goals have been partially met or when goals have not yet been met, two conclusions may be drawn:

- The care plan may need to be revised because the problem is only partially resolved. The revisions may need to occur during assessing, diagnosing, or planning phases, as well as interventions.
- The care plan does not need revision, because the client merely needs more time to achieve the

previously established goal(s). In order to make this decision, the nurse must assess why the goals are being only partially achieved, including whether the evaluation was conducted too soon.

Reviewing and Modifying the Nursing Care Plan

After drawing conclusions about the status of the client's problems, the nurse modifies the care plan as indicated. Depending on the agency, modifications may be made by drawing a line through portions of the care plan, using a Hi-Liter pen, or writing "Discontinued (dc'd)" and the date.

Whether or not goals were met, there are a number of decisions to make about continuing, modifying, or terminating nursing care for each problem. Before making modifications, the nurse must first determine why the plan was not completely effective. This requires a review of the entire care plan and a critique of the nursing process steps involved in its development.

CONSIDER . . .

- how a nurse can determine whether the achievement of outcomes is related to a specific nursing intervention.
- whether the nurse's attitude when performing a specific intervention might affect the client outcome. How might the nurse determine whether staff attitudes are negatively affecting client outcomes?

EVALUATING THE QUALITY OF NURSING CARE

Evaluating the quality of nursing care is an essential part of professional accountability. Other terms used for this measurement are quality assessment and quality assurance. **Quality assessment** is an examination of services only; **quality assurance** implies that efforts are made to evaluate *and* ensure quality health care.

Historical Perspective

Evaluation of the quality of care is not a new concept. Florence Nightingale's *Notes on Hospitals*, published in 1859, included an evaluation of medical and nursing care. Since that time, evaluation has progressed through a number of stages. Initially, it focused on

the environment; for example, whether equipment was available at the time it was needed. Later, organizational standards in agencies were developed; for example, the ratio of nurses to clients was evaluated in terms of clients' needs. Since 1952, the Joint Commission on Accreditation of Hospitals (JCAH), a voluntary organization, has surveyed hospitals. Objective criteria were applied to evaluate a client's record after discharge from the hospital. This was called a **retrospective audit.** (*Retrospective* means relating to a past event, and *audit* means an examination or review of records.) A **nursing audit** is a review of clients' charts to evaluate nursing competence or performance. In 1972 and 1973, the JCAH (now called the JCAHO) revised its standards to include the requirement that hospitals be subjected to medical and nursing audits before receiving accreditation.

In 1972, the United States government enacted legislation to control health care costs and evaluate the quality of health care services received by Medicare and Medicaid clients. Since that time, a national and statewide system of professional review organizations (PROs) has been established to develope standards and monitoring the quality of, cost of, and access to care. The objective of these procedures is to ensure that the care given under federal programs was necessary and that the appropriate facilities were chosen to provide the care.

The PROs are based on a concept of peer review. A **peer review** is an encounter between two persons equal in education, abilities, and qualifications, during which one person critically reviews the practices that the other has documented in a client's record. These evaluative processes may be **concurrent audits,** that is, reviews of present practices.

Approaches to Quality Evaluation

Three aspects of care—structure, process, and outcome—can be evaluated. Standards of care for each type of evaluation have been developed based on nursing and health-related research and expert opinion. A good evaluation needs to consider all three aspects of care.

The Structure in Which Client Care Takes Place

Structure evaluation focuses on the organization of the client care system, for instance, administrative and financial procedures that direct the provision of care, staffing patterns, management styles, availability of equipment, and physical facilities. Information about these support structures can be obtained easily. Quality care cannot be delivered without adequate staff and resources. However, adequate staffing patterns and adequate facilities do not ensure quality care.

The Process of Care

Process evaluation focuses on the activities of the nurse, that is, the performance of the caregiver in relation to the client's needs. The care given by the nurse is evaluated by talking with the client, auditing the client's record, and observing the nursing activities. Evaluators may seek answers to questions such as these: Are medications recorded correctly? Was client teaching documented? Is the care plan complete? This type of evaluation is time-consuming and requires the judgment of expert practitioners. The ANA *Standards of Clinical Nursing Practice* (1991) are process standards that provide the nursing profession with a framework for the delivery and evaluation of care.

Outcomes of the Care

The focus of *outcome evaluation* is the client's health status, welfare, and satisfaction, or the results of care in terms of changes in the client. Its advantage is that outcomes may be easily observed, especially in relation to medical care, which focuses on disease entities. In nursing, however, outcomes are more difficult to determine, because nursing takes a more holistic view of the client. Defining emotional, social, and behavioral outcomes is complex. In addition, client outcomes cannot be wholly attributed to nursing care. The client's own physical and psychologic mechanisms and contributions by support persons and other health professionals collectively produce outcomes. Outcome evaluation can focus on the client's change in behavior toward goal achievement prior to discharge (concurrent audit), or the client's record may be reviewed after discharge for evidence of goal attainment (retrospective audit).

READINGS FOR ENRICHMENT

Carpenito, L. J. (1995). *Nursing diagnosis: Application for clinical practice* (6th ed.) Philadelphia: Lippincott.

This book provides detailed coverage of nursing diagnoses—their development, types and components, issues and controversies, and how they are derived. The diagnoses are organized alphabetically. The author provides information about each diagnosis, including its definition, defining characteristics, related factors, focus assessment criteria, principles and rationale for nursing care, outcome criteria, and nursing interventions.

McCloskey, J. C. & Bulechek, G. M. (1996). *Iowa Intervention Project: Nursing Interventions Classification (NIC)* 2nd ed. St. Louis: Mosby-Yearbook, Inc.

The Nursing Intervention Project represents an effort to define and classify the treatments that are performed by nurses. The authors discuss the importance of an intervention classification system for nursing and the development of a three level taxonomy of nursing interventions for use in the delivery of nursing care. The top level consists of 6 domains; the second level consists of 27 classes; and the third level

consists of 433 interventions that have been linked to the NANDA diagnoses. The first two levels are shown in Table 14–10 on page 278 of this textbook. Each intervention has a label name and unique number (to facilitate computerization), a definition, and a list of appropriate direct and indirect care activities that might be selected for the care of a specific client.

Null, S., Richter-Abt, D., & Kovac, J. (1995, March). Development of a perioperative nursing diagnosis flow sheet. *AORN Journal*, 61, 547–557.

Nurses on the perioperative and postoperative units at the DePaul Health Center in St. Louis recognized that documentation tools both lacked nursing diagnoses terminology and failed to allow nurses to document the related nursing interventions. A nursing diagnosis task force was formed, which led to the development, implementation, and universal use of a perioperative nursing diagnoses flowsheet within the surgical services department. Eleven nursing diagnoses were chosen. For each diagnosis, the form includes a desired outcome and interventions that can be recorded throughout the perioperative period.

READINGS FOR ENRICHMENT   *continued*

Richard, J. E., & Stern, P. N. (1991, Fall). How primary nurses operationalize accountability. *Canadian Journal of Research*, 23(3), 49–66.

Primary nursing is believed to promote individualized care, higher quality care, continuity of nursing care, professional practice, and accountability. This study was conducted to determine what 24-hour accountability means to nurses and how they put it into practice. The population sample was composed of 21 registered nurses working in medical, surgical, and psychiatric units of two large teaching hospitals in Montreal, Quebec. These nurses reported that they achieve accountability through a process of communicating *each aspect of the nursing process* with clients, families, peers, and the health care members.

The authors provide two schematics. One illustrates the communicating process that maintains 24-hour

accountability; the other illustrates concepts related to accountability in primary nursing.

You make the diagnosis: Care Studies. (1995). *Nursing Diagnosis*. January/March 1993 through January/March 1996 (all issues).

This series of case studies prepared by various authors provide clinical examples of situations for which the reader is asked to make nursing diagnoses based on the data presented. The authors who submit the case studies provide an analysis of diagnoses they would select. The author's analysis is followed by a commentary by another nurse author. *Nursing Diagnosis* grants permission for users to copy the case studies and analyses for educational purposes.

SUMMARY

The nursing process is a systematic, rational method of planning and providing individualized nursing care for individuals, families, groups, and communities. It is organized into five interrelated, interdependent phases: assessing, diagnosing, planning, implementing, and evaluating. The goals of the nursing process are to identify a client's actual or potential health care needs, to establish plans to meet the identified needs, and to deliver and evaluate specific nursing interventions to meet those needs. The nursing process can be used in all health care settings; it is cyclic and dynamic, client centered, interpersonal and collaborative, and universally applicable. It provides a framework for nurses' accountability and responsibility.

Assessing involves collecting, organizing, verifying, and recording data. Assessment involves active participation by the client and nurse in obtaining subjective and objective data about the client's health status. Data must be validated. Subjective data can be used to validate objective data, and vice versa. Primary and secondary data can also be used to validate each other. Nursing models provide frameworks for collecting and organizing client data. Data must be recorded in a factual manner, without interpretation or inferences. The nursing assessment must be complete and accurate, because nursing diagnoses and interventions are based on this information.

Diagnosis is a reasoning process utilizing critical thinking. The nurse makes a clinical judgment (nursing

diagnosis) about a client's potential or actual health problems. The critical-thinking skills used in diagnosing include analysis, synthesis, inductive reasoning, deductive reasoning, and decision making. The three phases of the diagnostic process are data analysis; identification of the client's health problems, health risks, and strengths; and formulation of nursing diagnoses. In data analysis and processing the nurse compares data against standards to identify significant cues, clusters the data, and identifies gaps and inconsistencies. Significant cues are those that (a) point to change in a client's health status or pattern, (b) vary from norms of the client population, or (c) indicate a developmental delay. The end product of the diagnostic process is a nursing diagnosis or a clinical judgment about the client's responses to actual and potential health problems or life processes. The basic format for a nursing diagnostic statement is "Problem related to etiology." However, there are several variations on this format. A nursing diagnosis provides the basis for selecting independent nursing interventions to achieve outcomes for which the nurse is accountable.

Prognostic judgments are made at the end of the diagnostic phase and before the planning phase of the nursing process. Nursing prognoses, like medical prognoses, influence goals, nursing interventions, and evaluative data. They have three components: prognostic variables or indicators, outcomes, and trajectory.

Planning is the process of designing nursing strategies required to prevent, reduce, or eliminate a client's health problems. Five activities of planning are setting priorities, establishing client goals, planning nursing strategies, writing nursing orders, and writing a nursing care plan. Client goals/outcome criteria are derived from the first *clause of the nursing diagnosis. Outcome criteria describe specific and measurable client responses and help the nurse evaluate the effectiveness of the nursing intervention. Nursing strategies are focused on the etiology or* second *clause of the nursing diagnosis. The nursing care plan provides direction for individualized care of the client. Preprinted, standardized care plans should be adapted and used with handwritten plans to meet individual client needs. Planning involves the nurse, the client, support persons, and other caregivers. The nurse consults with other nurses or health professionals to verify information, implement changes, or obtain additional knowledge to aid in client goals.*

Implementing is putting planned nursing strategies into action. It incorporates all of the activities performed to promote health, prevent complications, treat present problems, and facilitate the client's coping with chronic alterations in health status. Cognitive, interpersonal, and technical skills are used to implement nursing strategies. More specifically, implementing activities include communicating, caring, teaching, counseling, leading, managing, and acting as a client advocate and change agent. Reassessing occurs simultaneously with the implementing phase of the nursing process. The implementing phase terminates with the documentation of the nursing activities and client responses.

Evaluating is the process of comparing client responses to preselected outcomes to determine whether goals have been met. It includes review and modification of the care plan. Evaluating may be ongoing, intermittent, or terminal. It is purposeful and organized. The expected outcomes formulated during the planning phase serve as criteria for evaluating client progress and improved health status. They determine the data that must be collected to evaluate the client's health status. Professional standards of care hold that nurses are responsible and accountable for implementing and evaluating the plan of care.

SELECTED REFERENCES

American Nurses Association. (1991). *Standards of nursing practice.* Kansas City, MO: Author.

Briody, M. E., Jones, D. A., & Fitzpatrick, J. J. (1992, July/Sept.). Toward further understanding of nursing diagnosis: An interpretation. *Nursing Diagnosis, 3*(3), 124–128.

Carnevali, D. L., & Thomas, M. D. (1993). *Diagnostic reasoning and treatment decision making in nursing.* Philadelphia: Lippincott.

Carpenito, L. J. (1995). *Nursing diagnosis: Application to clinical practice* (6th ed.). Philadelphia: Lippincott.

Dobrzyn, J. (1995, Jan./March). Components of written diagnostic statements. *Nursing Diagnosis, 6*(1), 29–36.

Durand, M., & Prince, R. (1993, April-June). A glance back in time. Nursing diagnosis: Process and decision. *Nursing Forum, 28*(2), 25–32.

Eisenhauer, L. A. (1994, Winter). A typology of nursing therapeutics. *Image: Journal of Nursing Scholarship, 26*(4) 261–264.

Gordon, M. (1994). *Nursing diagnosis: Process and application* (3rd ed.). St. Louis: Mosby.

Guzzetta, C. (1987, Nov.). Nursing diagnoses in nursing education: Effect on the profession. Part 1. *Heart and Lung, 16,* 629–635.

Iowa Intervention Project. McCloskey, J., & Bulechek, G. (eds). (1993). The NIC taxonomy structure. *Image: Journal of Nursing Scholarship, 25*(3), 187–192.

Joint Commission on Accreditation of Healthcare Organizations. 1992. *Accreditation Manual for Hospitals.* Chicago: Joint Commission on Accreditation of Healthcare Organizations, Nursing Services.

Kerr, M. E., Fitzpatrick, J. J., Warren, J. J., Carpenito, L. J., et al. (1992, April/ June). Development of definitions for Taxonomy II. *Nursing Diagnosis, 3*(2), 65–71.

Kerr, M., Hoskins, L., Fitzpatrick, J., Hurley, M., Mills, W., Rottkamp, B., Warrne, J., & Carpenito, L. J. (1991, July/Sept.). From Taxonomy I to Taxonomy II. *Nursing Diagnosis, 2*(3), 131–135.

Kim, M. J., McFarland, G. K., & McLane, A. M. (eds.). (1984). *Classification of nursing diagnoses: Proceedings of the fifth national conference.* St. Louis: Mosby.

McCloskey, J. C., & Bulechek, G. M. (eds.). (1996). *Nursing interventions classification (NIC)* (2nd ed.). St. Louis: Mosby-Year Book.

Mundinger, M. O. (1980). *Autonomy in nursing.* Gaithersburg, MD: Aspen Publishers.

Newland, P. L. (1994, Sept./Oct.). A guide for care planning. *Nurse Educator, 19*(5), 9.

Nightingale, F. 1957. *Notes on Nursing.* Philadelphia: Lippincott. (Originally published 1860).

North American Nursing Diagnosis Association. (1990). *Taxonomy I, revised—1990.* St. Louis: Author.

North American Nursing Diagnosis Association. (1992). *NANDA nursing diagnoses: Definitions and classifications, 1992.* St. Louis: Author.

Null, S., Richter-Abt, D., & Kovac, J. (1995, March). Development of a perioperative nursing diagnoses flowsheet. *AORN Journal, 61,* 547–557.

Yura, H., & Walsh, M. B. (1983). *Human Needs 3 and the Nursing Process.* Norwalk, CT: Appleton-Century Crofts.

Yura, H., & Walsh, M. B. (1988). *The nursing process: Assessing, planning, implementing, evaluating* (5th ed.). Norwalk, CT: Appleton & Lange.

Weber, G. (1991, Oct.). Making nursing diagnosis work for you and your client. A step-by-step approach. *Nursing and Health Care, 12,* 424–430.

Wilkinson, J. (1996). *Nursing process: A critical thinking approach* (2nd ed.). Redwood City, CA: Addison-Wesley Nursing.

Zander, K. (1988a, Jan.). Managed care within acute care settings: Design and implementation via nursing case management. *Health Care Supervisor, 6*(2), 27.

Zander, K. (1988b, Sept.) Nursing case management: Resolving the DRG paradox. *Nursing Clinics of North America, 23,* 503–520.

Zander, K. (1992). Focusing on patient outcome: Case management in the 90's. *Dimensions of Critical Care Nursing, 11*(3), 127–129.

Group Process

OBJECTIVES

- Describe essential facts about groups, including types and stages of group development.

- Explain the features of effective groups.

- Describe essential characteristics of group dynamics.

- Analyze group interactions to determine effective group processes.

"The quality of peoples' lives often depends on their ability to perform effectively in the groups to which they belong."
—Carolyn Chambers Clark, 1994

Nurses belong to a variety of professional groups, ranging from **dyads** (two-person groups) to large professional associations. In these groups the nurse may fill a variety of roles including leader, advisor, elaborator, encourager, and so on.

- People are usually born into a family group and interact with others at all stages of their lives through societal, cultural, and religious socialization.
- A **group** consists of two or more people who share needs and goals and who take each other into account in their actions.
- Groups are important in peoples' lives. The family provides for socialization, while other groups (e.g., peer, social, religious, work, political), are vehicles for learning and satisfaction.
- **Group dynamics,** or **group process,** is the study of a group's functioning and its effectiveness or ineffectiveness.

GROUPS

Groups exist to help people achieve goals that might be unattainable by individual effort alone. By pooling the ideas and expertise of several individuals, groups can often solve problems more effectively than one person. Information can be disseminated to groups more quickly and with more consistency than to individuals. In addition, groups often take greater risks than do individuals. Just as responsibilities for actions are shared by group members, so are the consequences of actions.

In the clinical setting, nurses work in groups as they collaborate with other nurses, other health care professionals, clients, and support persons when planning and providing care. Nurses also work in groups when joining professional and specialty organizations and civic and community groups to promote the goals of nursing on professional, civic, and political levels. Group skills are therefore important for nurses in all settings.

Types of Groups

Groups are classified as either primary or secondary, according to their structure and type of interaction.

A **primary group** is a small, intimate group in which the relationships among members are personal, spontaneous, sentimental, cooperative, and inclusive. Examples are the family, a play group of children, informal work groups, and friendship groups. Members of a primary group communicate with each other largely in face-to-face interactions and develop a strong sense of unity or "oneness." What belongs to one person is often seen as belonging to the group. For example, a success achieved by one member is shared by all and is seen as a success of the group.

Primary groups set standards of behavior for the members but also support and sustain each member in stresses he or she would otherwise not be able to withstand. Expectations are informally administered and involve primarily internal constraints imposed by the group itself. To its members, the primary group has a value in itself, not merely as a means to some other goal. The group has a sense of "we" and "our" to it, in contrast to "I" and "mine." Affective relationships are stressed.

The role of the primary group, particularly the family, in health care is increasingly recognized. It is to the primary group that people turn for help and support when they have health problems. Treatment and health care of individuals therefore are developing an expanded focus that includes the family.

A **secondary group** is generally larger, more impersonal, and less sentimental than a primary group. Examples are professional associations, task groups, ad hoc committees, political parties, and business groups. Members view these groups simply as a means of getting things done. Interactions do not necessarily occur in face-to-face contact and do not require that the members know each other in any inclusive sense. Thus, there is little sentiment attached to such relationships. Expectations of members are formally administered through impersonal controls and external restraints imposed by designated enforcement officials. Once the goals of the group are achieved or change, the interaction is discontinued.

Functions of Groups

Sampson and Marthas (1990, pp. 3–21) describe eight functions of groups. See Table 15–1. Any one group generally has more than one function, and it may serve different functions for different group members. For example, for one member a group may provide support; for another, information.

TABLE 15-1 **Functions of Groups**

Function	Description
Socialization	Primary socialization in growth and development.
	Professional socialization into nursing or to a change in position.
	Socialization into the culture of an organization (i.e., new customs and beliefs) when a hospital is taken over by a corporate organization.
Support	Provision of social support for the members, a source of collegiality, and a source of help when needed.
Task completion	Complete tasks that are beyond the scope of any one individual.
	Each person may bring specialized knowledge and skills.
	Cooperation is important in task completion.
Camaraderie	Provision of goodwill among the members, thereby providing moments of pleasure.
Information	Provide a context for defining social reality, for setting performance goals, for establishing priorities, and for sharing special knowledge.
Normative function	Develop definitions and standards and enforce those standards, thereby encouraging compliance and discouraging deviations.
Empowerment	Empowering people and thereby encouraging change. A group often has more power than any individual.
Governance	Groups are often active in making decisions and serving as a source of governance within an organization.

Source: Adapted from *Group Process for Health Professions* (3rd ed.) by E. E. Sampson and M. Marthas, 1990, Albany, NY: Delmar.

Levels of Group Formality

Groups may be classified as formal, semiformal, or informal.

Formal Groups

The most common example of the formal group is the work organization. People become familiar with many different formal work groups during their lifetimes and spend a major part of their working hours in such groups. Formal groups usually exist to carry out a task or goal rather than to meet the needs of group members. Traditional features of formal groups are shown in the box on the following page.

Semiformal Groups

Examples of semiformal groups include churches, lodges, social clubs, PTAs, and some labor unions. Many of an individual's social and ego needs are often satisfied by membership in these groups. The groups are similar in form to formal groups, but exhibit slight differences. Features of semiformal groups are shown in the box on the following page.

Informal Groups

Most people, from childhood on, have membership in numerous informal groups. These groups provide much of a person's education and develop most cultural values. Five types of groups are representative of the numerous informal groups in existence:

- *Friendship groups.* The first groups formed in life are friendship groups. They are often formed on the basis of common interests. Many arise out of semiformal group interactions or are formed spontaneously from the work organization.
- *Hobby groups.* Hobby groups bring together people from all walks of life. Differences in members' personalities and backgrounds are largely ignored in the interests of the hobby itself.
- *Convenience groups.* Many examples of convenience groups are found both in and out of the work setting. Two examples are the carpool and the childcare group organized by mothers.
- *Work groups.* Informal work groups can make or break an organization. Managers need to be sensitive to such groups and cultivate their cooperation

Characteristics of Formal Groups

- Authority is imposed from above.
- Leadership selection is assigned from above and made by an authoritative and often arbitrary order or decree.
- Managers are symbols of power and authority.
- The goals of the formal group are normally imposed at a much higher level than the direct leadership of the group.
- Fiscal goals have little meaning to the members of the group.
- Management is endangered by its aloofness from the members of the work group.
- Behavioral **norms** (expected standards of behavior), regulations, and rules are usually superimposed. The larger the turnover rate of members, the greater the structuring of rules.
- Membership in the group is only partly voluntary.
- Rigidity of purpose is often a necessity for protection of the formal group in the pursuit of its objectives.
- Interactions within the group as a whole are limited, but informal subgroups are generally formed.

Characteristics of Semiformal Groups

- The structure is formal.
- The hierarchy is carefully delineated.
- Membership is voluntary but selective and difficult to achieve.
- Prestige and status are often accrued from membership.
- Structured, deliberate activities absorb a large part of the group's meeting time.
- Objectives and goals are rigid; change is not recognized as desirable.
- In many cases, the leader has direct control over the choice of a successor.
- The day-to-day operating standards and methods (group norms) are negotiable. Because most people become bored at quibbling about norms, people can often "railroad" acceptance of a list of norms they desire.

Characteristics of Informal Groups

- The group is not bound by any set of written rules or regulations.
- Usually there is a set of unwritten laws and a strong code of ethics.
- The group is purely functional and has easily recognized basic objectives.
- Rotational leadership is common. The group recognizes that only rarely are all leadership characteristics found in one person.
- The group assigns duties to the members best qualified for certain functions. For example, the person who is recognized as outgoing and sociable will be assigned responsibilities for planning parties.
- Judgments about the group's leader are made quickly and surely. Leaders are replaced when they make one or more mistakes or do not get the job done.
- The group is an ideal testing ground for new leadership techniques, but there is no guarantee that such techniques can be transferred effectively to a large, formal organization.
- Behavioral norms are developed either by group effort or by the leader and adopted by the group.
- Deviance by one member from the group's behavioral norms is more threatening to the perpetuation of small, informal groups than to large, formal, heterogeneous groups. Conformity and group solidarity are important for the protection and preservation of small groups.
- Group norms are enforced by **sanctions** (punishments) imposed by the group of those who violate a norm. Different values are placed on norms in accordance with the values of the leader. One leader may regard the action as a gross violation, whereas another leader may find it quite acceptable.
- Interpersonal interactions are spontaneous.

and good will. Friendships often arise between a new member and the person who makes him or her feel a welcome addition to the group.

- *Self-protective groups.* Self-protective groups can be found anywhere but are particularly common in work organizations. They arise spontaneously out of a real or perceived threat. For example, a supervisor may approach a worker too strongly and find a group of workers organizing a united front against the threat. Such groups dissipate as soon as the threat has subsided.

The main features of informal groups are shown in the box on page 292.

Group Development

The phases of group development have been variously described. Clark (1994, pp. 59–63) divides group development into three phases: orientation, working, and termination. In the *orientation phase*, group members seek to be accepted, and to find out how similar and different each one is from the other. Anxiety is often high during this period. The group is more likely viewed as a group of individuals than as a unified whole. Uncertainty and insecurity are often present in the group; safe topics are discussed.

In the *working phase*, group members feel more comfortable with one another, and group goals are established. Decisions are more likely to be made by consensus rather than by vote. Problem solving takes place, and frustration is often replaced by cautious optimism. Differences that are present are handled by adapting and problem solving rather than conflict. Disagreements are dealt with openly.

During the *termination phase*, the focus is on evaluating and summarizing the group experience. Feelings vary from frustration and anger to sadness or satisfaction, depending on whether the group has achieved its goals and attained group cohesion (group unity).

Tuckman and Jensen (1977) identified six stages of group (team) development. Each group member should be aware of these stages and of the process of development. See Table 15–2.

TABLE 15–2 Stages of Team Development

Stage	Team Behaviors	Leadership Behaviors
Orientation	Uncertainty Unfamiliarity Mistrust Nonparticipator	Directive style Outline purpose Negotiate schedules Define the team's mission
Forming	Acceptance of each other Learning communication skills High energy, motivated	Plan/focus on the problem Positive role modeling Actively encourage participation
Storming	Team spirit developed Trust developed Conflict may arise Impatience, frustration	Evaluate group dynamics Focus on goals Conflict resolution Establish goals and objectives
Norming	Increased comfort Identify responsibilities Effective team interaction Resolution of conflicts	Focus on goals Attend to process and content Supportive style
Performing	Clear on purpose Unity/cohesion Problem solve and accept actions	Act as a team member Encourage increased responsibility Follow-up on action plans Measure results
Terminating	Members separate Team gains closure on objectives	Reinforce successes Celebrate and reward

SOURCE: "Quality Work Improvement Groups: From Paper to Reality" by G. B. Smith and E. Hukill, July 1994, *Journal of Nursing Care Quality, 8*, p. 5. Used with permission.

Features of Effective Groups

To be effective, a group must achieve three main functions: accomplish its goals, maintain its cohesion, and develop and modify its structure to improve its effectiveness.

See Table 15–3 for comparative features of effective and ineffective groups.

CONSIDER . . .

- the number and types of groups to which nurses belong. Identify primary and secondary groups and formal, semiformal, and informal groups in which nurses commonly participate. How does membership in these groups enhance the individual nurse and the goals of professional nursing?

- your own involvement in groups. How many groups do you participate in? Which groups fulfill personal goals? Which groups fulfill professional goals? Which groups are specific to fulfilling work goals? How does the organization of your different groups relate to the characteristics of the various types of groups described in this chapter?

- whether there could be situations where the nurse may experience conflict as a result of participating in two or more different groups. What conflicts might result, and what are the alternatives to resolving such conflicts?

TABLE 15–3   Comparative Features of Effective and Ineffective Groups

Factor	Effective Groups	Ineffective Groups
Atmosphere	Informal, comfortable, and relaxed. It is a working atmosphere in which people demonstrate their interest and involvement.	Obviously tense. Signs of boredom may appear.
Goal setting	Goals, tasks, and objectives are clarified, understood, and modified so that members of the group can commit themselves to cooperatively structured goals.	Unclear, misunderstood, or imposed goals may be accepted by members. The goals are competitively structured.
Leadership and member participation	Shift from time to time, depending on the circumstances. Different members assume leadership at various times, because of their knowledge or experience.	Delegated and based on authority. The chairperson may dominate the group, or the members may defer unduly. Members' participation is unequal, with high-authority members dominating.
Goal emphasis	All three functions of groups are emphasized—goal accomplishment, internal maintenance, and developmental change.	One or more functions may not be emphasized.
Communication	Open and two-way. Ideas and feelings are encouraged, both about the problem and about the group's operation.	Closed or one-way. Only the production of ideas is encouraged. Feelings are ignored or taboo. Members may be tentative or reluctant to be open and may have "hidden agendas" (personal goals at cross-purposes with group goals).
Decision making	By consensus, although various decision-making procedures appropriate to the situation may be instituted.	By the highest authority in the group, with minimal involvement by members; or an inflexible style is imposed.
Cohesion	Facilitated through high levels of inclusion, trust, liking, and support.	Either ignored or used as a means of controlling members, thus promoting rigid conformity.

TABLE 15-3   *continued*

Factor	Effective Groups	Ineffective Groups
Conflict tolerance	High. The reasons for disagreements or conflicts are carefully examined, and the group seeks to resolve them. The group accepts unresolvable basic disagreements and lives with them.	Low. Attempts may be made to ignore, deny, avoid, suppress, or override controversy by premature group action.
Power	Determined by the members' abilities and the information they possess. Power is shared. The issue is how to get the job done.	Determined by position in the group. Obedience to authority is strong. The issue is who controls.
Problem solving	High. Constructive criticism is frequent, frank, relatively comfortable, and oriented toward removing an obstacle to problem solving.	Low. Criticism may be destructive, taking the form of either overt or covert personal attacks. It prevents the group from getting the job done.
Self-evaluation as a group	Frequent. All members participate in evaluation and decisions about how to improve the group's functioning.	Minimal. What little evaluation there is may be done by the highest authority in the group rather than by the membership as a whole.
Creativity	Encouraged. There is room within the group for members to become self-actualized and interpersonally effective.	Discouraged. People are afraid of appearing foolish if they put forth a creative thought.

SOURCE: Psychiatric Nursing (5th ed.) by H. S. Wilson and C. R. Kneisl, 1996, Redwood City, CA: Addison-Wesley Nursing, p. 736.

GROUP DYNAMICS

Every group has its own characteristics and way of functioning. Seven aspects of group dynamics follow.

Commitment

The members of effective groups have a **commitment** (agreement, pledge, or obligation to do something) to the goals and output of the group. Because groups demand time and attention, members must give up some autonomy and self-interest. Inevitably conflicts arise between the interests of individual members and those of the group. However, members who are committed to the group feel close to each other and willingly put themselves out for the group. Some indications of group commitment are shown in the accompanying box.

Leadership Style

Leadership style refers to "the typical ways in which a person takes on the leadership role within a group" (Sampson & Marthas, 1990, p. 186). See Chapter 10.

Indications of Group Commitment

- Members feel a strong sense of belonging.
- Members enjoy each other.
- Members seek each other for counsel and support.
- Members support each other in difficulty.
- Members value the contributions of other members.
- Members are motivated by working in the group and want to do their tasks well.
- Members express good feelings openly and identify positive contributions.
- Members feel that the goals of the group are achievable and important.

Decision-Making Methods

Making sound decisions is essential to effective group functioning. Effective decisions are made when:

1. The group determines which decision method to adopt.

2. The group listens to all the ideas of members.

3. Members feel satisfied with their participation.

4. The expertise of group members is well used.

5. The problem-solving ability of the group is facilitated.

6. The group atmosphere is positive.

7. Time is used well; that is, the discussion focuses on the decision to be made.

8. Members feel committed to the decision and responsible for its implementation.

For additional information about decision making, see Chapter 12.

Three decision-making aids are described by McMurray (1994, pp. 62–65): brainstorming, the nominal group technique, and the Delphi technique. The idea behind **brainstorming** is that the interaction of several people in a group can generate more ideas about a subject than could the individuals by themselves. According to McMurray, there is evidence that brainstorming groups produce more ideas than individuals acting alone. For brainstorming, (1) the individuals in the groups must have a level of trust, (2) there must be a criticism-free atmosphere that allows ideas to flow freely, and (3) all ideas receive initial approval and are critically examined thereafter.

Nominal group technique (NGT) is also an aid to decision making. In this instance the individuals meet as a group, but they write their responses without discussion. The ideas are then collected and open discussion proceeds.

The **Delphi technique** was originally used for technologic forecasting. It has been used for decisions that require more time or need responses from people in disparate locations. The participants maintain their anonymity, which eliminates peer pressure. Data is gathered through interviews or questionnaires in a series of rounds in which an initial question is posed. Once the responses are returned, they are compiled and redistributed. The participants do not know who said what: The comments or ratings are gathered for a compiled listing and are rated through averaging or statistical analysis. With the Delphi technique, agreement is reached as the process continues either by consensus, voting, or mathematical average (McMurray, 1994, p. 64). See Table 15–4 for a comparison of brainstorming, nominal group technique, and the Delphi technique.

Member Behaviors

The degree of input by members into goal setting, decision making, problem solving, group evaluation, and so on, is due in part to the group structure and leadership style, but members, too, have responsibilities for group behavior and participation. Each member participates in a wide range of **roles** (assigned or assumed functions) during group interactions. Individuals may perform different roles during interactions in the same group or may vary roles in different groups. These roles have been categorized as (a) task roles, (b) maintenance or building roles, and (c) self-serving roles.

A *task role* is related to the task of the group. Its purpose is to enhance and coordinate the group's movement toward achievement of its goals. For example, a member may suggest ideas, critically evaluate ideas, help pull ideas together, seek facts, summarize decisions, question group accomplishments, maintain minutes, or stimulate group action.

The *maintenance role* is related to maintaining or building the group's continuity, cohesion, and stability. For example, a person might offer praise and agree with other members, mediate conflicts and disagreements, seek compromise, or promote open communication.

Self-serving roles often present obstacles to effective group functioning. The self-serving role is aimed at satisfying the individual's needs and does not enhance group effectiveness. As an example, a member can act negatively towards other members, express negative points of view, call attention to personal activities, use the group to gain sympathy, or assert authority and manipulate others.

Interaction Patterns

Interaction patterns can be analyzed by using a **sociogram,** a diagram of the flow of verbal communication within a group during a specified period, for example, 5 or 15 minutes. This diagram indicates who speaks to whom and who initiates the remarks. Ideally the interaction patterns of a small group would indicate verbal interaction from all members of the group to all members of the group (Figure 15–1). In reality, not all communication is a two-way

TABLE 15–4 **Comparison of Brainstorming, Nominal Group Technique, and Delphi Technique**

Brainstorming	Nominal Group Technique	Delphi Technique
Group activity, open discussion.	Group activity; initial silent interaction with later discussion.	No personal interaction; input is anonymous.
Can be conducted in one session.	Can be conducted in one session.	Takes place over three to four rounds of data collection and analysis.
Relaxed, noncritical atmosphere is essential.	Non-critical atmosphere desirable in discussion stage.	No interaction; responses are anonymous.
Largely unstructured format.	Structured format; sequential steps or stages to be followed.	Structured format; requires "rounds" of interaction.
Easy to conduct; requires little preparation or understanding.	Easy to conduct; requires little preparation or understanding.	Requires coordination of responses, can be time-consuming.
Promotes more ideas than do individuals acting alone.	Promotes more and better quality ideas than does brainstorming.	Promotes many high-quality ideas.
Possible influence of results by peer pressure.	Peer influence likely only in discussion phase.	Little peer pressure noted.

SOURCE: "Three Decision-Making Aids: Brainstorming, Nominal Group and Delphi Technique" by A. R. McMurray, March/April 1994, *Journal of Nursing Staff Development, 10,* 62–65. Used with permission.

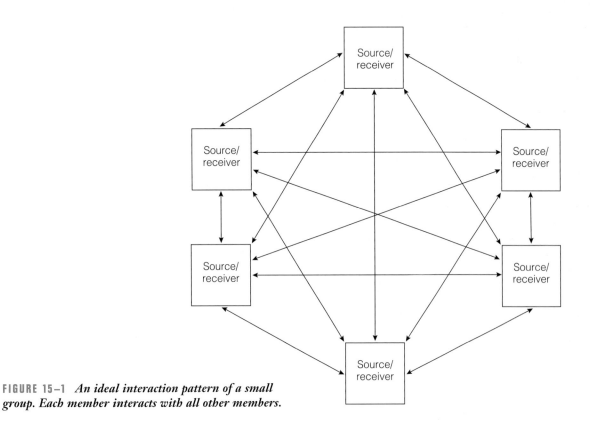

FIGURE 15–1 *An ideal interaction pattern of a small group. Each member interacts with all other members.*

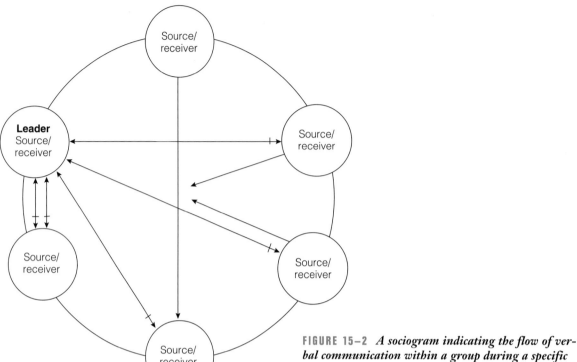

FIGURE 15–2   *A sociogram indicating the flow of verbal communication within a group during a specific period. Note that five questions or comments calling for a response were directed at the leader.*

process. In the sociogram shown in Figure 15–2, the lines with arrowheads at each end indicate that the statement made by one person was responded to by the recipient; a short cross-line drawn near one of the arrowheads indicates who initiated the remark. One-way communication is indicated by lines with an arrowhead at only one end. Remarks made to the group as a whole are indicated by arrows drawn to only the middle of the circle. By using a sociogram, nurses can analyze strengths and weaknesses in a group's interaction patterns. Used in conjunction with member behavior tools, this can offer considerable data about the group's dynamics.

Cohesiveness

Groups that have the characteristic of **cohesiveness** possess a certain group spirit, a sense of being "we," and a common purpose. Groups lacking cohesiveness are unstable and more prone to disintegration. See the accompanying box for some of the attitudes and behaviors that reflect group cohesiveness.

Power

Patterns of behavior in groups are greatly influenced by the force of power. **Power** can be defined as the ability to influence another person in some way or the ability to do something, whether it is to decide the fate of a nation or to decide that a certain change in policy or practice is necessary.

Many people have a negative concept of power, likening it to control, domination, and even coercion of others by muscle and clout. However, power can be viewed as a vital, positive force that moves people toward the attainment of individual or group goals. The overall purpose of power is to encourage cooperation and collaboration in accomplishing a task. For more about power, see Chapter 22.

CONSIDER...

- groups in which you are a participant. What level of commitment do the various group members exhibit? How does the level of commitment exhibited by the individual group members affect the goal attainment of the group?
- the leaders of the various groups in which you are a participant. What are their leadership styles, and what decision-making methods do they use to achieve the group goals? How do the leader's style and decision-making method affect the goal attainment of the group?

Attributes of Group Cohesiveness

Members' Attitudes and Behaviors

- Like each other, trust one another, and are friendly and willing to interact.
- Receive support from the group and praise one another for accomplishments.
- Have similar attitudes and beliefs.
- Are loyal to the groups and defend it against outside criticism.
- Readily accept assigned roles and tasks.
- Influence each other and value being influenced by others.
- Feel satisfied and secure.
- Stay in the group and value group goals.

Group Characteristics

- Goals are valued and are consistent with the goals of individuals.
- Activities are handled by group action.
- Actions are interdependent and cooperative.
- Goals that are difficult to achieve are met by persistent efforts.
- Participation is high.
- Commitment is high.
- Communication is high.
- "We" is frequently heard in discussions.
- Productivity is high.
- Norms are adhered to and protected.

Group Process Skills

- Active listening.
- Focusing discussions on the purpose.
- Checking perceptions of the group.
- Reflecting—the ability to convey the essence of what a group member has said so that others can understand it.
- Clarifying—focusing on key underlying issues and sorting out confusing and conflicting feelings and thinking.
- Summarizing—restating, reflecting, and summarizing major ideas and feelings by pulling important ideas together and establishing a basis for further discussion. Summarize points of agreement and disagreement among group members.
- Facilitating—assisting the members to express their feelings and thoughts openly and actively working to create a climate of openness and acceptance in which members trust one another and therefore engage in a productive exchange of ideas, opinions, and perceptions.
- Interpreting—offering possible explanations.
- Questioning—be careful not to overuse, because members can become frustrated and annoyed with continued questions.
- Confirming—restating a member's basic ideas by emphasizing the facts and encouraging further discussion.
- Encouraging—as a leader, don't agree or disagree with a member's ideas. Use noncommittal words with a positive tone of voice. Examples: "I see …"; "Uh-huh …"; "That's interesting …".

- the interaction patterns demonstrated in groups in which you participate. How do the interaction patterns affect the goal attainment of the group? What strategies might have been used to improve the interaction of the group members?

FACILITATING GROUP DISCUSSION

A group leader can use certain techniques to facilitate group discussion. Smith and Hukill (1994, pp. 8–9) suggest the following:

- Ask open-ended questions to begin discussions and to probe for details from individuals and from the group.
- Encourage questions from group members.
- Respond with positive statements or a summary each time a participant makes a contribution.
- Reinforce participant's contributions by giving them your full attention.
- Do no make negative comments about group members' contributions. Instead, summarize or restate them and ask other team members for their thoughts about the idea.
- Avoid taking sides on issues. Instead, summarize differences of opinion, stress that issues can be

viewed from many different perspectives, and emphasize relative consensus.

- When monitoring small break-out work groups, avoid becoming involved in any of the groups. Participants tend to expect the group leader to intervene, rather than focusing on the task themselves or seeking input from each other.
- Seek equal contribution from all group members.

In order to conduct an effective group process, a leader needs to have certain skills. Some of these skills are listed in the box on page 299.

GROUP PROBLEMS

Problems that occur in groups include monopolizing, conflict, scapegoating, silence and apathy, and transference and countertransference.

Monopolizing

Because most group meetings have time restraints, domination of the discussion by one member seriously deprives others of their chances to participate. A sense of injustice develops, and ultimately members may direct their frustration and anger toward the group leader, who they think should do something to stop the monopolizer's behavior.

There may be several reasons for monopolizing behaviors, including anxiety, a need for attention, recognition, and approval. Whatever the reason, the goal of the leader is to assist the person to moderate his or her participation in the group. Often, compulsive talkers are unaware of their behavior and its effect on others and need help to recognize their behavior and its consequences.

Four strategies for dealing with monopolizing follow:

- *Interrupt simply, directly, and supportively.* This strategy is an initial attempt to .get the person to hear others.
- *Reflect the person's behavior.* This strategy is an attempt to help the person become aware of the monopolizing behavior.
- *Reflect the group's feelings.* This strategy is an attempt to help the person become aware of the effects of his or her behavior on others.
- *Confront the person and/or the group.* This strategy can be directed toward the individual or toward the group to help members realize their own responsibility for the problem.

Conflict

Sampson and Marthas write that conflict is a normal stage in group development (1990, p. 242). Conflict refers to disagreement, impatience, and argument among members. It can be either productive or nonproductive, and group leaders need to distinguish destructive conflict from constructive conflict. Conflict is productive and beneficial when members feel involved, when the issue being discussed is important to them, and when they are working intensively on a problem. Productive conflict contributes to problem solving as long as the goal is clearly understood.

Nonproductive conflict leads the group astray and hinders the achievement of group goals. There are three common reasons for this type of conflict (Bradford, Stock, & Horwitz, 1974, p. 38):

1. The group has been given an impossible task, or the task is not clear. Members are frustrated because they feel unable to meet the demands on them.

2. The main concern of members is to find status in the group and to deal with their personal and individual tasks rather than the group problem.

3. Members are operating from unique, unshared points of view and may have competing loyalties to and conflicting interests in outside groups.

The nurse leader should intervene early rather than later. In some instances, the nonproductive conflict is best avoided or played down rather than confronted.

If the leader decides it is more beneficial for the group to face the issue directly, the leader can employ the following strategies (Sampson and Marthas 1990, pp. 245–246):

- *Interpreting.* The leader explains her or his view of the problem. For example, the leader might say, "I think the group is having trouble making a decision because there are some distinct conflicts among several group members. Before we try to accomplish any other task I think we had better take some time and look at those conflicts."
- *Reflecting.* With this strategy, the leader points out certain behaviors of the members or points out his or her own feelings. To *reflect behavior* the leader may say, "I've noticed that several persons have been very quiet for some time, that others are talking a great deal but usually at cross-purposes, and that as a group we seem to be unable to focus our efforts on anything except disagreeing."

To *reflect feeling* the leader may say, "I'm not sure how anyone else feels, but I'm feeling frustrated and annoyed over the constant bickering. I know we have a job to do, and I'd like to get on with it."

- *Confronting.* With this strategy, the leader calls the group's attention to what she or he perceives is taking place with one or more of the members. For example, the leader may say, "Mrs. Purple, I think you are angry because…, and you seem to feel…. Is that why you are so distressed?" or "I think that Mr. Black and Ms. White are each trying to gain some points in this discussion, but this is not helping us deal with the task at hand. I wonder if you two could either cool it for a while or let us all explore your behavior with you?"

- *Voicing the unmentionable.* Here the leader states a belief or feeling which will be uncomfortable for the listener, for example, "I think you are afraid of losing power on your unit, and that is why you are disagreeing with everything that is being said without listening to the others."

Scapegoating

Scapegoating is a process in which one or two members are singled out and agree, consciously or unconsciously, to be targets for group hostility or advice (Clark, 1994, p. 97). Scapegoating is a convenient method people use to negate any responsibility for what occurs in a group. By scapegoating, individuals can decrease their own anxiety. By also focusing on another's weakness, scapegoaters can minimize their own feelings of ineptitude.

For leaders to deal with scapegoating, they must be alert to its development and be prepared to accept anger when they confront the scapegoaters.

Silence and Apathy

Nonparticipation or **apathy** of one or more group members is sometimes best handled by nonintervention. Sometimes such silences are not a reflection of something in the immediate group setting but rather of some past experience. For example, after expressing an idea previously, this person may have been told, "That was a stupid thing to say." Having been hurt once in a group, such persons feel insecure about their views and are reluctant to express themselves again in groups.

Continued nonparticipation or apathy, however, needs to be dealt with by the leader, after a careful assessment of whether the apathy is a reflection of leadership style, task issues, or interpersonal conflicts.

For apathy reflecting the members' opinions that the task is unimportant, the leader may suggest, "I think there is general boredom with today's task. Do people feel that what we are doing is not really relevant or important?" After members have responded, the leader needs to ask, "What things would you prefer the group to do?"

For apathy related to members' feelings of inadequacy about handling the task or lack of the structure and organization needed for problem solving, the leader may ask, "Are people feeling generally that the group is not up to handling the task we are facing?" or "I think, because we're not really sure of what to do or how to go about dealing with the task facing us, that it may be helpful if we break up the task into smaller parts, decide what the important issues are, and develop a method for dealing with each part."

For apathy based on an interpersonal issue such as anger or fear and expressed by silence, the leader needs to decide whether to let the silence simply pass or intervene. If generally responsive group members suddenly become silent, it is important to note which issue or topic immediately preceded the silence. Sometimes a conflict among a few members has been uncovered or the group has been pushed into discussing a topic considered irrelevant or threatening. In this situation the leader may say, "I am wondering whether people are angry at what I've done," or "Are some of you anxious about bringing up that topic, since it may bring out bad feelings?" For apathy in response to an autocratic leadership style, the leader must implement measures to change the style and assist the group to work through and change their relationship with the leader.

Transference and Countertransference

Transference is the transfer of feelings that were originally evoked by parents or significant others to people in the present setting. An example is a group member who acts toward the leader as she or he would act toward a parent. In addition, members of a group can transfer to others in the group personal feelings of love, guilt, or hate.

When leaders respond to group members because of reactions from earlier relationships, they are engaging in **countertransference.** For example, if a group member reminds a leader of a teacher who was menacing and demanding, the leader is likely to react with anxiety and may become unreasonably fearful. It is therefore important that leaders recognize the possibility of overreaction because of countertransference and that it is not an unusual reaction among nurses, who are highly involved in helping others.

CONSIDER...

- what personal goals may be achieved by a group member who exhibits monopolizing, scapegoating, or apathetic behaviors. How might the leader or other group members intervene to redirect such blocking behaviors?
- the effect of problem behaviors in an individual group on the goals of the organization as a whole. How might such problem behaviors in groups composed of nurses be viewed by non-nurses within an organization? How might this affect the role of nursing in the organization?

TYPES OF HEALTH CARE GROUPS

Much of a nurse's professional life is spent in a wide variety of groups, ranging from dyads to large professional organizations. As a participant in a group, the nurse may be required to fulfill different roles: member or leader, teacher or learner, adviser or advisee, and so on.

Common types of health care groups include task groups, teaching groups, self-help groups, self-awareness/growth groups, therapy groups, work-related social support groups, and professional nursing organizations. There are similarities and differences among the characteristics of these various types of groups and the nurse's role.

Task Groups

The task group is one of the most common types of work-related groups to which nurses belong. Examples are health care planning committees, nursing service committees, nursing team meetings, nursing care conference groups, and hospital staff meetings. The focus of such groups is the completion of a specific task, and the format is defined at the outset by the leader and/or members. The methods used to perform the task vary according to the task to be performed.

The leader of a task group, usually called the *chairperson*, must be accepted by the members as an appropriate leader and therefore should be an expert in the area of task emphasis. The chairperson's role is to identify the specific task, clarify communication, and assist in expressing opinions and offering solutions. *Committee members* are generally selected in terms of their individual functional role and employment status, rather than in terms of their personal characteristics. Member participation is determined by the task. A target date for termination of the group is usually set in advance.

RESEARCH NOTE

Can Groups Change Ineffective Behavioral Patterns?

In one study, researchers used focus group interviews to promote development of a program designed to reduce AIDS-related risk behaviors in minority populations. When performed in a nonthreatening group environment, the focus group interview permits investigation of a number of perceptions regarding the problem. This type of interview reveals attitudes and perceptions that relate to needs. The main advantage of this technique is the spontaneous revelation of thoughts and attitudes.

In this particular study, findings revealed that African-American women who practiced high-risk activities regarding AIDS, especially those who were homeless,

experienced serious environmental restraints that led to feelings of powerlessness. It therefore became evident that health care professionals needed to understand the concerns and stresses of these people and to include strategies which would enhance feelings of control. Implications: The use of focus group interviews can provide direction for nursing practice and for creating an environment that optimizes learning and behavior change.

SOURCE: "Focus Group Interview: A Research Technique for Informed Practice" by A. Nyamathi and P. Shuler, Nov. 1990, *Journal of Advanced Nursing, 15*, 1281–1288.

Teaching Groups

The major purpose of teaching groups is to impart information to the participants. Examples of teaching groups include group continuing education and client health care groups. Numerous subjects are often handled via the group teaching format: childbirth techniques, exercise for middle-aged and older adults, and instructions to family members about follow-up care for discharged clients. A nurse who leads a group in which the primary purpose is to teach or learn must be skilled in the teaching-learning process discussed in Chapter 9.

Self-Help Groups

A **self-help group** is a small, voluntary organization composed of individuals who share a similar health, social, or daily living problem (Rollins, 1987, p. 403). These groups are based on the helper-therapy principle: those who help are helped most. A central belief of the self-help movement is that persons who experience a particular social or health problem have an understanding of that condition which those without it do not. Positive aspects of these groups are outlined in the accompanying box.

Self-Awareness/Growth Groups

The purpose of self-awareness/growth groups is to develop or use interpersonal strengths. The overall aim is to improve the person's functioning in the group to which they return, whether job, family, or community. From the beginning, broad goals are usually apparent, for example, to study communication patterns, group process, or problem solving. Because the focus of these groups is interpersonal concerns around current situations, the work of the group is oriented to reality testing with a here-and-now emphasis. Members are responsible for correcting inefficient patterns of relating and communicating with each other. They learn group process through participation and involvement and guided exercises.

Therapy Groups

Therapy groups work toward self-understanding, more satisfactory ways of relating or handling stress, and changing patterns of behavior toward health. Members are referred to as clients or, in some settings, as patients. They are selected by health professionals after extensive selection interviews that consider the pattern of personalities, behaviors,

---

Positive Aspects of Self-Help Groups

- Members can experience almost instant kinship, because the essence of the group is the idea that "you are not alone."

- Members can talk about their feelings and listen to the concerns of others, knowing they all share this experience.

- The group atmosphere is generally one of acceptance, support, encouragement, and caring.

- Many members act as role models for newer members and can inspire them to attempt tasks they might consider impossible.

- The group provides the opportunity for people to help as well as to *be* helped—a critical component in restoring self-esteem.

SOURCE: "Self-Help" by V. J. Gilbey, April 1987, *Canadian Nurse, 83*, p. 25.

---

needs, and identification of group therapy as the treatment of choice. Duration of therapy groups is not usually set. A termination date is usually mutually determined by the therapist and members.

Work-Related Social Support Groups

Many nurses experience some of the high levels of vocational stress, for example, hospice, emergency, and critical care nurses. Social support groups can help reduce stress for such nurses if various types of support are provided to buffer the stress. Group members who know about the work of others can encourage and challenge members to be more creative and enthusiastic about their work and to achieve more. For example, a nurse may help another team member consider alternative strategies for intervention. Members also can share the joys of success and the frustration of failure through active listening without giving advice or making judgments. This type of social support is best given *outside* the work-related support group.

Professional Nursing Organizations

Professional nursing organizations function as groups and through smaller groups composed of organization members to promote quality health care for all and support the needs of nurses. Professional nursing organizations can serve as task groups, teaching groups, self-help groups, and support groups. The effectiveness of professional nursing organizations is related to the commitment and effectiveness of their members.

CONSIDER . . .

- the various health care groups in your practice setting. Identify specific task groups, teaching groups, self-help groups, self-awareness groups, therapy groups, and work-related groups in your practice setting. What are the purposes of these various groups? In what way are nurses actively involved in these groups? If nurses are not involved in the various groups, how might the lack of their participation affect the perception of professional nursing? How might nurses become involved in these groups?

- the various health care groups in your community. Identify specific task groups, teaching groups, self-help groups, self-awareness groups, therapy groups, and work-related groups in your community. What are the purposes of these various groups? In what way are nurses actively involved in these groups? If nurses are not involved in the various groups, how might that affect the perception of professional nursing? How might nurses become involved in these groups?

- the various professional nursing organizations in your community. How effective are these organizations in promoting quality health care for the community?

SUMMARY

Groups can be classified as primary or secondary, according to their structure or their type of interaction. Groups can assume any one or more of eight functions:

READINGS FOR ENRICHMENT

Abraham, I. L., Niles, S. A., Thiel, B. P., Siarkowski, K. I., & Cowling, W. R. III. (1991, Sept.). Therapeutic group work with depressed elderly. *Nursing Clinics of North America, 26,* 635–650.

This article focuses on therapeutic group work for depressed older adults. Group work with older adults requires adaptations of the general principles of group interventions and additional leadership characteristics described in the article. In the study, researchers adapted seven principles to address cognitive errors predominant among older adults: overgeneralizing, "awfulizing," exaggerating self-importance, placing excessive demands on others, mind reading, self-blame and unrealistic expectations. The authors also explain focused visual imagery.

Davidhizar, R., & Bowen, M. (1991, Dec.). Understanding people in groups. *Today's OR Nurse, 13,* 34–36.

Davidhizar describes three behaviors of group members that facilitate accomplishing group tasks: encouraging or supporting others, negotiating or compromising, and actively contributing to group problem solving or task completion. The author also discusses eight behaviors that block group work: personal preoccupation, misdirected communication, monopolization, belligerent and hostile attitude, pseudo-intellectualization, reminiscence, delayed response, and

overly agreeable opinions. Guidelines for intervention follow the discussion of the blocking behaviors.

Davis, L. L., & Cox, R. P. (1994, Jan./Feb.). Looking through the constructivist lens: The art of creating nursing work groups. *Journal of Professional Nursing, 10,* 38–46.

Davis and Cox provide an overview of group work through a social constructivist perspective. Constructivist-based approaches to groups promote consensus, cohesion, and cooperation in nursing work groups. Social constructivism supports the belief that what is known, thought, or perceived is primarily a social invention achieved through social interaction and discourse with others.

Constructivist perspectives provide individuals with the freedom to consider ideas that can be discussed and changed rather than unchangeable truths.

This article provides examples of constructivist-based suggestions for managers and nursing groups. This approach contrasts with linear patterns of communication, in which, for example, groups are appointed, tasks are assigned, and expectations are established. The employment of constructivism by nurse managers is thought to improve decision making and group outcomes. New solutions to problems are created by the group members and nurse managers working together.

socialization, support, task completion, camaraderie, information, normative function, empowerment, and governance. They can also be described according to their formality, that is, as formal, semiformal, or informal.

According to Clark (1994) groups develop in three stages: orientation, working, and termination. Tuckman and Jensen (1977) describe six stages: orientation, forming, storming, norming, performing, and terminating. Effective groups produce outstanding results, succeed in spite of difficulties, and have members who feel responsible for the output of the group.

Group dynamics (group process) are forces in the group situation that determine the behavior of the group and its members. Factors in group dynamics include commitment, leadership style, decision-making methods, member behavior, interaction patterns, cohesiveness, and power. Three decision-making aids are brainstorming, the nominal group technique, and the Delphi technique. Interaction patterns within a group can be assessed through the use of sociograms. Cohesive groups possess a common purpose and a group spirit. Groups lacking in cohesiveness are prone to disintegration.

Group discussion can be facilitated in eight ways, including asking open-ended questions and seeking equal contributions from all group members. Group leaders need certain skills to conduct an effective group process. A number of group problems commonly occur: monopolizing, conflict, scapegoating, silence and apathy, and transference and countertransference.

Nurses often serve as members of task groups, teaching groups, self-help groups, self-awareness groups, work-related social support groups, and professional nursing organizations.

SELECTED REFERENCES

Anderson, L. K. (1993, Sept.). Teams: Group process, success, and barriers. *Journal of Nursing Administration, 23*, 15–19.

Benne, K. D., & Sheats, P. (1974). Functional roles of group members. In L. P. Bradford (Ed.), *Group development*. La Jolla, CA: University Associates.

Bradford, L. P. (Ed.). (1974). *Group development*. La Jolla, CA: University Associates.

Bradford, L. P., Stock, D., & Horwitz, M. (1974). How to diagnose group problems. In L. P. Bradford (Ed.), *Group development*. La Jolla, CA: University Associates.

Burnside, I. (1994, Jan.). Group work with older persons. *Journal of Gerontological Nursing, 20*, 43–45.

Clark, C. C. (1994). *The Nurse as Group Leader* (3rd ed.). New York: Springer.

Corbin, D. E. (1983, May/June). Self-help groups: What the health educator should know. *Health Values, 7*, 10–14.

Davis, L. L., & Cox, R. P. (1994, Jan./Feb.). Looking through the constructivist lens: The art of creating nursing work groups. *Journal of Professional Nursing, 10*, 38–46.

Dawn, A. L. (1993, Nov.). Cohesion vs. collusion: Maintaining group direction. *Nursing Management, 24*, 90–91.

Farkas, M. (1990). Utilizing the nursing process in the development of a medication group on an inpatient psychiatric unit. *Perspectives in Psychiatric Care, 26*(3), 12–17.

Fisher, D. W. (1985, Jan.). Guidelines to effective group functioning. *Point View, 22*, 6–8.

Gilby, V. J. (1987, April). Self-help. *Canadian Nurse, 83*, 23, 25.

Jensen, D. B. (1993, March). Interpretation of group behavior. *Nursing Management, 24*, 49–50, 52–54.

McCann, G. (1993, Dec.). Relatives support groups in a special hospital: An evaluation study. *Journal of Advanced Nursing, 18*, 1883–1888.

McMurray, A. R. (1994, March/April). Three decision-making aids: Brainstorming, nominal group and Delphi technique. *Journal of Nursing Staff Development, 10*, 62–65.

Miller, D. (1991, Dec.). Group dynamics: Handling subgroups. *Nursing Management, 22*, 33–35.

Nyamathi, A., & Shuler, P. (1990, Nov.). Focus group interview: A research technique for informed nursing practice. *Journal of Advanced Nursing, 15*, 1281–1288.

Rollins, J. A. (1987, Nov./Dec.). Self-help groups for parents. *Pediatric Nursing, 13*, 403–409.

Sampson, E. E., & Marthas, M. S. (1990). *Group process for the health professions* (3rd ed.). New York: Delmar.

Smith, G. B., & Hukill, E. (1994, July). Quality work improvement groups: From paper to reality. *Journal of Nursing Care Quality, 8*, 1–12.

Tuckman, B. W., & Jensen, M. A. (1977). Stages of small group development revisited. *Group and Organization Studies, 2*, 419–427.

Wilson, H. S., & Kneisl, C. R. (1996). *Psychiatric nursing* (5th ed.). Redwood City, CA: Addison-Wesley Nursing.

UNIT

4

Elements of Professional Practice

CHAPTERS

16

CHAPTER

Promoting Health of Individuals and Families

by Suzanne Phillips and Sandra Lobar

OBJECTIVES

- Differentiate theoretical frameworks as they apply to the health promotion of individuals and families across the life span.

- Identify essential data required by the nurse to plan health promotion activities for individuals and families.

- Discuss factors that impact the development, implementation, and evaluation of health promotion plans for individuals and families.

"The essence of humanness is not only to exist but to experience growth toward increasing richness and complexity throughout the life span. Such growth presupposes a life style that is health producing and energy generating."

—Nola Pender, 1987

Recent societal changes have significantly impacted the health promotion role of the professional nurse.

- The health care delivery system has undergone a dramatic increase in the number of managed care corporations that profit by keeping individuals healthy and out of acute and chronic care institutions. Many of these individuals and their families are increasingly aware of the importance of healthy life-styles in preventing illnesses and are actively seeking sources of health promotion care within their communities.

- Societal changes have impacted both nursing education and nursing services. Current nursing education increasingly is emphasizing the acquisition of knowledge and skills in promoting health across the life span. Educational institutions are also supporting nurse researchers in developing and empirically testing theories that describe and explain health behaviors as well as various interventions and strategies used in health promotion (see Chapter 8).

- In nursing services, demand for nurses in primary and community settings is increasing. Nurses are interacting with individuals and families as clients in maintaining health through anticipatory guidance, counseling, and education; using illness prevention interventions through immunizations and screenings; and providing leadership in health protection programs, such as sports, playground, and vehicle safety.

- A discussion of the theoretical bases of wellness, health promotion, health prevention and health protection, and the role of the nurse can be found in Chapters 3 and 8. This chapter focuses on health promotion assessment tools and intervention strategies.

PERSPECTIVES OF INDIVIDUALS AND FAMILIES

Concept of Individuality

Each individual is a unique human being with a different genetic makeup, life experiences, and environmental interactions. Dimensions of individuality include the person's total character, self-identity, and perceptions. The person's *total character* encompasses behaviors, emotional state, attitudes, values, motives, abilities, habits, and appearances. The person's *self-identity* encompasses perception of self as a separate and distinct entity alone and in interactions with others. The person's *perceptions* encompass the way the person interprets the environment or situation, directly affecting how the person thinks, feels, and acts in any given situation.

When providing health promotion care, nurses need to focus on the client within both a total care and an individualized care context. In the total care context, the nurse considers all the principles and areas that apply when taking care of any client of that age and condition. In the individualized care context, the nurse becomes acquainted with the client as an individual, referring to the total care principles and using those principles that apply to this person at this time. For example, a nurse who is advising the mother of a preschooler understands that the child's desire to explore his world is a developmental stage that all preschoolers experience. However, the preschooler diagnosed with attention deficit disorder with hyperactivity who is interacting with his environment may have an increased risk of accidents and injuries due to his impulsivity and poor self-control.

Roles and Functions of the Family

The **family** is a basic unit of society. There has been a resurgence of interest in the family unit and its impact on the health, values, and productivity of individual family members. In the nursing profession, this interest in the family as a unit has been expressed by the emergence of **family-centered nursing:** nursing that considers the health of the family as a unit in addition to the health of individual family members.

As the structure of the family has become more diverse, it has been necessary to define the family more broadly to encompass the wide variety of family forms seen in today's society. See types of families next in this chapter.

To provide flexibility in the study of families, Mallinger (1989, p. 26) defines a family as "composed of one or more individuals closely related by blood, marriage, or friendship." A family of parents and their offspring is known as the **nuclear family.**

The relatives of nuclear families, such as grandparents or aunts and uncles, comprise the **extended family.** In some families, members of the extended family live with the nuclear family. Although members of the extended family may live in different areas, they are a frequent source of support and companionship for the family.

The family's major roles are to protect and socialize its members. Among the many functions it serves, of prime importance is the role the family plays in providing emotional support and security to its members through love, acceptance, concern, and nurturing. This affective (emotional) component holds families together, gives family members a sense of belonging, and develops a sense of kinship.

In addition to providing an emotionally safe environment for members to thrive and grow, the family is also a basic unit of physical protection and safety. This is accomplished by meeting the basic needs of its members: food, clothing, and shelter. Provision of a physically safe environment requires knowledge, skills, and economic resources.

In modern society, the economic resources needed by the family are secured by adult members through employment or government programs. The family also protects the physical health of its members by providing adequate nutrition and health care services. Nutritional and life-style practices of the family not only influence the health of family members but also directly affect the developing health attitudes and life-style practices of the children.

In addition to providing an environment conducive to physical growth and health, the family creates an atmosphere that influences the cognitive and the psychosocial growth of its members. Children and adults in healthy, functional families receive support, understanding, and encouragement as they progress through predictable developmental stages, as they move in or out of the family unit, and as they establish new family units. In families where members are physically and emotionally nurtured, individuals are challenged to achieve their potential in the family unit. As individual needs are met, family members are able to reach out to others in the family and the community, and to society.

The family is a major educator of its members. Parents are often called a child's first teachers. This early learning plays an influential part in the development of a child's attitudes about family, education, health, work, and recreation. These attitudes persist throughout their lives. In addition, families play a major role in the transmission of religious, cultural, and societal values. As the family socializes its new members to the expectations of home, community, and society, it provides a place of warmth, acceptance, and nurturing that insulates its members from the demands of society.

Families from different cultures are an integral part of North America's rich heritage. Each family has values and beliefs (*cultural heritage*) that are unique to their culture of origin and that shape the family's structure, methods of interaction, health care practices, and coping mechanisms. These factors interact to influence the health of families. Families from different cultures may cluster to form mutual support systems and to preserve their heritage; however, this practice may isolate them from the larger society.

Becoming acculturated is a slow, stressful process of learning the language and customs of a new country. Children in cultural clusters often have greater contact with the world around them than adults; through school, children become more proficient in language and more comfortable with new customs and behaviors. Sometimes children create conflict in the family when they bring home new ideas and values. For more information about cultural aspects of health of individuals and families, see Chapter 18.

Types of Families in Today's Society

Traditional Family

The traditional family is viewed as an autonomous unit in which both parents reside in the home with their children, the mother assuming the nurturing role and the father providing the necessary economic resources. In today's society, both males and females are less bound to traditional role patterns. For example, fathers are more likely to be involved with the household chores, their children, and family life.

Two-Career Family

In two-career (or dual career) families, both the husband and wife are employed. They may or may not have children. Two-career families have steadily increased since the 1960s because of increased career opportunities for women, a desire to increase their standard of living, and economic necessity. Finding quality, affordable child care is one of the greatest stresses faced by working parents.

Single-Parent Family

Today it is estimated that over 50% of North American children live in a single-parent home. There are many reasons for single parenthood, including death of a spouse, separation, divorce, birth of a child to an unmarried woman, or adoption of a child by a single man or woman. Nearly 90% of single parent families are headed by a female. The stresses of single parenthood are many: child care concerns, adequate financial resources, role overload and fatigue in managing daily tasks, and social isolation.

Adolescent Family

A growing proportion of infants are born each year to adolescent parents, especially those of minority racial or ethnic groups. These young parents are developmentally, physically, emotionally, and financially ill prepared to undertake the responsibility of parenthood. Adolescent pregnancies frequently interrupt or stop formal education. Children born to an adolescent are often at greater risk for health and social problems, and they have few role models to assist in breaking out of the cycle of poverty.

Blended Family

Existing family units who join together to form new families are known as blended (or reconstituted) families. Families with children living with a birth and nonbirth parent are commonly called *step families*. Family reintegration requires time and effort. Stresses occur as blended families get acquainted with each other, respect differences, and establish new patterns of behavior.

Cohabiting Family

Cohabiting (or communal) families consist of unrelated individuals or families who live under one roof. Reasons for cohabiting may be a need for companionship, a desire to achieve a sense of family, testing a relationship or commitment, or sharing expenses and household management. Cohabiting families illustrate the flexibility and creativity of the family unit in adapting to individual challenges and changing societal needs.

Gay and Lesbian Family

A number of homosexual adults in today's society have formed gay and lesbian families based on the same goals of caring and commitment seen in heterosexual relationships. Children raised in these family units develop sex role orientations and behaviors similar to children in the general population. The greater danger to children in these families is the prejudice and ridicule expressed by others in society.

Single Adults Living Alone

Individuals who live by themselves represent a significant portion of today's society. Singles include young self-supporting adults who have recently left the nuclear family as well as the older adults living alone. Older adults find themselves single through divorce, separation, or the death of a spouse. Single adults frequently maintain contacts with other family members, such as parents, siblings, adult children, and grandchildren.

APPLYING THEORETICAL FRAMEWORKS

A variety of theoretical frameworks provide the nurse with a holistic overview for health promotion of the individual and families across the life span. Major theoretical frameworks that nurses use in promoting the health of the *individual* are needs theories, developmental stage theories, and systems theories. Major theoretical frameworks that nurses use in promoting the health of the *family* are developmental stage theories, systems theories, and structural-functional theories.

Needs Theories

In needs theories, (e.g., Maslow's hierarchy of needs) human needs are ranked on an ascending scale according to how essential they are for survival. Physiologic needs are most crucial for survival; self-actualization needs (developing one's maximum potential) can be met only after all other needs at each level are met. Throughout their lifetimes, individuals strive to meet needs. A person's perception of a need and his or her response to satisfy a need may be influenced by ethnocultural standards, by external and internal stimuli (e.g., hunger), and by self-determined priorities (e.g., stopping smoking). Positive factors that affect the satisfying of needs are an individual's healthy position on the wellness-illness continuum, the presence of supportive relationships, a good self-concept, and the satisfactory achievement of developmental stages. For example, if an infant achieves the developmental task of learning to trust, then the basic needs of feeling loved and secure are readily resolved.

Knowledge of the theoretical bases of human needs assists nurses in responding therapeutically to a client's behaviors and in understanding themselves and their own responses to needs. Human needs serve as a framework for assessing behaviors, assigning priorities to outcome criteria, and planning nursing interventions. For example, an adult with poor self-esteem would have difficulty in accomplishing self-actualization. Therefore, nursing interventions would focus on increasing the client's self-esteem.

Developmental Stage Theories

Developmental stage theories related to individuals categorize a person's behaviors or tasks into approximate age ranges or in terms that describe the features of an age group. The age ranges of the stages do not take into account individual differences; however, the categories do describe characteristics associated with the majority of individuals at periods when distinctive developmental changes occur and with the specific tasks that must be accomplished. Because human development is highly complex and multifaceted, developmental stage theories describe only one aspect of development, such as cognitive, psychosexual, psychosocial, moral, and faith development. Stage theories emphasize a definite, predictable sequence of development that is orderly and continuous. Each stage is affected by those stages preceding it and affects those stages that follow. For example, an adolescent who is unable to establish a stable sense of personal identity may have difficulty in later developmental stages with adult roles and career aspirations.

Developmental stage theories allow nurses to describe typical behaviors of an individual within a certain age group, explain the significance of those behaviors, predict behaviors that might occur in a given situation, and provide a rationale to control behavioral manifestations. Individuals can be compared with a representative group of people at the same point in time or compared at different points in time. During health promotion care, the nurse's knowledge of stage theories can be utilized in parental and client education, counseling, and anticipatory guidance.

Developmental stage theories view *families* as ever-changing and growing. Crucial, yet predictable, tasks occur at each level or stage of development. Achievement of tasks appropriate at one level is a prerequisite for successfully achieving the tasks expected at the next level. A major task of the family, from a developmental perspective, is to create an environment where the family can master critical developmental tasks. This ensures orderly progression through the stages of the family life cycle.

Systems Theories

Human systems theories assert that the individual is an open system in constant interaction with a changing environment. The human being is a complex system with multiple subsystems. Because individuals are biopsychosocial beings, their physiologic, psychologic, social, and ethnocultural, developmental, and spiritual components can be regarded as systems with hierarchic subsystems. All parts of human systems are interrelated, and the whole system responds to changes in one of its subsystems. This interrelatedness is the basis for nursing's holistic view of individuals. For example, a person under stress may exhibit both physiologic and psychologic symptoms, such as changes in cardiac function and reacting with anger to a work situation.

Open systems function through the quality and quantity of input (information, material, energy coming into the system), throughput (processing of that information, material, energy), and output (information, material, energy given out). Persons interact with the environment by adjusting themselves to it or adjusting it to themselves. Constant input into the system and feedback to it maintains the system in a state of dynamic equilibrium (homeostasis). This premise directs the nurse to look at environmental factors influencing the system and to plan nursing interventions to help the client maintain homeostasis. For example, the individual who is experiencing severe anxiety may be taught a variety of stress management techniques.

Table 16–1 on page 314 summarizes selected theoretical frameworks for individuals. It describes major theory types, the names and author(s), age ranges or stages, general descriptions, strengths and weaknesses, and applications in health promotion.

The family unit can also be viewed as a system. Its members are interdependent, working toward specific purposes and goals. Many families are described as *open systems*, for they are continually interacting and influenced by other systems in the community. Boundaries regulate the input from other systems that interact with the family system; they also regulate output from the family system to the community or to society. Boundaries protect the family from the demands and influences of other systems. Open families are likely to welcome input from without, encouraging individual members to adapt beliefs and practices to meet the changing demands of society. Such families are more likely to seek out health care information and use community resources. These families are adaptable and therefore better prepared to cope with changes in life-style needed to restore, maintain, or promote health.

Family systems also can be described as *closed systems*. Closed families are self-contained units resistant to outside interaction or influence. Such families may be suspicious of others and are content with the status quo. They are less likely to change values and practices; they tend to exert more control over the lives of their members and distrust recommendations made by nonfamily members. It is more difficult for closed family systems to use community resources that may be helpful in dealing with a family health crisis or to incorporate new behaviors that may promote a healthier family. The boundaries of most families, however, are permeable and flexible, regulating input and output according to family needs, values, and developmental stage.

Structural-Functional Theories

The structural functional theory, as the name implies, focuses on family structure and function. The structural component of the theory addresses the membership of the family and the relationships among family members. Intrafamily relationships are complex because of the numerous relationships that exist within the family structure—mother-daughter, brother-sister, husband-wife, and so on. These relationships are constantly evolving as children mature and leave the family nest and adults age and become more dependent on others to meet their daily needs.

The functional aspect of the theory examines the effects of intrafamily relationships on the family system, as well as their effects on other systems. Some of the main functions of the family include developing a sense of family purpose and affiliation, adding and socializing new members, and providing and

distributing care and services to members. A healthy family organizes its members and resources in meeting family goals; it functions in harmony, working toward shared goals.

Nurses generally use a combination of theoretical frameworks in promoting the health of individuals and families. For example, the nurse may provide education for the mother of a toddler who is struggling to accomplish Erikson's (1963) developmental stage of autonomy. Simultaneously, the nurse may also provide guidance for the toddler's family who is undergoing a stressful "transition period" between developmental stages (described by Duvall & Miller, 1985) as their older school-age child becomes an adolescent. Table 16–2 on page 318 summarizes selected theoretical frameworks for families. The table describes the major theory types, the names and author(s), stages, general descriptions, strengths and weaknesses, and applications in health promotion.

CONSIDER . . .

- how the various theoretical frameworks for individuals and families described in Tables 16–1 and 16–2 may apply to your area of nursing practice. Compare and contrast the various theories as they relate specifically to nursing.
- the interrelationship of the various theoretical frameworks. Where are there similarities between the different theories or theory types? Where are there specific differences?
- whether the theorists or their theories support the inclusion of nursing in the provision of health promotion activities for individuals and families.

ASSESSING THE HEALTH OF INDIVIDUALS

A thorough assessment of the individual's health status is basic to health promotion. Components of this assessment are the health history and physical examination, physical fitness assessment, health risk appraisal, life-style assessment, health beliefs review, and life-stress review (Pender, 1987, p. 103). As nurses move toward greater autonomy in providing client care, expanded assessment skills are essential to provide the meaningful data needed for health planning.

TABLE 16-1   Health Promotion: Applying Selected Theoretical Frameworks to Individuals

Theory Type	Theory Name/Author	Age Range	Description
Needs theories	**Hierarchy of needs** Maslow (1970) Kalish (1983)	All ages Five to six levels of needs: from physiologic to self-actualization	Needs motivate the behavior of an individual. Human needs are ranked according to how crucial to survival they are. Needs at one level must be met before needs on next level can be met.
Developmental stage theories	**Developmental tasks** Peck (1968)	Two sequential stages: middle age through old age in adulthood	Developmental tasks focus on adults coming to terms with decreasing physical capacities while maintaining or increasing mental and social capacities.
	Havighurst (1972)	Six sequential stages: infancy/childhood through adulthood	Describes developmental tasks that individuals learn or strive to accomplish during their lifetimes.
	Psychosexual development Freud (1962)	Five sequential stages: infancy through adolescence and beyond	Psychosexual development is a lifelong struggle between instinctual pleasures (id), reality expectations (ego), and moral values (superego).
	Psychosocial development Sullivan (1953)	Seven sequential stages: infancy through adulthood	Focuses on the self-concept as key to development, emphasizing reduction of tension as pivotal in personality development.
	Erikson (1963, 1976)	Eight sequential stages: infancy through adulthood	Psychosocial development is an interactive process in which the individual struggles between opposing results (crises).
	Gould (1972)	Seven sequential stages: adolescence through adulthood	Central theme is transformation. The path to adult maturity is the acceptance of each stage as a natural progression of life.
	Cognitive development Piaget (1963)	Four sequential stages: infancy/toddler through adolescence and beyond	Cognitive development is a result of the individual's interaction with the environment together with maturation.
	Moral development Kohlberg (1976)	Seven sequential stages in three levels: infancy/toddler through adulthood	Identifies morality with justice and the relationships of liberty, equality, and reciprocity and contracts between persons. Adults may not reach later stages.

Strengths/Limitations of Theory	Nursing Applications for Health Promotion
Strengths. Provides a framework for prioritizing human needs and supporting individuals in moving toward higher levels. Acknowledges role of motivation. *Limitations.* Simplistic. Does not explain complex human interactions, behaviors, and responses that may cross levels.	Provides the nurse with a knowledge of human needs to help individuals develop and grow. For example, the nurse can assist clients in moving toward self-actualization by helping them find meaning in and control during a stressful event in their life.
Strengths. Acknowledges opposing psychosocial responses to developmental tasks in adulthood. Emphasizes healthy aspects of aging. *Limitations.* Individual and ethnocultural differences are not addressed.	Provides nurses with guidelines for an adult's positive resolution of tasks. For example, to accomplish "ego differentiation," the nurse can assist the retired adult in replacing work with other satisfying activities.
Strengths. Provides a framework for predicting readiness and evaluating an individual's accomplishments. *Limitations.* Some adolescent tasks may be unrealistic in view of the extended adolescence found in today's society.	Individuals have "teachable moments" during which they have increased readiness to learn a task. For example, a new mother is receptive to learning about infant care.
Strengths. Establishes the role of childhood experiences and the environment in personality development. *Limitations.* Theory was built on study of maladjusted patients and focuses on single motivating factor: satisfying sexual and aggressive needs. Suggests females are inferior (i.e., narcissistic, passive).	Parental education: Meet child's pleasure-focused needs. For example, toilet training should be an experience that provides the toddler with satisfaction and a sense of control, fostering a creative and productive personality.
Strengths. Recognizes the importance of the environment—social approval and disapproval—in the formation of the self-concept. Has some predictive value. *Limitations.* Does not recognize the maturation process.	Parental education: Provide social experiences that foster and maintain a positive self-concept. For example, at all ages discipline should target the misbehavior, not the child.
Strengths. Emphasizes a healthy personality but makes allowances for development to move in either direction. *Limitations.* Individual and ethnocultural differences in development are not addressed.	Parental education: Provide experiences that assist children in a positive resolution of a developmental crisis. For example, to promote "industry," school-age children should be given opportunities to create and complete short projects.
Strengths. Expands on adult development, providing a basis for assessing adults at specific ages. *Limitations.* Individual and ethnocultural differences are not addressed.	Provides nurses with a framework in assessing the adult. For example, adults aged 35–43 may be going through a period of self-reflection, questioning values and realizing that time is finite.
Strengths. Some theoretical predictions have been tested through research. *Limitations.* Ignores motivation and its impact on behavior. Theory tends to underestimate a preschooler's abilities and overestimate adolescent abilities. Individual differences are not addressed.	Parental education. Provide experiences that foster a child's cognitive abilities. For example, play "peek-a-boo" with an infant to encourage development of object permanence.
Strengths. Allows for variations in moral thinking. *Limitations.* Studies have not supported invariable sequential development of moral reasoning. Discrepancies occur between what individuals say and their actual behavior. Theory is based on studies of young males, limiting its predictive power to others.	Parental education: Emphasize rights and needs of others, and set realistic standards of right and wrong. Individuals at all ages need opportunities to explore the elements of moral/ethical problems and the possible solutions.

TABLE 16–1   **Health Promotion: Individuals** *continued*

Theory Type	Theory Name/Author	Age Range	Description
	Moral development *continued* Gilligan (1982)	Three sequential stages: no age range identified	Goal of moral maturity is a blending of perspectives on the ethic of care (based on nonviolence, typically female) and ethic of justice (based on fairness, typically male).
	Faith development Aden (1976)	Eight sequential stages: infancy through adulthood	Faith is a gift from a higher power. Faith is initially manifested as trust in caregivers and finally as acceptance in decline of one's physical abilities.
	Westerhoff and Willimon (1980)	Four sequential stages: infancy/early adolescence through adulthood/old age	Faith is a way of being and behaving. Faith evolves from the experienced faith of infancy and childhood which is guided by significant persons to an owned faith internalized in adulthood.
	Fowler (1981)	Eight sequential stages: infancy through adulthood	Faith is universal, a way of viewing life in holistic images (inner representations) and an individual's actions and feelings about the meaning of life and relationships.
Systems theory	**General systems theory:** von Bertalanffy (1968) Nursing theorists oriented toward systems theory: Johnson (1980); King (1981); Roy and Andrews (1991); Orem (1995); Neuman (1995)	All ages	Individuals are open systems, constantly interacting with a dynamic changing environment. Input and feedback into the system assist in maintaining a state of dynamic equilibrium or homeostasis.

Health History and Physical Examination

The health history and physical examination provide a means for detecting any existing problems. The age of the individual must be considered when collecting data. For example, an environmental safety assessment and immunization history must be appropriate to the person's age. A nutritional assessment is an important part of the health history. The nurse must consider both age and body build of the client when gathering information on dietary patterns.

Physical Fitness Assessment

During an evaluation of physical fitness, the nurse assesses several components of the body's physical functioning: muscle strength and endurance, joint flexibility, body composition, and cardiovascular endurance. Specific guidelines for obtaining measurements and the optimal values for men, women, and children can be found in physical fitness texts.

Strengths/Limitations of Theory	Nursing Applications for Health Promotion
Strengths. Provides an explanation as to why women typically score lower on moral development scales which have a male emphasis of individualism and autonomy. *Limitations.* Theory is based on studies of adult women, limiting its predictive value in men and children.	Provides nurses with an alternative framework for assessing moral reasoning, especially for women who tend to be more concerned with the concepts of caring and responsibility.
Strengths. Congruent with other developmental stage theorists, such as Erikson and Piaget. *Limitations.* Research studies based on this theoretical framework are limited, decreasing its predictability.	Provides nurse with a theoretical basis for assessing and intervening. For example, for the individual who is under great physical or emotional stress, faith—in whatever source of a higher authority—provides strength.
Strengths. Provides a framework for assessment of faith development in individuals. *Limitations.* Theory was based largely on Westerhoff's own interpretation of his life experiences, reducing predictability to other individuals.	See nursing application for Aden.
Strengths. Provides a useful framework in describing an individual's faith development in the past, present and future. *Limitations.* Subjects studied were not randomized, decreasing predictive power of theory. Also, Eastern religious groups were underrepresented in studies.	See nursing application for Aden.
Strengths. Applicable to all ages and all human conditions. *Limitations.* In complex systems, cause-and-effect relationships between subsystems may be difficult to determine. The concept of homeostasis has been challenged; some authors feel that individuals are an ever-changing, ever-growing system.	Provides a framework for the nurse to identify environmental factors that may influence a client's system(s) as well as looking at ways the client handles changing situations in the internal and external environments.

Muscle Strength and Endurance

A common test for muscle strength and endurance is performing *sit-ups with knees bent* (bent-knee sit-ups) for 1 to 2 minutes. The number of sit-ups performed during that time is compared to standardized charts.

Joint Flexibility

Range of motion in joints can be assessed quickly by asking the person to touch the toes several times.

The average touch point is 1 to 3 inches in front of the toes.

Body Composition

Body composition indicates the ratio of body fat to muscle mass and is estimated through girth and skinfold measurements. *Girth measurements* are obtained through measuring the girth of the chest, waist, hips, upper arm (biceps), thigh, calf, and ankle. *Skinfold measurements* are obtained by grasping the skinfold (skin layers and subcutaneous fat) between

TABLE 16–2   Health Promotion: Applying Selected Theoretical Frameworks to Families

Theory Type	Theory Name/Author	Age Range	Description
Developmental stage theories	**Traditional families** Duvall and Miller (1985) Carter and McGoldrick (1989) Friedman (1992)	From between families to later years: eight, six, and nine stages, respectively	Describes family developmental tasks that are to be accomplished in each stage. Transitions to the next stage can be a time of stress. Successful completion of a transition leads to growth and creativity.
	Single families Hill (1986)	Similar to two-parent families	Tasks differ in the number, timing, and length of transitions and in support, childrearing, companionship, and gender role modeling.
	Divorced families Ahrons and Rodgers (1987) Peck and Manocharian (1989)	Decision to divorce through post divorce	Divorce is an interruption and disruption of the traditional family life cycle, compounding the complexity of developmental tasks.
	Step-parent families Mills (1984)	Entering relationship through re-marriage	Remarriage is a disruptive transitional process, impeding the family's movement through and completion of developmental tasks.
	Adoptive families Hajal and Rosenberg (1991) Reitz and Watson (1992)	Decision to adopt through post adoption	Developmental tasks differ in the timing and length of transitions and the amount of societal support.
Systems theories	Kanto and Lehr (1975) McCubbin and Dahl (1985) Nursing theorists oriented toward family systems: Fawsett (1975); King (1981); Roy and Andrews (1991); Orem (1995); Neuman (1995)	All ages	The family is viewed as a social system with boundaries and self-regulatory mechanisms, interacting with a variety of subsystems and macrosystems within the environment.
Structural-functional theories	Parsons and Bales (1955) Leslie and Korman (1989)	All ages	The family consists of a social system with members who have specific roles and functions. The theory focuses on the inter-relatedness, interdependence and integration between the family structure, family functioning, and wider society.

Strengths/Limitations of Theory	Nursing Application for Health Promotion
Strengths. Addresses both changes within the family and changes in the family as a social group over its life history. Anticipates potential stresses that normally accompany transitions to various stages. *Limitations*. Not easily applied to nontraditional family units, such as divorced or step families.	Assists nurses in anticipatory guidance and educational strategies. For example, the nurse can support child-bearing family with anticipatory guidance strategies for integrating a new baby into the existing family unit.
Strengths. Acknowledges the differences that occur in family developmental tasks when the second parent is absent. *Limitations*. Reasons for single parenting (death/divorce of a parent) may influence developmental tasks.	Assists nurses in providing guidance for managing stressful family transitions. For example, the nurse can refer a family to an association provides male and female role models for children.
Strengths. Acknowledges the impact of divorce on the whole family. Has some predictability. *Limitations*. Limited to families coping with divorce.	The nurse can provide parental education on how children of different ages are affected by a divorce.
Strengths. Acknowledges the impact of remarriage on the whole family. Has some predictability. *Limitations*. Limited to step families.	For a mother who is considering remarriage, the nurse can provide anticipatory guidance and intervention strategies for children's typical reactions.
Strengths. Acknowledges the impact of adoption on the whole family. Has some predictability. *Limitations*. Tasks differ between an infant and older child adoption.	Assists nurses in providing parental education and anticipatory guidance for new adoptive parents.
Strengths. Applicable for the family in normal everyday life as well as family dysfunction and pathology. Useful for families of varying structures and various stages of the life cycle. *Limitations*. More difficult to determine cause-and-effect relationships. Some authors have suggested that families are not homeostatic systems but rayher ever-changing and ever-adapting systems.	The nurse may be able to effect change in a family by identifying and working through several subsystems and macrosystems. For example, a repeat pregnancy in an adolescent may be avoided by utilizing peer group counseling, engaging family relatives for support, and referring the teen to a health care system clinic for contraception.
Strengths. Considers interplay within the family as well as the larger social system, such as the school and workplace. Provides a comprehensive perspective for assessing the family. *Limitations*. Strong emphasis on family stability and maintaining status quo.	The nurse can utilize the structural-functional theoretical framework to assess dual career families in their management of combining work with family roles and responsibilities.

the thumb and forefinger and measuring the skin-fold with special calipers.

Cardiovascular Functioning

One test for cardiovascular functioning is the *step test*. Individuals step up and down on a 17-inch step for 3 minutes at a prescribed rate. After the test, the client sits in a chair while the nurse assesses the pulse rate at several determined intervals.

Life-Style Assessment

Life-style assessment focuses on the personal life-style and habits of the client as they affect health. Categories of life-style generally assessed are physical activity, nutritional practices, stress management, and such habits as smoking, alcohol consumption, and drug use. Other categories may be included. The goals of life-style assessment tools are to provide an opportunity for clients to assess the

---

Circle the category that most closely answers the question.

(Rarely, Sometimes, Very Often)

1. I am conscious of the ingredients of the food I eat and their effect on me. R, S, VO
2. I avoid overeating and abusing alcohol, caffeine, nicotine, and other drugs. R, S, VO
3. I minimize my intake of refined carbohydrates and fats. R, S, VO
4. My diet contains adequate amounts of vitamins, minerals, and fiber. R, S, VO
5. I am free from physical symptoms. R, S, VO
6. I get aerobic cardiovascular exercise. R, S, VO (Very Often is at least 12–20 minutes 5 times per week vigorously running, swimming, or bike riding)
7. I practice yoga or some other form of limbering/stretching exercise. R, S, VO
8. I nurture myself. R, S, VO (Nurturing means pleasuring and taking care of oneself, for example, massages, long walks, buying presents for self, "doing nothing," sleeping late without feeling guilty, etc.)
9. I pay attention to changes occurring in my life and am aware of them as stress factors. R, S, VO (See Life-Change Index—a score of over 300 is considered very stressful)
10. I practice regular relaxation. R, S, VO (Suggested 20 minutes a day "centering" or "letting go" of thoughts, worries, etc.)
11. I am without excess muscle tension. R, S, VO
12. My hands are warm and dry. R, S, VO
13. I am both productive and happy. R, S, VO
14. I constructively express my emotions and creativity.   R, S, VO
15. I feel a sense of purpose in life and my life has meaning and direction.   R, S, VO
16. I believe I am fully responsible for my wellness or illness. R, S, VO

Using your answers at the left to guide you, you can synthesize a graphic picture of your wellness. Each numbered pie-shaped segment of the circle below corresponds to the same numbered question on the preceding page. (They are divided into quarters representing four major dimensions of wellness.) Color in an amount of each segment corresponding to your answer to the question with the same number. The inner broken circle corresponds to "rarely," the next one to "sometimes," and third to "very often." You don't need to restrict yourself to these categories, however, and can fill in any amount in between. You may use different colors for each section if you like.

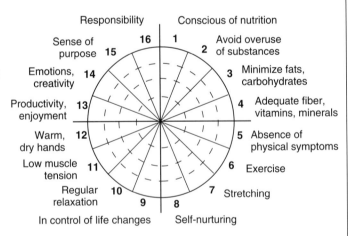

Now look at the shape of your index. Is it lopsided or balanced? This should provide beginning suggestions for improving your lifestyle and health habits.

FIGURE 16–1 *Wellness Index.*

Source: Reprinted from *Wellness Workbook* ©1981, 1988 by John W. Travis, M.D. and Regina Sara Ryan with permission of Ten Speed Press, Berkeley, CA.

impact of their present life-style on their health and to provide a basis for decisions related to desired behavior and life-style change.

Several tools are available to assess life-style. These instruments are most appropriate for the adolescent or adult; however, studies have shown that there is a direct relationship between health behaviors of adult parents and those of their children (Blecke, 1990, p. 284; Gillis, 1994, p. 13). See Appendix A. Ryan and Travis (1981) have developed an assessment form called the Wellness Index. This tool may be used for initial assessments when client time is limited. See Figure 16–1.

Health Risk Appraisal

A **health risk appraisal (HRA)** or *health hazard appraisal (HHA)* is an assessment and educational tool that indicates a client's risk for disease or injury over the next 10 years by comparing the client's risk with the mortality risk of the corresponding age, sex, and racial group. The client's health behavior and demographic data are compared to behaviors of and data about a large national sample. The principle behind risk appraisal is that each person, as a member of a specific group, faces certain quantifiable health hazards and that average risks are applicable to a client if the health professional knows the client's characteristics and the mortality of a large group of cohorts with similar characteristics (Pender, 1996, p. 123). The objectives of most HRAs are twofold:

1. To assess risk factors that may lead to health problems. A **risk factor** is a phenomenon (e.g., age or life-style behavior) that increases a person's chance of acquiring a specific disease such as cancer. The concept of at-risk aggregate is increasingly being used in community nursing practice. An *at-risk aggregate* is a subgroup within the community or population that is at greater risk of illness or poor recovery.

2. To change health behaviors that place the client at risk of developing an illness.

Many HRA instruments are available today. Recently, HRAs have begun to reflect a broader approach to health. The new focus is on the assessment of life-style factors and health behaviors. Risk factors may be categorized according to (a) age, (b) genetic factors, (c) biologic characteristics, (d) personal health habits, (e) life-style, and (f) environment. Clients cannot control some of the risk factors appraised, such as age, sex, and family history; others, such as blood pressure, stress, and cigarette smoking, can be partially or totally controlled.

Health Care Belief

Clients' health care beliefs need to be clarified, particularly those beliefs that determine how they perceive control of their own health care status.

Locus of control (see Chapter 3) is a measurable concept that can be used to predict which people are most likely to change their behavior. Wallston, Wallston, and DeVellis (1978) have developed two Multi-dimensional Health Locus of Control (MHLC) instruments to assess perceptions of health control. See Figure 16–2 for one such instrument. Assessment of clients' health care beliefs provides the nurse with an indication of how much the clients believe they can influence or control health through personal behaviors.

Researchers have not been able to validate a significant association between a person's health beliefs and behaviors (Muhlencamp, Brown & Sands, 1985, p. 327). Cox developed a measure of motivation called the Health Self-Determination Index (HSDI) for adults (Cox, 1985, p. 178) and children (Cox, Cowell & Marion, 1990, p. 237). She believes that motivation is multidimensional, that is, based on many factors. The process of choosing between behaviors is a primary factor.

Life-Stress Review

There is abundant literature about the impact of stress on mental and physical well-being. A variety of stress-related instruments have been found in the literature. For example, Holmes and Rahe (1967, p. 213) developed a Life-Change Index, a tool that assigns numerical values to life events (e.g., divorce, pregnancy). A similar instrument has been developed for children (Heisel, Ream & Raitz, 1973, p. 119). Studies have shown that a high score is associated with an increased possibility of illness in an individual.

CONSIDER . . .

- the various instruments included in this chapter for the appraisal of the individual's wellness and health risk. What conclusions do you make when you apply these instruments to your own life-style? Is your life-style one that is healthy or one that places you at risk for health alterations?

This questionnaire is designed to determine the way in which different people view certain important health-related issues. Each item is a belief statement with which you may agree or disagree. Beside each statement is a scale that ranges from strongly disagree (1) to strongly agree (6). For each item we would like you to circle the number that represents the extent to which you disagree or agree with the statement. The more strongly you agree with a statement, the higher will be the number you circle. The more strongly you disagree with a statement, the lower will be the number you circle. Please make sure that you answer every item and that you circle *only one* number per item. This is a measure of your personal beliefs; obviously, there are no right or wrong answers.

Please answer these items carefully, but do not spend too much time on any one item. As much as you can, try to respond to each item independently. When making your choice, do not be influenced by your previous choices. It is important that you respond according to your actual beliefs and not according to how you feel you should believe or how you think we want you to believe.

1 = Strongly Disagree;   2 = Moderately Disagree;
3 = Slightly Disagree;   4 = Slightly Agree;
5 = Moderately Agree;   6 = Strongly Agree.

1. If I become sick, I have the power to make myself well again.   1 2 3 4 5 6
2. Often I feel that no matter what I do, if I am going to get sick, I will get sick.   1 2 3 4 5 6
3. If I see an excellent doctor regularly, I am less likely to have health problems.   1 2 3 4 5 6
4. It seems that my health is greatly influenced by accidental happenings.   1 2 3 4 5 6
5. I can only maintain my health by consulting health professionals.   1 2 3 4 5 6
6. I am directly responsible for my health.   1 2 3 4 5 6
7. Other people play a big part in whether I stay healthy or become sick.   1 2 3 4 5 6
8. Whatever goes wrong with my health is my own fault.   1 2 3 4 5 6
9. When I am sick, I just have to let nature run its course.   1 2 3 4 5 6
10. Health professionals keep me healthy.   1 2 3 4 5 6
11. When I stay healthy, I'm just plain lucky.   1 2 3 4 5 6
12. My physical well-being depends on how well I take care of myself.   1 2 3 4 5 6
13. When I feel ill, I know it is because I have not been taking care of myself properly.   1 2 3 4 5 6
14. The type of care I receive from other people is what is responsible for how well I recover from an illness.   1 2 3 4 5 6
15. Even when I take care of myself, it's easy to get sick.   1 2 3 4 5 6
16. When I become ill, it's a matter of fate.   1 2 3 4 5 6
17. I can pretty much stay healthy by taking good care of myself.   1 2 3 4 5 6
18. Following doctor's orders to the letter is the best way for me to stay healthy.   1 2 3 4 5 6

FIGURE 16–2 *Multidimensional health locus of control scale (Form B).*

SOURCE: "Development of Multidimensional Health Locus of Control (MHLC) Scales" by K. A. Wallston, B. S. Wallston, and R. DeVellis, Spring 1978, *Health Education Monographs*, 6, 164–165. Reprinted by permission of John Wiley & Sons, Inc.

ASSESSING THE HEALTH OF FAMILIES

The information gathered during assessment is the basis for planning and delivering nursing care to family members or to the family as a whole. The nurse must consider a number of factors in selecting a family assessment tool or in developing a tool that meets the demands of the families served in a particular practice setting.

A family assessment tool should be holistic, eliciting information about a wide variety of family characteristics, beliefs, and behaviors. The tool should be understandable and acceptable to both the family and the nurse. In other words, the nurse must use terminology comprehensible to a wide range of clients, and the tool should be quickly and easily administered. The instrument should also yield clinically relevant data about the family—information useful in formulating nursing diagnoses and planning nursing interventions that promote the health of families.

Overall Family Assessment

The purpose of family assessment is to determine the level of family functioning, to clarify family interaction patterns, to identify family strengths and weaknesses, and to describe the health status of the family and its individual members.

Important are family living patterns, including communication, child rearing, coping strategies, and health practices. An overall family assessment gives an overview of the family process and helps the nurse identify areas that need further assessment. Nurses carry out a more detailed assessment in specific target areas as they become more acquainted with the family and begin to understand family needs and strengths more fully. In planning interventions, nurses need to focus not only on problems but also on family strengths and resources as part of the nursing care plan. Appendix B lists selected family assessment tools developed by nurses. The box below shows the short form of the Friedman Family Assessment Model.

The **family APGAR** is a screening tool that reveals how family members perceive the level of functioning of the family unit as a whole (Smilk-

stein, 1978) (Figure 16–3 on page 324). Open-ended questions assess family functioning in the areas of adaptation, partnership, growth, affection, and resolve. The nurse then elicits information on family satisfaction with each of the functional components of family functioning. The information gained provides basic data about the level of family functioning and gives the nurse an idea about which areas need more detailed assessment and intervention and about family strengths that can be mobilized in solving other family problems.

Health Appraisal

The *health appraisal* begins with a complete health history. The nurse focuses first on the family unit and then on the individuals in that family. The health history is one of the most effective ways of identifying existing or potential health problems. The history is followed by physical assessment of

---

Friedman Family Assessment Model (Short Form)

Identifying Data
1. Family name
2. Address and phone
3. Family composition
4. Type of family form
5. Cultural (ethnic) background
6. Religious identification
7. Social class status
8. Family's recreational or leisure-time activities

Developmental Stage and History of Family
9. Family's present developmental stage
10. Extent of developmental stage fulfillment
11. Nuclear family history
12. History of family of origin of both parents

Environmental Data
13. Home characteristics
14. Characteristics of neighborhood and larger community
15. Family's geographic mobility
16. Family's associations and transactions with community

17. Family's social support network

Family Structure
18. Communication patterns
19. Power structure
20. Role structure
21. Family values

Family Functions
22. Affective function
23. Socialization function
24. Health care function

Family Coping
25. Short- and long-term familial stressors
26. Family's ability to respond, based on objective appraisal of stress-producing situations
27. Coping strategies utilized
28. Areas/situations where family has achieved mastery
29. Dysfunctional adaptive strategies utilized

SOURCE: Adapted from *Family Assessment: Theory and Practice* (3rd ed.) by M. Friedman, 1992, Norwalk, CT: Appleton & Lange, pp. 409–411. Used with permission.

family members. If further evaluation is indicated, referral is made to the appropriate health care professional. When the focus is on health, the appraisal includes information on life-style behaviors and health beliefs. The nurse uses data from the health appraisal to formulate a health profile. The health profile provides the data necessary to determine wellness or to establish a nursing diagnosis and to plan appropriate nursing interventions to promote optimal health through life-style modification.

Health Beliefs

To promote health, the nurse must understand the health beliefs of individuals and families. Health beliefs may reflect a lack of information or misinformation about health or disease. They may also include folklore and practices from different cultures. Because of the many advances in medicine and health care during the last few decades, many clients have out-dated information about health, illness, treatment, and prevention. The nurse is frequently in a position to give information or correct misconceptions. This function is an important component of the nursing care plan. For additional information on health beliefs, see Chapter 3.

Family Communication Patterns

The effectiveness of family communication determines its ability to function as a cooperative, growth-producing unit. Messages are constantly being communicated among family members, both verbally and nonverbally. The information transmitted influences how members work together, fulfill their assigned roles in the family, incorporate family values, and develop skills to function in society. **Intrafamily communication** plays a significant role in the development of self-esteem, which is necessary for the growth of personality.

Families who communicate effectively transmit messages clearly. Members are free to express their feelings without fear of jeopardizing their standing in the family. Family members support one another and have the ability to listen, empathize, and reach out to one another in times of crisis. When the needs of family members are met, they are more able to reach out to meet the needs of others in society.

When patterns of communication among family members are dysfunctional, messages are often communicated unclearly. Verbal communication may be incongruent with nonverbal messages.

Family APGAR Questionnaire

	Almost always	Some of the time	Hardly ever
I am satisfied that I can turn to my family* for help when something is troubling me.	_____	_____	_____
I am satisfied with the way my family talks over things with me and shares problems with me.	_____	_____	_____
I am satisfied that my family accepts and supports my wishes to take on new activities or directions.	_____	_____	_____
I am satisfied with the way my family expresses affection and responds to my emotions, such as anger, sorrow, and love.	_____	_____	_____
I am satisfied with the way my family and I share time together.	_____	_____	_____

Scoring: The patient checks one of three choices, which are scored as follows: "Almost always (2 points). "Some of the time" (1 point), or "Hardly ever" (0) The scores for each of the five questions are then totaled. A score of 7 to 10 suggests a highly functional family. A score of 4 to 6 suggests a moderately dysfunctional family. A score of 0 to 3 suggests a severely dysfunctional family.

*Family is defined as the individual(s) with whom you usually live. If you live alone, your "family" consists of persons with whom you now have the strongest emotional ties.

FIGURE 16–3 *Family APGAR questionnaire.*

SOURCE: *The APGAR Questionnaire. Screening for Social Support: Family, Friends, and Work Associates* by G. Smilkstein, M.D., and W. R. Moore, Professor, May 1988, Department of Family Practice, University of Louisville, Louisville, KY, p. 33. Used with permission.

Power struggles may be evidenced by hostility, anger, or silence. Members may be cautious in expressing their feelings because they cannot predict how others in the family will respond. Many things remain unsaid to preserve family unity and tranquility. When family communication is impaired, the growth of individual members is stunted. Members often turn to other systems to seek personal validation and gratification.

The nurse needs to observe intrafamily communication patterns closely. Nurses should pay special attention to who does the talking for the family, which members are silent, how disagreements are handled, and how well the members listen to one another and encourage the participation of others. Nonverbal communication is important because it gives valuable clues about what people are feeling. For additional information about interaction patterns in groups, see Chapter 15.

Family Coping Mechanisms

Family coping mechanisms are the behaviors families use to deal with stress or changes. Coping mechanisms can be viewed as an active method of problem solving developed to meet life's challenges. The coping mechanisms families and individuals develop reflect their individual resourcefulness. Families may use the same coping patterns rather consistently over time or may change their coping strategies when new demands are made on the family. Coping is a basic function that helps the family meet demands imposed both from within and without. The success of a family depends on how well it copes with the stresses it experiences.

Nurses working with families realize the importance of assessing coping mechanisms as a way of determining how families relate to stress. Also important are the resources available to the family. Internal resources, such as knowledge, skills, effective communication patterns, and a sense of mutuality and purpose within the family, assist in the problem-solving process. In addition, external support systems promote coping and adaptation. These external systems may be extended family, friends, religious affiliations, health care professionals, or social services. The development of social support systems is particularly valuable today, when many families, due to stress, mobility, or poverty, are isolated from resources that would help them cope.

Identifying Families at Risk for Health Problems

Risk assessment helps the nurse identify individuals and groups at higher risk than the general population of developing specific health problems, such as stroke, diabetes, and lung cancer. Risk may be related to genetic factors; for example, persons who have a family history of diabetes are at greater risk of developing diabetes than persons with no family history of diabetes. Certain practices also increase the risk of health problems; for instance, cigarette smokers are at greater risk of developing lung cancer than nonsmokers. Environmental factors, such as air pollution or exposure to toxic chemicals, increase the risk of certain health problems.

Risk reduction among individuals and groups identified as at risk poses a special challenge to health care professionals. The nurse's role is to plan and implement interventions to reduce health risks or to optimize the current health status of those individuals or groups when risks cannot be reduced. The vulnerability of family units to health problems may be based on family developmental level, age of family members, heredity or genetic factors, sociologic factors, and life-style practices. The goal of the nurse is to promote optimal family health and functioning.

Developmental Factors

Newly formed families entering the childbearing and childrearing phases of development experience many changes in roles, responsibilities, and expectations. These changes occur when adult family members are attempting to establish financial security. The many, often-conflicting demands on the young family cause stress and fatigue, which may impede growth of family members and the functioning of the group as a unit.

Adolescent mothers, because of their developmental level and lack of knowledge about parenthood, and single-parent families, because of role overload experienced by the head of the household, are more likely to develop health problems. Moreover, the elderly are at risk of developing degenerative and chronic health problems. Many elderly persons feel a lack of purpose and decreased self-esteem. These feelings in turn reduce their motivation to engage in health-promoting behaviors, such as exercise or community and family involvement.

Hereditary Factors

Persons born into families with a history of certain diseases, such as diabetes or cardiovascular disease, are at greater risk of developing these conditions. A detailed family health history, including genetically transmitted disorders, is crucial to the identification of persons and families at risk. These data are used not only to monitor the health of individual family members but also to recommend modifications in health practices that potentially reduce the risk, minimize the consequences, or postpone the development of genetically related conditions.

Other family units or family members may be at risk of developing a disease by reason of sex or race. Males, for example, are at greater risk of having cardiovascular disease at an earlier age than females, and females are at greater risk of developing osteoporosis, particularly after menopause. While at times it is difficult to separate genetic factors from cultural factors, certain risk factors seem to be related to race. Some diseases are more prevalent among whites than blacks, and vice versa. Sickle-cell anemia, for example, is a hereditary disease limited to blacks of African descent. Native Americans and Asians seem more susceptible to certain diseases and less susceptible to others than the general population.

Life-Style Factors

It has become clear that many diseases are preventable, the effects of some diseases can be minimized, or the onset of disease can be delayed through life-style modification. Cancer, cardiovascular disease, adult-onset diabetes, and tooth decay are among the life-style diseases. The incidence of lung cancer, for example, would be greatly reduced if people stopped smoking. For example, good nutrition, dental hygiene, and use of fluoride—in the water supply, in toothpaste, as a topical application, or as supplements—have been shown to reduce dental decay or caries, one of America's most prevalent health problems.

Other important life-style considerations are exercise, stress management, and rest. Today, health professionals have the knowledge to prevent or minimize the effects of some of the main causes of disease, disability, and death. The challenge is to disseminate information about prevention and to motivate families to make life-style changes prior to the onset of illness. An important question is: Will people take the time to be responsible for their own health?

Sociologic Factors

Poverty is a major problem that affects not only the family but also the community and society. Poverty is a real concern among the rising number of one-parent families headed by a female, and, as the number of these families increases, poverty will affect a large number of growing children.

When ill, the poor are likely to put off seeking services until the illness reaches an advanced state and requires longer or more complex treatment. Although the health of the American people has improved significantly over the past century, it is clear that this progress has not benefited all segments of society, particularly the poor.

CONSIDER . . .

- the various instruments included in this chapter and Appendices A and B for the appraisal of the family's wellness and health risk. What conclusions do you make when you apply these instruments to your family? Is your family at risk for health alterations?
- the relationship between individual life-style assessment data and family assessment data. How do the data obtained from the individual's life-style assessment affect the results of their family assessment? In what ways do the life-style risks of one family member influence family health?
- whether nurses are currently utilizing individual and family theoretical frameworks to provide holistic health promotion services. Are you using a theoretical framework to guide your practice?

DEVELOPING AND IMPLEMENTING PLANS FOR HEALTH PROMOTION

Following assessment, validation, and summarizing of data, nursing diagnoses are identified. **Wellness nursing diagnoses,** or *strength-oriented diagnoses,* can be applied at all levels of prevention but are particularly useful in primary care settings such as schools, industries, clinics, and community health facilities. When the nurse and client conclude that the client has positive function in a certain pattern area, such as adequate nutrition or effective coping, the nurse can use this information to help the client reach a higher level of functioning. As mentioned in Chapter 14, there are currently four one-part NANDA wellness diagnoses. Other wellness diagnoses can be written as "Potential for enhanced" followed by the desired higher level of wellness (for example, **Potential for enhanced parenting**). NANDA diagnoses written as *potential* or *risk* diagnostic statements can also direct activities related to health promotion. See examples of diagnoses in the accompanying box.

The client then determines a health promotion plan. Health promotion plans need to be developed according to the needs, desires, and priorities of the client. The client decides on health promotion goals, the activities or interventions to achieve these goals, the frequency and duration of the activities, and the method of evaluation. During the planning process the nurse acts as a resource person rather than as an adviser or counselor. The nurse provides information when asked, emphasizes the importance of small steps to behavioral change, and reviews the client's goals and plans to make sure they are realistic, measurable, and acceptable to the client.

NANDA Nursing Diagnoses Related to Health Promotion

- Health-seeking behaviors related to new role as parent

- Health-seeking behaviors related to optimal nutrition for age and body size

- Risk for altered health maintenance related to insufficient finances

- Risk for altered growth and development related to school-related stressors

- Risk for diversional activity deficit related to postretirement status

- Risk for ineffective individual coping related to new parenting role

- Risk for decisional conflict related to college and career choices

- Risk for injury related to knowledge deficit of environmental hazards

- Risk for impaired adjustment related to divorce and inadequate support from family members

- Risk for activity intolerance related to lack of motivation

Steps in Planning

Pender (1996, pp. 147–161) outlines several steps in the process of health promotion planning, which are carried out jointly by the nurse and the client:

1. *Identify health care goals.* The client selects two or three top priority goals or areas of improvement. Common goals follow:
   a. To reduce the risk of cardiovascular disease
   b. To achieve or maintain a desired weight
   c. To increase knowledge of safety practices in the home

2. *Identify behavioral or health outcomes.* For each of the selected goals or areas in step 1, determine what specific behavioral changes are needed to bring about the desired outcome. For example, to reduce the risk of cardiovascular disease, the client may need to change behaviors such as stop smoking, lose weight, and increase activity level.

3. *Develop a behavior change plan.* A constructive program of change is based on client "ownership" of the behavior changed (Pender, 1996, p. 153). Clients may need to be assisted in examining value-behavior inconsistencies and in selecting behavioral options that are most appealing and that they are most willing to try. The client's priorities will reflect personal values, activity preferences, and expectations for success.

4. *Reiterate benefits of change.* The benefits will probably need to be reiterated even though the client is committed to the change. The health-related and non–health-related benefits should be kept before the client as central motivating factors.

5. *Address environmental and interpersonal facilitators and barriers to change.* Environmental and interpersonal factors that support positive change should be used to reinforce the client's efforts to change life-style. All people experience barriers, some of which can be anticipated and planned for, thereby making the change more likely to occur.

6. *Determine a time frame for implementation.* By developing a time frame, the appropriate knowledge and skills can be developed before a new behavior is implemented. The time frame may be several weeks or months. Scheduling short-term goals and rewards can offer encouragement to achieve long-term objectives. Clients may need help to be realistic and to deal with one behavior at a time.

7. *Make a commitment to goals of behavior change.* In the past, commitments to changing behaviors have usually been verbal. Increasingly, a formal, written behavioral contract is being used to motivate the client to follow through with selected actions. Motivation to follow through is provided by a positive reinforcement or reward stated in the contract. Contracting is based on the belief that all people have the potential for growth and the right of self-determination, even though their choices may be different from the norm.

Exploring Available Resources

Another essential aspect of planning is identifying support resources available to the client. These may be community resources, such as a fitness program at a local gymnasium, or educational programs, such as stress management, breast self-examination, nutrition, smoking cessation, and health lectures. The nurse, too, may meet some of the client's educational needs. A major nursing role is to support the client. The nurse can contact the client or be available at specified intervals to review the contract and to assist with problem solving.

Providing and Facilitating Support

A vital component of life-style change is ongoing support that focuses on the desired behavior change and is provided in a nonjudgmental manner. Support can be offered by the nurse on an individual basis or in a group setting. The nurse can also facilitate the development of support networks for the client, such as family members and friends.

Individual Counseling Sessions

Counseling sessions may be routinely scheduled as part of the plan or may be provided if the client encounters difficulty in carrying out interventions or meets insurmountable barriers to change. In a counseling relationship, the nurse and client share ideas. In this sharing relationship, the nurse acts as a facilitator, promoting the client's decision making regarding the health promotion plan.

Telephone Counseling

Regular telephone sessions may be provided to the client to help in answering questions, reviewing goals and strategies, and reinforcing progress. The client may find that scheduling a weekly telephone session is helpful or may wish to initiate a call if a problem occurs. The client is asked, "Is your plan working?" If the plan is not working, the nurse asks, "What would you like to do?" The client may wish to continue or may wish to change the plan to a more realistic one. Telephone support is efficient for the busy client who may not have the time for regular, in-person sessions.

Group Support

Group sessions provide an opportunity for participants to learn the experiences of others in changing behavior. Group contact gives individuals a renewed commitment to their goals. Groups can be scheduled at monthly or less frequent intervals for over a year.

Facilitating Social Support

Social networks, such as families and friends, can facilitate or impede the efforts directed toward health promotion and prevention. The nurse's role is to assist the client to assess, modify, and develop the social support necessary to achieve the desired change. In order to provide the necessary support, families must communicate effectively, be aware of and support each other's needs and goals, and provide help and assistance to one another to achieve those goals. The client may wish the nurse to meet with the family or significant others and help in enlisting their understanding and support.

Providing Health Education

Health education programs on a variety of topics can be provided to groups, individuals, or communities. Group programs need to be planned carefully before they are implemented. The decision to establish a health promotion program must be based on the health needs of the people; also, specific health promotion goals must be set. After the program is implemented, outcomes must be evaluated.

In the evaluation of health promotion programs, the client's understanding must be ascertained. Simply asking clients if they understand may be inappropriate (Byham & Vickery, 1988, p. 10). In some cases, the client may understand the information but may not be able to apply it or may have anxiety about doing a particular task. For instance, a new parent may understand all the principles of giving an infant a bed bath but have considerable anxiety about safely managing the procedure. Giving clients ample opportunity to demonstrate or practice routines and procedures, asking them to repeat important steps or information, and clarifying any unclear statements allows the nurse to evaluate the clients' knowledge and competence more fully.

Nurses may offer an abundance of information less formally. To do so, however, nurses need up-to-date knowledge, the ability to assess learning needs, and effective teaching skills. See Chapter 9 for detailed information. For example, nurses often disseminate information about parenting, breast and testicular self-examination, prevention of sexually transmitted disease, nutritional needs, and monitoring blood pressure and pulse rates.

Health fairs are being used to disseminate information to the public about health promotion and disease prevention and early detection. Nurses are often the initiators of health fairs and may provide participants of all age groups with information, teaching, counseling, or screening. Health fairs are usually offered in convenient locations such as shopping malls, schools, hospitals, and business settings to encourage maximum participation.

Enhancing Behavior Change

Whether people will make and maintain changes to improve health or prevent disease depends on many interrelated factors. See the section on assessing health care beliefs, earlier in this chapter. Murphy (1982, p. 427) says that the distances between wanting to change, attempting to change, and being able to change can be enormous. She emphasizes this statement by pointing out the difficulty many people have in acquiring regular dental flossing habits. When a client succeeds in making healthy behavior changes because of information the nurse has provided, the nurse feels satisfied and pleased. When, however, the client does not succeed in planned behavioral changes, the nurse tends to feel frustrated and often describes the person as "resistant," "uninterested," "unmotivated," or "noncompliant."

Murphy (1982) says the nurses are erroneously inclined to believe (a) that change will occur simply by bringing unhealthy behavior to the client's attention and (b) that when the client does not change, the desire to change is absent.

To help clients succeed in implementing behavior changes, the nurse needs to understand the process of change and the nature of the client's motivation or the client's current situation. An application of Lewin's stages of change (Lewin 1951) can help the nurse recognize the client's needs. See Chapter 13 for additional information on Lewin's stages.

The response of the nurse to lack of change in the client is generally to provide more information or to withdraw from the interaction after concluding that there is no point wasting time on people who do not want to change. Both responses deny such clients the opportunity to improve their health. By providing more information to the client, the nurse assumes that the client lacks knowledge. If,

RESEARCH NOTE

What are the Health Concerns of Adolescent Girls?

Researchers conducted a study to assess adolescent females' health concerns. An anonymous self-reporting questionnaire was designed and administered to 1416 female students in grades 7–10 from 38 schools in northwestern Ontario. Results indicated that the future and personal appearance were the students' greatest concerns. Factor analysis of the items grouped concerns into four factors: risk-taking behaviors (such as substance abuse and sexuality), appearance (such as figure, weight, and hair), health promotion/future orientation (such as healthy diet and adequate sleep and exercise) and psychologic functioning (such as nervousness and feeling "blue"). In comparing the four factors, the researchers found that concern about risk-taking behaviors and psychologic functioning did not change as the child aged.

Concern about appearance increased as the grade increased. Concern about health promotion/future orientation issues decreased as the grade increased.

Implications: This study provides the nurse with information that can be used in targeting the health promotion needs of adolescent females. Gender and age should be taken into consideration in planning health promotion services. The study also suggests that health promotion services should not be limited to the "traditional areas" of substance abuse and teenage pregnancy but should be broad in scope to reach all participants.

SOURCE: "Health Concerns of Adolescent Girls" by L. McKay and E. Diem, February 1995, *Journal of Pediatric Nursing*, 10(1), 19–27.

Clinical Guidelines

Enhancing Behavior Change

- Recognize that motivation is the basis of all behavior whether it is healthy or unhealthy, good or bad.

- Recognize that people are motivated by their needs.

- Avoid labeling people as unmotivated. The label simply means that the person does not comply with the wishes of the nurse who applies the label.

- Focus on the sources or factors that motivate the person's behavior rather than on the presence or absence of motivation.

- Remember that resistance is a normal part of change and a healthy response to a threat.

- Understand that a client may choose to keep unhealthy habits for many reasons.
  a. The habit may be a culturally learned response such as cigarette smoking and alcohol consumption. In North America, these habits were once associated with a glamorous or sophisticated life-style and a certain kind of satisfaction.
  b. The client may be directing all available energies to meet other needs. A person who is grieving the loss

of a loved one, or a recently divorced person, for example, may not have the energy to follow a weight-loss diet.
  c. The conditions required to change may be absent. For example, clients need help first to "unlearn" or "unfreeze" old habits and recognize the benefits of new habits before they can consider or undertake action.

- Cast aside the idea that the client *must* change. This attitude is not conducive to a helping relationship with the client and does not convey respect for the client. The client who does not change is entitled to the nurse's interest and nonjudgmental response.

- Measure your competence in terms of how well you understand clients' needs and implement clients' care rather than by the extent to which clients change their behavior.

SOURCE: "Why Won't They Shape Up? Resistance to the Promotion of Health" by M. M. Murphy, Nov./Dec. 1982, *Canadian Journal of Public Health, 73,* 427–430.

---

however, the client has understood the information, repeating or amplifying the information more than likely will annoy the client. The nurse has failed to identify the problem clearly. Withdrawal from clients who have difficulty changing implies that the nurse's health promotion efforts will be directed toward persons who readily and willingly comply. Such people, however, are probably the ones who least need the nurse's help. Additional guidelines for assisting the client toward behavior change are offered in the accompanying box.

Modeling

Modeling consists of observing the behavior of other people who have successfully achieved the goal that clients have set for themselves (Pender, 1996, pp. 174–175). Modeling is not imitating. Through observing a model, the client acquires ideas for behavior and coping strategies for specific problems. The client is not expected to mimic the sequence of actions or behavior patterns of the model.

The nurse and client should mutually select models with whom the client can identify, since the

cultural and ethnic backgrounds of the nurse and client often differ. Models should be frequently available during the early learning and change stages of unfreezing and moving. Models should also be people the client respects.

Nurses should serve as models of wellness. In order to model effectively, nurses need to have a philosophy and life-style that demonstrate good health habits. In many colleges and universities, undergraduate nursing students work with faculty and college health services to develop a wellness program. Through such a plan, students can assess their own life-styles, develop a health promotion plan, and actually carry out the implementation strategies. The college years offer access to facilities and health services that may not be available when students begin their working life. Once students have had a firsthand experience with creating a health promotion plan and with the difficulties involved with behavior change, they will be able to work more effectively with peers and clients. Clients are more likely to respect and trust the nurse who can tell them what worked in the nurse's personal situation.

CONSIDER...

- what national local changes have influenced health promotion strategies for individuals and families in your community.
- what specific health problems in your community lend themselves to change through prevention and other health promotion activities.
- what resources are available in your community for the health promotion of individuals and families.
- the changing emphasis on health promotion strategies in nursing curricula. How much content on health promotion was included in your basic nursing program? Compare your findings with other nurses who were educated either before or after you.

EVALUATING THE HEALTH PROMOTION PLAN

Evaluation takes place on an ongoing basis, both during the attainment of short-term goals and after the completion of long-term goals. During evaluation, the client may decide to continue with the plan, reorder priorities, change strategies, or revise the health promotion contract. Evaluation of the plan is a collaborative effort between the nurse and the client. Goals are written during the planning phase and a date determined for attaining the specific results or behaviors that are desired to promote health or prevent illness.

Using the nursing process for promotion of health and prevention of illness assumes that the client is a motivated, self-directed, responsible consumer. The nurse's role is to assist clients in achieving their goals. The nurse is available to lend expertise in the assessment of health, the implementation of a health promotion plan, and the evaluation of the goals. The nurse also enhances the potential for client success in goal achievement by using strategies such as teaching, counseling, support, and the modeling of good health behaviors.

CONSIDER...

- whether nurses are effective role models of healthy life-styles. Do you have a philosophy and life-style that demonstrates good health habits? How does your life-style influence your nursing practice, your clients, and your colleagues?

- whether nurses have the academic and experiential preparation to take leadership positions in coordinating available resources for health promotion of individuals and families.

READINGS FOR ENRICHMENT

Edelman, C. L., & Mandle, C. L. (1994). *Health promotion throughout the lifespan* (3rd ed.). St. Louis: Mosby.

Edelman and Mandle note that encouraging positive health changes has been a major effort of health professionals, the government, and society in general. Nurses today must have a better understanding of interventions to promote health as well as interventions to protect health and prevent disease and injury. Their book discusses the foundations of health promotion, assessment of individuals and families, intervention strategies, and applying health promotion to the developing individual. Edelman and Mandle also address the nurse's role in health promotion for the year 2000 and beyond.

Griffen, H. M., & Rahman, M. I. (1994, Oct.). Implementing the Put Prevention into Practice program. *Nurse Practitioner*, *19*(10), 12, 15–16, 18–19.

Put Prevention into Practice (PPIP) is a national program designed to improve delivery of preventive care to clients by primary care health professionals. PPIP covers the full range of preventive services, such as immunizations and screening tests. The program involves clients, clinic/office staff and systems, and health care providers, such as nurse practitioners. The authors found that successful implementation of the PPIP program included a high level of administrative support, "ownership" by all players in the process, a designated person responsible for the program, and an evaluation process that provided feedback to the health care providers.

Pender, N. J. (1996). *Health promotion in nursing practice* (3rd ed.). Norwalk, CT: Appleton & Lange.

Nola Pender has written extensively in the nursing and health-related literature about health promotion issues. She developed a model for health-promoting behavior (described in her book) that has been used as a theoretic framework for research studies. She discusses the nurse's role in the quest for health as well as nursing strategies for preventing illness and injury and promoting the health of individuals, families, and communities. Dr. Pender's leadership in health promotion issues has enhanced the competence of nurses who are assisting clients in moving toward their maximum health potential.

SUMMARY

The goal of health promotion is to raise the level of health of individuals and families. The family is the basic unit of society. In working with the wide variety of family forms in today's society, the nurse must be aware of many factors that affect the health of families. Family-centered nursing addresses the health of individual family members as well as the family as a unit.

There are a variety of social, psychologic, and nursing theoretical frameworks that provide the nurse with a holistic overview for health promotion of individuals and families across the life span. Theoretical frameworks that can be used to view individuals include needs theories, developmental stage theories, and systems theories. Theoretical frameworks that provide a holistic view of families include developmental stage theories, systems theories, and structural-functional theories.

A complete and accurate assessment of the individual's health status is basic to health promotion. Wellness and life-style assessment tools give clients the opportunity to assess the impact of their present life-style behaviors on their health and to make decisions about specific life-style changes. Health risk or hazard appraisals provide the data that often spur the individual to adopt healthier life behaviors. The individual's beliefs and values about health provide the nurse with an indication of how much the person believes he or she can control health through personal behaviors.

Because the individual is a member of the family unit, it is important to assess the family's health patterns. Through family assessment, the nurse determines the level of family functioning, clarifies interaction patterns, identifies strengths and weaknesses, and describes the health status of the family and its individual members. The nurse also identifies health beliefs and practices that influence the wellness of the family.

Organizing assessment data from individual and family assessment enables the nurse to make wellness-oriented nursing diagnoses that identify client strengths, recognize self-care abilities, and enhance health promotion goals. The nurse explores the motivating sources of the client's behavior. Health promotion activities are directed toward developing the resources of the individual and family that maintain or enhance well-being. The nurse provides ongoing support and supplies additional information and education in order to help individuals and their families change their life-styles or health behaviors. During the evaluation phase of the health promotion process, the nurse assists clients in determining whether they will continue with the plan, reorder priorities, or revise the plan.

As role models for their clients, nurses should develop attitudes and behaviors that reflect healthy life-styles. Nurses can identify their own attitudes, beliefs, and practices related to healthy life-style behaviors by completing one or more life-style or health risk appraisal instruments. An awareness of personal life-style behaviors and of the difficulty in changing unhealthy behaviors enables the nurse to better understand client reactions to the results of these assessment tools.

SELECTED REFERENCES

Aden, L. (1976, Summer). Faith and the developmental cycle. *Pastoral Psychology, 24*(2), 215–230.

Ahrons, C., & Rodgers, R. H. (1987). *Divorced families: A multidisciplinary developmental view.* New York: Norton.

Blecke, J. (1990, July). Exploration of children's health and self-care behavior within a family context through qualitative research. *Family Relations, 39*(3), 284–291.

Bomar, P. J. (1989). *Nurses and family health promotion: Concepts, assessment, and interventions.* Philadelphia: W. B. Saunders.

Byham, L. D. & Vickery, C. E. (1988, July/August). Compliance and health promotion. *Health Values, 12*(4), 5–12.

Carter E. A., & McGoldrick, M. (Eds.). (1989). *The changing family life cycle: A framework for family therapy* (2nd ed.). Boston: Allyn and Bacon.

Clark, C. (1986). *Wellness nursing: Concepts, theories, research, and practice.* New York: Springer.

Cox, C. L. (1985, May/June). The health self-determination index. *Nursing Research, 34*(3), 177–183.

Cox, C. L., Cowell, J., Marion, L., & Miller, E. (1990, July/Aug.). The health self-determination index for children. *Research in Nursing and Health, 13*(4), 237–246.

Danielson, C. B., Hamel-Bissell, B., & Winstead-Fry, P. (1993). *Families, health, and illness: Perspectives on coping and intervention.* St. Louis: Mosby-Year Book.

Davies, B. (1995, Oct.) Windows on the family. *Canadian Nurse, 91*, 37–41.

Duvall, E., & Miller, B. (1985). *Marriage and family development* (6th ed.). New York: Harper and Row.

Erikson, E. (1963). *Childhood and society* (2nd ed.). New York: Norton.

Erikson, E. (1976). *Adulthood.* New York: Norton.

Fawsett, J. (1975, July/Aug.). The family as a living open system: An emerging conceptual framework for nursing. *International Nursing Review, 22*(4), 113–116.

Feetham, S., & Humenick, S. (1982). Feetham family functioning survey. In S. Humenick (Ed.), *Analysis of current assessment strategies in the health care of young children and childbearing families* (pp. 259–269). Norwalk, CT: Appleton & Lange.

Fowler, J. W. (1981). *Stages of faith: The psychology of human development and the quest for meaning.* San Francisco: Harper and Row.

Friedman, M. M. (1992). *Family nursing: Theory and practice* (3rd ed.). Norwalk, CT: Appleton & Lange.

Gilligan, C. (1982). *In a different voice: Psychological theory and women's development.* Cambridge, MA: Harvard University Press.

Gillis, A. J. (1994, Summer). Determinants of health-promoting lifestyles in adolescent females. *Canadian Journal of Nursing Research, 26*(2), 13–20.

Gould, R. L. (1972, Nov.). The phases of adult life: A study in developmental psychology. *American Journal of Psychiatry, 129*(5), 521–531.

Grandine, J. (1995, Oct.). Embracing the family. *Canadian Nurse, 91,* 31–36.

Hajal, F., & Rosenberg, E. (1991, Jan.). The family life cycle in adoptive families. *American Journal of Orthopsychiatry, 61*(1), 78–85.

Havighurst, R. J. (1972). *Developmental tasks and education* (3rd ed.). New York: David McKay.

Hill, R. (1986, Jan.). Life cycle stages for types of single parent families: Of family development theory. *Family Relations, 35*(1), 19–29.

Holmes, T. H., & Rahe, R. H. (1967, Aug.). The social readjustment rating scale. *Journal of Psychosomatic Research, 11,* 213–218.

Holt, S., & Robinson, T. (1979, May). The school nurse's family assessment tool. *American Journal of Nursing, 79*(5), 950–953.

Houdin, A., Saltstein, S., & Ganley, K. (1987). *Nursing diagnosis for wellness.* Philadelphia: Lippincott.

Johnson, D. E. (1980). The behavioral system model for nursing. In J. P. Riehl and C. Roy (Eds.). *Conceptual models for nursing practice* (2nd ed.). Norwalk, CT: Appleton-Century-Crofts.

Kalish, R. A. (1983). *The psychology of human behavior* (5th ed.). Monterey, CA: Brooks/Cole.

Kantor, D., & Lehr, W. (1975). *Inside the family: Toward a theory of family process.* San Francisco: Jossey-Bass.

King, I. M. (1981). *A theory for nursing: Systems concepts, and process.* New York: Wiley.

Kohlberg, L. (1976). Moral stages and moralization: The cognitive developmental approach. In T. Lickona (Ed.). *Moral development and behavior.* New York: Holt, Rinehart, and Winston.

Leslie, G. R., & Korman, S. K. (1989). *The family in social context* (3rd ed.). New York: Oxford University Press.

Lewin, K. (1951). *Field theory in social science.* New York: Harper and Row.

Mallinger, K. M. (1989). The American family: History and development. In P. J. Bomar (Ed.). *Nurses and family health promotion: Concepts, assessment, and interventions.* Baltimore: Williams and Wilkins.

Maslow, A. H. (1970). *Motivation and personality* (2nd ed.). New York: Harper and Row.

McCubbin, H., & Dahl, B. (1985). *Marriage and family: Individuals and life cycles.* New York: Wiley.

Mischke-Burkey, K., Warner, P., & Hanson, S. (1989). Family health assessment and intervention. In P. Bomar (Ed.), *Nurses and family health promotion: Concepts, assessment, and intervention* (pp. 139–154). Philadelphia: W. B. Saunders.

Mills, D. M. (1984, July). A model for stepfamily development. *Family Relations, 33*(3), 365–372.

Muhlenkamp, A. F., Brown, N. J., & Sands, D. (1985, Nov./Dec.). Determinants of health promotion activities in nursing clinic clients. *Nursing Research, 34*(6), 327–332.

Murphy, M. M. (1982, Nov./Dec.). Why don't they shape up? Resistance to the promotion of health. *Canadian Journal of Public Health, 73*(6), 427–430.

National Wellness Institute. (1988). *Wellness assessment questionnaire.* Stevens Point, WS: Author.

Nettle, C., et al. (1993, Jan.). Family as client: Using Gordon's health pattern topology. *Journal of Community Health Nursing, 10*(1), 53–61.

Neuman, B. (1989). The Neuman nursing process format: Family. In J. P. Riehl-Sisca (Ed.). *Conceptual models for nursing practice* (3rd ed.). Norwalk, CT: Appleton & Lange.

Neuman, B. (1995). *The Neuman systems model* (3rd ed.). Norwalk, CT: Appleton & Lange.

Nightingale, F. (1894). *Health and local government.* [Pamphlet]. Aylesbury: Pouton and Co., Printers, Bucks Advertising Office. As cited in L. A. Monteiro, 1985, Florence Nightingale on public health nursing. *American Journal of Public Health, 75,* 181–185.

Orem, D. E. (1995). *Nursing: Concepts of practice* (5th ed.). New York: McGraw-Hill.

Parsons, T., & Bales, R. F. (1955). *Family socialization and the interaction process.* New York: Free Press.

Peck, R. (1968). Psychological developments in the second half of life. In B. L. Neugarten (Ed.). *Middle age and aging.* Chicago: University of Chicago Press.

Peck, J. S., & Manocharian, J. R. (1989). Divorce in the changing family life cycle. In B. Carter and M. McGoldrick (Eds.). *The changing family life cycle* (2nd ed.). New York: Allyn and Bacon.

Pender, N. J. (1996). *Health promotion in nursing practice* (3rd ed.). Norwalk, CT: Appleton & Lange.

Piaget, J. (1963). *The origins of intelligence in children.* New York: Norton.

Reitz, M., & Watson, K. W. (1992). *Adoption and the family system.* New York: Guildford Press.

Roy, C. (1983). Analysis and application of the Roy adaptation model. In I. Clements and F. Roberts (Eds.). *Family health: A theoretical approach to nursing care.* New York: Wiley.

Roy, C., & Andrews, H. A. (1991). *The Roy adaptation model: The definitive statement.* Norwalk, CT: Appleton & Lange.

Smilkstein, G. (1978). Assessment of family function. *Journal of Family Practice, 6,* 1231–1239.

Stanhope, M., & Lancaster, J. (1992). *Community health nursing: Process and practice for promoting health* (3rd ed.). St. Louis: Mosby.

Sullivan, H. S. (1953). *The interpersonal theory of psychiatry.* New York: Norton.

Travis, J. W., & Ryan, R. S. (1988). *Wellness workbook* (2nd ed.). Berkeley, CA: Ten Speed Press.

von Bertalanffy, L. (1968). *General systems theory: Foundations, development, applications.* New York: Braziller.

U. S. Department of Health and Human Services, Office of Health Information, Health Promotion, Physical Fitness, and Sports Medicine. (1985). *Self-test for health style.* Washington, DC: U. S. Government Printing Office.

Walker, S., Secrist, K., & Pender, N. (1987, March/April). The health-promoting lifestyle profile: Development and psychometric characteristics. *Nursing Research, 36*(2), 76–81.

Wallston, K. A., Wallston, B. S., & DeVellis, R. (1978, Spring). Development of the Multidimensional Locus of Control (MHLC) scales. *Health Education Monographs, 6,* 164–165.

Westerhoff, J., & Willmon, W. H. (1980). *Liturgy and learning through the life cycle.* New York: Seabury Press.

Wright, L., & Leahey, M. (Eds.). (1994). *Nurses and families: A guide to family assessment and intervention* (2nd ed.). Philadelphia: F. A. Davis.

Providing Care in the Home and Community

by Suzanne Phillips and Sandra Lobar

OBJECTIVES

- Describe the roles of the home health and community health nurse.

- Compare differences in applying the nursing process in the home setting versus the hospital setting.

- Describe characteristics of a healthy community.

- Discuss various elements and settings for community health nursing practice.

- Apply the nursing process to the community as client.

- Discuss the interrelationship between the home health and community health nurse.

"The cornerstone of nursing's plan for reform is the delivery of primary health care services to households and individuals in convenient, familiar places. If health is to be a true national priority, it is logical to provide services in the places where people work and live."
— Nursing's Agenda for
Health Care Reform, 1991

In the past decade there has been an observable increase in the delivery of nursing services in home and community settings. A number of factors have contributed to this trend, among them rising health care costs, an aging population, and a growing emphasis on managing chronic illness and stress, preventing illness and enhancing the quality of life.

- Concepts important to home and community nursing practice are health promotion, disease prevention, health maintenance, and health restoration.
- Increasing access to preventive health services is a goal of Healthy People 2000. This goal can best be achieved by delivering services where people reside, in their homes and communities. More information about the goals of Healthy People 2000 can be found in Chapter 3 and Chapter 8.
- For the home health care nurse, nursing care generally focuses on the individual and support persons and the client.
- For the community health nurse, there are three general types of clients: individuals, families, and groups. Groups may be communities, at-risk aggregates, or persons with similar problems and needs.
- Home health nursing practice and community health nursing practice differ from nursing in acute care settings in many ways. For example, home and community health nurses assume a higher degree of autonomy and independence.

HOME HEALTH NURSING

Historically, nurses who provided direct services in the home were strong generalists who focused on long-term preventive, educational, remedial, and rehabilitative outcomes. Today, **home health** services center on individualized, episodic care with curative, short-term outcomes. Many home health care nurses are generalists or specialists possessing high-technology skills that were formerly used only in acute care settings. For example, nurses provide a variety of intravenous therapies in the home setting and monitor clients who are dependent on technologically complex medical equipment, such as ventilators and central lines. These nurses collaborate with physicians and other health care professionals in providing care; usually, third-party payors pay for their services.

Home nursing care is one of the fastest growing sectors of the health care system. The U.S. Department of Health and Human Services (1991) predicts that by the year 2000 there will be a significant shortage of home health care nurses. Several factors have contributed to the growth of home health care. These factors include (1) the increase in the older population, who are frequent recipients of home care; (2) third-party payors who favor home care to control costs; (3) the ability of agencies and institutions to successfully deliver high-technology services in the home; and (4) consumers who prefer to receive care in the home rather than an institution (Stulginsky, 1993a, p. 402).

Definitions of Home Nursing

The delivery of nursing services in the home has been called by a variety of terms, including home health nursing, home care nursing, and visiting nursing. Spradley and Allender (1996, p. 484) define home health care as "all the services and products provided to clients in their homes to maintain, restore, or promote their physical, mental, and emotional health." Stanhope and Lancaster (1996, p. 806) add that "home health care cannot simply be defined as 'care at home' but includes an arrangement of disease prevention, health promotion, and episodic illness–related services provided to people in their places of residence." This suggests that home health nursing services might be provided in long-term care facilities, residential hospices, residential shelters for abused women and children and the homeless, and adult congregate living facilities (ACLFs). According to the American Nurses Association (1992), home health nursing is a "synthesis of community health nursing and selected technical skills from other nursing specialties," including medical-surgical nursing, psychiatric-mental health nursing, gerontologic nursing, parent-child nursing, and community health nursing. The Department of

Health and Human Services presented a more comprehensive definition of home health care in 1980 (Warhola, 1980). The USDHHS states that:

> home health care is that component of a continuum of comprehensive health care whereby health services are provided to individuals and families in their places of residence for the purposes of promoting, maintaining or restoring health, or of maximizing the level of independence while minimizing the effects of disability and illness, including terminal illness. Services appropriate to the needs of the individual patient and family are planned, coordinated, and made available by providers organized for the delivery of home care through the use of employed staff, contractual arrangements, or a combination of the two patterns.

The focus then of home health care nursing is individuals and their families. This differs somewhat from the focus of community health nursing, which focuses on the health of the community as a whole. This difference will be discussed in more detail later in this chapter.

Perspectives of Home Health Nursing

Stulginsky (1993a) interviewed home health care nurses who identified their practice as "meeting the acute and chronic care needs of patients and their families in the home environment" (p. 404). These nurses maintained that care centers on the client and that their role is to advocate for the client despite possible conflict in the opinions and needs of various care providers. Because the home is the family's territory, power and control issues in delivering nursing care differ from those in the institution. For example, entry into a home is granted, not assumed; the nurse must therefore establish trust and rapport with the client and family. Families also may feel more free to question advice, to ignore directions, to do things differently, and to set their own priorities and schedules.

Home health care nurses have identified significant advantages in caring for individuals and families in the home. The home setting is intimate; this intimacy fosters familiarity, sharing, connections, and caring between clients, families, and their nurse. Behaviors are more natural, cultural beliefs and practices are more visible, and multigenerational

interactions tend to be displayed. Home health care nurses become realistic about what they can remedy and learn how to provide various supports and use creative interventions for what they cannot remedy (Stulginsky, 1993b, pp. 477–480).

Home health care nurses have also identified issues that negatively impact care in the home. More than any other care providers, these nurses have first-hand knowledge and experience about the burden of caregiving. In the interest of cutting health care costs, policy makers, third-party payors, and medical providers are placing increasingly complex responsibilities on clients' families and significant other(s). Caregiving demands may go on for months or years, placing the caregivers themselves (many of whom are older adults) at risk for physiologic and psychosocial problems. Additionally, nurses enter homes where the living conditions and support systems may be inadequate. When additional support or improved caregiving cannot be obtained for the client, home health care nurses face difficult decisions (Stulginsky, 1993a, p. 406).

Because home health care nurses must function independently in a variety of home settings and situations, employers generally prefer that the nurse be prepared at the baccalaureate level or above. In 1995, the American Nurses Credentialing Center (ANCC) approved a certification for clinical specialist in home health nursing. This certification requires a master's degree in nursing and recognizes the need for home health clinical specialists who can provide direct care, manage client care, and engage in consulting, education, administrative, and research activities ("ANCC approves," 1995, p. 11). As employment opportunities for registered nurses decrease in acute care institutions, the growth of home health care is providing nurses with additional career choices and career opportunities.

Hospice nursing is often considered a subspecialty of home health nursing as hospice services are frequently delivered to terminally ill clients in their residence. See the box on page 338 for an interview of a hospice nurse.

What is the future for home health care? Experts in the home health care industry have identified some trends:

1. Establishing ethics committees to handle ethical issues that arise in the home. These committees may be necessary for agencies to receive accreditation through the Joint Commission on

the Accreditation of Healthcare Organizations (JCAHO).

2. Providing third-party reimbursement for community clinic nurse specialists and psychiatric nurse specialists. These advanced practice nurses can provide education, support, counseling, and therapy for clients and their families.

3. Providing third-party reimbursement for social workers. Social workers can assist clients and their families in the home with financial and household problems, freeing the nurse to focus on nursing care.

4. Utilizing nurse pain specialists to assess and manage pain in the home, thus avoiding costly hospitalizations and procedures.

5. Obtaining a separate Medicare certification to provide hospice care. Medicare-certified hospices receive per diem allotments rather than fees for each visit, thus making this care more economical.

6. Providing pet care for clients who may become too ill to care for them. Clients can make arrangements for the care of a pet if they are hospitalized or die.

7. Utilizing electronic home visits. A computerized phone system can obtain information, such as blood pressure readings, allowing case managers to review a client's progress ("Home health," 1995, p. 58).

Applying the Nursing Process in the Home

The application of the nursing process is focused on the needs of individual clients and their caregivers. According to the American Nurses Credentialing Center (1995, p. 12), "the framework of home health practice is care management, which includes: the use of the nursing process to assess, diagnose, plan, and evaluate care; performing nursing interventions, including teaching; coordinating and using referrals and resources; providing and monitoring all levels of technical care; collaborating with other disciplines and providers; identifying clinical problems and using research knowledge; supervising ancillary personnel; and advocating for the client's right to self-determination."

Assessing McFarland and McFarlane (1993, pp. 308–317) state that the nurse "must assess not only the health care demands of the patient and family but also the home and community environment." The home health nurse obtains a health history from the client, reviews documents from the referral agency, examines the client, observes the client and caregiver relationship, and assesses the home and community environment. Parameters of assessment of the home environment include client and caregiver mobility, client ability to perform self-care, the cleanliness of the environment, the availability of caregiver support, safety, food preparation, financial supports, and emotional status of the client and caregiver.

Diagnosing In addition to nursing diagnoses specific to the client's health needs, nursing diagnoses related to the home environment may be identified. An example of a nursing diagnosis appropriate for home care is **Impaired Home Maintenance Management,** which is defined by Carpenito (1992,

---

INTERVIEW

Hospice Nurse

Jace Martinson, RN, BSN, MSN

Why did you choose this practice setting? I worked in an intensive care unit in Alaska and found that I was very comfortable and effective in dealing with families before and after their loved one died. I also liked the flexible schedule and autonomy that hospice nursing offers.

What qualities do you think are necessary to be a nurse in this setting? The most important quality is compassion. Additionally, it is important to be truly empathetic and sympathetic but also therapeutic during interactions with families.

What has been your most gratifying moment as a nurse in this setting? Hospice nursing is the only job I ever had where I entered my client's home as a stranger and two hours later emerged as part of the family. I watched families come together, become prepared, and know what to expect before and after their family member's death.

What encouragement would you give a nurse considering practice in your setting? I would encourage nurses to be well aware of their feelings about death and their own mortality. I would tell them that the job is very satisfying, and that the client and family really do benefit from the service.

p. 479) as the "state in which an individual or family experiences or is at risk to experience a difficulty in maintaining self or family in a home environment." Impaired home maintenance management may be related to impaired cognition, immobility, fatigue, or financial constraints (McFarland & McFarlane 1993, p. 313).

Planning and Intervention Planning and intervention, done in collaboration with the client and caregivers, focuses on establishing a realistic plan for home health management, teaching the client and family the techniques of home care, and identifying appropriate resources to assist the client and family in maintaining self-sufficiency.

Evaluating Evaluation can be done by the nurse on subsequent home visits by observing the same parameters assessed on the initial home visit. The nurse can also teach caregivers parameters of evaluation so that they can obtain professional intervention if needed.

CONSIDER...

* the differences in professional autonomy between the home health care nurse and the hospital nurse. What are the legal and ethical implications of the independence experienced by the home health care nurse?
* the different roles of the professional nurse. What differences might there be in the practice of the nurse's professional roles between the home health care nurse and the hospital nurse?
* how the availability of computer technology might assist the home health care nurse in providing and documenting better nursing care.

COMMUNITY HEALTH NURSING

The goal of many public and private efforts is to develop and maintain healthy communities. Characteristics of a healthy community are described in the accompanying box. Nursing, as a caring profession, exists because individuals, families, and groups (and, therefore, communities) are not always healthy or self-sufficient. The focus in community nursing is the *community:* it is a practice that is comprehensive and continuous, takes place in a wide variety of set-

> ### Ten Characteristics of a Healthy Community
>
> *A healthy community:*
>
> * Is one in which members have a high degree of awareness that "we are a community."
> * Uses its natural resources while taking steps to conserve them for future generations.
> * Openly recognizes the existence of subgroups and welcomes their participation in community affairs.
> * Is prepared to meet crises.
> * Is a problem-solving community; it identifies, analyzes, and organizes to meet its own needs.
> * Possesses open channels of communication that allow information to flow among all subgroups of citizens in all directions.
> * Seeks to make each of its systems' resources available to all members.
> * Has legitimate and effective ways to settle disputes that arise within the community.
> * Encourages maximum citizen participation in decision making.
> * Promotes a high level of wellness among all its members.
>
> SOURCE: Adapted from *Community Health Nursing: Concepts and Practice* (4th ed.), 1996, by B. W. Spradley and J. A. Allender. Philadelphia: Lippincott, p. 206.

tings, is directed toward all age groups, and commands the utilization of all professional nursing roles. Spradley and Allender (1996, pp. 4–5) state that "community health nurses are an integral part of community health practice. Their roles and activities are so varied that it is impossible to describe the 'typical' community health nurse."

The **community health nurse specialist** is prepared in graduate nursing programs at universities and colleges. These programs usually prepare the nurse for leadership and coordinating functions in the community. The many roles of the community health nurse can include care provider, client advocate, consultant, coordinator, manager, educator, collaborator, and researcher. See the interview box on page 340 for a community health nurse specialist's description of her practice.

INTERVIEW

Community Health Nurse
Mary Jorda, ARNP, BSN, MPH

Why did you choose this practice setting? After a year of working in a poor public hospital in Honduras (when I was in the Peace Corps), I noticed that the same patients were returning frequently with the same problems. I began to think that a more effective solution would be to provide education and health promotion in the community.

What qualities do you think are necessary to be a nurse in this setting? Working in the community requires patience, persistence, understanding, and flexibility. The clients set the agenda and priorities; we as health care workers are "guests" in assisting communities to realize their goals in improving health.

What has been your most gratifying moment as a nurse in this setting? While I was working in a refugee camp in Honduras, we transported a young girl who was very ill to a makeshift hospital. She was diagnosed with typhoid fever and started on IV antibiotics. The next morning I found her back in her hut. Her brother reported that "spirits" had entered her body through the IV. I realized that she had been delirious, but her family would not return her to the hospital. I conferred with the family and neighbors and we developed a plan to care for the girl in the camp. I administered antibiotics and bathed her, and her family gave her fluids. Some neighbors prayed; others boiled water. I also provided continuing education in the camp on the transmission of the disease. She survived. It was gratifying to see her well again and to realize the important role the family and community played in her recovery.

What encouragement would you give a nurse considering practice in your setting? If you believe in preventing health problems before they arise, then community health nursing is the place to be.

Five Functions of a Community

1. *Production, distribution, and consumption of goods and services.* These are the means by which the community provides for the economic needs of its members. This function includes not only the supplying of food and clothing but also the provision of water, electricity, and police and fire protection and the disposal of refuse.

2. *Socialization.* Socialization refers to the process of transmitting values, knowledge, culture, and skills to others. Communities usually contain a number of established institutions for socialization: families, churches, schools, media, voluntary and social organizations, and so on.

3. *Social control.* **Social control** refers to the way in which order is maintained in a community. Laws are enforced by the police; public health regulations are implemented to protect people from certain diseases. Social control is also exerted through the family, church, and schools.

4. *Social interparticipation.* **Social interparticipation** refers to community activities that are designed to meet people's needs for companionship. Families and churches have traditionally met this need; however, many public and private organizations also serve this function.

5. *Mutual support.* **Mutual support** refers to its ability to provide resources at a time of illness or disaster. Although the family is usually relied on to fulfill this function, health and social services may be necessary to augment the family's assistance if help is required over an extended period.

Definitions of a Community and Community Nursing

To understand community health nursing one must first define the word community and other terms associated with community health. A **community** is a collection of people who share some attribute of their lives. It may be that they live in the same locale, attend a particular church, or even share a particular interest, such as painting. Groups that constitute a community because of common member interests are often referred to as a *community of interest* (e.g., religious and ethnic groups). A community can also be defined as a *social system* in which the members interact formally or informally and form networks that operate for the benefit of all people in the community. Five of the functions of the community are described in the accompanying box. In community health, the community may be viewed as having a common health problem, for example, populations where there is a high incidence of infant mortality or communicable disease, such as tuberculosis or HIV infection.

Stanhope and Lancaster (1996, p. 1086) define **community health nursing** as "the synthesis of nursing and public health practice applied to promoting and preserving the health of populations.

The practice is general and comprehensive, with the dominant responsibility being to the population as a whole." For many, this definition is more appropriately used to describe the practice of public health nursing, and the term community health nursing "refers more broadly to nursing in the community" (Spradley & Allender 1996, p. 77). Spradley and Allender (1996, p. 77) suggest that the "distinction between the two terms might be that community health nursing is the beginning level of specialization and public health nursing is an advanced level of practice."

Elements of Community Health Nursing Practice

There are six basic elements of community health practice: (1) promotion of healthful living, (2) prevention of health problems, (3) remedial care for health problems, (4) rehabilitation, (5) evaluation, and (6) research (Spradley & Allender, 1996, p. 13).

Promotion of Healthful Living

The promotion of the health of individuals and groups has long been recognized as an important aspect of community health nursing. Health promotion programs are provided to raise the levels of wellness of individuals, families, groups, and the entire community. At the individual level, programs may include smoking cessation, reduction of alcohol and drug abuse, exercise and fitness, and stress management. At the family level, preventive health services such as family planning, pregnancy and infant care, immunizations, and information about sexually transmitted diseases may be offered. At the group level, occupational safety and health, and accidental injury may be considered. At the community level, toxic agent control, fluoridation of water supplies, and infectious agent control are of significance. See Chapters 8 and 16 for additional information on health promotion.

Prevention of Health Problems

Health protection activities are highly varied. They may include the prevention of nutritional deficiency, accidents at work and at home, communicable diseases, cardiovascular disease, lung cancer, child abuse, poisoning, pollution, and so on. Three levels of prevention were first discussed by Leavell and Clark in the 1950s. Their concept was based on public health concepts. See Chapter 8 for details.

Remedial Care for Health Problems

Community health care nurses provide direct and indirect services to individuals with chronic health problems. A variety of health care services provide **direct services,** such as home visits for the assessment and monitoring of health problems, dietary planning, administration of injections, personal care, homemaking services, and information about equipment resources (e.g., bath seats, wheelchairs, canes, walkers, syringes, dressing materials, and so on). **Indirect services** focus on assisting people with health problems to obtain treatment. For example, a community health nurse may assist a person to get a physician's appointment after eliciting data about an elevated blood pressure, a persistent cough, or vaginal bleeding. In other instances, the nurse may refer an individual or family to other agencies that provide information and/or therapy such as (a) a family therapy and counseling program, (b) a self-help group or association, or (c) a chemical dependency counseling and treatment center.

On a community level, individual community members and health workers may lobby for the development of programs to remedy unhealthy situations or to initiate services that are lacking. Examples of unhealthy situations are an inadequate school lunch program, inhumane conditions in a nursing home, and excessive pollution of water supplies from industrial wastes. Examples of new initiatives are increased shelters for abused women, low-cost housing for the elderly, the establishment of nursing services on the streets, and provision of health care to the homeless.

Rehabilitation

Rehabilitation services that focus on reducing disability and/or restoring function are provided at the individual, family, and community level. At the individual level, a community health nurse in conjunction with other allied health workers (e.g., physical and occupational therapists) may assist physically disabled persons (e.g., those with cerebrovascular accidents, heart conditions, amputations, or paralysis) regain some degree of lost function, prevent further disability, and develop new skills that enable them to assume an appropriate vocation or degree of independence. Many rehabilitative community groups are available to assist families and individuals with chronic health problems. Examples are colostomy clubs, postmastectomy groups, halfway houses for the discharged mentally ill, and Alcoholics Anonymous. The community health nurse can be instrumental in informing clients of available services.

Evaluation

Ongoing evaluation of health and health care services at the individual, national, and international levels is an essential component of community health practices. Its aim is to (a) determine the effectiveness of current activities, (b) determine needs, and (c) develop improved services. For example, evaluation of services available for rape victims may reveal a need for more comprehensive counseling programs.

Research

Research, a critical component of community health care practice, provide the means to identify problems and examine improved methods of providing health services. Research occurs at all levels—from federal agencies such as the U.S. Public Health Service to state and municipal groups. Researchers may investigate (a) patterns of illness and health, (b) possible causes and means of preventing specific problems such as child abuse, suicide, homicide, trauma, and substance abuse, (c) deficiencies in services such as day care centers or services for the elderly, (d) the effectiveness of treatment programs such as weight reduction, stress management, or substance abuse programs, (e) the effect of societal and environmental changes on existing services, and (f) utilization of existing health services.

Settings for Community Health Nursing Practice

Community health nursing is practiced in diverse settings, including community centers, schools and the workplace, among others.

Community Centers

Community health nurses utilize a variety of community sites for practice. In community centers, the client is usually a group of individuals with common needs or interests. Nurses may provide health-related education and influenza immunizations for older adults in an adult day-care center, offer blood pressure screenings and nutritional counseling at a community health fair, lead a discussion in stress management at a local church, and teach cardiopulmonary resuscitation (CPR) in a school. Community

health nurses also staff stationary or mobile clinics that provide primary care and health screening services for the medically indigent or disadvantaged. Using clinics increases nurse efficiency and decreases nurse travel time. Community health nurses may also collaborate with other community professionals, such as environmental health professionals who regulate day-care facilities. This collaboration provides opportunities for the nurse to educate day-care staff on managing ill children, identifying children who are neglected or abused, preventing injuries, and promoting normal growth and development (Stanhope & Lancaster, 1996, p. 614).

Schools

Community schools reflect the society they are part of. Today, school systems are encountering increasingly complex health-related morbidities in children, such as substance abuse and pregnancies; dealing with major environmental risks, such as violence and poverty; and accommodating children with significant physical and psychosocial impairments. The core components of a **school health**

INTERVIEW

School Nurse
Nancy Humbert, ARNP, MSN

Why did you choose this practice setting? I chose school health in order to participate in holistic, family-centered, and multidisciplinary nursing practice.

What qualities do you think are necessary to be a nurse in this setting? To function effectively in a school health setting, a nurse must have clinical expertise in public health and pediatrics. The school health nurse must be flexible, patient, creative, and culturally competent.

What has been your most gratifying moment as a nurse in this setting? My most gratifying moment as a school health nurse was when I helped empower an adolescent to overcome a severe case of bulimia.

What encouragement would you give a nurse considering practice in your setting? I would encourage any nurse to consider the school health practice setting after first developing strong basic nursing skills. School health is by far the most rewarding and challenging setting I've ever encountered. One must love change, challenge, and children.

program are health services, health education, and a healthy environment (Stanhope & Lancaster, 1996, p. 884). Nursing services are an integral part of the school health program. School nurses provide direct care in school clinics, manage immunization programs, provide health education in classrooms, offer health-related expertise during student conferences, coordinate student health services, promote safety, and advocate for student health programs at the local and state level. Although the health needs of today's children have increased, many school systems have cut support for school health programs in order to cut costs. Other school systems recognize

that providing health services today is an investment in children's future, and they directly or indirectly support health services at school sites by, for example, maintaining primary care clinics. Nurses who wish to pursue a specialty and certification in school nursing will find a variety of graduate programs that provide advanced degrees in this field. See the interview box on the previous page, in which a school nurse describes her role.

Occupational Health

Occupational health nurses consider an organization's needs as well as workers' needs (Stanhope & Lancaster, 1996, p. 908). The primary functions of the occupational nurse are to provide emergency treatment and promote worker health and safety; however, rapid changes in technology, the health care system, and societal expectations have expanded the nurse's role and made it increasingly complex. Occupational health nurses may now develop and carry out health promotion, health maintenance, and risk management programs and consult with their employers in reducing health-related costs. They may offer direct care to employees, manage program evaluation, and analyze work-related injuries and illnesses. In companies where management positions have been pared, the occupational health nurse may assume expanded responsibilities in job analysis, safety, and benefits management. Specialization in the field is often a requirement for additional responsibilities. Nurses who wish to pursue specialization and certification in occupational health will find a number of graduate programs that offer advanced education in this field. See the accompanying interview box, in which an occupational health nurse describes her practice.

CONSIDER...

- organizations within your community where health care is currently delivered or where health and nursing services could be delivered. What are the advantages to delivering health care in these various settings?
- whether nursing and health services are better provided to the traditionally underserved (e.g., the poor, older adults, minorities) by providing that care in the community and in the home.
- which nursing services can be effectively delivered in the home and community. Are there any nursing services that can be delivered only in the hospital? If yes, which services and why?

INTERVIEW

Occupational Health Nurse
Ethel Oatman, RN, BSN, MS

Why did you choose this practice setting? I found that I enjoyed working with adults in an ambulatory setting. There is so much to offer in the field of occupational health. The workplace is a natural environment for building a rapport with employees. Even though there is treatment of injuries and illnesses, much more can be done through employee health education, especially in the areas of health promotion and disease and injury prevention.

What qualities do you think are necessary to be a nurse in this setting? It is helpful to have medical-surgical and emergency nursing skills and be able to work independently. To be credible and effective, occupational health nurses must possess skills and knowledge in the areas of workers' compensation, health education, counseling, and human relations. Good verbal and written skills are also required.

What has been your most gratifying moment as a nurse in this setting? The focus of many of our clinics is on prevention and early detection of disease. I was coordinating a skin cancer clinic and three malignant melanomas were found. Since all of the melanomas were in the early, treatable stage, I feel I saved three lives that day.

What encouragement would you give a nurse considering practice in your setting? In order to stay in business, companies must address health cost containment, usually through managed care. Occupational health nurses have opportunities to assume leadership roles in ensuring high-quality, appropriate health care while remaining a client advocate.

Are there nursing services that are more effectively delivered in the home or community? If yes, which services and why?

APPLYING THE NURSING PROCESS IN THE COMMUNITY

Assessing

Nurses assess community health by using epidemiologic studies and by using an established community assessment framework or tool.

Epidemiologic Studies

"**Epidemiology** is the study of the distribution of states of health and of the causes of deviations from health in populations and the application of this study to control the health problems" (Stanhope & Lancaster 1996, p. 1090). Epidemiologic studies provide health professionals with information about the health and illness patterns of a specified population, the people involved, and any causal factors. Most health problems are currently thought to be the result of multiple causes. That is, a multiplicity of factors interact to result in coronary heart disease or teenage pregnancy, for example.

Epidemiologists use three types of studies: analytic, descriptive, and experimental. In *analytic studies*, the epidemiologist uses prospective (forward-looking) and retrospective (backward-looking) and/or experimental studies to test hypotheses about health and illness. In a *prospective study*, the epidemiologist determines the variables and the investigation method and establishes possible hypotheses. Data are then collected to see whether the hypothesis is supported. For example, a nurse may establish a hypothesis about the relation of dietary habits to weight, then follow a group of people, collecting data regarding their diet. In a *retrospective study* the investigator goes back over existing records to collect data that may or may not support a hypothesis. For example, when studying weight loss patterns among a group of people, a nurse might refer to records about the activity and diet of these people.

Descriptive studies rely primarily on existing data. The epidemiologist describes the people most likely to be affected by a disease, the geographic region in which it will occur, when it will occur, and its overall effect.

Experimental studies are often conducted to determine the effectiveness of a particular therapeutic modality. Subjects are assigned to one of two groups: the experimental group of the control group. People in the experimental group are, for example, exposed to a condition thought to improve health, to prevent disease, or to influence a person's health status in some manner, such as walking for a half hour each day. The members of the matched control group are not exposed to the experimental condition. Any subsequent differences in the health patterns between the two groups are then attributed to the manipulated factor.

Two types of rates are commonly used when describing health patterns in a population: the incidence rate and the prevalence rate. The **incidence rate** reflects the number of people with a particular health problem or characteristic over a given unit of time, such as a year.

The **prevalence rate** describes a situation at a given point in time. For example, if 63 students in a school have chickenpox, the number of students who have the disease is divided by the number of students in the school.

Community Assessment Framework

There are many sources for obtaining data for community assessment (see the accompanying box). Stewart (1985) proposes a general systems theory as a framework for community assessment. She identifies nine subsystems of the community for analysis: health, communication, economy, education, law, politics, recreation, religion, and social life. See Table 17–1 for details about assessment data for these subsystems.

Assessment of the **health subsystem** of a community includes collecting data about population size, rate of growth, density, and composition; life expectancy; overall health status of individuals; health care facilities and services and accessibility to the facilities; and quantity and types of caseloads of health professionals. The **communication subsystem** is an important part of the health of a community since a community relies on the abilities of individuals and groups to exchange ideas and feelings and work toward common goals. The **economic subsystem** or economic status of the community significantly affects the physical and emotional health of its citizens. Successful industries and high income and employment levels provide financial support for health, education, and recreational services. The **education subsystem** promotes intellectual development and socialization of

Sources of Community Assessment Data

- City maps to locate community boundaries, roads, churches, schools, parks, hospitals, and so on.
- State or provincial census data for population composition and characteristics.
- Chamber of Commerce for employment statistics, major industries, and primary occupations.
- Municipal, state or provincial health departments for location of health facilities, occupational health programs, numbers of health professionals, numbers of welfare recipients, and so on.
- City or regional health planning boards for health needs and practices.
- Telephone book for location of social, recreational, and health organizations, committees, and facilities.
- Public and university libraries for district social and cultural research reports.
- Health facility administrators for information about employee caseloads, prevalent types of problems, and dominant needs.
- Recreational directors for programs provided and participation levels.
- Police department for incidence of crime, vandalism, and drug addiction.
- Teachers and school nurses for incidence of children's health problems and information on facilities and services to maintain and promote health.
- Local newspapers for community activities related to health and wellness, such as health lectures or health fairs.
- On-line computer services that may provide access to public documents related to community health.

the community's youth. Communities that expend a great deal of energy on educational, social, and cultural activities achieve a higher level of development than those whose energies are directed toward law enforcement and economic concerns (Hanchett 1979). The **law subsystem** ensures social order and the safety of a community and thus preserves the emotional and physical security of its members. In regard to the **political subsystem,** "political jurisdictions identify the formal boundaries of many of a community's subsystems such as school, health, and police districts" (Stewart 1985, p. 371). Local and other governments carry specific responsibilities for

all community subsystem services that directly and indirectly affect the health of a community. The **recreational subsystem** provides facilities and activities that are essential for the physical, emotional, and social health of individuals and families. The **subsystem of religion** functions to promote the spiritual health of citizens. It is often a pervading force in providing support to individuals and families in times of crisis. **Social life** as a subsystem consists of all the social, economic, and ethnic classes of people in the community and the social clubs and organizations that function to promote cohesiveness of all members of the community.

TABLE 17–1 Systems Framework for Community Assessment

System	Assessment Data	Rationale
Health	Size	Size influences the number and size of health care agencies.
	Rate of growth or decline	Rapid growth may place excessive demands on health care services.
	Density	Density affects the availability of health care services.
	Composition	Composition may identify the types of health care needs.
	Life expectancy	Life expectancy indicates the need for services for the aged or the physically and mentally incapacitated.

TABLE 17–1 Systems Framework for Community Assessment *continued*

System	Assessment Data	Rationale
Health continued	Health status, including nutritional status	This reflects the overall physical, emotional, and social health of the members of the community.
	Health care facilities and services, including resource allocation and utilization, health programs, and age groups served	These indicate the degree to which the health needs of the community are being met.
	Geographic, economic, and cultural accessibility to health care services	Accessibility to health care services is considered a basic right by many people regardless of economic status, ethnic origin, or geographical location.
	Consumer participation in health care programs	Consumer participation reflects people's interest in and values about health maintenance and promotion.
	Number, type, and routine caseloads of health professionals (e.g., community health nurses, nutritionists, dental hygienists, family physicians and specialists, public health inspectors)	Caseload numbers and types indicate physical and emotional health problems prevalent in the community.
	Sources of health knowledge	This identifies information about agencies and available services for consumers.
	Levels of immunization among children	This information reflects the citizens' knowledge and values about disease prevention.
	Ambulance services	The availability of emergency services indicates the ability of the community to respond to life-threatening situations.
	Sanitation services	Quality sanitation services prevent disease.
	Opinions about community health services	Satisfaction with current services and proposed improvements can be determined.
	Environmental conditions of air, water, and soil	The state of the environment can affect physical and emotional health.
Communication	Existence and frequency of public forums	Public forums enable inputs or feedback to the system, thus enhancing satisfaction with and survival of the system.
	Telephone services	Telephones promote communication among members and ability to contact health services.
	Newspapers and television	Newspapers and television provide an ongoing flow of information about community activities and health care.
	Transportation and road networks	Transportation influences access to health care facilities and programs, as well as to recreational and educational facilities that indirectly affect health.
Economy	Industries and occupations	A strong industrial base in a community provides financial support for health, education, and recreational facilities.
	Number or percentage of population employed or attending school	Social health problems such as stress, depression, drug abuse, and crime are frequently widespread where there are economic problems such high unemployment.

TABLE 17–1 *continued*

System	Assessment Data	Rationale
Economy continued	Income levels and quality and types of housing (private dwellings, apartments, mobile homes, and so on)	Overcrowded and poor-quality dwellings may affect the health of residents.
	Occupational health programs	The presence of occupational health programs can help workers maintain health and prevent accidents.
Education/schools	School health facilities, services, and personnel	Quality health facilities and services can provide information and assistance to maintain and promote health.
	Existence of nutritious lunch programs, extracurricular sports activities, libraries, and counseling services	These services contribute to children's physical, emotional, and social health.
	Number and types of health problems handled by the school nurse	The number and types of problems reflect individual and family health problems in the community.
	Adjunctive services (e.g., resource teachers, community volunteers) for individuals with physical and mental disabilities	Available services and resources for the disabled indicate the attitudes of the community toward these citizens.
	Type of continuing education or evening extension classes provided	Continuing education programs can affect the development of a community, the literacy of its adults, and its overall health values.
	Parent-teacher associations and the extent of parental involvement in the schools	Maximum parental involvement in the schools can indicate minimal individual and family health problems such as school dropouts, teenage pregnancies, drug abuse, vandalism, etc.
Law	Caseloads of police force and lawyers	These caseloads identify the social problems of a community (e.g., child abuse, vandalism, drug addiction, alcoholism, juvenile crime, etc.). Such problems reflect the social order of the community, the safety of the citizens, and the need for special programs such as youth recreation, arts and crafts for older adults, and child abuse programs.
Politics	Responsibilities of local and other governments and community councils for all community subsystem services (e.g., health and welfare councils, housing authorities, transportation authorities, sanitation authorities	Formal political channels and authority to direct use of the health care dollar are reflected in government responsibilities.
	Political leaders or other influential people in community affairs	This helps the nurse determine and recognize the power framework and perhaps leaders' issues of concern.
	Election issues and average election turnout	Election turnouts can indicate the degree of citizen involvement, community cohesiveness, and desire to influence change.
Recreation	Location of *inexpensive* recreational services for all age groups, including use made of schools and other vacant buildings	Recreational activities provide physical and emotional outlets and intellectual stimulation that promote and maintain health.

→

TABLE 17–1 Systems Framework for Community Assessment *continued*

System	Assessment Data	Rationale
Recreation continued	Number of playgrounds, pools, sports fields, and parks and utilization of them	Existence and use of recreational facilities indicates the community system's goals and values about them.
	Participation levels in fitness programs	Low participation levels may indicate the need to provide inexpensive programs for certain age groups, such as senior citizens.
	Number of family-centered programs	Family-centered programs assist in the maintenance of family health and cohesiveness.
	Persons responsible for developing and maintaining playgrounds and parks	Knowledge of those responsible for playgrounds and parks helps the citizens provide direct input about any problems.
Religion	Number and types of churches and religious programs	Church members provide support to individuals and families, particularly in times of crisis.
	Level of participation in various church programs	Church programs help people grow spiritually and morally, both of which are important influencing factors in the development and maintenance of a healthy self-concept.
Social life	Predominant social classes, racial and ethnic makeup, language, values, and childrearing practices	The community's classes, cultures, and values affect its health and its ability to make use of input from the environment.
	Number and type of social committees, organizations, and clubs, and kinds of services offered	These groups promote cohesiveness of the system's citizens. Such groups, whether formal government agencies or informal friendship groups, often provide financial assistance, emotional support, counseling, and rehabilitation services to the handicapped and to senior citizens.
	Number of persons who belong to social groups and participate in volunteer activities	The level of participation and numbers of volunteers are indicators of community health.

SOURCE: Modified from "Community and Aggregates: Systematic Community Health Assessment" by M. Stewart, J. Innes, S. Searl, and C. Smillie, *Community Health Nursing in Canada*, 1985, Toronto, Ontario: Gage Educational Publishing, pp. 363–377.

Diagnosing

After assessing, validating, and summarizing data, the nurse identifies nursing diagnoses for the community. NANDA diagnoses have largely focused on individual and family responses. McCloskey and Bulechek (1996, p. 704) identify three community-focused NANDA nursing diagnoses:

- **Ineffective community coping:** a pattern of community activities for adaptation and problem solving that is unsatisfactory for meeting the demands or needs of the community (McCloskey & Bulechek, 1996, p. 618).

- **Potential for enhanced community coping:** a pattern of community activities for adaptation and problem solving that is satisfactory for meeting the demands or needs of the community but can be improved for management of current and future problems/stressors (McCloskey & Bulechek, 1996, p. 619).
- **Ineffective Community Management of Therapeutic Regimen:** a pattern of regulating and integrating into the community processes programs for treatment of illness and the sequelae of illness that are unsatisfactory for meeting health-related goals (McCloskey & Bulechek, 1996, p. 619).

Planning and Implementing

Planning community health may be oriented toward improved crisis management, disease prevention, health maintenance, or health promotion. The responsibility for planning at the community level is usually broadly based. The exact resources and skills of members of the community will often be dependent on the size of the community. A broadly based planning group is most likely to create a plan that is acceptable to members of the community. Also, people who are involved in planning become educated about the problems, the resources, and the interrelationships within the system relative to health and problems.

When setting priorities, health planners must work with consumers, interest groups, or other involved persons to prioritize health problems. The priority areas established in *Healthy People 2000* can be used as a guide in this stage (USDHHS 1990). See Chapter 8. It is important to take into consideration the values and interests of community members, the severity of the problems, and the resources available in order to identify and act on the problems. Because any plan will probably result in change, members of the planning group should be cognizant of and employ planned change theory. See Chapter 13.

Establishing goals also requires consumer participation. The goals should reflect a desirable state—for example, to reduce infant mortality 15%. National statistics and/or *Healthy People 2000* goals may be helpful in keeping goals realistic (see Chapter 3). Among the many other factors that must be considered are the traditions of people in the community, vested interests, current organizations, and resources, all of which may be barriers to change. An example of a goal of a community would be to reduce the incidence of infectious disease in a school.

Outcome criteria or objectives are specific, measurable targets. An example of such an objective is an increase in immunization levels by 20%, to be achieved by September 1998.

Implementing nursing strategies in community health is generally a collaborative action. According to Spradley (1990), nurses are also frequently catalysts and facilitators in implementation of plans. The primary goal in community health nursing is to help people help themselves.

McCloskey and Bulechek (1996) through the Nursing Intervention Classification (NIC) Project, describe three specific interventions appropriate to the management of community health problems: **environmental management: community, health policy monitoring,** and **health education.** In implementing health education (NIC 5510) as an intervention, the nurse "develops and provides instruction and learning experiences to facilitate voluntary adaptation of behavior conducive to health in individuals, families, groups, or communities." See Chapter 9 for more information about the nurse as a health educator. In promoting community environmental management (NIC 6486), the nurse "monitors and influences the physical, social, cultural, economic, and political conditions that affect the health of groups and communities" through the following activities (McCloskey & Bulechek, 1996, p. 258):

- Initiating screening for health risks from the environment.
- Participating in multidisciplinary teams to identify threats to safety in the community.
- Monitoring the status of known health risks.
- Participating in community programs to deal with known risks.
- Collaborating in the development of community action programs.
- Promoting governmental policy to reduce specified risks.
- Encouraging neighborhoods to become active participants in community safety.
- Coordinating services to at-risk groups and communities.
- Conducting educational programs for targeted risk groups.
- Working with environmental groups to secure appropriate governmental regulations.

McCloskey and Bulechek also describe the nurse's role in political advocacy in the nursing intervention health policy monitoring (NIC 7970), which is defined as the "surveillance and influence of government and organization regulations, rules, and standards that affect nursing systems and practices to ensure quality care of patients." The nurse does this by carrying out the following activities (McCloskey & Bulechek, 1996, p. 310):

1. Reviewing proposed policies and standards in organizational, professional, and governmental literature, and in the popular media.

2. Assessing implications and requirements of proposed policies and standards for quality client care.

3. Comparing requirement of policies and standards with current practices.

4. Assessing negative and positive effects of health policies and standards on nursing practice, client, and cost outcomes.

5. Identifying and resolving discrepancies between health policies and standards and current nursing practice.

6. Acquainting policy makers with implications of current and proposed policies and standards for client welfare.

7. Lobbying policy makers to make changes in health policies and standards to benefit clients.

8. Testifying in organizational, professional, and public forums to influence the formulation of health policies and standards that benefit clients.

9. Assisting consumers of health care to be informed of current and proposed changes in health policies and standards and the implications for health outcomes.

See Chapter 22 for more information about the nurse as a political activist.

Evaluating

In community health, evaluation determines whether the planned interventions have led to the achievement of the established goals and objectives; for example, was the immunization rate of preschool children improved. Because community health is usually a collaborative process between health providers, including nurses, community leaders, politicians, and consumers, all may be involved in the evaluation process. Often the community health nurse is the agent of evaluation in collecting and assessing the data that determines the effectiveness of implemented programs. Evaluation data may include community statistics related to changes in disease incidence rates, mortality and morbidity rates, the costs to provide programs and the availability of required financial and other resources, and citizen program utilization and satisfaction rates. Leaders must decide whether the benefits of a program merit the costs in money, time, and other resources. Based on such evaluation, effective programs may be continued, ineffective programs may be discontinued, existing programs may be modified, or new programs might be implemented.

CONSIDER...

• the responsibility and role of the hospital-based nurse in promoting community health. What activities can all nurses pursue to promote community health?

• the value of collaboration among various health professionals in promoting community health. How can health professionals influence legislators and policy makers, who have little or no knowledge and experience related to health care, to make wise and effective decisions regarding community health?

INTEGRATION OF HOME AND COMMUNITY NURSING

"Home care has been an organized system of care in the United States for approximately 100 years. Home care was developed in response to (a) the needs and preferences of families to care for ill and infirm members at home and (b) limitations and costs of institutional care" (Barkauskas 1990, p. 394). The focus of home nursing has always been on the individual client, and their family. Community nursing has an equally prestigious history as nurses focused on the health needs of the community as a whole. In many ways the roles and practice settings of the home health care nurse and the community health nurse are separate and distinct. For example, the home health care nurse works exclusively in the client's residence. Community nurses may work in the home but are more frequently found in clinics, immigrant and refugee centers, public health centers, community nursing centers, and other community-based providers of care outside the home or hospital. The home health care nurse is usually providing care to a client who is recovering from illness or injury; the community health nurse is usually working in areas of health promotion and illness prevention.

The home health care nurse is the care provider, teacher, and advocate for the client and their family. The nurse may intervene to mobilize the resources of the community or the hospital to meet the client's identified needs, but the focus remains the client and family. The community nurse may work with the individual client and their family but often must subjugate the needs of the individual to the needs of the community. For example, a client with a highly communicable disease may have their freedom of movement restricted in order to protect the community, or a client diagnosed with a sexually transmitted disease may have to defer their right of confidentiality for the identification and treatment of their contacts.

Some consider home health nursing an aspect of community nursing as the client's residence is within his or her community and the strengths and weaknesses of the community impact on the client's ability to stay well or recover from illness in the home. While the issue of whether home health nursing is community nursing may be debated, it is more important that nurses recognize the wide range of professional opportunities for nurses to influence the health of individuals, families, and communities.

CONSIDER...

• what academic and experiential qualifications a nurse should have to practice in the home or community setting. What are the differences in knowledge and skill required to become certified as a home care nurse of a community health nurse?

• the differences in autonomy in decision making and practice between the hospital nurse, the home care nurse, and the community nurse. Does one type of nurse have greater autonomy than another, or are there simply differences in the types of independent decision making and practice?

READINGS FOR ENRICHMENT

Deal, L. W. (1994, Oct.). The effectiveness of community health nursing interventions: A literature review. *Public Health Nursing, 11* (5), 315–323.

In this era of increasingly limited health care resources, it is imperative that community health nurses document the effectiveness of their interventions. This article describes a variety of interventions community health nurses provide in response to needs of high-risk families, specific geographical communities, and other vulnerable population groups. The effectiveness of these interventions is based on available literature. Descriptive analyses and outcome evaluation studies are used to support the effectiveness of home-based and community-centered nursing interventions and to provide a basis for eliciting local, state, and national support.

Lusk, S. L., Ronis, D. L., Kerr, M. J., & Atwood, J. R. (1994, May/June). Test of the Health Promotion Model as a causal model of workers' use of hearing protection. *Nursing Research, 43*(3), 151–157.

An estimated 14 million workers in the United States are exposed to hazardous noise levels at work. This study utilized Pender's Health Promotion Model as a causal model to predict workers' use of hearing protection. The theoretical model was an excellent fit and accounted for approximately half of the variance in behavior. Self-efficacy, value of use, and barriers had the strongest effects. These findings support the rationale for use of Pender's Health Promotion Model to predict this protective behavior.

May, K. M., & Evans, G. G. (1994, Fall/Winter). Health education for homeless populations. *Journal of Community Health Nursing, 11*(4), 229–237.

Fifty volunteer instructors, including nurses, provided a health education program for the homeless in 13 urban shelters and treatment sites. Approximately 50 health topics were discussed in 176 classes. The program was evaluated through a client survey. Clients found the classes helpful and provided suggestions for future topics, such as stress management and increasing self-esteem. Their perceived ability to discuss issues was related to group size and gender composition. Survey results provided feedback for program development.

Spradley, B. W. (1991). *Readings in Community Health Nursing* (4th ed.). Philadelphia: Lippincott.

This anthology of reprinted articles is designed to provide insights into the nature of community health nursing in today's world. The articles present important contemporary aspects of health care and community health nursing in an interesting and meaningful manner. The book discusses topics related to community health nursing: the issues, trends, and mission; assessment and health planning; tool utilization; nursing populations, groups, and families; cultural dimensions; and ethical and political influences.

SUMMARY

Because of changing demographics and a need for health care cost containment, the focus of health care has shifted from hospital-based illness treatment to community-based health promotion and disease prevention in home and community settings. While not new nursing practice settings, this shift in focus has created new opportunities for nurses to impact the health of individuals, families, and communities.

Home health care nursing is a rapidly growing industry providing a wide range of nursing services to clients in their places of residence. It may include the administration of physician prescribed treatments, independent nursing interventions, and high-tech therapies including chemotherapy and dialysis. The home health care nurse assesses the care needs of clients in their home; plans, implements, and supervises that care; teaches clients and their families self-care; and mobilizes the resources of hospitals, physicians, and community agencies in meeting the needs of the clients and their families.

Community health nurses may provide nursing services in the home, but are more frequently found in clinics, schools, and other community-based settings. Community health nurses focus on the health needs of the community as a whole, providing health education, illness prevention through immunization programs, and communicable disease follow-up.

Both home health care nurses and community health nurses are essential components of a health care delivery system that ensures access to quality health care at an affordable cost.

SELECTED REFERENCES

American Nurses Association. (1992). *A statement on the scope of home health nursing practice.* Washington, DC: Author.

American Nurses Credentialing Center. (1995). *1995 Certification Catalog.* Washington, DC: Author.

ANCC approves new certification program for clinical specialist in home health nursing. (1995, July 4). *Vital signs: The pulse of Florida's health care opportunities,* p. 11.

Barkauskas, V. H. (1990). Home health care: Responding to need, growth, and cost containment. In N. L. Chaska (Ed.), *The Nursing Profession: Turning Points* (pp. 394–405). St. Louis: Mosby.

Carpenito, L. J. (1992). *Nursing diagnosis: Application to clinical practice* (4th ed.). Philadelphia: Lippincott.

Hegyvary, S. T. (1990, Jan./Feb.). Education: Redefining community. *Journal of Professional Nursing, 6,* 7.

Home health care update 95. (1995, July). *Nursing 95, 7,* 57–59.

Kalisch, P. A., & Kalisch, B. J. (1995). *The advance of American nursing* (3rd ed.). Philadelphia: Lippincott.

Leavell, H. R., & Clark, E. G. (1965). *Preventive medicine for the doctor in his community* (3rd ed.). New York: McGraw-Hill.

McCloskey, J. C., & Bulechek, G. M. (1996). *Iowa Intervention Project: Nursing interventions classification (NIC)* (2nd ed.). St. Louis: Mosby.

McFarland, G. K., & McFarlane, E. A. (1993). *Nursing diagnosis and intervention: Planning for patient care* (2nd ed.). St. Louis: Mosby.

McFarland, G. K., & McFarlane, E. A. (1995). *Mosby's home health nursing pocket consultant.* St. Louis: Mosby.

Spradley, B. W. (1990). *Community health nursing: Concepts and practice* (3rd ed.). Glenview, IL: Scott, Foresman.

Spradley, B. W. (1991). *Readings in community health nursing* (4th ed.). Philadelphia: Lippincott.

Spradley, J. W., & Allender, J. A. (1996). *Community health nursing: Concepts and practice* (4th ed.). Philadelphia: Lippincott.

Stanhope, M., & Lancaster, J. (1996). *Community health nursing: Promoting health of aggregates, families, and individuals* (4th ed.). St. Louis: Mosby.

Stewart, M. (1985). Community and aggregates: Systematic community health assessment. In M. Stewart, J. Innes, S. Searl, & C. Smillie (Eds.), *Community health nursing in Canada* (pp. 363–377). Toronto, Ontario: Gage Educational Publishing.

Stulginsky, M. M. (1993a, Oct.). Nurses' home health experience. Part 1: The practice setting. *Nursing & Health Care, 14*(8), 402–407.

Stulginsky, M. M. (1993b, Nov.). Nurses' home health experience. Part 2: The unique demands of home visits. *Nursing & Health Care, 14*(9), 476–485.

U.S. Department of Health and Human Services. (1990, Sept.). *Healthy People 2000: National health promotion and disease prevention objectives.* (DHHS No. PHS 91-50212). Washington, DC: U.S. Government Printing Office.

U.S. Department of Health and Human Services. (1991). *Health personnel in the U.S.: Eighth report to Congress.* (DHHS No. HRS P-00-92-1). Rockville, MD: U.S. Government Printing Office.

Warhola, C. (1980, Aug.). *Planning for home health services: A resource handbook.* (Pub No. HRA 80-14017). Washington, DC: USDHHS, Public Health Service.

Supporting Cultural Needs

OBJECTIVES

- Identify components of Leininger's Sunrise Model.

- Identify concepts pertaining to cultural diversity in nursing.

- Discuss components of culture pertinent to nursing care.

- Identify guidelines to foster culturally sensitive health care.

- Assess clients from a cultural perspective and plan culturally competent client care.

"What the people need most to grow, remain well, avoid illness and survive or to face death is human caring. Care is the essence of nursing and the distinct, dominant, central, and unifying, focus of nursing; caring is the "heart and soul" of nursing and what people seek most from professional nurses and in health care services; nurses are therefore challenged to gain knowledge about cultural care values, beliefs, and practices, and to use this knowledge to care for well and sick people."

— Madeleine Leininger, 1991

Nurses need to become informed about and sensitive to culturally diverse subjective meanings of health, illness, caring, and healing practices. A transcultural care perspective is now considered essential for nurses and other health care professionals to deliver quality health care to all clients.

- North America is a continent of many cultural groups. It has been called a "melting pot" of peoples: however, the term "cultural mosaic" may be a more accurate description of the way in which many people of different cultures maintain the cultural values, beliefs, traditions, and practices of their "homeland" for many generations.
- In addition to the indigenous peoples (Native Americans and Aboriginals), there is much diversity in immigrant groups in North America.
- It is important for nurses to understand their own cultural beliefs and biases.
- Health care professionals are not expected to know and understand *all* cultures of the world; it is possible, however, for health care professionals to develop an in-depth understanding of three or four cultures and to learn about other cultures through time (Leininger, 1993, p. 32).
- It is important for nurses to be aware that although people from a given ethnic group share certain beliefs, values, and experiences, often there is also widespread intra-ethnic diversity. Major differences within ethnic groups may be due to such factors as age, sex, level of education, socioeconomic status, religious affiliation, and area of origin in the home country (rural or urban). Such factors influence the client's beliefs about health and illness, health and illness practices, help-seeking behaviors, and expectations of health professionals (Anderson, Waxler-Morrison, Richardson, Herbert & Murphy, 1990, p. 246). For these reasons, nurses should make special effort to avoid ethnic stereotyping.

- In 1991, the American Nurses Association (ANA) stated that "culture is one of the organizing concepts upon which nursing is based and defined" (ANA, 1991, p. 1). Nurses need to understand how cultural groups understand life processes, how cultural groups define health and illness, what cultural groups do to maintain wellness, what cultural groups believe to be the causes of illness, how healers cure and care for members of cultural groups, and how the cultural background of the nurse influences the way in which the nurse provides care. Because the nurse is expected to provide individualized care based on an assessment of the client's physiologic, psychologic, and developmental status, the nurse must understand how the client's cultural beliefs and practices can affect the client's health and illness (ANA, 1991, p. 1).

CONCEPTS RELATED TO CULTURE

All groups of people face similar issues in adapting to their environment: providing nutrition and shelter, caring for and educating children, division of labor, social organization, controlling disease, and maintaining health. Humans adapt to varying environments by developing cultural solutions to meet these needs. An understanding of the cultural dimension of people is the focus of the field of anthropology. Cultural anthropologists attempt to understand culture by studying both similarities and differences among human groups. Nurses use the cultural information gained by cultural anthropologists to understand and help clients (individuals, their families, or groups) to achieve optimum health.

Culture is a universal experience, but no two cultures are exactly alike. Two important terms identify the differences and similarities among peoples of different cultures. **Culture-universals** are the commonalities of values, norms of behavior, and life patterns that are similar among different cultures. **Culture-specifics** are those values, beliefs, and patterns of behavior that tend to be unique to a designated culture and do not tend to be shared with members of other cultures. For example, most cultures have ceremonies to celebrate the passage from childhood to adulthood; this practice is a culture-universal. However, different cultural groups celebrate this important life event in very different ways. In Latin or Hispanic cultures, the "quince" or "quinceañero" party, which celebrates a girl's fifteenth birthday, signifies that the young girl has now become a woman. In the Jewish tradition, the bar mitzvah (for boys) and the bat mitzvah (for girls) are celebrations of the passage to adulthood.

Anthropologists have also traditionally divided culture into material and nonmaterial culture. **Material culture** refers to objects (such as dress, art, religious artifacts, or eating utensils) and ways these are used. **Nonmaterial culture** refers to beliefs, customs, languages, and social institutions.

The terms *culture, diversity, ethnicity,* and *race* are often used interchangeably, but they are not synonymous. **Culture** is defined as "the learned, shared, and transmitted values, beliefs, norms, and lifeway practices of a particular group that guide thinking, decisions, and actions in patterned ways" (Leininger, 1988, p. 158).

Because cultural patterns are learned, it is important for nurses to note that members of a particular group may not share identical cultural experiences. Thus, each member of a cultural group will be somewhat different from his or her own cultural counterparts (Waxler-Morrison, et al., 1990 p. 6). For example, white Roman Catholics will have cultural patterns and beliefs different from those of white Seventh-Day Adventists. Third-generation Japanese Americans, or *Sansei,* will differ in cultural understandings from first-generation Japanese, or *Issei.*

Large cultural groups often have cultural subgroups or subsystems. A **subculture** is usually composed of people who have a distinct identity and yet are also related to a larger cultural group. A subcultural group generally shares ethnic origin, occupation, or physical characteristics with the larger cultural group. Examples of cultural subgroups include occupational groups (e.g., nurses), societal groups (e.g., feminists), and ethnic groups (e.g., Cajuns, who are descendants of French Acadians).

Bicultural is used to describe a person who crosses two cultures, life-styles, and sets of values (Giger & Davidhizar, 1991, p. 51). For example, a young man whose father is Cherokee and whose mother is European American may maintain his traditional Cherokee heritage while also being influenced by his mother's cultural values.

Diversity refers to the "fact or state of being different" (Steinmetz & Braham, 1993, p. 141). Many factors account for differences: race, gender, sexual orientation, culture, ethnicity, socioeconomic status, educational attainment, religious affiliation, and so

on. Diversity therefore occurs not only between cultural groups but also within a cultural group.

The term **ethnic** refers to a group of people who share a common and distinctive culture and who are members of a specific group. The **ethnic group** shares a common social and cultural heritage that is passed on to successive generations (Giger & Davidhizar, 1991, p. 51). The characteristics of the group give an individual a sense of **cultural identity. Ethnicity** has been defined as "a consciousness of belonging to a group that is differentiated from others by symbolic markers (culture, biology, territory). It is rooted in bonds of a shared past and perceived ethnic interest" (Sprott, 1993, p. 190). Other factors that help to define ethnicity are religion and geographic background of the family.

Race is the classification of people according to shared biologic characteristics, genetic markers, or features. They have common characteristics such as skin color, bone structure, facial features, hair texture, and blood type. Different ethnic groups can belong to the same race, and different cultures can be found within the same ethnic group. For example, the term *Caucasian* and *European American* describe the race of people whose origins are in Europe. Whereas British Americans are a subgroup of European Americans, Scottish Americans (an ethnic subgroup of British Americans) may share different cultural practices than other British Americans. It is important to understand that not all people of the same race have the same culture. Culture should not be confused with either race or ethnic group.

It is helpful to differentiate the terms *acculturation* and *ethnic identity.* **Acculturation** is often defined in terms of such observable factors as dress, food, language, and values. Individuals who are acculturated may no longer eat foods associated with their culture or always wear traditional dress (Lynam, 1992, p. 151). **Ethnic identity,** in contrast, refers to a subjective perspective of the person's heritage and to a sense of belonging to a group that is distinguishable from other groups. Thus, people may be visibly acculturated to the mainstream culture but may retain an identity that differs from the mainstream.

The cultural beliefs and practices regarding the health and illness of North America's many different ethnic and cultural groups are important considerations for nurses in planning nursing care. Nursing ethnoscientists study the health beliefs of cultures so that nurses can provide culturally competent care to clients of different cultures. Madeleine Leininger, a nurse anthropologist, described **transcultural nursing** as the study of different cultures and subcultures with respect to nursing and health illness caring practices, beliefs, and values (1978, p. 493). The goal of transcultural nursing is to provide culture-specific and culture-universal nursing care. Cultural awareness and cultural sensitivity are prerequisite to the provision of culturally competent nursing care. **Cultural awareness** is the conscious and informed recognition of the differences and similarities between different cultural or ethnic groups. Cultural awareness is not knowledge derived solely from myths and stereotypes. **Cultural sensitivity** is the respect and appreciation for cultural behaviors based on an understanding of the other person's perspective. **Cultural competence** is "knowing, utilizing, and appreciating the culture of another in assisting with the resolution of a problem" (DeSantis & Lowe 1992, p. 1). The culturally competent nurse, therefore, works within the cultural belief system of the client to resolve health problems. To provide culturally competent care, nurses need data about the client's personal and cultural views regarding health and illness. To make valid assessments, nurses need to try to see and hear the world as their clients do. When developing care plans, nurses need to consider the client's world and daily experiences. Although a client's needs and behaviors can be better understood when particular cultural health norms are identified, nurses must take care to avoid stereotyping clients by culture norms. This allows for individualized care.

Culture shock can occur when members of one culture are abruptly moved to another culture or setting. **Culture shock** is the state of being disoriented or unable to respond to a different cultural environment because of its sudden strangeness, unfamiliarity, and incompatibility to the stranger's perceptions and expectations (Leininger, 1978, p. 490). For example, when immigrants first enter the United States or Canada, language and behavior differences may initially cause them difficulty in carrying out normal activities. People can also experience culture shock when they are abruptly thrust into the health care subculture. Nursing students, for example, may experience culture shock when they enter nursing school and must learn medical terminology (a new language) and provide care for clients in clinical environments with which they are unfamiliar. Expressions of culture shock can range from silence and immobility to agitation.

Not uncommonly, people of a minority group assume the attitudes, values, beliefs, and practices of the dominant or host society, resulting in a new blended cultural pattern. This process is referred to as cultural **assimilation** or **acculturation**.

CONSIDER . . .

- the various cultural and ethnic groups in your community. Is cultural difference valued? If cultural and ethnic difference is valued, in what ways is this value manifested in your community, the nation, and the world? In what ways are negative responses to cultural difference manifested in your community, the nation, the world?

Characteristics of Culture

Culture exhibits several characteristics.

- *Culture is learned.* It is neither instinctive nor innate. It is learned through life experiences from birth.
- *Culture is taught.* It is transmitted from parents to children over successive generations. All animals can learn, but only humans can pass along culture. Verbal and nonverbal communication patterns are the transmitters of culture.
- *Culture is social.* It originates and develops through the interactions of people: families, groups, and communities.
- *Culture is adaptive.* Customs, beliefs, and practices change as people adapt to the social environment and as biologic and psychologic needs of people change. Some traditional forms in a culture may cease to provide satisfaction and are eliminated. For example, in many cultures it is customary for family members of different generations to live together (extended family); however, education and employment considerations may require children to leave their parents and move to other parts of the country. In such cases, the extended family norm may change.
- *Culture is satisfying.* Cultural habits persist only as long as they satisfy people's needs. Gratification strengthens habits and beliefs. Once they no longer bring gratification, they may disappear.
- *Culture is difficult to articulate.* Members of a specific cultural group often find it difficult to articulate their own culture. Many of the values and behaviors are habitual and are carried out subconsciously.

- *Culture exists at many levels.* Culture is most easily identified at the material level. For example, art, tools, and clothes usually reveal aspects of a culture relatively readily. More abstract concepts, such as values, beliefs, and traditions, are often more difficult to find out about. Nurses may need to ask culture-sensitive questions of the client or support persons to obtain this information.

Components of Culture

Cultures are very complex. They consist of facets that relate to all aspects of life: language, art, music, values systems (beliefs, morals, rules), religion, philosophy, family interaction, patterns of behavior, childrearing practices, rituals or ceremonies, recreation and leisure activities, festivals and holidays, nutrition, food preferences, and health practices. Many facets of culture (e.g., health and illness practices, attitudes about touch, territory and privacy, childbirth, and death and dying practices) have an impact on nursing practice.

Religious values are part of the cultural values of groups that have one dominant religion. For example, the roles of men and women in Islamic cultures is clearly defined by the Koran. The tenets of Roman Catholicism dictate the value for life and family and influence both laws and customs in many Roman Catholic cultures around the world. Culture and religion are deeply intertwined among many Jews, most notably in the nation of Israel, which is founded on Jewish beliefs and traditions.

Religions values associated with any culture influence many facets of life, including dietary restrictions, family planning, use of blood transfusions, and death-related practices, such as autopsy, organ donation, cremation, and prolonging life.

CONSIDER...

- your own cultural values, beliefs, and practices. How do you describe yourself culturally? What meaning does your cultural identification have for you? How do you celebrate your cultural identification? How do your cultural beliefs and practices influence your religious or spiritual beliefs and practices? How do your religious or spiritual beliefs and practices influence your cultural beliefs and practices?

CULTURE AND HEALTH CARE

Two transcultural health care systems generally exist side by side with limited awareness by practitioners of both systems: an indigenous health care system and a professional health care system (Leininger, 1993, p. 36). The *indigenous health care system* refers to traditional folk health care methods, such as folk medicines and other home treatments. The modern *professional health care system* refers to a structured system maintained by individuals who have engaged in a formal program of study. The indigenous system is the older system and has often provided health care long before a professional system enters the culture. According to Leininger, few professional health care workers are knowledgeable about the indigenous health care system or its practitioners. Some professionals regard the indigenous system as unscientific or "primitive," or even as "quackery." Leininger emphasizes that the goal of health care should be to use the best of both systems and that health professionals need to consider ways to interface with the two systems for the benefit of the people served. "Every culture has health, caring, and curing processes, techniques, and practices viewed as important to the people" (1993, p. 38).

Leininger's Sunrise Model

Leininger produced the Sunrise Model to depict her theory of cultural care diversity and universality (Figure 18–1). This model emphasizes that health and care are influenced by elements of the social structure, such as technology, religious and philosophical factors, kinship and social systems, cultural values, political and legal factors, economic factors, and educational factors. These social factors are addressed within environmental contexts, language expressions, and ethnohistory. Each of these systems is part of the social structure of any society; health care expressions, patterns, and practices are also integral parts of these aspects of social structure (Leininger, 1993, p. 35).

Technologic factors, such as the availability of technical and electrical equipment, greatly determine what health equipment will be used. For example, many European Americans regard resuscitative equipment as essential. The *economic* system determines the quality of health care within a culture, for example, the availability of funds for health care services materially affects the health of the culture's

Sunrise Model

Leininger's Sunrise Model to Depict Theory of Cultural Care
Diversity and Universality
Cultural Care
World View
Cultural & Social Structure Dimensions

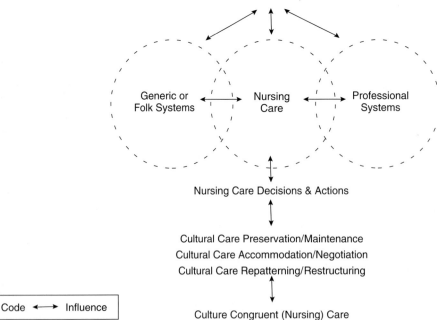

Cultural
Values &
Lifeways

Kinship &
Social
Factors

Environmental Context
Language & Ethnohistory

Political &
Legal
Factors

Religious &
Philosophical
Factors

Influences
Care Expressions
Patterns & Practices

Economic
Factors

Technological
Factors

Health (Well Being)

Educational
Factors

Individuals, Families, Groups, Communities & Institutions
in Diverse Health Systems

Generic or
Folk Systems

Nursing
Care

Professional
Systems

Nursing Care Decisions & Actions

Cultural Care Preservation/Maintenance
Cultural Care Accommodation/Negotiation
Cultural Care Repatterning/Restructuring

Code ◄──► Influence

Culture Congruent (Nursing) Care

FIGURE 18–1 *Leininger's Sunrise Model.*

SOURCE: *Culture Care Diversity and Universality: A Theory of Nursing* by M. Leininger, 1991,
New York: National League for Nursing Pub. No. 15-2402, p. 43. Reprinted with permission.

infants and aged. The *political* system is a major determinant of what health programs will be available and which health practitioners may provide health services. *Legal* aspects govern the roles, functions, and standards of health professionals within cultures. *Kinship and the social system* often influence who will or will not receive health care and how promptly it will be provided. For example, in some cultures a person of high status (e.g., tribal leader, CEO, or king) may receive prompt care; a person of lower status (e.g., a peasant, housewife, or child) may experience a considerable waiting period for care. Because of male dominance in many cultures, men may receive care before a wife or female child. *Cultural, educational, religious,* and *philosophical* factors are closely related. They influence the type, quality and quantity of health care considered desirable, appropriate, or acceptable to the culture. *Environmental* and *demographic* factors relate to the health needs of the culture and which strategies of care can be used in the setting.

CULTURALLY SENSITIVE CARE

Kittler and Sucher (1990) suggest a four-step process to improve cultural sensitivity:

1. *Become aware of one's own cultural heritage.* Nurses should identify their own cultural values and beliefs. For example, does the nurse value stoic behavior in relation to pain? Are the rights of the individual valued over and above the rights of the family? Only by knowing one's own culture (values, practices, and beliefs) can a person be ready to learn about another's.

2. *Become aware of the client's culture as described by the client.* It is important to avoid assuming that all people of the same ethnic background have the same culture. When the nurse has a knowledge of the client's culture, mutual respect between client and nurse is more likely to develop.

3. *Become aware from the client of adaptations made to live in a North American culture.* During this interview, a nurse can also identify the client's preferences in health practices, diet, hygiene, and so on.

4. *Form a nursing care plan with the client that incorporates his or her culture.* In this way, cultural values, practices, and beliefs can be incorporated with care and judgment.

Barriers to Cultural Sensitivity

Many factors can be barriers to providing culturally sensitive or culturally congruent care to clients and their support persons. These factors can also affect communication and working relationships with other health care personnel. Ethnocentrism, stereotyping, prejudice, and discrimination are some of these factors.

Ethnocentrism refers to an individual's belief that his or her culture's beliefs and values are superior to those of other cultures. In the health care area, ethnocentrism means that the only valid health care beliefs and practices are those held by the health care culture. Nurses who take a transcultural view, however, value their own beliefs and practices while respecting the belief and practices of others. It is important for nurses to realize that although many people of differing racial and religious backgrounds have combined their traditional health practices with Western health practices, other people may be unable to do so.

Most people are gradually exposed to the cultural beliefs, values, and practices over a period of years starting at birth. Ethnocentrism is thought to result from lack of exposure or knowledge of cultures other than one's own. **Ethnorelativity** is the ability to appreciate and respect other viewpoints different from one's own.

Stereotyping is assuming that all members of a culture or ethnic group are alike. For example, a nurse may assume that all Italians express pain volubly or that all Chinese people like rice. Stereotyping may be based on generalizations founded in research, or it may be unrelated to reality. For example, research indicates that Italians are likely to express pain verbally; however, an Italian client may not verbalize pain. Stereotyping that is unrelated to reality may be either positive or negative and is frequently an outcome of racism or discrimination.

It is important for nurses to realize that not all people of a specific group will have the same health beliefs, practices, and values. It is therefore essential to identify a specific client's beliefs, needs, and values rather than assuming they are the same as those attributable to the larger group.

Prejudice is strongly held opinion about some topic or group of people. A prejudice may be positive or negative. A positive prejudice often stems from a strong sense of ethnocentrism (Eliason, 1993, p. 226), that is, beliefs that one's cultural group are vastly superior to the beliefs held by others. One example is that American nursing education is superior to European nursing education. Prejudice may also derive from ignorance, misinformation, past experience, or fear. Other types of negative prejudice are ageism, which includes negative attitudes toward older adults; sexism, meaning negative attitudes toward women; and homophobia, which is negativism toward lesbians and gay men.

Banks and Banks (1989, p. 327) define **discrimination** as "the differential treatment of individuals or groups based on categories such as race, ethnicity, gender, social class, or exceptionality." For example, a nurse takes a child who is waiting in an emergency department ahead of another child. The child taken ahead appears clean, is neatly dressed, and is smiling; the other child appears dirty, is wearing worn clothes, and is angry. **Racism** is a form of discrimination related to ethnocentrism where a person believes that race is the primary determinant of human traits and capacities and that racial differences produce an inherent superiority of a particular race.

Conveying Cultural Sensitivity

It is important for nurses to be culturally sensitive and to convey this sensitivity to clients, support persons, and other health care personnel. Some of the ways to do so follow.

- Always address clients by their last names (e.g., Mrs. Aylia, Dr. Rush) until they give you permission to use other names. In some cultures, the more formal style of address is a sign of respect, whereas the informal use of first names may be considered disrespect. It is important to ask clients how they wish to be addressed.
- When meeting a person for the first time, introduce yourself by name, and, when appropriate, explain your position. This helps establish a relationship and provides an opportunity for both clients and nurses to clarify pronunciation of one another's names, and so on.
- Be authentic with people, and share your lack of knowledge about their culture.
- Use language that is culturally sensitive; for example, say "gay," "lesbian," or "bisexual" rather than "homosexual"; do not use "man" or "mankind" when referring to a woman; "African American" and "Latino" are currently preferred over "black" or "Hispanic." "Asian" is more acceptable than "Oriental" (Eliason, 1993, p. 228).

However, nurses need to keep up with language changes.

- Find out what the client knows about his or her health problems, illness, and treatments. Assess whether this information is congruent with the dominant health care culture. If the beliefs and practices are incongruent, establish whether this will have a negative effect on the client's health.
- Do not make any assumptions about the client, and always ask about anything you don't understand.
- Respect the client's values, beliefs, and practices, even if they differ from your own or from those of the dominant culture. If you don't agree with them, it is important to respect the client's right to hold these beliefs.
- Show respect for the client's support people. In some cultures males in the family make decisions affecting the client, while in other cultures females make the decisions.
- Make a concerted effort to obtain the client's trust, but do not be surprised if it develops slowly or not at all.

SELECTED CULTURAL PARAMETERS FOR NURSING

This section outlines selected cultural and ethnic phenomena of significance to nursing.

Health Beliefs and Practices

Andrews and Boyle (1995, pp. 22–29) describe three health belief views: magico-religious, scientific, and holistic. In the **magico-religious health belief view,** health and illness are controlled by supernatural forces. The client may believe that illness is the result of "being bad" or opposing God's will. Getting well is also viewed as dependent on God's will. The client may make statements such as, "If it is God's will, I will recover," or "What did I do wrong to be punished with cancer?" Some cultures believe that magic can cause illness. A sorceror or witch may put a spell or hex on the client. Some people view illness as possession by an evil spirit. Although these beliefs are not supported by empirical evidence, clients who believe that such things can cause illness may, in fact, become ill as a result. Such illnesses may require magical treatments in addition to scientific treatments. For example, a man who experiences gastric distress, headaches, and hypertension after being told that a spell has been placed on him may recover only if the spell is removed by the culture's healer.

The scientific or **biomedical health belief view** is based on the belief that life and life processes are controlled by physical and biochemical processes that can be manipulated by humans (Andrews & Boyle, 1995, p. 23). The client with this view will believe that illness is caused by germs, viruses, bacteria, or a breakdown of the human machine, the body. This client will expect a pill, or treatment, or a surgery to cure health problems.

The **holistic health belief view** holds that the forces of nature must be maintained in balance or harmony. Human life is one aspect of nature that must be in harmony with the rest of nature. When the natural balance or harmony is disturbed, illness results. The Medicine Wheel is an ancient symbol used by Native Americans of North and South America to express many concepts. Related to health and wellness, the Medicine Wheel teaches the four aspects of the individual's nature: the physical, the mental, the emotional, and the spiritual. Each of the dimensions must be in balance to be healthy. The Medicine Wheel can also be used to express the individual's relationship with the environment as a dimension of wellness. The concept of yin and yang in the Chinese culture and the hot/cold theory of illness in many Spanish cultures are examples of holistic health beliefs. When the client has a yin illness or a "cold" illness, the treatment will need to include a yang or "hot" food. For example, a Chinese client who has been diagnosed with cancer, a yin disease, will want to eat cultural foods that have yang properties. What is considered as hot or cold varies considerably across cultures. In many cultures, the mother who has just delivered a baby should be offered warm or hot foods and kept warm with blankets, because childbirth is seen as a "cold" condition. Conventional scientific thought recommends cooling the body to reduce a fever. The physician may order liquids for the client and cool compresses to be applied to the forehead, the axillae, or the groin. Galanti (1991, p. 97) states that many cultures believe that the best way to treat a fever is to "sweat it out." Clients from these cultures may want to cover up with several blankets, take hot baths, and drink hot beverages. Giger and Davidhizar (1995, p. 84) state that the nurse must keep in mind that a treatment strategy that is consistent with the client's beliefs may have a better chance of being successful. For example, the Mexican-American client who avoids "hot" foods when he has a stomach disturbance such as an ulcer may be eating foods consistent with the bland diet that is normally prescribed by physicians for clients with ulcers.

Sociocultural forces, such as politics, economics, geography, religion, and the predominant health care system, can influence the client's health status and health care behavior. For example, people who have limited access to scientific health care may turn to folk medicine or folk healing. **Folk medicine** is defined as those beliefs and practices relating to illness prevention and healing which derive from cultural traditions rather than from modern medicine's scientific base. The student may recall special teas or "cures" that were used by older family members to prevent or treat colds, fevers, indigestion, and other common health problems. For example, many people continue to use chicken soup as a treatment for "flu."

Why do individuals use these nontraditional folk healing methods? Folk medicine, in contrast to biomedical health care, is thought to be more humanistic. The consultation and treatment takes place in the community of the recipient, frequently in the home of the healer. It is less expensive than scientific or biomedical care, because the health problem is identified primarily through conversation with the client and the family. The healer often prepares the treatments, for example, teas to be ingested, poultices to be applied, or charms or amulets to be worn. A frequent component of treatment is some ritual practice on the part of the healer or the client to cause healing to occur. Because folk healing is more culturally based, it is often more comfortable and less frightening for the client.

It is important for the nurse to obtain information about folk or family healing practices that may have been used prior to the client's seeking Western medical treatment. Often clients are reluctant to share home remedies with health care professionals for fear of being laughed at or rebuked. The nurse should remember that treatments once considered to be folk treatments, including acupuncture, therapeutic touch, and massage are now being investigated for their therapeutic effect.

CONSIDER...

- nursing situations in your experience that reflect each of the health belief views as described by Andrews and Boyle: the magico-religious health belief view, the biomedical health belief view, and the holistic health belief view. Describe culturally competent nursing interventions that would be appropriate to each of your nursing situations.

Family Patterns

The family is the basic unit of society. Cultural values can determine communication within the family group, the norm for family size, and the roles of specific family members. In some families the man is usually the provider and decision maker. The woman may need to consult her husband prior to making decisions about her medical treatment or the treatment of her children (Galanti, 1991, p. 63). Some families are matriarchal; that is, the mother or grandmother is viewed as the leader of the family and is usually the decision maker. The nurse needs to identify who has the "authority" to make decisions in a client's family. If the decision maker is someone other than the client, the nurse needs to include that person in health care discussions.

The value placed on children and elderly within a society is culturally derived. In some cultures, children are not disciplined by spanking or other forms of physical punishment. Rather, children are allowed to interact with their environment and to learn from their environment while caregivers provide subtle direction to prevent harm or injury. In other cultures, the elderly are considered the holders of the culture's wisdom and are therefore highly respected. Responsibility for caring for elder relatives is determined by cultural practices. In many cultures, older relatives who cannot live independently often live with a married daughter and her family.

Cultural sex-role behavior may also affect nurse-client interaction. In some countries, the male dominates and women have little status. The male client from these countries may not accept instruction from a female nurse or physician but be receptive to the same instruction given by a male physician or nurse (Galanti, 1991, pp. 66–78). In some cultures, there is a prevailing concept of machismo, or male superiority. The positive aspects of machismo require that the adult male provide for and protect his family, including extended family members. The woman is expected to maintain the home and raise the children.

Cultural family values may also dictate the extent of the family's involvement in the hospitalized client's care. In some cultures, the nuclear and the extended family will want to visit for long periods of time and participate in care. In other cultures, the entire clan may want to visit and participate in the client's care (Galanti, 1991, p. 55). This can cause concern on nursing units with strict visiting policies. The nurse should evaluate the positive benefits of family participation in the client's care and modify visiting policies as appropriate.

Cultures that value the needs of the extended family as much as those of the individual may hold the belief that personal and family information must stay within the family. Some cultural groups are very reluctant to disclose family information to outsiders, including health care professionals. This attitude can present difficulties for health care professionals who require knowledge of family interaction patterns to help clients with emotional problems.

In many cultures naming systems differ from those in North America. In some cultures (e.g., Japanese and Vietnamese) the family name comes first and the given name second. One or two names may or may not be added between the family and given names. Other nomenclature may be used to delineate sexual, child, or adult status. For example, in traditional Japanese culture, adults address other adults by their surname followed by *san*, meaning *Mr.*, *Mrs.*, or *Miss*. An example is Murakami san. The children are referred to by their first names followed by *kun* for boys and *chan* for girls. Sikhs and Hindus traditionally have three names. Hindus have a personal name, a complimentary name, and then a family name. Sikhs have a personal name, then the title *Singh* for men and *Kaur* for women, and lastly the family name. Names by marriage also vary. In Central America, a woman who marries retains her father's name and takes her husband's. For example, if Louisa Viccario marries Carlos Gonzales she becomes Louisa Viccario de Gonzales. The connecting *de* means "belonging to." A male child will be Pedro Gonzales Viccario. Nurses need to become familiar with appropriate ways to address clients. In many cultures, using a client's first name is considered patronizing.

Communication Style

Communication and culture are closely interconnected. Through communication, the culture is transmitted from one generation to the next, and knowledge about the culture is transmitted within the group and to those outside the group. Communicating with clients of various ethnic and cultural backgrounds is critical to providing culturally competent nursing care. There can be cultural variations in both verbal and nonverbal communication.

Verbal Communication

The most obvious cultural difference is in verbal communication: vocabulary, grammatical structure, voice qualities, intonation, rhythm, speed, pronunciation, and silence (Giger & Davidhizar, 1995, p. 23). In North America, the dominant language is English; however, immigrant groups who speak English still encounter language differences, because English words can have different meanings in different English-speaking cultures. For example, in the United States a boot is a type of footwear that comes to the ankle or higher; in England, a boot can also be the trunk of a car. Spanish is spoken by people in several regions of the world: Spain, South America, Central America, Mexico, the Caribbean, and the Philippines. It is the second most commonly spoken language in the United States. Nevertheless, each cultural group that speaks Spanish may use different vocabulary, apply rules of grammar differently, and use different pronunciation, so that often two people of different Latino cultures, speaking Spanish together, may not completely understand each other.

Initiating verbal communication may be influenced by cultural values. The busy nurse may want to complete nursing admission assessments quickly. The client, however, may be offended when the nurse immediately asks personal questions. In some cultures, it is believed that social courtesies should be established before business or personal topics are discussed. Discussing general topics can convey that the nurse is interested in the client and has time for the client. This enables the nurse to develop a rapport with the client before progressing to more personal discussion.

Verbal communication becomes even more difficult when an interaction involves people who speak different languages. Both clients and health professionals experience frustration when they are unable to communicate verbally with each other. For clients who have limited knowledge of English, the nurse should avoid slang words, medical terminology, and abbreviations. Augmenting spoken conversation with gestures or pictures can increase the client's understanding. The nurse should speak slowly, in a respectful manner and at a normal volume. Speaking loudly does not help the client

understand and may be offensive. The nurse must also frequently validate the client's understanding of what is being communicated. The nurse must be wary of interpreting a client's broad smiling and head nodding to mean that the client understands; the client may only be trying to please the nurse and not understand what is being said.

For the client who speaks a different language, a translator may be necessary. Galanti (1991, p. 16) states that cultural rules often dictate who can discuss what with whom. Guidelines for using an interpreter are shown in the accompanying box.

Translators should be objective individuals who can provide accurate translation of the client's information and of the health professional's questions, information, and instruction. Many institutions that are located in culturally diverse communities have translators available on staff or maintain a list of employees who are fluent in other languages. Embassies, consulates, ethnic churches (e.g., Russian Orthodox, Greek Orthodox), ethnic clubs (e.g., Polish-American Club, Italian-American Club) or telephone communication companies may also be able

---

Using an Interpreter

- Avoid asking a member of the client's family, especially a child or spouse, to act as interpreter. The client, not wishing family members to know about his or her problem, may not provide complete or accurate information.

- Be aware of gender and age differences; it is preferable to use an interpreter of the same sex as the client to avoid embarrassment and faulty translation of sexual matters.

- Avoid an interpreter who is politically or socially incompatible with the client. For example, a Bosnian Serb may not be the best interpreter for a Muslim, even if he speaks the language.

- Address the questions to the client, **not** to the interpreter.

- Ask the interpreter to translate as closely as possible to the words used by the nurse.

- Speak slowly and distinctly. Do **not** use metaphors, for example, "Does it swell like a grapefruit?" or "Is the pain stabbing like a knife?"

- Observe the facial expressions and body language that the client assumes when listening and talking to the interpreter.

to provide translating services. Nursing and other health personnel can use pictures and gestures to augment verbal communication. Some schools of nursing and health care institutions do not permit nursing students to translate for a procedure consent because a lack of knowledge about the procedure may lead the student to give inaccurate information. The student should check the institution's policy prior to agreeing to translate for institutional staff and physicians.

Nurses and other health care providers must remember that clients for whom English is a second language may lose command of their English when they are in stressful situations. It is not uncommon for clients who have used English comfortably for years in social and business communication to forget and revert back to their primary language when they are ill or distressed. It is important for the nurse to assure the client that this is normal and to promote behaviors to facilitate verbal communication.

Nonverbal Communication

To communicate effectively with culturally diverse clients, the nurse needs to be aware of two aspects of nonverbal communication behaviors: what nonverbal behaviors mean to the client and what specific nonverbal behaviors mean in the client's culture. It is not required that the nurse be knowledgeable about the nonverbal behavior patterns of all cultures; however, before the nurse assigns meaning to nonverbal behavior, the nurse must consider the possibility that the behavior may have a different meaning for the client and the family. Furthermore, to provide safe and effective care, nurses who work with specific cultural groups should learn more about cultural behavior and communication patterns within those cultures.

Nonverbal communication can include the use of silence, touch, eye movement, facial expressions, and body posture. Some cultures are quite comfortable with long periods of silence, whereas others consider it appropriate to speak before the other person has finished talking. Many persons value silence and view it as essential to understanding a person's needs or use silence to preserve privacy. Some cultures view silence as a sign of respect, whereas to other persons silence may indicate agreement (Giger & Davidhizar, 1995, p. 28).

Touch and touching is a learned behavior that can have both positive and negative meanings. In the American culture, a firm handshake is a recog-

nized form of greeting that conveys character and strength (Giger & Davidhizar, 1995, p. 28). In some European cultures, greetings may include a kiss on one or both cheeks along with the handshake. In some societies, touch is considered magical and because of the belief that the soul can leave the body on physical contact, casual touching is forbidden. In the Hmong culture, only certain elders are permitted to touch the head of others, and children are never patted on the head. Nurses should therefore touch a client's head only with permission (Rairdan & Higgs, 1992, p. 55). The sex of the person touching and being touched often has cultural significance. Galanti (1991, p. 82) describes a situation in which an Orthodox Jewish husband could not touch his wife during labor and delivery; to Orthodox Jews, the blood of both menstruation and birth render a woman unclean, and her husband is forbidden to touch her during those times.

Cultures also dictate what forms of touch are appropriate for individuals of the same sex and opposite sex. In many cultures, for example, a kiss is not appropriate for a public greeting between persons of the opposite sex, even those who are family members; however, a kiss on the cheek is acceptable as a greeting among individuals of the same sex. The nurse should watch interaction among clients and families for cues to the appropriate degree of touch in that culture. The nurse can also assess the client's response to touch when providing nursing care, for example, by noting the client's reaction to the physical examination or the bath.

Facial expression can also vary between cultures. Giger and Davidhizar (1995, p. 31) state that Italian, Jewish, African-American, and Spanish-speaking persons are more likely to smile readily and use facial expression to communicate feelings, whereas Irish, English, and northern European persons tend to have less facial expression and are less open in their response, especially to strangers. Facial expressions can also convey the opposite meaning of what is felt or understood. For example, clients who have difficulty understanding English may smile and nod their heads as though they understood what is being said, when, in fact, they do not understand at all, but do not want to displease the caregiver.

Eye movement during communication has cultural foundations. In Western cultures, direct eye contact is regarded as important and generally shows that the other is attentive and listening. It conveys self-confidence, openness, interest, and

Strategies for Communicating with Clients from Different Cultures

- Consider the cultural component of communication, and integrate it into the relationship.

- Encourage the client to communicate cultural interpretations of health, illness, treatments, and planned care. Incorporate this into the plan of care so that it is congruent with the client's life-style and needs as the client views them.

- Understand that respect for clients and their communicated needs is crucial to the effective helping relationship.

- Use an open and attentive approach so that the client knows you are really listening.

- Relate to the client in an unhurried manner that considers the social and cultural amenities. Give the client time to answer. Engage in appropriate social conversation prior to discussing more intimate or personal details.

- Use validation techniques while communicating to check that the client understands. Note that big smiles and frequent head nodding may indicate merely that the client is trying to please you, not necessarily that the client understands you.

- Sexual concerns may be difficult for clients to discuss. Try to have a nurse of the same sex as the client discuss sexual matters.

- Use alternative methods of communication for clients who do not speak English: foreign language dictionaries or phrase books, interpreter, gestures, pictures, facial expressions, tone of voice.

- Learn key phrases in languages that are commonly spoken in the community. For example, medical phrase books are available in Spanish and French.

honesty. Lack of eye contact may be interpreted as secretiveness, shyness, guilt, lack of interest, or even a sign of mental illness. Other cultures may view eye contact as impolite or an invasion of privacy. In the Hmong culture, continuous direct eye contact is considered rude, but intermittent eye contact is acceptable (Rairdan & Higgs, 1992, p. 53). The nurse should not misinterpret the character of the client who avoids eye contact.

Body posture and gesture are also culturally learned. Finger pointing, the "V" sign with the index and middle fingers, and the "thumbs up" sign may have different meanings. For example, the "V" sign means victory in some cultures, while it may be an offensive gesture in other cultures (Galanti, 1991, p. 22). In the Hmong culture, bowing the head slightly when entering the room where an elder is present or using both hands to give something to someone are considered signs of respect (Rairdan & Higgs, 1992, p. 52).

Communication is an essential part of establishing a relationship with a client and their family. It is also important for developing effective working relationships with health care colleagues. To enhance their practice, nurses can observe the communication patterns of clients and colleagues and be aware of their own communication behaviors. The accompanying box provides strategies for communicating with clients from different cultures. The same strategies can be used in communication with professional colleagues.

CONSIDER . . .

- your own values, beliefs, and practices related to verbal and nonverbal communication. How might your values, beliefs, and practices related to communication conflict with those of people from the different cultural groups in your community?

Space Orientation

Space is a relative concept that includes the individual, the body, the surrounding environment, and objects within that environment. The relationship between the individual's own body and objects and persons within space is learned and is influenced by culture. For example in nomadic societies space is not owned; it is occupied temporarily until the tribe moves on. In Western societies people tend to be more territorial, as reflected in phrases such as "This is my space" or "Get out of my space." In Western cultures, spatial distances are defined as the intimate zone, the personal zone, and the social and public zones. The intimate zone is the smallest area of space around the individual, the public zone the largest area. The size of these areas may vary with the specific culture. Nurses move through all three zones as they provide care for clients. The nurse needs to be aware of the client's response to movement toward the client. The client may physically withdraw or back away if the nurse is perceived as being too close. The nurse will need to explain to the client why there is a need to be close to the client. To assess the lungs with a stethoscope, for example, the nurse needs to move into the client's intimate space. The nurse should first explain the procedure and await permission to continue.

Clients who reside in long-term care facilities, or are hospitalized for an extended time, may want to personalize their space. They may want to arrange their space differently and control the placement of objects on their bedside cabinet or over-bed table. The nurse should be responsive to clients' needs to have some control over their space. When there are no medical contraindications, clients should be permitted and encouraged to wear their own clothing and have objects of personal significance. Wearing cultural dress or having personal and cultural items in one's environment can increase self-esteem by promoting not only one's individuality but also one's cultural identity. Of course, the nurse should caution the client about responsibility for loss of personal items.

Time Orientation

Time orientation refers to an individual's focus on the past, the present, or the future (Galanti, 1991, p. 29). Most cultures combine all three time orientations, but one orientation is more likely to dominate. The American focus on time tends to be directed to the future, emphasizing time and schedules (Smith, 1992, p. 27). Nursing students know what times they "must" be in class or clinical. They know what courses they will take in future semesters. European Americans often plan for next week, their vacation, or their retirement. Other cultures may have a different concept of time. Leininger (1987, pp. 256, 262) describes the Navajo emphasis as "on the flow of life within the natural environment without specific time boundaries." For example, a Navaho mother may not become upset if her child does not achieve a specific developmental milestone, such as walking or toileting, on schedule.

The culture of nursing and health care values time. Appointments are scheduled, and treatments are prescribed with time parameters (e.g., changing a dressing once a day). Medication orders include how often the medicine is to be taken and when (e.g., digoxin 0.25 mg, once a day, in the morning). Nurses need to be aware of the meaning of time for clients. Giger and Davidhizar (1995, p. 109) state that when caring for clients who are "present-oriented," it is important to avoid fixed schedules. The nurse can offer a time range for activities and treat-

ments. For example, instead of telling the client to take digoxin every day at 10:00 AM, the nurse might tell the client to take it every day in the morning, or every day after getting out of bed.

Nutritional Patterns

Most cultures have staple foods, that is, foods that are plentiful or readily accessible in the environment. For example, the staple food of Asians is rice; of Italians, pasta; and of Eastern Europeans, wheat. Even clients who have been in the United States or Canada for several generations often continue to eat the foods of their cultural homeland.

The way food is prepared and served is also related to cultural practices. For example, in the United States, a traditional food served for the Thanksgiving holiday is stuffed turkey; however, in different regions of the country the contents of the stuffing may vary. In Southern states, the stuffing may be made of cornbread; in New England, of seasoned bread and chestnuts.

The ways in which staple foods are prepared also varies. For example, some Asian cultures prefer steamed rice; others prefer boiled rice. Southern Asians from India prepare unleavened bread from wheat flour rather than the leavened bread of Anglo-Americans.

Food-related cultural behaviors can include whether to breast feed or bottle feed infants, and when to introduce solid foods to them. Food can also be considered part of the remedy for illness. Foods classified as "hot" foods or foods that are hot in temperature may be used to treat illnesses that are classified as "cold" illnesses. For example, corn meal (a "hot" food) may be used to treat arthritis (a "cold" illness). Each culture group defines what it considers to be hot and cold entities.

Religious practice associated with specific cultures also affects diet. Some Roman Catholics avoid meat on certain days, such as Ash Wednesday and Good Friday, and some Protestant faiths prohibit meat, tea, coffee, or alcohol. Both Orthodox Judaism and Islam prohibit the ingestion of pork or pork products. Orthodox Jews observe Kosher customs, eating certain foods only if they are inspected by a rabbi and prepared according to dietary laws. For example, the eating of milk products and meat products at the same meal is prohibited. Some Buddhists, Hindus, and Sikhs are strict vegetarians. The nurse must be sensitive to such religious dietary practices.

CONSIDER . . .

- the nutritional content of the foods of various cultures. Identify the food preferences of cultural groups in your community. How do these diets fulfill nutritional requirements? What nutritional deficiencies exist in these diets?

Pain Responses

It has been demonstrated that beliefs about and responses to pain vary among ethnic/racial groups. Cultural response to pain must be viewed in relation both to the actual perception of pain and to the meaning or significance of pain to the client and family. In some cultures, pain may be considered a punishment for bad deeds; the individual is, therefore, to tolerate pain without complaint in order to atone for sins. In other cultures, self-infliction of pain is a sign of mourning or grief. In other groups, pain may be anticipated as a part of the ritualistic practices of passage ceremonies, and therefore tolerance of pain signifies strength and endurance. In yet other cultures, the expression of pain elicits attention and sympathy, while in other cultures, boys especially are taught "to take pain like a man" and "big boys don't cry."

Cavillo and Flaskerud (1991, p. 16) found that nurses and clients assess pain differently. In a study of Mexican-American clients with pain, they found that nurses and physicians tend to underestimate and undertreat their client's pain in relation to the client's expression of pain. Client responses to pain should be assessed within the context of their culture. If the client does not complain of pain, it should not be assumed that the client is not experiencing pain. The nurse must be aware of what conditions are likely to cause pain and offer clients pain relief as appropriate.

Treatment for pain may also vary with culture. In European-American cultures, medication is typically used for pain relief. In other cultures, heat, cold, relaxation, or other techniques and treatments may be used.

Death and Dying Practices

Death is a universal experience, and people want to die with dignity. Various cultural and religious traditions and practices associated with death, dying, and the grieving process help people cope with these experiences. Nurses are often present through the dying process and at the moment of death, especially when it occurs in a health care facility. Knowledge of the client's religious and cultural heritage helps nurses provide individualized care to clients and their families, even though they may not participate in the rituals associated with death.

Dying in solitude is generally unacceptable in most cultures. In many cultures, people prefer a peaceful death at home rather than in the hospital. Some ethnic groups may request that health professionals not reveal the prognosis to dying clients. They believe the person's last day should be free of worry and pain. People in other cultures prefer that a family member (preferably a male in some cultures) be told the diagnosis so that the client can be tactfully informed by a family member in gradual stages or not be told at all. Nurses also need to determine whom to call, and when, as the impending death draws near.

Beliefs and attitudes about death, its cause, and the soul also vary amongst cultures. Unnatural deaths, or "bad deaths," are sometimes distinguished from "good deaths." The death of a person who has behaved well in life is considered less threatening because that person will be reincarnated into a good life next time.

Beliefs about preparation of the body, autopsy, organ donation, cremation, and prolonging life are closely allied to the person's religion. *Autopsy*, for example, may be prohibited, opposed, or discouraged by Eastern Orthodox religions, Muslims, Jehovah's Witnesses, and Orthodox Jews. Some religions prohibit the removal of body parts and dictate that all body parts be given appropriate burial. *Organ donation* is prohibited by Jehovah's Witnesses and Muslims, whereas Buddhists in America consider it an act of mercy and encourage it. *Cremation* is discouraged, opposed, or prohibited by the Mormon, Eastern Orthodox, Islamic, and Jewish faiths. Hindus, in contrast, prefer cremation and cast the ashes in a holy river. *Prolongation of life* is generally encouraged; however, some religions, such as Christian Science, are unlikely to use medical means to prolong life, and the Jewish faith generally opposes prolonging life after irreversible brain damage. In hopeless illness, Buddhists may permit euthanasia.

Nurses also need to be knowledgeable about the client's death-related rituals, such as last rites and administration of Holy Communion, chanting at the bedside, and other rituals, such as special procedures for washing, dressing, positioning, and shrouding the dead. For example, certain immigrants may wish to retain their native customs, in which family members of the same sex wash and prepare the body for burial and cremation. Muslims also customarily turn the body toward Mecca. Nurses need to ask family members about their preference and verify who will carry out these activities. Burial clothes and other cultural or religious items are often important symbols for the funeral. For example, faithful Mormons are often dressed in their "temple clothes." Some Native Americans may be dressed in elaborate apparel and jewelry and wrapped in new blankets with money The nurse must ensure that any ritual items present in the health care agency be given to the family or to the funeral home.

CONSIDER...

- cultural beliefs and practices related to death and dying among people of the different cultural groups in your community. How can the nurse support the client and family in the performance of death and dying practices?

Childbirth and Perinatal Care

Prenatal Care

In North America, emphasis is placed on regular prenatal medical visits, dental care, prenatal classes for both parents, and avoidance of communicable disease. These practices are accepted in varying degrees by people of other cultures. To some for example, regular medical checkups are often avoided because they are equated with problems or abnormalities. Traditionally, these women will see a physician only if there is a problem. Many immigrants may also prefer not to attend prenatal classes for a variety of reasons. Some of these relate to language problems or discomfort and embarrassment about doing exercises in front of others, discussing sexual matters, or seeing movies about childbirth.

Because in many cultures pregnancy and childbirth are considered the exclusive realm of women, some women prefer to have a female friend or relative attend prenatal classes and the birth rather than the husband. Nurses need to respect this choice. However, some new immigrant husbands, in the absence of a mother, mother-in-law or other female, may indicate interest in attending prenatal classes and the birth, if only to act as interpreters for their wives.

Prenatal practices vary in regard to safeguarding the health of the fetus and mother. People in several cultures (e.g., Mexican Americans, Asians, Chinese) emphasize the equilibrium model of health—that is, balancing yin and yang or hot and cold—during pregnancy. Pregnant women therefore avoid too much "hot" or "cold" food as determined by their culture. Some women believe that hot foods during the first trimester of pregnancy can cause miscarriage or a premature delivery; as a result, they emphasize the ingestion of cool foods, such as some fruit, coconut, buttermilk, and yogurt, and the avoidance of hot foods, such as meat, nuts, and eggs, during this period (Waxler-Morrison, et al., 1990, p. 168).

Labor and Delivery

In some cultures, pregnant women traditionally return to their parents' home for the delivery of the first child and, sometimes, subsequent births. Births in the home are usually managed by a midwife, with the assistance of the woman's mother, mother-in-law, or married sister. Traditionally, the husband is not present. In other cultures, childbirth takes place in homes, hospitals, and clinics and is attended by physicians and certified midwives.

Positions used for delivery vary from the standard lithotomy position of North Americans. For example, squatting, kneeling, sitting, or standing, may be preferred.

Responses to labor pain vary. Some women of certain cultures tolerate considerable pain and stoically accept pain for many reasons. They may, for example, want to avoid showing weakness or calling undue attention to themselves for fear of shaming themselves and their families, or they may act accordingly simply because it is expected behavior within their culture. In other cultures, women express pain and anguish more freely. For example, screaming and sobbing are acceptable and expected responses. It is important for the nurse to know that the absence of crying and moaning does not necessarily mean that pain is absent, nor does the presence of crying and moaning necessarily mean that pain relief is desired at that moment. With clients from some cultures, nurses may use touching and the support of others (husband, female relative, or friend) to decrease pain during labor. Various other cultures may or may not value the same comfort measures. Pain relief medications may also be used, but some clients are hesitant to request it.

Postpartum Care

Most cultures emphasize certain postpartal routines or rituals for mother and baby. These are frequently designed to restore harmony or the hot-cold balance of the body. In many cultures, the mother's health status is classified as cold due to stress and the loss of blood. Thus, people take care to warm the body and to avoid cold after birth. This prohibition includes cold air and wind, as well as designated foods and fluids. Showers, tub baths, and shampoos are restricted, often until the lochia stops or longer, to avoid chilling. Sponge baths may be taken using warm water and/or special products that have medicinal properties. Foods considered "hot" by the specific culture are provided, whereas foods considered "cold" are avoided. Some women may wear binders around the abdomen and perineum not only to protect the body from cold but also to aid the uterus to return to its normal size. Mexican Americans may also cover the head, body, and feet to avoid cold air, infection, and other problems, such as sterility.

Confinement periods also vary and in many cultures are considerably longer than that of the health care system of North America. For example, traditional Chinese practice a "sitting in" period for 1 month to avoid cold winds. This confinement also applies to the newborn. New Mexican-American mothers may remain in bed for 3 days following delivery, begin to walk inside the home after 1 week and may go outside after 2 weeks.

For most cultures, the extended family frequently plays an essential role during the postnatal period. A grandmother, mother, mother-in-law, aunt, or married sister may be the primary helper for the mother and newborn. This gives the new mother time to rest as well as access to someone who can help with problems and concerns as they arise.

The Newborn

Breast-feeding is the traditional feeding method in most cultures. However, bottle feeding is becoming more common among women who are employed. The current emphasis in North America on breast-feeding is confusing to some new immigrants because effective advertising campaigns have convinced women of the superiority of bottle feeding; they believe babies grow faster on the formulas. Nurses need to provide additional encouragement and clear explanations for these women.

In some cultures, newborn babies may have a coin placed on the umbilicus or their waist tied with a belly band to prevent a protruding umbilicus or hernia (Waxler-Morrison, et al., 1990, p. 60). Islamic practice requires a family member to pray in the newborn's ear as soon as possible after birth. Circumcision is mandatory according to some religious doctrines and cultural practices. However, in many cultures, circumcision is not performed.

It is important to remember that younger members of a specific cultural group may have been acculturated to the dominant culture and no longer follow traditional practices. In other instances, they follow some practices but not others. Sensitive nurses can work toward a blending of old and new behaviors to meet the goals of all concerned.

PROVIDING CULTURALLY COMPETENT CARE

All phases of the nursing process are affected by the client's and the nurse's cultural values, beliefs, and behaviors. As the client's culture and the nurse's culture come together in the nurse-client relationship, a unique cultural environment is created that can improve or impair the client's outcome. Self-awareness of personal biases can enable nurses to develop modifying behaviors or (if they are unable to do so) to remove themselves from situations where care may be compromised. Nurses can become more aware of their own culture through a values clarification (see Chapter 5). The nurse must also consider the cultural values of the health care setting because they, too, may influence the client's outcome.

To obtain cultural assessment data, the nurse uses broad statements and open-ended questions that encourage clients to express themselves fully. The important principle to remember when conducting an assessment is that "the client is the teacher and expert regarding his or her culture, and the nurse is the learner" (Rosenbaum, 1995, p. 188). At this stage, the nurse makes no conclusions but obtains information from the client.

There are many cultural assessment tools available. The nurse needs to use a tool appropriate to the situation and adapt it as required. For example, a nurse in an emergency department of an urban hospital may need a different format than a nurse working in a home care setting. Tripp-Reimer, Brink, and Saunders (1984, p. 78) note that it is unnecessary to complete a total cultural assessment for every client. Instead, nurses need to collect enough basic cultural data to identify patterns of behavior that may either facilitate or interfere with a nursing strategy or treatment plan.

Anderson et al. (1990, pp. 256–262) emphasize the following points relevant to cultural assessment.

- A cultural assessment takes time and usually needs to extend over several time periods.
- Recognition of one's own ethnicity and social background is essential. Even when the nurse and client share the same ethnic background, the nurse should expect differences in beliefs and values.
- The *process* of assessment is important. How and when questions are asked requires sensitivity and clinical judgment.
- The timing and phrasing of questions needs to be adapted to the individual. Timing is important in introducing questions. Sensitivity is needed in phrasing questions.
- Trust needs to be established before clients can be expected to volunteer and share sensitive information. The nurse therefore needs to spend time with the clients, introduce some social conversation, and convey a genuine desire to understand their values and beliefs.

Before a cultural assessment begins, the nurse determines what language the client speaks and the client's degree of fluency in the English language. The nurse can also learn about the client's communication patterns and space orientation by observing both verbal and nonverbal communication. For example, does the client speak for self or defer to another? What nonverbal communication behaviors does the client exhibit (e.g., touching, eye contact)? What significance do these behaviors have for the nurse-client interaction? What is the client's proximity to other people and objects within the environment? How does the client react to the nurse's movement toward the client? What cultural objects within the environment have importance for health promotion/health maintenance?

For the initial cultural assessment, regardless of the approach used, nurses should ask themselves the following questions (Grant, 1994, pp. 180–181):

- What does the client think about the nature of the illness? What does the client believe to be its cause? How does the client usually deal with the problem? How can others help?
- What support systems are available to the client? Is support from family, religious, community, or ethnic groups available to the client during and after treatment? Does the client need assistance contacting these individuals?
- What treatments is the client using to maintain health and fight illness? Are nontraditional healers involved? What remedies or treatments are ongoing or under consideration? What assistance will be needed from the health care institution or staff to accommodate a combined approach to the problem?
- What biologic and social factors should the nurse consider when planning client care? What health care risks and individual needs characterize the client's culture? What communication problems might occur?
- What does the client want from traditional medicine? What problems are foreseeable? What decisions can be anticipated? How might any legal or ethical problems be addressed?

As the client answers these questions, the sensitive nurse will identify other concerns and issues that can be queried. Examples of open-ended questions to elicit cultural data are shown in the accompanying box.

To provide *culturally congruent care* that benefits, satisfies, and is meaningful to the people nurses serve, Leininger (1991, pp. 41–42) conceptualizes three major modes to guide nursing judgments, decisions, and actions:

1. *Cultural care preservation and/or maintenance.* The nurse accepts and complies with the client's cultural beliefs. For example, the nurse provides herbal tea to ease a "nervous stomach," a practice the client says has worked well in the past.

2. *Cultural care accommodation and/or negotiation.* The nurse plans, negotiates, and accommodates the client's culturally specific food preferences, religious practices, kinship needs, child care practices, and treatment practices.

3. *Cultural care repatterning or restructuring.* The nurse is knowledgeable about culture care and develops ways to repattern or restructure nursing care.

Cultural care preservation may involve, for example, encouraging the use of cultural health care practices, such as ingesting herbal tea, chicken soup, or "hot foods" to the ill client. Accommodating the client's viewpoint and negotiating appropriate care require expert communication skills, such as responding empathetically, validating information,

---

Examples of Open-Ended Questions for a Cultural Assessment

Cultural Affiliation

I am interested in learning about your cultural heritage. Can you tell me about your cultural group, where you were born, and how long you have lived in this country?

Beliefs About Current Illness

What do you call your problem? What name do you give it? What do you think has caused it? Why did it start when it did? What does your sickness do to your body? How severe is it? What do you fear most about your sickness? What are the chief problems your sickness has caused for you personally, for your family, and at work?

Health Care Practices

What kinds of things do you do to maintain health? For example, what types of food do you eat to maintain health? What foods do you eat during illness, and how is food prepared? What other activities do you or your family do to keep people healthy (e.g., wearing amulets, religious or spiritual practices)? How do you know when you are healthy?

Illness Beliefs and Care Practices

What kind of things do you do to treat illness? Do you use traditional healers (shaman, curandero, priest, spiritualist, minister, monk)? Who determines when a person is sick? How would you describe your past experiences with cultural healers and Western health professionals? What

special remedies are generally used for the illness you have? What remedies are you currently using (e.g., herbal remedies, potions, massage, wearing of talismans, copper bracelets, or charms)? What remedies have you used in the past, and which did you find helpful? What remedies or treatments are you considering now, and how can we help?

Family Life and Support System

I would like to learn about your family. Who are the members of your family? What family duties do women and men usually perform in your culture? Whom do you consult when making health care decisions (e.g., other family member, cultural or religious leader)? Who will be able to help you during and after treatment? Do you need help to contact these people?

SOURCES: *Transcultural Concepts in Nursing Care* (2nd ed.) by M. M. Andrews and J. S. Boyle, 1995, Philadelphia: Lippincott, pp. 439–444; *Cross Cultural Caring. A Handbook for Health Professionals in Western Canada* by N. Waxler-Morrison, J. Anderson, and E. Richardson (Eds.), 1990, Vancouver, BC: UBC Press, pp. 245–267; "A Cultural Assessment Guide: Learning Cultural Sensitivity" by J. N. Rosenbaum, April 1991, *Canadian Nurse, 88*, pp. 32–33; and "Culture, Illness and Care" by A. Kleinman, L. Eisenberg, and B. Good, 1978, *Annals of Internal Medicine, 88*, pp. 251–258.

---

and effectively summarizing content. Negotiation is a collaborative process. It acknowledges that the nurse-client relationship is reciprocal and that differences exist between the nurse and client about notions of health, illness, and treatment. The nurse attempts to bridge the gap between the nurse's (scientific) and the client's (cultural) perspectives. During the negotiation process, the nurse first elicits the client's views and acknowledges these views and then, if appropriate, provides relevant scientific information. If the client's views reveal that certain behaviors would not affect the client's condition adversely, then the nurse incorporates these views in planning care. If the client's views can lead to harmful behaviors, then the nurse attempts to shift the client's perspectives to the scientific view. Negotiation therefore occurs when cultural treatment practices conflict with those of the health care system and when the cultural practices are considered

harmful to the client's well-being. The nurse must determine precisely how the client is managing the illness, what practices could be harmful, and which practices can be safely combined with Western medicine. For example, reducing dosages of an antihypertensive medication or replacing insulin therapy with herbal measures may be detrimental. In situations where harm may occur, the nurse needs to inform the client about possible outcomes. When a client chooses to follow only cultural practices and refuses all prescribed medical or nursing interventions, the nurse needs to adjust the client's goals. Anderson et al. (1990, p. 264) point out that monitoring the client's condition to identify changes in health state and to recognize impending crises before they become irreversible may be all that is realistically achievable. At a time of crisis, the nurse may then have the opportunity to renegotiate the original care approach.

RESEARCH NOTE

Is There a Relationship between Ethnic Group, Ethnic Identity, and Health in Middle Eastern Immigrants?

One study examined the relationship between the health, ethnic group, and ethnic identity of Middle Eastern immigrants. Five groups of subjects were selected. The sample included Egyptian (18), Yemen (24), Iranian (16), Armenian (14), and Arabian (16); 59% were females, and 41% were males. Ages ranged from 20 to 76 years. Seventy-eight percent were Muslims. In this report, *ethnic group* refers to country or culture of origin. *Ethnicity* denotes the characteristics commonly associated with an ethnic group, such as symbols, language, ways of greeting, and dress, that differentiate one group from another. *Ethnic identity* is defined as a *subjective* sense of social boundary of a self-definition that answers the question "Who am I?" Ethnic identity variables include cultural attitudes, social integration, family orientation, social attitudes, and perceived ethnic identity.

This study yielded four significant findings: (a) the five ethnic groups showed significant differences in ethnic identity; (b) there were significant group differences in health variables; (c) ethnic identity was significantly related to health variables; and (d) the longer the person had been living in the United States, the weaker the person's identification with the native country and the fewer reported total symptoms. In summary, ethnic group accounted for a significant percentage of variance in positive morale and perceived health status. Ethnic identity accounted for a significant proportion of variance in physical symptoms. Subjects who perceived themselves to be more traditionally ethnic tended to have more physical symptoms and less positive morale.

Implications: Nurses need to differentiate clients' ethnic groups and ethnic identities. For purposes of health assessment, the nurse can elicit ethnic identity by asking clients how strongly they identify with their ethnic group. Simply assigning a person to an ethnic group by last name or race may be misleading. Culturally appropriate care requires that health care professionals learn more than just an immigrant's country of birth or ethnic group; they need to be aware of the profound effects of immigration, which, even under ideal circumstances, influence health and illness status.

SOURCE: "Ethnicity and Health among Five Middle Eastern Groups" by A. I. Meleis, J. G. Lipson, and S. M. Paul, March/April 1992, *Nursing Research, 41,* 98–103.

Transcultural nursing care is challenging. It requires discovery of the meaning of the client's behavior, flexibility, creativity, and knowledge to adapt nursing interventions. For example, a culturally sensitive nurse knows that a Chinese woman who has just given birth and refuses to eat fruit and vegetables, refuses to drink the cold water at her bedside, stays in bed, and refuses to take sitz baths, baths, or showers needs to increase the return of yang forces. The nurse will make plans to adapt nursing interventions accordingly.

Nurses also need to identify community resources that are available to assist clients of different cultures. Nurses should try to learn from each transcultural nursing situation they encounter to improve the delivery of culture-specific care to future clients. The accompanying box offers suggestions for providing culturally competent nursing care.

Providing Culturally Competent Care to Families

- Learn the rituals, customs, and practices of the major cultural groups with whom you come into contact. Learn to appreciate the richness of diversity as an asset rather than a hindrance in your practice.

- Identify personal biases, attitudes, prejudices, and stereotypes.

- Incorporate culture practices into care. Recognize that cultural symbols and practices can often bring a client comfort.

- Include cultural assessment of the client and family as part of overall assessment.

- Recognize that it is the client's (or family's) right to make their own health care choices.

- Provide the services of an interpreter if one is needed.

- Convey respect and cooperate with traditional healers and caregivers.

CONSIDER...

- resources (e.g., churches, synagogues, or mosques; civic groups; embassies or consulates; and so on) available in your community that will assist health care providers in delivering culturally competent care.

- the value of learning the language of culturally different clients in your community. What resources are available in your community for nurses to learn different languages or phrases related to health care?

READINGS FOR ENRICHMENT

Professional Literature

Bell, R. (1994, May). Prominence of women in Navajo healing beliefs and values. *Nursing and Health Care, 15,* 232–240.

This nurse describes her experiences in the Indian Health Service of the U. S. Public Health Service in Arizona, where she grew to understand that "the Navajo views of health are closely related to traditional beliefs and values in a harmonious relationship with all living things."

Candle, P. (1993, Dec.). Providing culturally sensitive health care to Hispanic clients. *Nurse Practitioner, 18,* 40–51.

It is projected that Hispanics will constitute the largest minority in the United States by the year 2000. She discusses prevalent health problems, lack of care resources for Hispanics, and the implications for nursing practice.

Giger, J. N., & Davidhizar, R. (1990, Fall). Developing communication skills for use with black patients. *The ABNF Journal, 1,* 33–35.

These authors believe that the nurse who works with African-American clients must develop sensitivity to communication variances that exist between and within various ethnic and cultural groups. To help nurses communicate better with African-American clients, the authors delineate the conceptual and historical development of Black English and describe the variations in its pronunciation.

O'Hara, E. M., & Zhan, L. (1994, Oct.). Cultural and pharmacologic considerations when caring for Chinese elders: Knowledge of traditional Chinese medicine is necessary. *Journal of Gerontological Nursing, 20,* 11–16.

These authors state that to provide effective care for Chinese elders, nurses should be familiar with the philosophical perspectives of Confucianism and with traditional Chinese medicine, including herbal treatments, diet therapy, and the use of animal secretions and organs. The authors also describe the effects of some common Chinese herbal medicines and other nursing implications of caring for this group of clients.

Wilson, S., & Billones, H. (1994, Aug.). The Filipino elder: Implications for nursing practice—knowledge of heritage essential. *Journal of Gerontological Nursing, 20,* 31–36.

This article provides information about five significant Filipino cultural values influencing health behaviors: bahala, na, pakikisamu, hiya, amor propio, and utang na loob. The authors also discuss the immigration experience, changes in life-style patterns of immigrants, and nursing implications.

Contemporary Literature

African American

Angelou, M. (1969). *I Know Why the Caged Bird Sings.* New York: Bantam Books.

Ellison, R. (1947). *Invisible Man.* New York: Vintage.

Walker, A. (1982). *The Color Purple.* New York: Washington Square Press.

Asian

Buck, P. (1931). *The Good Earth.* New York: Washington Square Press.

Tan, A. (1989). *The Joy Luck Club.* New York: Vintage.

Hispanic

Marquez, G. G. (1967). *One Hundred Years of Solitude.* New York: Avon Books.

Marquez, G. G. (1985). *Love in the Time of Cholera.* New York: Penguin Books.

SUMMARY

North Americans come from a variety of ethnic and cultural backgrounds, and many North Americans retain at least some of their traditional values, beliefs, and practices. Many groups in North America are bicultural; that is, they embrace two cultures: their original ethnic culture and a North American culture. An individual's ethnic and cultural background can influence values, beliefs, and practices. Through acculturation, most ethnic and cultural groups in North America modify some of their traditional cultural characteristics. Personal characteristics also modify an individual's cultural values, beliefs, and practices.

Health beliefs and practices, family patterns, communication style, space and time orientation, nutritional patterns, pain response, death and dying practices, childbirth and perinatal care, and ethnic-related health problems influence the relationship between the nurse and the client who have different cultural backgrounds.

When assessing a client, the nurse considers the client's cultural values, beliefs, and practices related to health and health care.

SELECTED REFERENCES

American Nurses Association. (1991). *Position statement on cultural diversity in nursing practice.* Washington, DC.: Author.

Anderson, J. M. (1990, May/June). Health care across the cultures. *Nursing Outlook, 38,* 136–139.

Anderson, J. M., Waxler-Morrison, N., Richardson, E., Herbert, C., & Murphy, M. (1990). Delivering culturally-sensitive health care. In N. Waxler-Morrison, J. Anderson, & E. Richardson, *Cross cultural caring: A handbook for health professionals in Western Canada* (pp. 245–267). Vancouver, BC: UBC Press.

Andrews, M. M., & Boyle, J. S. (1995). *Transcultural concepts in nursing* (2nd ed.). Philadelphia: Lippincott.

Banks, J., & Banks, C. (1989). *Multicultural education and perspectives.* Boston: Allyn & Bacon.

Baye, A. L. (1995, Summer/Fall). A lesson in culture. *Minority Nurse,* pp. 35–38.

Bernal, H. (1993, Dec.). A model for delivering culture-relevant care in the community. *Public Health Journal, 10,* 228–232.

Bushy, A. (1992, April). Cultural considerations for primary health care: Where do self-care and folk medicine fit? *Holistic Nursing Practice, 6,* 10–18.

Calvillo, E. R., & Flaskerud, J. H. (1991, Winter). Review of literature on culture and pain of adults with focus on Mexican Americans. *Journal of Transcultural Nursing, 2,* 16–23.

DeSantis, L., & Lowe, J. (1992). Moving from cultural sensitivity to cultural competence in nursing practice: Pitfalls and progress. *Paper presented at the 18th Annual Transcultural Nursing Society Conference, Miami, FL, October 22–24, 1992.*

DeSantis, L., & Thomas, J. T. (1990, Summer). The immigrant Haitian mother: Transcultural nursing perspective on preventive health care for children. *Journal of Transcultural Nursing, 2,* 2–15.

Diaz-Gilbert, M. (1993, Oct.). Caring for culturally diverse patients. *Nursing93, 23,* 44–45.

Eliason, M. J. (1993, Sept./Oct.). Ethics and transcultural nursing care. *Nursing Outlook, 41,* 225–228.

Galanti, G. (1991). *Caring for patients from different cultures.* Philadelphia: University of Pennsylvania Press.

Giger, J. N., & Davidhizar, R. (1990, Jan./Feb.). Transcultural nursing assessment: A method for advancing nursing practice. *International Nursing Review, 37,* 199–202.

Giger, J. N., & Davidhizar, R. (1995). *Transcultural nursing: Assessment and interventions* (2nd ed.). St. Louis: Mosby-Year Book.

Grant, A. B. (1994). *The professional nurse: Issues and actions.* Springhouse, PA: Springhouse.

Grossman, D., & Taylor, R. (1995, Feb.). Working with people: Cultural diversity on the unit. *American Journal of Nursing, 95,* 64, 65–67.

Kavanaugh, K. H., & Kennedy, P. H. (1992). *Promoting cultural diversity.* Newbury Park: Sage Publications.

Kittler, P. G., & Sucher, K. P. (1990, March/April). Diet counseling in a multicultural society. *Diabetes Educator, 16,* 127–134.

Lea, A. (1994, Aug.). Nursing in today's multicultural society: A transcultural perspective. *Journal of Advanced Nursing, 20,* 307–313.

Leininger, M. M. (1978). *Transcultural nursing: Concepts, theories, and practices.* New York: Wiley.

Leininger, M. M. (1988, Nov.). Leininger's theory of nursing: Cultural care diversity and universality. *Nursing Science Quarterly, 14,* 152–160.

Leininger, M. M. (Ed.). (1991). *Culture care diversity and universality: A theory of nursing.* New York: National League for Nursing Press. Pub. No. 15-2402.

Leininger, M. M. (1993, Winter). Towards conceptualization of transcultural health care systems: Concepts and a model. *Journal of Transcultural Nursing, 4,* 32–40.

Lynam, M. J. (1992, Feb.). Towards the goal of providing culturally sensitive care: Principles upon which to build nursing curricula. *Journal of Advanced Nursing, 17,* 149–157.

Outlaw, F. H. (1994, April). A reformulation of the meaning of culture and ethnicity for nurses delivering care. *Medical-Surgical Nursing, 3,* 108–111.

Price, J. L., & Cordell, B. (1994, July/Aug.). Cultural diversity and patient teaching. *Journal of Continuing Education in Nursing, 25,* 163–166.

Rairdan, B., & Higgs, Z. R. (1992, March). When your patient is a Hmong refugee. *American Journal of Nursing, 92,* 52–55.

Rosenbaum, J. N. (1991, April). A cultural assessment guide: Learning cultural sensitivity. *Canadian Nurse, 88,* 32–33.

Rosenbaum, J. N. (1995, April). Teaching cultural sensitivity. *Journal of Nursing Education, 34,* 188–189.

Smith, S. (1992). *Communications in nursing* (2nd ed.). St. Louis: Mosby-Year Book.

Spector, R. E. (1991). *Cultural diversity in health and illness* (3rd ed.). Norwalk, CT: Appleton-Century-Crofts.

Sprott, J. (1993). The black box in family assessments: Cultural diversity. In S. Feetham, S. Meister, J. Bell & C. Gilliss (Eds.), *The nursing of families: Theory, research, education, practice* (pp. 189–199). Beverly Hills, CA: Sage Publications.

Steinmetz, S., & Braham, C. G. (Eds.). (1993). *Random House Webster's Dictionary.* New York: Ballantine Reference Library.

Stringfellow, I. (1978). The Vietnamese. In A. L. Clark (Ed.), *Culture, childbearing, health professionals.* Philadelphia: F. A. Davis.

Thiederman, S. B. (1986, Sept.). Health care issues: Ethnocentrism: A barrier to effective health care. *Nurse Practitioner, 11,* 53–54, 59.

Tripp-Reimer, T., Brink, P. J., & Saunders, J. M. (1984, March/April). Cultural assessment: Content and process. *Nursing Outlook, 32,* 78–82.

Waxler-Morrison, N., Anderson, J., & Richardson, E. (Eds.). (1990). *Cross cultural caring. A handbook for health professionals in Western Canada.* Vancouver, BC: UBC Press.

Wenger, A. F. Z. (1993, Jan.). Cultural meaning of symptoms. *Holistic Nursing Practice, 7,* 22–23.

19

CHAPTER

Enhancing Healing

OBJECTIVES

- Explain the concepts of holism and holistic nursing.

- Identify essential aspects of theories related to bodymind healing.

- Explain various healing modalities discussed within this chapter.

- Identify essential aspects of alternative medical therapies.

"Nurses have come a long way in a few short decades. In the past our attention focused on physical, mental and emotional healing. Now we talk of healing your life, healing the environment, and healing the planet."

— Lynn Keegan, 1994

Although nurses have always been concerned with the client as a whole—that is, with the holistic person—they are increasingly embracing holistic healing. Nurses are learning how to become "healing" nurses and seeing themselves as "healers."

- Nurses are incorporating into their practice such alternative healing techniques as massage, imagery, meditation, acupressure, art and music therapy, breathing exercises, biofeedback, reflexology, tai-chi exercises, therapeutic touch, prayer, humor, and others.
- Today many people are pursuing alternative methods of health care with unprecedented enthusiasm. Nurses therefore have an opportunity to play a major role in providing healing interventions that complement not only Western medical therapies but also alternative methods as well.
- Keegan (1994, p. 217) contends that nursing centers will be primary sites for future health care delivery. These centers will become healing centers staffed by nurse healers, other professionals, and lay people who focus on personal responsibility for health and who view illness as an opportunity for growth. These centers will house modern technologic equipment such as biofeedback devices, flotation tanks, light and color therapy units, and quadraphonic sound relaxation units.
- In the next millenium, more and more holistic health care centers will emerge that will help clients seek alternative healthy, self-fulfilling behaviors and mobilize inner healing capacities.

CONCEPTS OF HOLISM AND HOLISTIC NURSING

The term **holism** was coined by Jan Smuts, a South African statesman, in his book *Holism and Evolution* (1926). Smuts theorized that nature tends to bring things together to form whole organisms and that the determining factors in nature and evolution are wholes, not their constituent parts. The concept attracted further interest in the 1940s and 1950s, when Dunbar (1945) a pioneer in psychosomatic medicine, published studies that related stress and personality type to physical illness, and Hans Seyle (1956) published his theory about the psychophysiology of stress. Nurse theorist Martha Rogers (1970) introduced her philosophy in the work *Science of Unitary Human Beings*, a landmark work that set the stage for holistic nursing theories to follow, such as those of Parse (1981), Newman (1986), and Watson (1988). These nursing theories are discussed in Chapter 2.

According to holistic theory, all living organisms are seen as interacting, unified wholes that are more than the mere sum of their parts. Viewed in this light, any disturbance in one part is a disturbance of the whole system; in other words, the disturbance affects the whole being. This concept of holism emphasizes the fact that nurses must keep the whole person in mind and strive to understand how the area of concern relates to the whole person. Therefore, when assessing one part of an individual, the nurse must consider how that part relates to all others. The nurse must also consider how the individual interacts with and relates to the external environment and to others.

A **holistic health belief view** holds that the forces of nature must be maintained in balance or harmony. Human life is one aspect of nature that must be in harmony with the rest of nature. When the natural balance or harmony is disturbed, illness results. Many cultures have held the holistic health belief view for centuries. See Chapter 18 for more information. **Holistic health,** then, involves the total person: the whole of the person's being and the overall quality of life-style. **Holistic health care** considers all the components of health: health promotion, health maintenance, health education and illness prevention, and restorative-rehabilitative care. Advocates of the holistic approach view all of these components with equal importance when identifying a client's needs, planning and implementing care, and evaluating the results.

Holistic nursing is described by the American Holistic Nurses' Association (1994) as nursing practice that has as its goal the healing of the whole person. Holistic nurses provide services that strengthen individuals and enable them to achieve the wholeness inherent within them. They recognize and emphasize the biopsychosocial and spiritual dimensions of each person and incorporate body-mind or biobehavioral-oriented therapies in all areas of nursing to treat the physiologic, psychologic, social, and spiritual sequelae of all illness.

Holistic health practitioners focus on *whole-brain thinking*, a blending of linear thought processes regulated by the left hemisphere of the brain and intuitive thought processes regulated by the right hemisphere. The left brain has consistently been referred to as the dominant hemisphere and valued by Western medicine because it regulates reason, logic, and verbal, mathematical, and calculative aspects of thinking. Intuitive processes, or right-brain function, regulate creativity, artistry, poetry,

and "knowing-without-knowing-why" aspects of cognition (Keegan, 1994, p. 218). Examples of beliefs underlying holistic practice are shown in the box at the left.

Men and women have both masculine and feminine aspects. These qualities are regarded as polarities that together comprise the whole of the process of being. Each polarity in itself is incomplete and depends on the manifestation of its opposite for full expression (Achterberg, 1990, p. 191). See the box below for examples of qualities usually associated with masculine and feminine traits. Holistic practitioners focus on developing both masculine and feminine properties within each person.

Beliefs Underlying Holistic Practice

- The mind, body, and spirit are interdependent. They share one consciousness.

- The human spirit is the core of the person.

- A person's attitude and beliefs toward life are major etiologic factors in health and disease.

- The self is empowered with the ability to create or maintain health or disease.

- Human beings are energy fields. These energy fields can become unbalanced in response to stress in any of the three domains of body, mind, and spirit.

- Each individual is an open system with the environment.

- Health means feeling whole with regard to body, soul, and spirit.

- Spiritual health is essential for physical, mental, and emotional well-being.

- Wellness is increasing openness (acceptance of diversity) and increasing harmony (coherent energy fields).

- Changes in health occur through experiential learning—learning that occurs as a result of living through an activity, situation, or event.

- Health involves a transformational change that encompasses the whole person.

- The client-practitioner relationship is a partnership, although the responsibilities of each partner may differ.

SOURCES: The Nurse as Healer by L. Keegan, 1994, Albany, NY: Delmar, pp. 211–212; and *Caring as Healing: Renewal Through Hope* by D. A. Gaut and A. Boykin (Eds.), 1994, New York: National League for Nursing Press, Pub. no. 14-2607, pp. 16–17.

CONSIDER...

- how your beliefs about nursing compare with those of holistic nursing.
- nurses whom you think exemplify holistic beliefs in their practice. What attitudes and behaviors do they have?

Examples of Qualities Usually Associated as Masculine or Feminine

Masculine	*Feminine*
Intellect	Intuition
Rational	Irrational
Knowledge	Wisdom
Power	Compassion
Analysis	Synthesis
Reason	Feelings
How	Why
Objectivity	Subjectivity
Doing to	Being with
Curing	Caring
Fixing	Nurturing
Form	Process
Competition	Collaboration
Expansive	Contained
Proactive	Reactive
Giving	Receiving
External/public	Internal/private
Technical	Natural
Physical world	Invisible realm
Decisive	Flexible

SOURCE: Adapted from *Woman as Healer* by J. Achterberg, 1994, Boston: Shambhala Publications, p. 191, with permission of Shambhala Publications, Inc. © 1990.

- healing practices or rituals you can add to your life to enhance your own well-being.

CONCEPTS OF HEALING

"Healing has been largely overlooked and is far less understood than the pathophysiology of disease" (Achterberg, 1990, p. 193). Until recently, the idea of curing rather than healing has dominated the Western mode of health care, with emphasis on technology, power, analysis, and the repair of damaged parts. Curing also implies that the person who offers the cure is active, whereas the person who receives the cure is passive.

Dossey's Eras of Medicine

The concept of healing has broadened dramatically in this century. Larry Dossey, chairman of the recently established Panel on Mind/Body Interventions of the Office of Alternative Medicine of the National Institutes of Health categorizes three different eras of medicine according to their approach to health, illness, and healing (Dossey, 1993, pp. 42–43):

Era I refers to "physical medicine," which originated in the late 1860s and remains influential and effective today. It focuses on the effects of "things" on the body and includes Western medical therapies such as drugs, surgery, radiation, and so on. Era I is guided by classical laws of matter and energy; the universe and body are viewed as a vast clock-like mechanism that functions according to causal, deterministic principles.

Era II refers to "mind-body" medicine, which arose in the mid 1950s and is still developing. Dossey marks the mid 1950s as the beginning of Era II medicine because it was at this time that mind-body approaches first began to spark attention among researchers. Perceptions, thoughts, emotions, attitudes, and images were found to affect the body profoundly and gained recognition as being therapeutic and important to healing. Mind-body therapies focus on helping individuals to use their minds to heal their own bodies and include relaxation techniques, most types of imagery therapies, biofeedback, hypnosis, and counseling.

Era III refers to "nonlocal" or "transpersonal" medicine. Dossey differentiates Era III therapies from Era II therapies as follows: Era I and Era II therapies are "local" in emphasis. They adhere to a classical time-space framework in which the mind is seen as localized to points in *space* (i.e., the brain) and *time* (i.e., the present moment). In contrast, Era III medicine does not regard the "mind" or "consciousness" as localized within the individual brain and confined to the present moment; rather it claims that the mind can escape the confines of the body and the present moment and can move through time and space. Thus Era III medicine is seen as nonlocal and transpersonal; the mind is seen as a factor that can effect healing *between* persons. Era III therapies always involve a sender, or healer, and a receiver, or person being healed. Therapies include noncontact therapeutic touch, intercessory prayer, transpersonal imagery, some types of shamanic healing, and all forms of distant healing.

Noncontact therapeutic touch and intercessory prayer are discussed later in this chapter. Empirical testing of transpersonal imagery, noncontact therapeutic touch, and intercessory prayer has already been undertaken. Results support this theory of transpersonal healing. Dossey (1993, pp. 47–49) reports the results of 13 studies on transpersonal imagery conducted by researchers William C. Braud and Marilyn Schlitz from the Mind Science Foundation in San Antonio, Texas. They sought to determine whether a person could use specific mental imagery to change the reactions of a distant person with whom he or she has no physical or sensory contact. Findings revealed a significant relationship between the use of calming or activating imagery of one person and electrodermal activity (physiologic arousal) of another isolated distant subject.

Another study by researcher Daniel Wirth evaluated noncontact therapeutic touch using a double-blind study involving 44 patients with full-thickness surgical wounds. By the eighth day, the wound sizes of patients in the treatment group were significantly smaller than those in the control group. See also the discussion of intercessory prayer on page 392 for experiments related to prayer and healing.

Bodymind Healing

Barbara Dossey and colleagues use the term **bodymind** to refer to a state of integration that includes body, mind, and spirit (Dossey et al., 1995, p. 88). The limbic-hypothalamic system, located within the brain and biochemically interconnected with all other parts of the body, is the primary connecting link between body and mind. Questions arise as to where the mind is located. Traditionally, the mind was believed to be located within the anatomic structure of the brain; current thinking, however, proposes that memories, thoughts, and behavior processes are stored throughout the body (Dossey, 1995, p. 93).

Theoretical bases for bodymind healing include information transduction, self-regulation theory, state-dependent learning and memory, and mind-modulation of the autonomic, endocrine, immune, and neuropeptide systems (Dossey, 1995, pp. 87–109).

Information transduction is the conversion or transformation of information or energy from one form to another. The mind is seen as nature's way of receiving, generating, and transducing information. Information (an idea or event) that is novel—that is, challenging, intriguing, or mysterious—has the highest information value. Such information evokes changes in the body and mind that prompt neural pathways and consciousness to connect to bring about information transduction. Two examples of transduction are the use of relaxation techniques and imagery. Relaxation techniques can effect decreases in blood pressure, heart rate, respiratory rate, and pain. Imagery transforms images or ideas into an act of relaxation and physiologic healing.

Self-regulation theory refers to an individual's ability to learn to process information to bring involuntary body responses under voluntary control. According to self-regulation theory, perception (or imagery) elicits mental and emotional responses that produce limbic, hypothalamic, and pituitary biochemical responses. These biochemical responses, in turn, bring about physiologic changes that are perceived and responded to, thus completing a cybernetic feedback loop. Any perception or image can become a cognitive device or blueprint that directs (a) the retrieval of stored information, (b) the focus of attention, and (c) resulting thoughts/images and behavior. Bodymind interventions enable a person to gain access to inner memories and internal healing resources. The new imagery patterns are then reinforced or reframed into patterns that may bring about positive changes at biochemical levels within the cells.

What a person learns and remembers depends on that person's psychologic state at the time of the experience. This is referred to as **state-dependent learning,** or **memory.** Memories are state-dependent because they are limited to the state in which

they are acquired (Rossi, 1993, p. 47). The mind stores both positive and negative memories. Body-mind methods function by gaining access to and reframing the state-dependent learning and memory that encode problems and symptoms. **Reframing** is identifying thoughts or behaviors and taking responsibility to add or substitute another, more creative, alternative for undesired behavior.

Mind modulation refers to the process by which the brain converts *neural messages* (i.e., thoughts, attitudes, feelings, and emotions) into neurohormonal *messenger molecules* and communicates them to all body systems that evoke states of health or illness (Dossey, 1995, p. 88). The mind modulates cellular biochemical activities within all major organ systems of the autonomic nervous system, endocrine system, immune system, and the neuropeptide system. All of these systems are closely related; none is separate from the other. Activity of any one of these systems can modulate the activity of the other systems.

Mind modulation by the *autonomic nervous system* involves transmission of images and thoughts from the frontal cortex through the limbic-hypothalamic system by *neurotransmitters* (chemicals that facilitate nerve transmission in the body, initiate information transduction, and activate biochemical changes within tissues and cells). These neurotransmitters—norepinephrine of the sympathetic nervous system and acetylocholine of the parasympathetic nervous system—attach to **receptors,** sites on cell surfaces that serve as points of attachment for various types of messenger molecules. Once attached, the neurotransmitters change the structure of the receptor. This change, in turn, creates changes in cell wall permeability that cause a shift of ions (e.g., potassium, sodium, calcium), activity of cell enzymes, and the basic metabolism of each cell.

Mind modulation by the autonomic nervous system can be applied to holistic therapies such as relaxation, imagery, meditation, and music therapy. These therapies encourage bodymind healing by decreasing a person's sympathetic response to stress, thus enabling the calming effect of the parasympathetic system to dominate (see the accompanying box). In all respects, the effects of the sympathetic nervous system are opposite those of the parasympathetic system, with one exception: The sympathetic nervous system stimulates the adrenal cortex and adrenal medulla, thus effecting the fight-or-flight response of the adrenal medulla and the initiation of

Effects of the Autonomic Nervous System

Parasympathetic Branch (Relaxation)	Sympathetic Branch (Activation)
Decreased pupil size	Increased pupil size
Decreased lacrimal gland secretion	Increased lacrimal gland secretion
Increased salivary flow	Decreased salivary flow
Decreased heart rate	Increased heart rate
Vasodilation	Vasoconstriction
Bronchoconstriction	Bronchodilation
Increased gastric motility and secretion	Decreased gastric motility and secretion
Increased pancreatic secretion	Decreased pancreatic secretion
	Increased adrenal secretions (epinephrine and cortisol)*
Increased intestinal motility	Decreased intestinal motility

* Increased adrenal secretions bring about the fight-or-flight response and/or the general adaptation syndrome.

the general adaptation syndrome (GAS) by the adrenal cortex.

Mind modulation by the endocrine system involves stimulation of the senses which activates specific hormones of the endocrine system. Neurotransmitter changes of the hypothalamus bring information from the limbic-hypothalamic system under the regulation of the pituitary gland. Pituitary hormones, the endorphins, and the enkephalins are known to modulate stress, pain, perception, addictions, appetite, learning, memory, and so on (Dossey, 1995, p. 101).

In relation to the *immune system* receptor sites on the surface of T and B lymphocytes are able to activate, direct, and modify immune function. Research has revealed a direct correlation between relaxation, imagery, and the function of the immune system.

The neuropeptide system is another key to understanding bodymind interconnections. **Neuropeptides** are amino acid messenger molecules produced at various sites throughout the body. When a neuropeptide attaches to a receptor site, it either facilitates or blocks a cellular response. Pert (1986, p. 14) refers to neuropeptides as "messenger molecules" that are responsible for connecting body and emotions. The autonomic, endocrine, and immune systems are the vehicles for the neuropeptides. Approximately 50 neuropeptides have been identified, which Pert believes are the key to understanding how mind and body are interconnected. In Pert's words, "[T]he more we know about neuropeptides, the harder it is to think in traditional terms of a mind and a body. It makes more and more sense to speak of a single integrated entity—a *bodymind*" (Pert, 1986, p. 14).

CONSIDER . . .

- how you might reframe your beliefs about healing after reading this section.
- times you set aside for reflection. Does this time increase your motivation, creativity, and spirituality?
- nursing experiences you have had that have shown how "caring" influences healing.

HEALING MODALITIES

To become effective holistic nursing practitioners or nurse healers, nurses need to develop certain attitudes and behaviors. Awareness of and development of one's own holism are important components to integrating holism into clinical practice.

To facilitate the process of healing in others, nurses need to become conscious of healers within themselves, that is, practice personal care. Nurses themselves do not create changes in others; they participate in the process. It is the person receiving the treatment or healing modality, be it medication, surgery, or "alternative" treatment who does the healing. Nurses as healers, therefore, have a twofold responsibility: (a) to understand a biopsychosocial-spiritual approach to care that facilitates a client's growth toward wholeness of mind, body, and spirit, and (b) to care for themselves to reveal the healers within (Wells-Federman, 1996, p. 14). The box on the following page lists methods nurses can use to foster their personal health and well-being.

There are many healing modalities nurses may use to enhance client holism and healing. Nurses may also choose to use some of these modalities for their own benefit. These include various touch therapies, mind-body therapies, aromatherapy, and

---

Self-Healing Methods for Nurses

- *Clarify values and beliefs.* Identify those things that are important, meaningful and valuable to you, and assess whether your actions are consistent with your beliefs. For example, do you value time spent with your children and time reading or listening to music?

- *Set realistic goals.* Identify long term goals and then short term goals that will assist you to meet them. For example, a long term goal might be to "Experience an increase in emotional and physical comfort" and a short term goal to "Take a 30-minute walk each evening".

- *Challenge the belief that others always come first.* Overinvolvement with clients leads to overwork and oversolicitous helping that neglects the client's responsibilities, autonomy, and resources. It leaves little time for fulfillment of personal needs. Identify behaviors that indicate overinvolvement such as saying "yes" much too often, a tendency to avoid conflict whenever possible, feeling selfish when not responding to someone else's needs, and always listening to others who need emotional support but seldom asking anyone to pay attention to your emotional needs. Assess whether you need to make personal readjustment in your perspective and behavior. Learn to ask for what you need; acknowledge that you are doing the best you can; and affirm that you can meet your own needs as well as care for others.

- *Learn to manage stress.* Stress management requires:
  1. Acknowledging the mind-body connection, that is, the relationship among thoughts, feelings, behaviors, and the physiologic response to stress.
  2. Monitoring stress warning signals and evoking the relaxation response on a regular basis such as once a day for 20 minutes or twice a day for 10 minutes. "Mini-relaxations" (e.g., taking several deep breaths and thinking about something pleasant such as your favorite pet) throughout the day can also be used to counter the tension and anxiety associated with stress.
  3. Developing the skill of *personal presence* (physically "being there" and psychologically "being with" a client or other person). To be available to others in this way the nurse needs to practice the skill of being present to his or herself. Avoid allowing yourself to be hurried, distracted, or fragmented. Focus full attention on the activity you are doing at the moment.

- *Maintain and enhance physical health.* Eat healthy, balanced meals, exercise regularly, and obtain adequate rest.

- *Develop a support network.* Fellow nurses can often provide perspectives and insights to help cope with commonly shared experiences.

SOURCE: Adapted from "Awakening the Healer Within" by C. L. Wells Federman. 1996. *Holistic Nursing Practice, 10,* 13–29.

---

transpersonal therapies. Nurses need specialized education to perform many of these therapies.

Touch Therapies

Healing through touch goes back to early civilization. One of the earliest written documents on this subject originated in Asia 5000 years ago. Also, Hippocrates wrote about the effects of therapeutic massage and manipulation when Greek civilization was at its height. Although most cultures have developed some type of touch therapy, attitudes toward touch vary widely from culture to culture.

Touch rituals involve various parts of the body, and touch is an important part of healing (Bushy, 1992, p. 14). One possible explanation is that touch stimulates the production of certain chemicals in the immune system that promote healing.

There are a number of touch therapies. Three of the most common are therapeutic massage, foot reflexology, and acupressure. For nurses to become skilled in these therapies, special courses of study are required.

Therapeutic Massage

Over the centuries nurses have provided back massage. It was thought to improve the circulation of the blood and assist in relaxation. More recently, the benefits have been more precisely identified and categorized as physical, mental-emotional, and spiritual.

Physically, massage relaxes muscles and releases the buildup of lactic acid that accumulates during exercise. It can also improve the flow of blood and lymph, stretch joints, and relieve pain and congestion. Massage is also thought to release body toxins and stimulate the immune system, thereby helping the body combat disease (Kahn & Saulo, 1994, p. 129).

In the mental-emotional area, massage can relieve anxiety and provide a sense of relaxation and well-being. Spiritually, it provides a sense of harmony and balance (Kahn & Saulo, 1994, p. 129). The individuals receiving a massage may enter a meditative state, thus relaxing and expanding their awareness.

A variety of massage strokes or movements may be used singly or in combination, depending on the outcome desired. These include **effleurage** (stroking), friction, pressure, **petrissage** (kneading or large, quick pinches of the skin, subcutaneous tissue, and muscle).

Foot Reflexology

Reflexology, also called zone therapy, can trace its origins to ancient Egypt. Modern foot reflexology is attributed to Dr. William H. Fitzgerald, who developed the theory in the early 1900s. His main contribution was his theory that there are ten equal longitudinal zones which run the length of the body from the top of the head to the tips of the toes with five closely associated zones on each arm (Kunz & Kunz, 1980, pp. 2–6). Each big toe is the start of a line that runs up the medial aspect of the body through the center of the face ending at the top of he head. Each zone (five on each side of the body) has a reflex area on the hand and the foot. According to the precepts of reflexology, more than 72,000 nerves in the body terminate in the feet (Keegan,

1995, p. 550). See Figure 19–1. When the flow of energy is blocked or becomes congested, massaging the reflex points can release the tension. Blockages in any part of the zone can affect the entire zone.

Reflexology is based on the principle that the hands and feet are mirrors of the body and that they have reflex points which correspond to each of the body's glands, structures, and organs. When a reflex area is massaged, it stimulates the corresponding organs in that zone. The actual massage technique varies depending on the purpose of the treatment.

In the 1930s, Eunice Ingram established that the feet are more responsive to reflexology treatments than the fingers. The main goal of foot reflexology is to provide relaxation by maintaining or restoring a state of health and relieving congestion or tension in the zone.

At this time, there is no research to validate the theory or healing properties of foot reflexology. However, it is believed that foot reflexology can stimulate relaxation, which affects the autonomic response, which in turn affects the endocrine, immune, and neuropeptide systems. Although reflexology is a relatively safe procedure, experienced reflexologists need to be consulted when there are circulatory disorders of the extremities (Booth, 1994, p. 39).

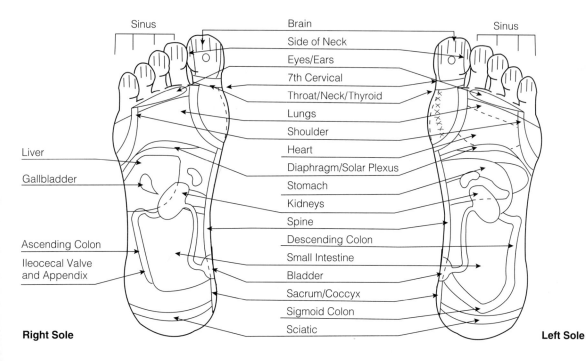

FIGURE 19-1 *Foot reflex areas.*

Acupressure

Acupressure is a form of healing in which the therapist exerts finger pressure on specific sites. According to the theory that underlies acupressure, there are 657 designated points that can be massaged. These points are similar to those used in acupuncture and shiatsu massage. The points run along 12 pathways or meridians that connect the points on each half of the body. The application of finger or thumb pressure is thought to restore balance in the flow of energy (Ki), and when energy can flow freely, the body can heal itself.

Acupressure can be used both to diagnose and to treat ailments. With the application of acupressure, the body is kept in harmony, thus terminating many minor ailments and preventing them from becoming major diseases.

Shiatsu is also based upon the same points that are used in acupuncture. Pressure is applied using the points of the thumbs, finger, *and the heel of the hand.* Shiatsu's main purpose is to maintain health rather than treat illness.

CONSIDER...

- clinical situations in which you have used your hands to soothe, comfort, and bring about a client's healing response. What form of touch did you use, and what was the client's response?
- clinical situations in which you could implement therapeutic massage.
- your attitude toward the use of reflexology and acupressure. Are there ways you can facilitate their use in your practice area?

Mind-Body Therapies

In mind-body therapies, individuals use their minds to heal their bodies. These therapies include progressive relaxation, biofeedback, imagery, yoga, meditation, prayer, music therapy, humor and laughter, and hypnosis.

Progressive Relaxation

Relaxation techniques have been used extensively to reduce high levels of stress and chronic pain. Using relaxation techniques enables the client to exert control over the body's responses to tension and anxiety. For many years, nurses on maternity units have encouraged women in labor to relax and breathe rhythmically.

Progressive relaxation requires that the client (a) tense and then relax successive muscle groups, and (b) focus attention on discriminating the feelings experienced when the muscle group is relaxed in contrast to when it was tense. Jacobsen (1938), the originator of the progressive relaxation technique, found that tension of a muscle group before its relaxation actually achieved a greater degree of relaxation than simply commanding oneself to relax. This technique can result in decreased body oxygen consumption, metabolism, respiratory rate, cardiac rate, muscle tension, and systolic and diastolic blood pressures.

Three requisites to relaxation are correct posture, a mind at rest, and a quiet environment. The client must be positioned comfortably, with all body parts supported, joints slightly flexed, and no strain or pull on muscles (e.g., arms and legs should not be crossed). To rest the mind, the client is asked to gaze slowly around the room (e.g., across the ceiling, down the wall, along a window curtain, around the

Guidelines for Progressive Relaxation

- Sit comfortably in a chair, with your feet flat on the ground.
- Tense and tighten your right fist. Focus on the feeling of tension as you do so.
- Allow the muscles in your right fist to relax. Contrast the difference in feeling from tension to relaxation.
- Repeat the above two steps for the left fist.
- Now tense and relax both your left and right fists.
- Focus on and relish the feeling of relaxation.
- Now tighten the muscles in both fists and both arms. Feel the tension, fully relax the muscles, and again focus on the sensation of relaxation.
- Progressively tighten and relax each muscle group in the body: toes, ankles, knees, buttocks and groin, stomach and lower back muscles, chest and upper back muscles, shoulders, forehead, jaw muscles.
- Couple deep breathing with progressive relaxation. While relaxing your muscles, inhale deeply, send the breath to the fist (or other muscle group), and exhale.
- The entire exercise should last a minimum of 10 minutes.

SOURCE: Adapted from *The Nurse as Healer* by L. Keegan, 1994, Albany, NY: Delmar, p. 156.

fabric pattern, and back up the wall). This exercise focuses the mind outside of the body and creates a second center of concentration.

Procedures for teaching progressive relaxation vary. The method for relaxing muscle groups, the specific muscle groups to be relaxed, the number of sessions involved, and the role of the instructor (taped versus live instructions) may differ. Tension of muscle groups is often maintained for a period of 5 to 7 seconds and is followed by relaxation of the muscle group at a predetermined cue. To achieve maximum relaxation, various positive and affirmative phrases are used, such as, "Let all the tension go" and "Enjoy the feelings as your muscles become relaxed and loose." Guidelines for progressive relaxation are outlined in the box on the previous page.

Biofeedback

Biofeedback is a technique that brings under conscious control bodily processes normally thought to be beyond voluntary command. In the past, most physiologic processes were considered involuntary.

However, it has been discovered that many of these processes are partially subject to voluntary control. Studies show that muscle tension, heartbeat, blood flow, peristalsis, and skin temperature, for example, can be controlled voluntarily. The feedback is usually provided through temperature meters that indicate skin temperature changes or an electromyogram (EMG) that shows the electric potential created by the contraction of muscles. Reduced EMG activity reflects muscle relaxation. Biofeedback teaches clients to achieve a generalized state of relaxation characterized by parasympathetic dominance and antagonistic to the pattern of physiologic arousal manifested in stress-related disorders.

Imagery

Imagery is the internal experience of memories, dreams, fantasies, and visions that serve as a bridge connecting body, mind, and spirit (Dossey, Keegan, Guzzetta & Kolkmeier, 1995, p. 610). Table 19–1 describes various types of imagery. Imagery sometimes involves one or more of the senses. It has also

TABLE 19–1 Selected Types of Imagery

Type	Description	Example
Active	The conscious formation of an image that is directed to a body part or activity.	A client visualizes a dragon eating up his tumor cells.
Correct biologic	Images that are biologically correct and appear as they do in real life as they would under a microscope.	A client visualizes white blood cells engulfing bacteria and normal blood flow to the hands and feet.
Customized	Images that contain personalized, unique information.	A client visualizes her heart bypass grafts as violet cylinders through which her blood flows without obstruction.
End-state	Images of a final healed state.	A client who has an injured shoulder visualizes playing tennis.
Generalized healing	Image of an event, light, sense of unity, universal power, or spirit.	A client describes being bathed with the warmth of the sun, or a white light penetrating the core of his being, or "an angel hovering over me."
Receptive	Images that enter the conscious mind but are not deliberately created; unexpected reception of an image.	A client describes feelings of tension in the back of the neck as a huge knot.
Guided	Access to the imagination through a guide (e.g., a nurse).	At the instructor's suggestion, a client visualizes a valley scene with its many shades of greenery.

SOURCE: Adapted from *Holistic Nursing: A Handbook for Practice.* (2nd ed.) by B. M. Dossey, L. Keegan, C. E. Guzzetta, & L. G. Kolkmeier, 1995, Gaithersburg, MD: Aspen.

been described as thoughts that draw on the senses (Achterberg, Dossey & Kolkmeier, 1994, p. 38). Messages (i.e., feelings, attitudes, and beliefs) are translated in the right hemisphere of the brain before they are understood by the autonomic nervous system. Then the stimuli pass to the left brain hemisphere, where an intellectual interpretation takes place.

Images can be either *concrete* or *symbolic*. A concrete image is one that is biologically correct; for example, a concrete image of body cells would resemble the way cells appear under a microscope. A person can also form symbolic images, which often replace concrete images. For example, a person may visualize pain in the abdomen as a grinder inside the abdomen. Similarly, a person receiving chemotherapy may visualize a dragon (representing the chemotherapeutic agent) traveling throughout the bloodstream eating cancer cells.

Imagery can assist clients to heal by moving them in a step-by-step process toward a specific goal; this is called *process imagery* (Dossey, 1995, p. 42). Process imagery can be used to focus on healing and to decrease anxiety, for example. To teach a client how to use healing imagery, the nurse can follow four steps:

1. Help the client identify the problem by explaining basic physiology about healing.

2. Start with several minutes of focused breathing, relaxation, or meditation.

3. Help the client develop images of the problem or disease, inner healing resources, belief systems, and external healing resources, such as surgery or medications.

4. Encourage the client to terminate each session with images of the desired state of health or well-being (Dossey, 1995, p. 43).

Other strategies to help clients with healing are shown in the accompanying box.

End-state imagery is imagining the healed final state. Achterberg et al. advise that end-state imagery be used after process imagery (1994, p. 46). For example, a client with a fractured femur might visualize walking unaided.

Yoga

The word **yoga,** derived from the Sanskrit root *yug*, meaning "to bind" or "to yolk," is the uniting of all the powers of the body, mind, and spirit. Yoga is an approach to living a balanced life based on ancient teachings found in Hindu spiritual treatises (Upanishads) written in 800–400 B.C. The great yogi Patanjali (500 B.C.) classified the teachings of the Upanishads into eight ways of being, referred to as Ashtanga Yoga, meaning integrated or eight-limbed yoga. The first two stages are the foundation of yoga. If a person does not practice them, the following six stages become meaningless. The remaining six stages set out practices that help a person to master the first two stages. The eight stages follow.

1. *Yama* (universal moral commandments). This refers to improvement in social behavior and is achieved by five noble practices: nonviolence (both physical and psychologic); truthfulness; refraining from stealing; self-restraint in every sphere of life; and refraining from hoarding.

2. *Niyama* (rules for daily conduct). These refer to improvement in personal behavior and are achieved by maintaining a purity of body and mind, developing a habit of contentment, practicing austerity in every sphere of life, studying relevant literature, and practicing dedication to God daily.

3. *Asanas* (physical postures). These consist of a series of 84 main postures (e.g., cobra posture and plough posture) intended to improve body health. The bending, stretching, and holding properties of the postures are designed to relax and tone the muscles and improve the function of

---

Supplemental Strategies to Assist with Imagery

- Speak slowly and calmly.

- Be creative with word choice. Vivid, unusual images occupy the individual's left brain, permitting intuitive, creative thoughts from the right brain to emerge.

- Help the client cross-sense, for example, "Can you see the warmth around you?"

- Assist the client to reframe negative images; for example, if a client describes his tumor as a round ball increasing in size, this image can increase both anxiety and pain. The nurse can suggest the client focus on one part of the ball and see it slowly decreasing in size.

SOURCE: Adapted from "Using Imagery to Help Your Patient Heal" by B. Dossey, June 1995, *American Journal of Nursing, 95,* 41–46.

various organs of the endocrine and nervous systems. People may assume 10 to 15 yogic postures, including stationary exercises, for all parts of the body for a period of about 15 minutes daily.

4. *Pranayama* (breath control). This stage includes eight main breath control techniques. Through the practice of various exercises, an individual learns not only to control breathing but also to restrain and quiet the flow of life force energy (*prana*). According to yogic philosophy, there is a direct relationship between life force activity and the rate of breathing. When the life force is operating smoothly, the breath is calm and regular, but when it is excited, breathing becomes erratic. Breath control is designed to still the mind and achieve transcendental awareness by controlling the life force. This is done by regulating and harmonizing the breath in particular patterns.

5. *Pratyahara* (controlling the senses). This aspect of yoga involves restraining the activities of all the sense organs with the ultimate goal of restraining the mind. It is achieved by minimizing the stimulation of the sense organs and leading as simple a life as possible.

6. *Dharana* (concentration of the mind on one point). Learning to avoid all distractions and concentrate on any object involves tremendous perseverance and willpower. Concentrating on an object of one's choice helps to calm any mental excitement and to induce tranquility and serenity of the mind.

7. *Dhayana* (meditation). This stage refers to meditation that occurs when a person's concentration has become one-pointed, enabling the person to unify consciousness completely and experience a state of transcendental awareness.

8. *Samadhi* (supraconsciousness). This stage refers to extension of conscious control over successively deeper realms of consciousness.

There are many different schools of yoga, including Hatha yoga, and Kundalini yoga, but the system of Ashtanga yoga is the core from which all other schools have evolved. Each school stresses a different technique, but all have as their goal the mastery of the self. For example, Hatha yoga is a series of gently stretching exercises using specific *asanas* (postures) and *pranayama* (breathing techniques). Translated, *Ha-Tha* means "sun/moon," a symbolic representation of the male and female energies in the body. The goal of Hatha yoga is to attain and maintain a balance between the sun and the moon, the masculine and feminine, the sympathetic and parasympathetic, the day and night, and the warm and the cool. Kundalini yoga is a more forceful, highly energizing form that focuses on pushing oneself to the limits. The breathing technique most commonly used in this type of yoga is the "breath of fire," a very deep, hard, and fast nostril breath.

Individuals interested in beginning yoga are advised to explore the specific program offered to ensure that it includes the techniques most suited to their needs.

Meditation

Meditation is a technique used to quiet the mind and focus it in the present and to release fears, worries, anxieties, and doubts concerning the past and the future (Kahn & Saulo, 1994, p. 75). It produces a state of deep peace and rest combined with mental alertness. Originally, meditation was viewed as a religious practice and is still practiced by many as a form of prayer. However, one does not need to be religious to meditate or to receive the benefits of meditation.

Meditation involves both relaxation and focused attention. Skill in meditation is enhanced when the person first masters the skills of breathing, progressive relaxation, and imagery (Keegan, 1994, p. 175).

Because many types of meditation exist, the techniques used to achieve the desired outcome vary widely. In one type of meditation, referred to as *concentrative meditation*, the person visualizes and focuses attention on one particular object (e.g., a candle or a flower) or repeats the words of a mantra so that all other objects and stimuli in the environment are excluded. The Sanskrit word *om* or *aum*, meaning "one," is a commonly used mantra. Hindus believe that *om* is the universal sound, and that its vibrational sound quality enhances a feeling of peace and deep meditation. People may, however, choose a word of phrase meaningful to them such as *Shalom*, *peace*, or "I am at one with God."

In another type of meditation, referred to as *"opening up"* or *"mindfulness"* meditation, the person attempts to remain open to all stimuli. Various types of meditation integrate elements of both techniques. For example, a person may focus on a breathing pattern (Zen meditation) or on a mantra (transcendental meditation) but be willing to allow other thoughts to "come up," watch those thoughts, and then return to the original focus.

Guidelines for meditating follow.

1. Create a special time and place for meditation. Ideally, choose the early morning or evening, and wait at least 2 hours after eating so that complete energy is devoted to meditation rather than to digestive demands. A quiet, comfortable place, devoid of distractions, is essential.

2. Sit either cross-legged on the floor or upright in a straight-backed chair, keeping the spine straight and the body relaxed. Avoid a lying position; this increases the tendency to fall asleep.

3. Support the palms on the thighs, and close the eyes.

4. Follow deep-breathing and/or progressive relaxation exercises.

5. Focus attention completely on either breathing or a chosen mental image. If using a mantra, repeat the word or phrase either aloud or silently while exhaling. When distracting thoughts appear, allow them to drift into and out of your mind without giving them undue attention; then refocus on your breathing or your mantra.

6. Practice this process daily for 10- to 15-minute periods.

Prayer

Prayer is similar to meditation but differs in that it generally involves communication with God, a saint, or some other being who answers the prayer. Prayer may be conducted individually or in groups and may even be conducted at a distance by individuals unknown to the person for whom the prayers of healing are made. (See also the discussion of intercessory prayer, later in this chapter.)

Music Therapy

The human body has a fundamental vibrating pattern. Musical vibrations that closely relate to the body's fundamental frequency or vibrating pattern can have a profound healing effect on the entire human body, mind, and spirit, bringing about changes in emotions, organs, hormones, enzymes, cells, and atoms. Theoretically, carefully selected music helps to restore regulatory functions that are out of tune during times of stress and illness. Music aligns the body, mind, and spirit with its own fundamental frequency. "It is from vibrations and rhythms of sound waves that our brain converts messages to neural impulses, to sensations, to feelings, to emotions, and then to aesthetic, spiritual, social, and healing meanings" (Keegan, 1994, p. 168).

Music therapy consists of listening, rhythm, body movement, and singing. It is used for a variety of reasons. Music can serve as a vehicle for altering ordinary levels of consciousness to achieve the mind's fullest potential. Individuals can move through various stages of consciousness: (a) normal waking state, (b) expanded sensory threshold, (c) daydreaming, (d) trance, and (e) meditative states.

Using music therapy, people can also shift their perception of time from actual time of hours, minutes, and seconds (which is perceived in the left cerebral hemisphere) to *experiential time*—that which is perceived through memory. Listeners can actually lose track of time for extended periods, enabling them to reduce anxiety, fear, and pain. Because music is nonverbal in nature, it appeals to the right cerebral hemisphere, which regulates the intuitive, creative, imaging way of processing information. It recognizes pitch, rhythm, style, and melody. Music does not need logic or analysis from the left brain. However, as a person's knowledge of music increases, left-brain functioning may dominate; musicians, for example, critique compositional techniques and other features of the music. To benefit from music therapy, such people need to learn to let go of these conditioned responses to integrate the functioning of both hemispheres of the brain.

Music therapy can be used in a variety of practice settings. Quiet, soothing music without words is often used to induce relaxation. Musical selections without words are preferred because clients may concentrate on the messages and meaning of words rather than allowing themselves to flow with the music. Music audiocassettes are often used to relax and distract clients in perioperative holding areas, cardiac care units, birthing rooms, counseling rooms, rehabilitation and physical therapy units, and sleep induction units. For individualized therapy, the nurse needs knowledge of the effects that particular types of music produce. Therapeutic music can include mood, choral, classical, Romantic, impressionist, country, soft rock-and-roll, opera, or New age Music. When selecting appropriate music, the nurse needs to consider the client's preferences as well as the goals of therapy. Additionally, the nurse must consider appropriate times for use and length of therapy sessions. For example, some peo-ple may wish to have a music session after a morning shower to balance the body-mind for the day's events. The usual duration of a session is about 20 minutes. Clients are encouraged to let the body respond to the music as it wishes; that is, to relax the muscles, lie down, hum, clap, or dance. Some clients may wish to make their own audiocassette of musi-cal selections they find appealing. The healing capa-bilities of music are intimately bound with personal experience and what can achieve inner quietness or other desired quality within that person.

Humor and Laughter

Health care professionals recently have focused on the positive effects of humor and laughter on health and disease. Humor involves the ability to discover, express, or appreciate the comical or absurdly incongruous, to be amused by one's own imperfec-tions or the whimsical aspects of life, and to see the funny side of an otherwise serious situation. Humor in nursing is defined as "facilitating the client to per-ceive, appreciate, and express what is funny, amusing or ludicrous in order to establish relationships, relieve tension, release anger, facilitate learning, or cope with painful feeling (McCloskey and Bulechek, 1992, p. 297). This definition includes the functions that humor serves in nursing situations.

- *Establishing relationships.* Humor decreases the social distance between persons and assists in putting persons at ease. When tension is decreased, a person can focus on the message and on other people rather than on his or her own feelings. Use of humor helps nurses establish rapport with clients, an important aspect of achieving success in nursing interventions.
- *Relieving tension and anxiety.* Freud (1905) stated that laughter releases psychic energy previously used to block expression of socially or personally unacceptable impulses. The effective use of humor relieves the tension of emotionally charged events. The personal nature of humor, for example, helps clients deal with the imper-sonal nature of wearing a hospital gown and numbered ID band and with embarrassing ques-tions and uncomfortable tests. People can also use humor prophylactically to decrease stress.
- *Releasing anger and aggression.* Humor helps indi-viduals act out impulses or feelings in a safe and nonthreatening manner. It dissipates feelings of anger and aggression by focusing on the comic elements of a situation.
- *Facilitating learning.* Many lectures and presenta-tions begin with a joke or cartoon. Humor not only reduces the presenter's anxiety, but also gains the audience's attention. People learn more when humor is used and anxiety levels are reduced (Parfitt, 1990, p. 114; Lamp, 1992, p. 92). People also recall more information when they associate information with a joke. Use of humor in instruction, however, needs to be carefully planned so that it will contribute to learning.
- *Coping with painful feelings.* People may use humor to blunt the immediate impact of situa-tions that are too painful, such as the impact of a threatening diagnosis or treatment. Humor diminishes anxiety and fear and reduces tension, thus enabling the person to confront and deal with the situation.

Humor also has physiologic benefits that involve alternating states of stimulation and relaxation. Laughter stimulates increases in respiratory rate, heart rate, muscular tension, and oxygen exchange. A state of relaxation follows laughter, during which heart rate, blood pressure, respiration, and muscle tension decrease. Humor stimulates the production of catecholamines and hormones. It also releases endorphins, thereby increasing pain tolerance.

Humor can be either verbal or situational. *Verbal humor* includes puns, jokes, comic verses, anecdotes, and satires. *Situational humor* includes practical jokes, tickling, impersonation, and sight gags. According to Cousins (1989), humor brings out and integrates people's "positive emotions": hope, faith, will to live, festivity, purpose, and determination. It therefore has healing properties.

To use humor effectively, nurses need to be aware of their own feelings as well as the feelings of others and cultural variations in what people consider humorous. Therapeutic humor is a two-way street: The person delivering the humor gains a height-ened view of life, while the person receiving the humor is amused and/or entertained. "Amusement has an aura of freedom, of surrender to relaxation" (Ditlow, 1993, p. 71).

Many health care settings are now displaying their interest in providing humor as a caring skill and are recognizing that "laughter is the best medicine." "Humor" rooms are being created for clients and staff that are supplied with games, funny audiotapes

SOURCE: "Laughing and Health: A Study Using Parse's Research Method" by R. R. Parse, *Nursing Science Quarterly*, 7(2), 55–63.

RESEARCH NOTE

Are Laughter and Health Integrally Intertwined?

One nurse researcher, R. R. Parse, believes that laughter is a chosen way of becoming; it yields a happy feeling and a sense of total well-being as a person lives a situation. See Parse's Human Becoming Theory in Chapter 2. To uncover a structure of the lived experience of laughing and health, Parse conducted a study of 20 English-speaking men and women over 65 years of age. When asked to talk about laughter and health in their lives, participants responded with statements such as "I laughed so much it made me feel good. I was down in the dumps," "[Laughter] feels good… it takes the pain away," "[Laughter is] a relief… it dissolves problems," "It gives you hope," and so on.

Implications: Participants clearly connected health with feeling good and considered laughter as something that prompted this good feeling. Nurses can contribute to such feelings by incorporating humor into their practice.

and videotapes, humorous books, collections of cartoons, and so on.

Hypnosis

Hypnosis is an altered state of consciousness in which an individual's concentration is focused and distraction is minimized. Hypnosis can be used to control pain, alter body functions, and change lifestyle habits. Scientists do not understand exactly how hypnosis relieves pain; however, one theory is that it prevents pain stimuli in the brain from penetrating the conscious mind. Hypnosis requires a client's active participation; clients can even learn to invoke their own hypnotic state. Hypnosis does not take away a person's self-control; in fact, people under hypnosis cannot be made to do anything that they consider immoral or dangerous. In a hypnotic trance, the client does not fall asleep but does become so sharply focused that minor distractions are ignored. A number of hypnosis techniques are used for clients, depending on the type of pain and

the preference of the client and the therapist. One of the most commonly used is symptom suppression, in which the client's awareness of the symptom (i.e. pain) is blocked and the client is distanced from it. The effectiveness of this type of hypnosis depends on the severity of the symptom and the client's ability to concentrate.

CONSIDER...

- clients or other individuals who are currently participating in some form of alternative therapy. Do they believe it is helpful? How?
- clinical situations in which you might use progressive relaxation to allay a client's anxiety or to induce sleep. How would you initiate, implement, and evaluate this therapy?
- attitudes and behaviors nurses need in order to assist clients with imagery. What characteristics do you need to develop?
- what alternative therapies you believe are most effective for individuals with a specific problem or illness (e.g., medically prescribed weight reduction or smoking cessation, impending surgical procedure, pain). Explain why you believe these therapies help.

Aromatherapy

Aromas are detected by the olfactory receptor cells in the nares. The stimuli travel along the olfactory nerve (cranial nerve I) to the olfactory bulb and then to the brain. From there they are thought to play a role in a variety of body functions, emotions and memory.

Aromatherapy involves the distillation of a plant to yield concentrated essential oils. These oils are the resin of the plant and are thought to contain its life force (Kostiuk, 1994, p. 45). Aromatherapy was first used by the early Egyptians to ease pain. As a more recent example, in the 1800s rosemary leaves were burned in hospitals for fumigation. In the past few years, there has been a resurgence of interest in using aromatherapy for a variety of purposes.

There are about 300 essential oils currently used in aromatherapy. They may be inhaled, massaged on the body, applied as compresses, or added to bath water. Examples are shown in Table 19–2.

Transpersonal Therapies

Transpersonal therapies are therapies that effect healing *between* persons. Two therapies are discussed

TABLE 19–2 Some Essential Oils and Some of Their Uses

Oil	Use
Birch	Anti-inflammatory agent, decongestant, relief for arthritis
Geranium	Mood modifier, antidiarrheal agent
Lavender	Relief for headache, stress, and insomnia
Peppermint	Relief for nausea, antipyretic, respiratory aid

Source: Adapted from "The Sweet Smell of Health" by C. Kostiuk, October 1994, *Canadian Nurse, 90*(9), p. 45.

in this chapter: noncontact therapeutic touch and intercessory prayer.

Noncontact Therapeutic Touch

Noncontact **therapeutic touch (TT)** is a process by which energy is transmitted or transferred from one person to another with the intent of potentiating the healing process of one who is ill or injured. It is derived from, but not the same as, the "laying on of hands" associated with some religious philosophies. Delores Krieger (1979), who coined the term *therapeutic touch*, refers to TT as a healing meditation.

Basic to therapeutic touch are the concepts that the human being is an energy field, known as a human field, and that energy can be intentionally channeled from one person to another. The human field extends beyond the level of the skin and is perceptible to the trained sense (primarily touch) of a healer. This energy field can be most clearly "felt" within several feet of the body. An everyday experience that may demonstrate this field phenomenon is the feeling of having one's space invaded when someone stands too close in a crowded elevator, even though there is no physical contact.

The body and the environment are considered open systems and constantly exchange energy and matter. The pattern and organization of the human field are constantly affected by the flow of energy to and from the environment. In a healthy person there is an equilibrium between the inward and outward flow of energy. In situations of disease, illness, or pain, the pattern and organization of the field are disrupted; there may be a loss of energy, a disruption

in the flow, an accumulation, or a blockage of energy flow (Wright 1987, p. 708).

The therapeutic touch process requires specialized education. It consists of the following four steps (Snyder, 1985, p. 203):

1. *Centering* is a meditative step in which the person directs attention inward to achieve a sense of detachment, sensitivity, and balance.

2. *Assessing* is a head-to-toe scanning process in which the nurse holds the palms of both hands 2 to 3 inches over the client's skin surface. This process can be performed by one nurse or two. One nurse scans the client's front while the second nurse simultaneously scans the client's back. The purpose of the assessment is to detect asymmetric differences in the client's energy flow, such as heat, cold, tingling, congestion, pressure, emptiness, or other sensations.

3. *Unruffling,* or *mobilizing,* is a process in which an identified congestive energy field is "unruffled," or mobilized, to make the client's energy field more receptive and to enhance the transfer of energy from the nurse to the client. The nurse accomplishes this step by moving the hands (palms facing the client) in a sweeping motion from the area where pressure was perceived down along the long bones of the body.

4. *Transferring energy* is the process in which the actual transfer of energy occurs from the nurse to the client. The nurse must know which form of energy to use, how to modulate energy, and where to apply energy. This assists the client to repattern his or her energy. The form of energy has different effects and is related to colors: Blue energy is sedating; yellow energy is stimulating and energizing; and green energy is harmonizing. The nurse modulates these energy forms by mentally visualizing the color, for example, by visualizing light through a blue stained-glass window. The nurse may apply energy directly over an identified area of congestion or to one of the *chakras* (special channels that serve as entry areas for energy from the environment). These are located in the thoracic or solar plexus. Energy transference helps restore the balance of the energy field and provides additional energy to promote self-healing.

Healing touch is defined as energy-based therapeutic touch. It influences a person's energy field and energy centers, thereby affecting physical, mental, and spiritual health as well as healing. In 1993 healing touch became a certificate program of the American Holistic Nurses' Association (AHNA).

Intercessory Prayer

Intercessory prayer refers to prayer offered in favor of another. The praying people are referred to as intercessors. In a chapter titled "Prayer and Healing: Reviewing the Research," Dossey (1993, pp. 179–180) describes a study designed by cardiologist Randolph Byrd to evaluate the role of prayer in healing.

In 1986, a carefully controlled 10-month study of 393 coronary care clients at San Francisco General Hospital revealed that clients who were prayed for daily did better on average than clients who did not receive prayer (Byrd, 1988). The researcher recruited people of various religious groups from across the country to pray for half the group. They were given the first names of the clients as well as a brief description of the diagnosis and condition. They were asked to pray daily but were offered no instructions on how to pray. The clients did not know who was being prayed for nor did the nurses and doctors. Findings revealed that those who were prayed for were five times less likely to need antibiotics and three times less likely to develop pulmonary edema. None needed ventilatory support (compared to 12 in the group not prayed for), and fewer died.

The study indicated that the effectiveness of *healing at a distance* is not restricted to one religion because there is no correlation between a person's private religious beliefs and the effect of the prayer. Anyone can pray for recovery from illness. Prayer is considered akin to the sending of information. The one common ingredient in healing prayer appears to be love. Compassion, empathy, and a deep sense of caring is often connected with a sense of oneness and unity between healer and healed.

Since publication, Byrd's work has come under sharp criticism. Other studies, however, corroborate Byrd's findings on both human subjects and nonhuman subjects, such as fungi, yeast, bacteria, plants, and mice (Benor, 1990, pp. 9–33; Braud, 1990, pp. 1–24; and Braud & Schlitz, 1993, p. 186). More recent studies are being conducted at St. Louis University and other research centers. Much more research is required to explore the benefits of intercessory prayer and healing.

ALTERNATIVE MEDICAL THERAPIES

Interest in alternative or complementary medical therapy is rapidly increasing as the public demands more choice in health care. Not only do alternative therapies appeal to people whose health care needs have not been met through traditional medicine, but some people believe they should have the freedom to choose for themselves the type of therapy they undergo.

In response to these concerns, some traditional medical practitioners are providing alternative medical modalities, such as acupuncture and herbal and homeopathic therapies.

Acupuncture

Acupuncture is an ancient Chinese practice based on a principle that energy is channeled through the body along specific pathways. In acupuncture, needles are inserted into the body at specific points along these internal channels, which are called meridians. The needles can be heated, attached to a mild electric current, or twirled continuously with the hand. The internal organs are believed to be connected to the skin points and to the meridians; the acupuncture helps to balance the energy that flows within them. It is therefore considered helpful in healing and for pain.

Studies have shown that acupuncture is effective for pain management. It is believed to exert its effects by releasing endogenous opioids that are produced in various parts of the central nervous system. These opioids combat the pain and promote deep muscle relaxation.

Chiropractic Therapy

Chiropractic therapy was founded by D. D. Palmer in 1895. Chiropractors believe that manipulation of the spinal column is effective in dealing with back pain. These adjustments also affect the nervous system and have a positive effect on the other areas of the body, such as the respiratory and gastrointestinal systems. Chiropractors believe that displacements of the spine can result in a variety of symptoms that can be cured by spinal manipulation. They are also concerned with maintaining the self-regulatory systems of the body. Chiropractors emphasize allowing the body to heal itself rather than intervening in the body's processes.

Practitioners study at a university for 3 years before being admitted to a 4-year course of studies in chiropractic medicine. Some medical doctors believe that the usefulness of chiropractice is limited to conditions of the back, such as muscle spasm.

Herbal Medicine

Since earliest times, herbs, also referred to as botanicals, have been used to treat illness. Herbal medicine is one of the fastest growing areas of alternative medicine. Herbal medicines are found today in drugstores and food stores as well as in specialty stores. The person who advises on herbs is referred to as an **herbalist,** although herbs are also recommended by naturopaths and physicians who engage in alternative medical practices. Herbs are used for a variety of ailments, including digestive problems, colds, immune system disorders, and cancer.

Herbal remedies are said to have three effects on the body: detoxification and elimination of waste, strengthening and healing, and the building up of organs (Trevelyan, 1993, p. 36). Remedies can be made from a single herb or a combination of herbs. They are given to the client in a variety of forms that include syrups, tinctures, liniments, salves, tablets, oils, flower waters, suppositories, infusions, douches, enemas, and poultices.

Most herbs are harmless. However, some can be toxic to the liver or cause digestive system problems. The content and quality of herbal medicine can vary with the brand, and some products can be contaminated with other substances.

Naturopathy

Naturopathic medicine involves herbal medicines, nutritional counseling, acupuncture, and homeopathy. Doctors of naturopathic medicine must complete 3 years of university study and a 4-year program.

Homeopathy

Homeopathy was founded in the late 18th century by a German physician, Samuel Hahnemann. It is based on the theory that the cure for the disease lies in the disease itself, much like the principle underlying vaccination. Therefore the sick are treated with highly diluted amounts of substances that, were they given in more concentrated amounts, would produce the same symptoms as the disease.

Although many studies have been conducted on homeopathy, only a few have shown any medicinal benefit. However, homeopathy is a fast growing alternative therapy. In Canada, homeopathic practitioners must complete a 3-year part-time course of study. A training program is offered through the International Academy of Homeopathy in Toronto, Ontario.

READINGS FOR ENRICHMENT

Burkhardt, M. A., & Nagai-Jacobson, M. G. (1994, March). Reawakening spirit in clinical practice. *Journal of Holistic Nursing, 12*(1), 9–21.

This article describes processes for incorporating spirituality into clinical nursing practice. Spirituality is expressed in the caring connections with oneself, others, nature, and God/life force. The authors make the point that nurturing the nurse's own spirit is essential for responding to the spirit in any interaction.

This article suggests processes through which nurses can more clearly identify spiritual issues. Spirit is understood to be a source and a manifestation of one's spirituality. It explains ways for living artfully in order to care for the soul. Some of the ways highlighted in the article include taking time for self, centering, meditation, and prayer.

Continuing Education Series on Complementary Modalities. Part One. Mackey, R. B. (1995, April). Discover the healing power of therapeutic touch. *American Journal of Nursing, 95,* 27–33. Part Two. Good, M. (1995, May). Relaxation techniques for surgical patients. *American Journal of Nursing, 95,* 39–43. Part Three. Dossey, B. (1995, June). Using imagery to help your patient heal. *American Journal of Nursing, 95,* 41–47.

Part 1 of this series outlines the basic principles of therapeutic touch, ways to center oneself, sensing energy fields, and what current research reveals. Part 2 discusses ways to manage anxiety and enhance the effectiveness of pain medications through the use of relaxation techniques such as muscle relaxation, jaw relaxation, slow breathing techniques, and music therapy. Part 3 focuses on receptive and active imagery and ways the nurse can guide clients' images in a positive direction.

Kahn, S., & Saulo, M. 1994. *Healing yourself: A nurse's guide to self-care and renewal.* Albany: Delmar.

The authors point out in the preface the importance that in order to take care of clients, nurses must first take care of themselves. The focus of this book is nurses, the stress they undergo, and ways in which

→

READINGS FOR ENRICHMENT

they can heal themselves. It includes information about such modalities as relaxation, foot reflexology, and nutrition as well as exercises and self-instruction techniques. The authors' purpose is to help nurses achieve and maintain harmony of the body, mind, and spirit.

McKivergin, M. J., & Daubenmire, M. J. (1994, March). The healing process of presence. *Journal of Holistic Nursing, 12*(1), 65–81.

The authors describe the concept of *presence*, review the related literature, and discuss the relationship between healing and presence. Presence involves "being with" as well as "doing with." It is described as a mode of being available or open in a situation with the wholeness of one's unique individual being. Levels of presence, that is, physical presence, psychological presence, and therapeutic presence, are differentiated.

SUMMARY

Healing is a concept that is gaining increased recognition. Holistic nursing practice encompasses all nursing practice that has healing the whole person as its goal. Holistic nurses recognize and emphasize the biopsychosocial and spiritual dimensions of each person and the integrity of these dimensions. They incorporate various healing therapies in all areas of nursing to treat the psychologic, social, and spiritual sequelae of all illness.

There are several theoretical bases for body-mind healing: information transduction, self-regulation theory, state-dependent learning and memory, and mind modulation of the autonomic, endocrine, immune, and neuropeptide systems. The limbic-hypothalamic system, located within the brain and biochemically interconnected with all other parts of the body, is considered the primary connecting link between body and mind.

Healing modalities include touch therapies, mind-body therapies, aromatherapy, and transpersonal therapies. Touch therapies have been used for centuries and include therapeutic massage, acupressure, and foot reflexology. In mind-body therapies, individuals use their minds to heal their bodies. These therapies include relaxation techniques, biofeedback, imagery, yoga, meditation, prayer, music therapy, humor, and hypnosis. In the past few years there has been a resurgence of interest in aromatherapy to serve a variety of purposes. Transpersonal therapies, those that effect healing between

persons, include noncontact therapeutic touch and intercessory prayer.

Several nontraditional medical therapies are receiving increasing acceptance. These therapies are chosen either to complement Western medical therapy or to replace them. They include acupuncture, chiropractic therapy, herbal medicine, naturopathic medicine, and homeopathic medicine.

Holistic nursing modalities can be used to complement both Western medicine or alternative medical therapies. As healers, nurses need to develop specific healing attitudes and behaviors. Development of a holistic self is a vital beginning.

SELECTED REFERENCES

Achterberg, J. (1990). *Woman as healer.* Boston: Shambhala Publications.

Achterberg, J., Dossey, B., & Kolkmeier, L. (1994). *Rituals of healing: Using imagery for health and wellness.* New York: Bantam Books.

American Holistic Nurses' Association. (1994). *Description of holistic nursing.* Raleigh, NC: Author.

Benor, D. J. (1990, Sept.). Survey of spiritual healing research. *Complimentary Medical Research, 4,* 9–33.

Booth, B. (1993, Oct. 6). Hypnotherapy. *Nursing Times, 89,* 42–45.

Booth, B. (1993, Nov. 17). Shiatsu. *Nursing Times, 89,* 38–40.

Booth, B. (1994, Jan. 5). Reflexology. *Nursing Times, 90,* 38–40.

Booth, B. (1994, Feb. 16). Naturopathy. *Nursing Times, 90,* 44–46.

Braud, W. G. (1990, Jan.). Distant mental influence of rate of hemolysis of human red blood cells. *Journal of the American Society for Phychical Research, 84,* 1–24.

Braud, W. G., & Schlitz, M. (1993). Effects of prayer on human beings. In Dossey, L., *Healing words: The power of prayer and the practice of medicine.* San Francisco: Harper, p. 186.

Bushy, A. (1992, April). Cultural considerations for primary health care: Where do self-care and folk medicine fit? *Holistic Nursing Practice, 6*(3), 10–18.

Byrd, R. (1988). Positive effects of intercessory prayer in a coronary care unit population. *Southern Medical Journal, 81,* 826.

Cousins, N. (1989). *Head first.* New York: Penguin.

Ditlow, F. (1993, March). The missing element in health care: Humor as a form of creativity. *Journal of Holistic Nursing, 11*(1), 66–79.

Dossey, B. (1995, June). Using imagery to help your patient heal. *American Journal of Nursing, 95,* 41–46.

Dossey, B. M., Keegan, L., Guzzetta, C. E., & Kolkmeier, L. G. (1995). *Holistic nursing: A handbook for practice* (2nd ed.). Gaithersburg, MD: Aspen.

Dossey, L. (1989). *Recovering the soul.* New York: Bantam Books.

Dossey, L. (1993). *Healing words: The power of prayer and the practice of medicine.* San Francisco: Harper.

Dunbar, F. (1945). *Psychosomatic diagnosis.* New York: Paul B. Haebar.

Eisenberg, D. M., Kessler, R. C., Foster, C., Norlock, F. E., Calkins, D. R., & Delbanco, T. L. (1993, Jan. 28). Unconventional medicine in the United States: Prevalence, costs, and patterns of use. *New England Journal of Medicine, 328,* 246–252.

Freud, S. (1960). *Jokes and their relation to the unconscious.* New York: Norton.

Gaut, D. A., & Boykin, A. (Eds.). (1994). *Caring as healing: Renewal through hope.* New York: National League for Nursing Press, Pub. no. 14–2607.

Hover, D. (1995). *Healing touch.* New York: Delmar.

Jacobsen, E. (1938). *Progressive relaxation.* Chicago: University of Chicago Press.

James, D. H. (1995, Sept.). Humor: A holistic nursing intervention. *Journal of Holistic Nursing, 13*(3), 239–247.

Kahn, S., & Saulo, M. (1994). *Healing yourself: A nurse's guide to self-care and renewal.* Albany, NY: Delmar.

Keegan, L. (1994). *The nurse as healer.* Albany, NY: Delmar.

Keegan, L. (1995). Touch: Connecting with healing power. In B. M. Dossey, L. Keegan, C. E. Guzzetta, & L. G. Kolkmeier, *Holistic nursing: A handbook for practice* (2nd ed.) (pp. 539–569). Gaithersburg, MD: Aspen.

Kostiuk, C. (1994, Oct.). The sweet smell of health. *Canadian Nurse, 90*(9), 45.

Krieger, D. (1975, May). Therapeutic touch: The imprimature of nursing. *American Journal of Nursing* 75:784–87.

Krieger, D. (1979). *The therapeutic touch: How to use your hands to help or heal.* Englewood Cliffs, N.J.: Prentice-Hall.

Krippner, S. (1972). *The highest state of consciousness.* New York: Doubleday.

Kunz, E., & Kunz, B. (1980). *The complete guide to foot reflexology.* Englewood Cliffs, N.J.: Prentice Hall.

Lachman, V. D. (1996, Jan.). Stress and self-care revisited: A literature review. *Holistic Nursing Practice, 10,* 1–12.

Lamp, J. (1992, March/April). Humor in postpartum education: Depicting a new mother's worst nightmare. *Maternal Child Nursing, 17,* 82–85.

Lauterbach, S. S., & Becker, P. H. (1996, Jan). Caring for self: Becoming a self-reflective nurse. *Holistic Nursing Practice, 10,* 57–68.

Mackey, R. B. (1995, April). Discover the healing power of therapeutic touch. *American Journal of Nursing, 95,* 27–32.

McCloskey, J., & Bulechek, G. (1992). *Nursing interventions classification (NIC).* St. Louis: Mosby.

Moyers, B. (1993). *Healing and the mind.* New York: Doubleday.

Newman, M. A. (1986). *Health as expanding consciousness.* St. Louis: Mosby.

Parfitt, J. (1990). Humorous perioperative teaching: Effect of recall on postoperative exercise routines. *AORN Journal, 52,* 114–120.

Parse, R. R. (1981). *Man-living-health: Theory of nursing.* New York: Wiley.

Pert, C. (1986). The wisdom of the receptors: Neuropeptides, the emotions, and bodymind. *Advances, 3*(3), 14–17.

Reichlin, S. (1993). Neuroendocrine-immune interaction. *New England Journal of Medicine, 7,* 1246–1253.

Rogers, M. E. (1970). *An introduction to the theoretical basis of nursing.* Philadelphia: FA Davis.

Rossi, E. (1993). *The psychobiology of mind-body healing.* New York: Norton.

Seyle, H. (1956). *The stress of life.* New York: McGraw-Hill.

Smuts, J. (1926). *Holism and evolution.* New York: Macmillan.

Sodergren, K. M. (1985). Guided imagery. In M. Snyder, *Independent nursing interventions* (pp. 103–124). New York: Wiley.

Treveleyan, J. (1994, Jan. 26). Homeopathy. *Nursing Times, 90,* 56–58.

Udupa, K. N. (1983). Yoga and meditation for mental health. In R. H. Bannerman, J. Burton, & C. Wen-Chieh (Eds.), *Traditional medicine and health care coverage.* Geneva: World Health Organization.

Watson, J. (1988). *Nursing: Human science and human care.* New York: National League for Nursing.

Wells-Federman, C. L. (1996, Jan.). Awakening the nurse-healer within. *Holistic Nursing Practice, 10,* 13–29.

Wooten, P. (1996, Jan.). Humor: An antidote for stress. *Holistic Nursing Practice, 10,* 49–56.

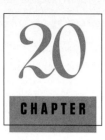

CHAPTER

Intervening in Crises

by Carol Ren Kneisl and Elizabeth A. Riley

OBJECTIVES

- Define *crisis* and *crisis intervention*.

- Identify the types of crises a person may experience.

- Trace the sequence of a crisis, and discuss its significance for the nursing care of clients in crisis.

- Explain the importance of crisis origins and balancing factors in the assessment phase of crisis management.

- Discuss three crisis intervention modalities for a person in crisis.

- Explain why the nurse may feel overwhelmed in caring for clients who are experiencing a crisis.

That I may not in blindness grope,
But that I may with vision clear
Know when to speak a word of hope
Or add a little wholesome cheer....
—S. E. Kiser

Nurses often are intimately connected with crises in their interactions with people who are facing new, frightening, and troublesome situations. Because of who they are, where they work, and their accessibility to individuals and families, nurses are in a position to offer supportive and therapeutic interventions that can change people's lives.

- Over the past two decades, there has been a dramatic surge of interest in the impact of stress, stressful life events, and disasters on individuals. Traumatic events are relatively common. However, the impact of the event on an individual is as unique as the individual.
- Although stress is not harmful in and of itself, it may precipitate a crisis state if the anxiety accompanying it exceeds the individual's ability to adapt. Anxiety that paralyzes or seriously interferes with usual functioning propels a person into crisis. It is impossible to predict who will or will not experience a crisis as a result of stress.
- Crisis intervention is not the specialty of any one professional group. People who intervene in crises come from the fields of nursing, medicine, psychology, social work, and theology. Police officers, teachers, school guidance counselors, rescue workers, and bartenders, among others, are often on the spot in moments of crisis. Crisis intervention can be the business of many different people.
- This chapter explores the period of time when an individual experiences an intolerable stressful event exceeding his or her usual coping resources, the resulting disorganization, and the variables that affect how an individual will respond.
- Beyond its negative effects, a state of crisis offers the individual or family great potential for growth and change.

CRISIS DEFINED

A **crisis** is an acute, time-limited state of disequilibrium resulting from situational, developmental, or societal sources of stress. The word *crisis* stems from the Greek *krinein*, "to decide." In Chinese, two characters are used to write the word; one is the character for *danger*, and the other the character for *opportunity*. A person in crisis is temporarily unable to cope with or adapt to the stressor by using previous methods of problem solving.

To understand the concept fully, it is helpful to describe what a crisis is *not*. Crisis is not stress. Everyone feels stress at various times, in a variety of forms. Stressful situations may demand attention and may be exhausting, but they are not crises. A crisis is not identical to an emergency. An emergency is a situation that often demands an immediate response to ensure the survival of an individual. Although an emergency is not itself a crisis, an emergency can ultimately precipitate a crisis. A crisis is not a mental disorder. A crisis can happen to someone who never had a mental disorder or to someone who is currently experiencing a mental disorder.

Crisis situations are turning points or junctures in a person's life. Successful negotiation of a crisis leads either to a return to the precrisis state or to psychologic growth and increased competence. Unsuccessful negotiation of a crisis leaves the person feeling anxious, threatened, and ineffective. Individuals may also respond to a crisis event with disturbed personal coping or frankly psychotic behavior.

Because a state of disequilibrium is so uncomfortable, a crisis is self-limiting. However, a person experiencing a crisis alone is more vulnerable to unsuccessful negotiation than a person working through a crisis with help. Working with another person increases the likelihood that the person in crisis will resolve it in a positive way.

Common characteristics of crises are shown in the box on the following page. Factors that place individuals at high risk for crisis follow:

- Intensity of exposure to the situation
- Low educational level
- Preexisting psychiatric symptoms and diagnosis
- Prior history of traumatic exposure
- Family history of psychiatric problems
- Early separation from parents
- Family history of anxiety and/or antisocial behavior
- Childhood abuse
- Poverty
- Cultural expectations that prohibit asking others for help
- Degree of threat to life involved in exposure to the situation (being on a plane that crashes versus watching a plane crash from a distance)

Common Characteristics of Crises

- All crises are experienced as sudden. The person is usually not aware of a warning signal, even if others could "see it coming." The individual or family may feel that they have little or no preparation for the event or trauma.

- The crisis is often experienced as ultimately life-threatening, whether this perception is realistic or not.

- Communication with significant others is often decreased or cut off.

- There may be perceived or real displacement from familiar surroundings or significant loved ones.

- All crises have an aspect of loss, whether actual or perceived. The losses can include an object, person, a hope, a dream, or any significant factor for that individual.

ORIGINS OF CRISES

In the contemporary view, the origin of a crisis is as important as the type of crisis. Hoff (1989, p. 37) points out that if nurses can determine how the crisis began, they have a better opportunity to intervene effectively. There are three categories of crisis origins:

1. Situational (traditional term: *unanticipated*)

2. Transitional (traditional terms: *maturational, anticipated*)

3. Cultural/social

Situational Crisis

Situational crises can originate from three sources: material or environmental sources (e.g., fire or natural disaster); personal or physical sources (e.g., heart attack, diagnosis of fatal illness, bodily disfigurement); and interpersonal or social sources (e.g., death of a loved one or divorce). These situations are usually unplanned and unexpected. Because the event leading to the crisis is usually unexpected, a person generally cannot do anything directly to prevent it. In a more indirect sense, a person can attempt to keep healthy and focus on the most effective methods of interacting with others. However, the complexity of the experience influences the person's ability to resolve the trauma. For instance, a

person coping with one traumatic incident is more likely to resolve the experience than someone faced with multiple traumas or factors.

An example of a situational crisis (whose origin is the husband's diagnosis of terminal cancer) follows:

> Sally, age 52, is a social worker at a local mental health clinic, who is feeling increasingly less able to function. She learned 3 days ago that her husband has a terminal form of cancer that is inoperable. They were married approximately one year ago. Many arrangements need to be made, including finding adequate medical treatment and doing appropriate evaluations on her husband. Sally has been unable to work for 2 to 3 days and now tells a psychiatric nurse that she can no longer function and doesn't know what to do. Sally has been unable to make any of the required phone calls, despite knowing she is the person who must coordinate all of this. She says she can't "think straight" and that she is becoming more frightened of talking to the doctors. She shakes her head and says, "Can you believe it? I do this all the time for others, but I can't do it now. Isn't that a joke?" She speaks of being overwhelmed. "What am I going to do without him?"

Transitional Crisis

There are two types of transitional crisis, universal and nonuniversal. *Universal transition states* are life cycle changes or normal transitions of human development. These are the traditional stages of human development that include infancy, childhood, puberty, adolescence, adulthood, middle age, and old age. During each stage, the individual is subject to unique stressors. Each stage of development is characterized by developmental tasks the individual must accomplish to progress to the next level. A failure at any one level compromises the next stage of development.

People in transition usually experience increased anxiety and tension as they move through each successive stage. For every stage, there are changes in expectations, roles, sense of self, body image, and attitudes toward others. Thus, the stages are predictable, and the nurse can help with preventive techniques, education in particular.

The second category of transition states, *nonuniversal transition states*, includes such changes as marriage, retirement, and the transition from student to worker. Crises associated with these states arise when the person enters a new area of development or functioning and cannot adapt to functioning at that level. Crises originating from these sources differ from situational crises. Nonuniversal transition states are like developmental transition states in that they can usually be anticipated and prepared for. Unlike developmental events or transitions, however, they are not experienced by everyone. An individual in a transitional state is at risk for experiencing a crisis. If the person experiences additional trauma or change, the risk increases. Whenever people experience more than two life changes or traumatic events, their coping capacity may be strained, and the potential for crisis becomes greater.

An example of a transitional crisis (whose origin is a decision to divorce) follows:

> Jennifer, age 31, is currently married with three children. Over the past 3 months, her husband has been drinking excessively. Over the same period, they have been evicted from two apartments, her husband has lost his job, and there is often little food available for the children. Jennifer has decided to divorce her husband. Two nights ago she took her clothes and belongings, put them in the car with her three children, and left home. Although she was hoping to drive to her sister's home in the next state, she was exhausted last night and fell asleep in the car for a few hours. Jennifer awoke when her husband pulled her out of the car, threw her into the street, and beat her with a bat. He threatened that if she did not come home, he "would finish the job." Jennifer has just come into the crisis unit after having been found by the police, crying, sobbing, and mumbling incoherently. The children accompany her and remain mute.

Crises that originate from situational and transitional states can be less complex and more easily treated than cultural/social crises.

Cultural/Social Crisis

Crises that have cultural and social sources include the loss of a job stemming from discrimination, being the victim of deviant acts of others, and behavior that violates social norms, such as robbery, rape, incest, marital infidelity, and physical abuse. These crises are never expected, but they are nonetheless somewhat predictable. Crises arising from sociocultural sources are less amenable to control by individuals. There is often a stronger component of community control or influence. Very often, cultural views or government action may be a component of either identification or the resolution of these crises.

An example of a cultural/social crisis follows. There is a threefold origin to this crisis:

1. The community's concern about the children who were abducted

2. The blaming of an African-American male

3. Subsequent information that the mother killed the children herself

> In late October 1994, the entire nation watched and worried with a young mother in South Carolina when she reported that her two children had been abducted during a carjacking. The mother described an African-American male as the person responsible for this terrible event. Worry and sadness turned to anger, shock, and disbelief within the community when 9 days later, the mother confessed to allowing the car with the children in it to roll into a lake. The children drowned in the submerged car. African-Americans expressed anger and outrage because allegations had been made against a black male. The small, close-knit community experienced two sources of disequilibrium: that one of their "own" people had killed her own children, and that racial tensions had further divided the community.
>
> Community and church leaders arranged for memorial services for the children and began the crucial task of restoring equilibrium in the community. All agree it will be a long time before things return to the way they were before the crisis occurred.

CONSIDER...

- how the experience of illness can result in crisis for ill clients, their families, and other support persons. What situational factors might influence the crisis response of ill clients and their families, either positively or negatively?

- how happy events, such as a wedding, anniversary, promotion, or birth of a child might precipitate a crisis response. What situational factors might influence the crisis response of someone experiencing a positive life event?

- how physiologic illness can be a manifestation of crisis events. What benefit does the occurrence of illness serve for the person experiencing crisis?

- factors in your own life experiences that place you at risk for a crisis response. Identify situational, transition, and cultural/social factors. What factors in your personal experience help you to cope with crisis?

CRISIS SEQUENCING

A crisis has three stages: precrisis, crisis, and postcrisis. One assumption in crisis theory is that all individuals are in a state of dynamic equilibrium with their environment. People strive to maintain this state of equilibrium by adapting or coping with the events of daily living.

At times in everyone's life, situations occur that have the potential to disrupt the equilibrium and result in a crisis. Factors that influence whether an individual enters or averts a crisis state are called balancing factors. These are described in a later section of this chapter.

Precrisis Stage

The *precrisis stage* is the stage in which the person maintains or attempts to maintain equilibrium. If the person's problem-solving methods are successful, the person avoids a crisis and reverts to a state of dynamic equilibrium. If the problem(s) are too severe or if the balancing factors are inadequate, equilibrium is not maintained, the problem is not solved, and a crisis results.

Crisis Stage

The *crisis stage* is the reaction to the event, problem, or trauma, not the event itself. Reactions to such events or traumas are highly individual. In this stage, the balancing factors have failed, and the individual is in a full crisis state. In this state of disequilibrium, the individual cannot apply previous methods of reducing tension and anxiety. Inner turmoil and intrapersonal conflict are great, as are anxiety and tension. The person may make erratic attempts to solve the problem. Significant others may observe a disorganization uncharacteristic of that person.

The crisis stage is so disruptive that an individual cannot maintain this state for long. Crisis stages are time-limited and do not last longer than 6 weeks.

Postcrisis Stage

Because the crisis stage is time-limited, everyone who experiences a crisis enters the *postcrisis stage*. During this stage, the person arrives at or develops a new equilibrium. This new equilibrium may be close to that of the precrisis state, or it may be a more positive or more negative state. If the new equilibrium is more positive, the person experiences growth and may now have a better social network, newfound problem-solving abilities, or an improved self-image. If the new equilibrium is more negative, the individual may lose skills, adopt a regressive stance, or develop socially unacceptable behaviors.

Not all people who are exposed to stress (even extreme stress) experience serious or prolonged problems. Approximately 80% of all people who are confronted with serious life experiences are able to work through these situations themselves with support from significant others. The remaining 20% have difficulties that require intervention and assistance.

Some applicable *psychiatric* diagnoses for people who experience a mental disorder following a crisis follow:

- Acute stress disorder
- Major depressive disorder
- Adjustment disorder with depressed mood
- Adjustment disorder with anxiety
- Adjustment disorder with disturbance of conduct
- Posttraumatic stress disorder
- Adjustment disorder with mixed disturbance of emotions and conduct
- Adjustment disorder with mixed anxiety and depressed mood
- Adjustment disorder not otherwise specified (NOS)

Acute stress disorder is a common postcrisis psychiatric diagnosis when symptoms occur within 1 month after exposure to an extreme traumatic stressor. The DSM-IV diagnostic criteria are given in the accompanying box. DSM-IV refers to a psychiatric diagnostic classification system published by the American Psychiatric Association (APA) in the *Diagnostic and Statistical Manual of Mental Disorders* (APA, 1994). The system includes five axes that provide a comprehensive biopsychosocial approach to assessment. This system has been adopted for use in many facilities in North America and around the world, and its multiaxial approach is significant for nurses. For further information, see H. S. Wilson

DSM-IV Diagnostic Criteria for Acute Stress Disorder

A. The person has been exposed to a traumatic event in which *both* of the following were present:
1. The person experienced, witnessed, or was confronted with an event or events that involved actual or threatened death or serious injury, or a threat to the physical integrity of self or others.
2. The person's response involved intense fear, helplessness, or horror.

B. Either while experiencing or after experiencing the distressing event, the individual has *three (or more)* of the following dissociative symptoms:
1. A subjective sense of numbing, detachment, or absence of emotional responsiveness.
2. A reduction in awareness of his or her surroundings (e.g., "being in a daze").
3. Derealization.
4. Depersonalization.
5. Dissociative amnesia (i.e., inability to recall an important aspect of the trauma).

C. The traumatic event is persistently reexperienced in at least one of the following ways: recurrent images, thoughts, dreams, illusions, flashback episodes, or a sense of reliving the experience; or distress on exposure to reminders of the traumatic event.

D. Marked avoidance of stimuli that arouse recollections of the trauma (e.g., thoughts, feelings, conversations, activities, places, people).

E. Marked symptoms of anxiety or increased arousal (e.g., difficulty sleeping, irritability, poor concentration, hypervigilance, exaggerated startle response, motor restlessness).

F. The disturbance causes clinically significant distress or impairment in social, occupational, or other important areas of function or impairs the individual's ability to pursue some necessary task, such as obtaining necessary assistance or mobilizing personal resources by telling family members about the traumatic experience.

G. The disturbance lasts for a *minimum of 2 days* and a *maximum of 4 weeks* and occurs *within 4 weeks* of the traumatic event.

H. The disturbance is not due to the direct physiological effects of a substance (e.g., a drug of abuse, a medication) or a general medical condition, is not better accounted for by Brief Psychotic Disorder, and is not merely an exacerbation of a preexisting Axis I or Axis II disorder.

SOURCE: *Diagnostic and Statistical Manual of Mental Health Disorders* (4th ed.) by the American Psychiatric Association, 1994, APA, pp. 429–430. Reprinted with permission.

and C. R. Kneisl, *Psychiatric Nursing* (5th ed.) (Redwood City, CA: Addison-Wesley Nursing, 1996), pp. 145–147 and Appendix B, pp. 934–949, or another psychiatric nursing textbook.

Although not every person experiencing a life change needs psychotherapy, most people benefit from information, support, and advice. A person's resiliency and vulnerability to stress are important.

BALANCING FACTORS

Many factors determine whether a person faced with a life change or traumatic event will enter a crisis period. The nature of the trauma or experience is one influence on the resolution of the crisis. In addition, the greater the number of balancing factors, the more effective the resolution. Aguilera (1994) indicates that three balancing factors are important to the successful resolution of a crisis:

- *Perception of the event:* how individuals perceive and understand the event/crisis in their lives. Are they being punished? Is this happening only to them and never to anyone else? How will the event affect their future? Do they see the situation realistically, or is it distorted?
- *Situational supports:* the availability of people who can help individuals in crisis solve the problem. Meaningful relationships with others give support and assistance during the crisis. Individuals with inadequate support are likely to experience a decrease in self-esteem. In turn, lowered self-esteem may make an event appear more threatening.
- *Coping mechanisms.* All people under stress use coping strategies to improve their situations. These coping strategies, or coping mechanisms, can be thought of simply as ways of getting along in the world. Because these behaviors have been successful in the past at relieving tension and anxiety, they become part of the person's behavior repertoire. These behaviors can be obvious (e.g., talking a problem out), or subtle (e.g., privately thinking a problem through).

It is unlikely that a crisis will result when individuals have a realistic perception of the event, adequate situational support, and adequate coping mechanisms.

CONSIDER...

- how one's cultural or spiritual background can influence one's response to crisis. How do cultural or spiritual belief systems serve as balancing factors in response to crisis?

- how nurses can intervene as a balancing factor for a client experiencing crisis.
- whether the nurse can be a negative factor in assisting a client to cope with crisis. What characteristics or behaviors of the nurse might interfere with the client's ability to cope with stress? What might be an appropriate action if the nurse identifies conflict in interacting with a client who is experiencing crisis?

CRISIS INTERVENTION

Crisis intervention as a therapeutic strategy is strongly humanistic. Central to the philosophy underlying crisis intervention is the belief that people are capable of personal growth and have the ability to influence and control their own lives. According to these concepts, the task of the person who intervenes in the crisis is to help the individual understand what combination of events led to the crisis and to guide the individual toward a resolution that will meet the person's unique needs and foster future growth and strength. Especially during the acute phase, the goal of crisis intervention is to restore the person to the pretrauma level of functioning as quickly as possible. This can be accomplished by taking advantage of rapid therapeutic gains that are possible when the person's normal defenses are relatively permeable or weakened. As the disequilibrium subsides, reorganization takes place. This state is generally seen as adaptive and integrative. However, it can also be maladaptive, and might result in further crises or even be destructive. Intervention prior to a maladaptive response is the goal of crisis intervention. The traditional steps of the nursing process correspond closely to the steps of crisis intervention.

Assessing

Assessment is the first phase of crisis intervention. The nurse or helper must focus on the person and the problem, collecting data about the client, the client's coping style, the precipitating event, the situational supports, the client's perception of the crisis, and the client's ability to handle the problem. This is an essential and critical step of crisis intervention. This information is the basis for later decisions about how and when to intervene, and whom to call.

The nurse also assesses and evaluates the client's suicide potential. (See Table 20–1 for lethality assessment.) During this time, a client may need to be hospitalized to ensure safety, and a referral to a psychiatrist, psychiatric nurse practitioner, or emergency room of the local hospital may be necessary. Part of the overall assessment is to determine what is necessary to return this client to a state of equilibrium; this may be different from what is necessary to solve the problem.

Often, the "symptom bearer" or "identified client" may really be seeking help for the entire family. The crisis may be a response to a family problem, as demonstrated in the following situation.

Kristen, age 13, was referred to the school nurse after talking openly in the classroom about suicide. Kristen lived with her mother, and she had changed schools three times during the school year because of her mother's recent hospitalization. Initially, it appeared that Kristen was reacting to the multiple moves and her mother's hospitalization. However, after further interviews with both mother and Kristen, the problem became much clearer. Kristen's father had not been able to see her despite her recent attempts to connect with him. He had been a source of support during her mother's absence. Kristen later said she was frightened that her mother would be rehospitalized and that no one would be there for her. Her parents continued to have a stormy relationship after their divorce, and often arguments would end in cold silences. Kristen said she was frightened and that she wanted and needed some attention. She mentioned being "terrified that I might be all alone." She thought her talk of suicide might make her parents stop fighting and bring them back together.

Common family crises include the death of a family member, the terminal illness of a family member, single parenting, divorce, drug/alcohol dependence, family violence, infidelity, remarriage, mental illness, incest, and "empty nest syndrome." These usually come under the heading of situational or transitional crises. To intervene effectively, the nurse meets with as many family members as possible to assess family resources, coping skills, and interpersonal styles. Very often, these crises accompany role changes or additional stress in families that do not have the resources to meet the challenge.

TABLE 20-1 Lethality Assessment Scale

Key to Scale	Danger to Self	Typical Indicators
1	No predictable risk of immediate suicide	Has no notion of suicide or history of attempts, has satisfactory social support network, and is in close contact with significant others.
2	Low risk of immediate suicide	Person has considered suicide using low-lethal method;* no history of attempts or recent serious loss; has satisfactory support network; no alcohol problems; basically wants to live.
3	Moderate risk of immediate suicide	Has considered suicide by means of highly lethal method† but no specific plan or threats; or has a plan to commit suicide by means of a low-lethal method; or has a history of low-lethal attempts, with tumultuous family history and reliance on diazepam (Valium) or other drugs for stress relief; is weighing the odds between life and death.
4	High risk of immediate suicide	Has current plan to commit suicide by means of a highly lethal method, obtainable means, history of previous attempts; has a close friend but is unable to communicate with him or her; has a drinking problem; is depressed and wants to die.
5	Very high risk of immediate suicide	Has current highly lethal plan with available means; history of highly lethal suicide attempts; is cut off from resources; is depressed and uses alcohol to excess, and is threatened with a serious loss, such as unemployment or divorce or failure in school.

* Low-Lethal Methods: Wrist cutting; house gas; nonprescription drugs (excluding aspirin and acetaminophen [Tylenol]); tranquilizers, such as diazepam (Valium), flurazepam (Dalmane)

† Highly Lethal Methods: Gun; jumping; hanging; drowning; carbon monoxide poisoning; barbiturates and prescribed sleeping pills; aspirin and acetaminophen (Tylenol) (high doses); car crash; exposure to extreme cold; antidepressants, such as amitriptyline (Elavil)

SOURCE: *People in Crisis* (3rd ed.) by L. A. Hoff, 1989, Redwood City, CA: Addison-Wesley, p. 209.

A critically important source of the meaning of an individual's response to stress or trauma is the broader sociocultural context in which the person lives. Lebowitz and Roth (1994) defined this sociocultural context as the ideas, beliefs, and metaphors that emerge from cultural productions and institutions (literature, media, religion, law, and so on), which can form a recognizable and coherent ideology and are relevant for a particular event. To be effective in sociocultural assessment, nurses must become aware of the influences and beliefs from their own experiences and be knowledgeable about other cultures. If unfamiliar with a client's culture,

the nurse asks respectful questions to help the client to fully express his or her distress, for example, "I want to understand how all of this might affect you. Can you tell me more about how you feel about this situation? Tell me how your neighbors might feel about it."

Children and Adolescents

Because the coping repertoire of children and adolescents is usually limited—their defenses are immature and they lack life experiences—they are particularly vulnerable to stress and stress responses. The reactions of children to disaster and to crisis are as varied as children themselves and may range from talking frankly about the crisis, complaining of somatic problems without a physical cause, having frightening nightmares, or becoming mute. A wide range of interventions is required. For the child who is in a crisis episode, the home and school are strong supports because of the child's dependence on family members and other adults to provide guidance. When assessing a child or an adolescent in crisis, review the individual factors as well as the resources of the family and the support network.

Webb (1991) points out five factors that should be assessed in the child or adolescent.

1. *Age and developmental level.* Specific developmental stages have corresponding expectations about a child's level of cognitive and moral development. Interventions for a 12-year-old will be quite different from interventions for a 4-year-old. Precrisis adjustment is an important factor in the assessment of children and adolescents. Information about how the children had been getting along at home and at school with peers prior to the crisis helps gauge the impact of the stress on the child.

2. *Coping style and ego assessment.* This area relates to the child's precrisis adjustment and temperamental style. It assesses particularly the child's current level of anxiety, ability to separate from parents, and ability to discuss the problem or crisis situation in the presence of symptoms. It also requires an assessment of the child's use of defenses.

3. *Past experience with crisis.* A review of the child's history helps the crisis evaluator understand and evaluate the current level of anxiety.

4. *Global assessment of functioning.* This is the DSM-IV Axis V scale of social, psychologic, and occupational functioning combined with the specific meaning of the crisis to the child. There may be differences in how the child can clarify the personal meaning of the crisis. When the conflict is close enough to the surface, the child might acknowledge it openly. At other times, it is not possible or desirable to seek information if it might be too threatening. However, it is understood that the underlying meaning of the crisis must be understood by the nurse so that the treatment goals can be appropriately established.

5. *Elements in the support system.* Elements in the support system of a child or adolescent include the nuclear and extended family, the school family, and community supports. Information about these areas makes it easier to incorporate potential resources in the child's network of church, friends, school, health care, and other institutions. It is important to note that with children and adolescents, as with adults, individual characteristics ultimately may determine how, or even whether, supports are used. Even though supports might be available, an individual who is in a vulnerable state or has had multiple past crises may be unable to cope.

Diagnosing

People in crisis may have a variety of problems and symptoms. They may appear overwhelmed, calm, or agitated. They may speak clearly or be psychotic. An individual's perception of the event and personal response will determine the nursing diagnoses. The most common nursing diagnoses for people in crisis are shown in the accompanying box.

Common Nursing Diagnoses for People in Crisis

- Ineffective individual coping
- Ineffective family coping
- Altered family processes
- Impaired adjustment
- Anxiety
- Spiritual distress
- Knowledge deficit
- Impaired verbal communication
- Post-trauma response
- Altered role performance
- Risk for violence: self-directed
- Risk for violence: directed to others
- Self-care deficit
- Hopelessness
- Fatigue
- Fear
- Chronic (or situational) low self-esteem
- Rape trauma syndrome

Planning and Implementing

Effective planning for crisis intervention must be

- Based on careful assessment.
- Developed in active collaboration with the person in crisis and the significant people in that person's life.
- Focused on immediate, concrete, contributing problems.
- Based on an understanding of human dependence needs.
- Appropriate to the person's level of thinking, feeling, and behaving.
- Consistent with the person's life-style and culture.
- Time limited, concrete, and realistic.
- Mutually negotiated and renegotiated.
- Organized to provide for follow-up.

Crisis Counseling

Crisis counseling is a type of brief therapy. Unlike therapies that focus on bringing about major personality changes, crisis counseling focuses on solving immediate problems. It lasts five or six sessions and involves individuals, groups, or families. The following techniques are used:

- Listen actively and with concern.
- Encourage the open expression of feelings.
- Help the client gain an understanding of the crisis.
- Help the client gradually accept reality.
- Help the client explore new ways of coping with problems.
- Link the client to a social network.
- Engage in decision counseling or problem solving with the client.
- Reinforce newly learned coping devices.
- Follow up the case after resolution of the crisis.

Telephone Counseling

Suicide prevention and crisis intervention centers rely heavily on telephone counseling by volunteers who have professional consultation available to them. Also known as hotlines and often available around the clock, they allow callers to remain anonymous and test what it feels like to ask for assistance. No appointment, travel time, or money is necessary, and help is immediately available. The volunteers usually work within a protocol that indicates what information they need from the client to assess the crisis. Their goal is to plan steps to provide immediate relief and then long-term follow-up if necessary.

The calls made to a hotline usually fall into one of four categories: crisis calls, ventilation calls, combinations of ventilation and information calls, or information-only calls. Calls that request information and ventilation are handled by supportive listening and the giving of information. Crisis calls need special techniques. A sample step-by-step protocol for volunteers to use on a hotline follows.

1. Always remain calm. Anxiety on your part can make the client's anxiety worse.

2. Assess the safety of the caller. Ask questions like
   a. Are you in a safe place to talk?
   b. Are you free of injury at this time?
   c. Do you need any emergency assistance?

3. Attempt to get the name, phone number, and address of the caller.
   a. Ask specific questions about whether guns or weapons are involved or available close by. Ask specific questions about the level and extent of prior violence in the home and with the individuals involved.
   b. Assess the involvement of vulnerable people or children.
      - Ask specific questions: Have the children been abused, threatened, or harmed in any way?
      - Remember that you may need to make a report to child protective services if there is any abuse or danger to a child.
   c. Use counseling tools to deepen the connection.
      - Use active listening skills.
      - Ask open-ended questions that allow the caller to give you more information.
      - Paraphrase what the caller has said to ensure that you understand what has been stated.
      - Allow feelings to emerge and be expressed.
      - Validate feelings.

4. Help the individual form an action plan.
   a. Determine whether direct action is needed, for example, to call the police or to get somebody to an emergency room.
   b. Develop a safety plan that will incorporate actions to take in the event that the danger reemerges.
   c. Give education and information about the particular problem the person is calling about. For example, if the call is about being

physically abused, give specific information about abuse and the cycle of violence.

d. Help the caller prioritize what he or she needs to do next.

e. Set realistic goals with the caller about what is possible to be done. For example, if there are multiple needs (financial or social support), remind the caller that it is going to take some time to get this accomplished.

f. Provide referrals to resources or individuals who have the potential to assist the person.

The following points are also important to consider in telephone counseling:

- If the caller is reluctant to give a name and location, do not press for this information. The caller may feel threatened and hang up.
- Listen for background noises that may give clues to the caller's location.
- Use a note pad to write messages to co-workers so that the conversation is not interrupted.
- Keep the caller talking. This gives you time to begin to develop a relationship, to trace the call, or to contact relatives or the police if necessary.
- Emphasize that you are available to talk as long as the caller needs to do so.
- Reinforce positive responses and actions, such as the fact that the caller is talking instead of acting-out hopeless feelings.
- Acknowledge that the caller feels distress, but explain that he or she does not need to inflict self-harm to emphasize it.
- Do not overuse reflection of feelings, which, in this setting, may sound uncaring or superficial. Instead, offer direction and solutions to problems.
- If the caller is threatening immediate harm to self or to others, notify the police, an area mental health crisis unit, or family members to intervene with the caller. Most hotlines have the ability to trace phone calls.
- To fully assess the client for suicide risk, perform a lethality assessment (see Table 20–1, page 403).

This type of intervention can be very stressful for the nurse/counselor. Remember that despite the nurse's efforts to communicate concern, the ultimate decision maker is the caller.

Home Crisis Visits

Home visits are made when telephone counseling does not suffice or when the crisis workers need to obtain additional information by direct observation or to reach a client who is unobtainable by telephone. Home visits are appropriate when crisis workers need to initiate contacts rather than waiting for clients to come to them—for example, when a telephone caller is assessed to be highly suicidal or when a concerned neighbor, physician, or clergyman informs the agency of clients in potential crisis.

Often these clients are too disorganized or distraught to seek help by themselves. The police may arrange for a home crisis visit to avoid imprisoning or hospitalizing a client. Problems commonly encountered are spousal abuse, child abuse, psychiatric emergencies, and medical emergencies.

The crisis workers are usually a team consisting of a man and a woman who are highly skilled and experienced in crisis intervention. The male-female team is generally perceived as less threatening than two men, two women, or a single person. Their goal is to defuse the situation with as little disruption and violence as possible and to engage the clients in longer-term treatment. They may also be members of mobile crisis units.

There are others who intervene in community crises as well. The public health nurse is in an excellent position to identify, assess, and intervene with clients experiencing a life crisis. Public health nurses often have access to community resources as well as informal communication lines, and they usually maintain contact with families and clients for longer periods of time than nurses in other settings. They are often recognized by the community as knowledgeable experts who are available for immediate assistance.

Emily, age 78, and her sister Frances, age 84, lived in a run-down part of town. Frances became seriously ill with pneumonia and became progressively weaker. Emily became more anxious about Frances's health when her sister refused to see a doctor. Emily was afraid her sister would die or need to go to a nursing home. Emily felt paralyzed and didn't know what to do. When the visiting nurse came by to visit Emily's neighbor, Emily asked the nurse to see Frances. Together they were able to persuade Frances to get medical care so that she could stay home.

Other Interventions

One-to-one interventions are important to an individual in crisis. However, nurses who work with people in crisis often need to use many nontraditional interventions, which can be as important as any verbal interventions. Nurses who work successfully with people in crisis must have a flexible, open view of what may be therapeutic with different individuals. They must have a full repertoire of skills and interventions that can be individualized to help all types of clients in crisis. Some examples of these interventions follow.

Assisting with Environmental Changes
- Finding shelter for a homeless person
- Obtaining shelter for an abused woman and her children
- Arranging for a home health aide to care for a family member

Assisting with Planned Events
- Discussing methods of contraception with adolescents or young men and women
- Preparing a child for a tonsillectomy
- Arranging for a volunteer from the Reach for Recovery Program to visit a woman who has had a mastectomy

Helping Develop Social Supports
- Introducing a woman whose husband is an alcoholic to Al-Anon groups in her community
- Referring a family with a terminally ill member to a local hospice
- Giving a rape victim the telephone number of the rape crisis hotline

Evaluating

Nurses in acute care or short-term settings may not see the long-term effects of their interventions. Typically, nurses in these settings need to evaluate the crisis, set up the plan, and begin implementing it.

In long-term settings, the nurse can evaluate the client or family response to the intervention by determining whether clients have resumed their precrisis level of functioning or show evidence of increased functioning (growth). A nurse in either a long-term or short-term setting may also have an opportunity to evaluate whether a similar problem might lead to another crisis for the client.

RESEARCH NOTE

How Do Helping Styles Compare Among Nursing Students, Psychotherapists, Crisis Interveners, and Untrained Individuals?

In one study, researchers Ryden, McCarthy, Lewis, and Sherman compared helping styles of nursing students with those of subjects in a prior study. In the prior study, the subjects comprised 17 psychotherapists, 12 crisis interveners, and 15 untrained people with a mean age of 24 years. Ryden et al. sought to assess whether nursing students use helping behaviors similar to those of psychotherapists. Subjects were 30 junior-year college students who were enrolled in the second part of a two-course sequence in interpersonal relations. Their mean age was 25.3 years. The subjects were videotaped in a 3-minute interaction with a simulated client. An experienced psychotherapist who was trained in the use of the Helping Skills Verbal Response System instrument rated each student.

Findings revealed that like the psychotherapists, the nursing students were able to focus on the client's perspective and placed minimal emphasis on giving advice and information. Like the crisis interveners, the nursing students took a structured approach; that is, they began the interview with the client by introducing themselves, giving personal information, and stating clearly their purpose in talking with the client. Also like the crisis interveners, the students directed the client toward action-oriented plans and talked more than the psychotherapists. The behaviors of the nursing students bore almost no resemblance to those of untrained individuals, who were highly verbose and directive and made little effort to modify their affect or weigh the content of their words.

Implications: The researchers state that "the nursing students' behaviors are compatible with values of the nursing profession, (i.e., the values of autonomy and empowerment of the client). Their approach is both empathetic (attending to client process), and directive (facilitating action plans). This type of approach seems appropriate since nurses typically have a short amount of time in which to establish client trust and work towards problem resolutions." Because the sample of nursing students was small and the role-playing was limited to 3 minutes, longer interactions need to be studied to determine whether nursing students maintain the approach identified in this study.

SOURCE: "A Behavioral Comparison of the Helping Styles of Nursing Students, Psychotherapists, Crisis Interveners, and Untrained Individuals" by M. B. Ryden, P. R. McCarthy, M. L. Lewis, and C. Sherman, June 1991, *Archives of Psychiatric Nursing*, 5(3), 185–188.

CONSIDER...

- how psychiatric diagnoses and DSM-IV diagnoses compare with nursing diagnoses. In which practice settings is it appropriate for the nurse to use psychiatric diagnoses? DSM-IV diagnoses? Nursing diagnoses? Is it possible that the nurse might use a combination of the different types of diagnoses to plan client care more effectively?
- what resources are available in your community to assist clients and families experiencing crisis. What services are provided by these resources? How are nurses in your community involved in the delivery or care for clients and families in crisis?

THE IMPACT OF CRISIS WORK ON NURSES

Working with people in crisis is stressful work. Nurses who work with clients in the highly disorganized crisis period or those who work with victims of rape, violence, or disaster may see the results of humankind at its worst.

It is important that nurses develop increased self-awareness and be able to handle their feelings so that they can intervene in a tense situation (see the accompanying box). Although nurses may not have all the answers, people in crisis will expect nurses to help them regain control of themselves, *not* to control them. The nurse's self-assurance and composure help the client to regain equilibrium. The nurse will become more skilled with experience.

Walker (1991, pp. 21–27) identified a number of attitudes and strategies that can help the nurse be effective in crisis work:

- Strive for balance between professional life and your personal life.
- Support people who have been victimized.
- Search for new knowledge, and challenge myths about victimization, trauma, and coping.
- Appreciate natural support systems.
- Be willing to create new support systems.
- Be willing to help unskilled clients.
- Be able to collaborate with other professionals.
- Develop support networks with co-workers and other professionals.
- Be willing to tolerate frustration.
- Respect each person's own unique timetable.
- Allow clients to make their own choices, even if

Working with People in Crisis

Ask yourself:

- Do I believe that people who are in crisis are helpless?
- How do I feel about providing help to people for short periods of time?
- Can I contain my own anxiety when I am working with someone who makes me anxious?
- How do I feel about not being in control in certain situations?
- How do I react to people who are frightened? Angry? Threatening to me?
- How do I feel to people who don't seem able to handle their own problems?
- How does my experience of my culture influence my thinking?
- Do I have ideas that will hinder my ability to help others? For example, do I believe any of the following: That women who are raped are asking for it; that men should be strong and not show emotions; that children should be seen and not heard?

---

they are believed to be misguided or wrong.
- Allow people to make mistakes without becoming angry with them.
- Receive regular supervision.

To remain effective and to continue to grow personally and professionally, the nurse should also pay attention to these important areas:

- Respect and believe in a person's capacity to grow and change.
- Be aware of the impact of repeatedly listening to horrible stories.
- Formulate an outlet for stress and anger.
- Be willing to be a role model.
- Deal with personal fears about violence and vulnerability to stress and conflict.
- Develop realistic expectations of what can be done for others.
- Involve administrative/supervisory individuals when making extensive intervention plans that call for more than the usual effort.

CONSIDER...

- your ability to work with people in crisis. What strengths do you possess that enhance your

ability to work with people in crisis? What weaknesses do you have that may interfere with your ability to work with people in crisis? How can you balance your strengths and weaknesses?
- the effects of working with people in crisis on your own health and wellness. What strategies do you use to minimize the negative effects of working with people in crisis?

READINGS FOR ENRICHMENT

Green, B. L., & Lindy, J. D. (1994, June). Post-traumatic stress disorder in victims of disasters. *Psychiatric Clinics of North America, 17*(2), 301–309.

The authors present a model of how various factors may combine to influence people's ability to adapt to natural and human-caused disasters. The authors note incidence and severity of post-traumatic stress disorder (PTSD) in disaster survivors and the persistence of the symptoms. The authors note characteristics that place a person at risk for PTSD and characteristics that promote recovery. Finally, the authors outline various ways in which the health professionals might intervene on behalf of disaster survivors.

Hayes, G., Goodwin, T., & Miars, B. (1990, Feb.). After disaster: A crisis support team at work. *American Journal of Nursing, 90,* 61–64.

After a school bus crash kills 24 children, a team of nurse volunteers (members of the Red Cross Crisis Support Nursing team, or CSNT) implement crisis intervention strategies to help the families deal with the tragedy. This article provides insight into what role the CSNT plays and how it got its start.

Lundin, T. (1994, June). The treatment of acute trauma: Post-traumatic stress disorder prevention. *Psychiatric Clinics of North America, 17*(2), 385–391.

According to the author of this article, "It is not quite clear that it is possible to prevent post-traumatic stress disorder (PTSD) by means of early psychological support, counseling, or psychotherapeutic treatment. Biologic and psychological risk factors might interfere with different kinds of treatment efforts. It is, however, a basic human duty to try to help our fellow human beings." The author discusses the role of treatment strategies, the protective function of cultural customs and rituals, and psychologic methods that may be used to prevent PTSD. The psychologic interventions include providing information, support, crisis intervention, and emotional first aid. Short-term psychotherapy and psychopharmacologic treatment are also described.

SUMMARY

Everyday living brings expected and unexpected changes that result in stresses and tensions. These stresses and tensions have the potential to become crises. A crisis is a self-limiting situation in which an individual's usual problem-solving and coping skills are inadequate to resolve the situation successfully. A crisis offers the opportunity for growth and change. By obtaining help from appropriate sources, a person undergoing a crisis is more likely to solve the crisis in a positive way. Nurses are often in key positions to help clients cope with and grow through the crisis experience.

Crises may originate from three sources: situational experiences (stressful life events that usually are unanticipated), transitional states (maturational experiences, which usually are anticipated), and cultural/societal sources (such as discrimination). The crisis episode may be understood as a sequence that involves three stages: precrisis, crisis, and postcrisis.

Crisis intervention as a therapeutic strategy is strongly humanistic in that it views people who are experiencing crisis not as helpless, but as capable of personal growth and able to control their own lives. Intervention strategies such as individual crisis counseling, crisis groups, family crisis counseling, telephone counseling, and home crisis visits are appropriate modes for dealing with either internal or external crisis.

SELECTED REFERENCES

Aguilera, D. C. (1994). *Crisis intervention: Theory and methodology* (7th ed.). St. Louis: Mosby.

AJN News. (1993, April). A Trade Center bombing puts New York RNs to the test. *American Journal of Nursing, 93,* 101–102.

Allodi, F. A. (1994). Post-traumatic stress disorder in hostages and victims of torture. *Psychiatric Clinics of North America, 17*(2), 279–288.

American Psychiatric Association. (1994). *Diagnostic and statistical manual of mental disorders* (4th ed.). : Author.

Bowler, R. M., Mergier, D., Huel, G., & Cone, J. F. (1994). Psychological, psychosocial and psychophysiological sequelae in a community affected by a railroad chemical disaster. *Journal of Traumatic Stress, 7*(4), 601–624.

Green, B. L., & Lindl, J. D. (1994). Post-traumatic stress disorder in victims of disasters. *Psychiatric Clinics of North America, 17*(2), 301–309.

Hayes, G., Goodwin, J., & Miars, B. (1990, Feb.). After disaster: A crisis support team at work. *American Journal of Nursing, 90,* 61–64.

Hodgkinson, P. E., & Shepherd, M. A. (1994). The impact of disaster support work. *Journal of Traumatic Stress, 7*(4), 587–600.

Hoff, L. A. (1989). *People in crisis: Understanding and helping* (3rd ed.). Redwood City, CA: Addison-Wesley.

Lebowitz, L., & Roth, S. (1994). "I felt like a slut": The cultural context and women's response to being raped. *Journal of Traumatic Stress, 7*(3), 363–390.

Lundin, T. (1994). The treatment of acute trauma: Post-traumatic stress disorder prevention. *Psychiatric Clinics of North America, 17*(2), 385–391.

Meyer, M. U., & Graeter, C. J. (1995, May). Health professionals' role in disaster planning. *AAOHN Journal, 43*, 251–262.

Phifer, J. F. (1990). Psychological distress and somatic symptoms after natural disaster: Differential vulnerability among older adults. *Psychology and Aging, 5*(3), 412–420.

Walker, L. (1991). PTSD in women: Diagnosis and treatment of the battered woman syndrome. *Psychotherapy, 28*(1), 21–27.

Webb, N. B. (1991). *Play therapy with children in crisis: A casebook for practitioners.* New York: Guilford Press.

Weisaeth, L. (1993). Disasters: Psychological and psychiatric aspects. In L. Goldberger & S. Breznitz (Eds.), *Handbook of stress: Theoretical and clinical aspects.* New York: Free Press.

Wilson, H. S., & Kneisl, C. R. (1996). *Psychiatric nursing* (5th ed.). Menlo Park, CA: Addison-Wesley Nursing.

Managing Family Violence

OBJECTIVES

- Define family violence.

- Recognize the incidence of violence within the family.

- Discuss theoretical perspectives of violence.

- Identify essential aspects of assessing victims of family violence.

- Explain the nurse's role in assisting victims of family violence.

- Discuss methods to prevent family violence.

Pain and suffering... are both essentially private experiences, even though we can often observe their effects. Pain [is] a distressing, hurtful sensation in the body. Suffering, by contrast, is... a sense of anguish, vulnerability, loss of control, and threat to the integrity of the self.... There can be pain without suffering, and suffering without pain. In either case, only I can experience it, and only I can be relieved of it.

—Daniel Callahan,
Director of the Hastings Center

Violence and abusive behavior have become major health problems in North America.

- In the United States, at least 30 of each 1000 women undergo severe physical abuse by their male partner each year (United States Department of Health and Human Services [US-DHHS], 1989).

- In the United States, one in six pregnant women are physically abused during pregnancy (McFarlane, Parker, Soeken & Bullock, 1992; Bullock, 1993). One in five pregnant teenagers are abused (Parker, McFarlane, Soeken, Torres & Campbell, 1993).

- In Canada, one in eight women will be physically and/or sexually abused by a husband, an ex-husband, or a live-in partner each year (Greene, 1991, p. 6).

- Half the women killed in the United States each year die at the hands of a male partner or ex-lover (American Medical Association, Council on Scientific Affairs, 1992).

- Of every 1000 women, 108 are raped each year. It is estimated that one of every four women and at least one of every ten men will be sexually assaulted by age 21 (USDHHS, 1989, pp. 17–19).

- Homicide is the leading cause of death in infants under 2 after the first 6 weeks (USDHHS, 1989).

- Of every 1000 children, 25 are physically, sexually, or emotionally abused or neglected each year by their parents (USDHHS, 1989).

- It is estimated that between 1 and 2 million older Americans are victims of elder abuse (Simon, 1992).

FAMILY VIOLENCE AND ABUSE

National health care policy makers have now taken the stand that violence is a health problem, not just a criminal justice problem. Violent and abusive behavior is one of the 22 priority areas of *Healthy People 2000* (USDHHS, 1990). This document outlines 18 categories related to violent and abusive behavior, including homicide, suicide, child abuse and neglect, partner abuse, rape, weapon-related deaths, and so on. The American Nurses Association (ANA, 1991) has issued a position statement on physical violence against women. This statement produces the framework and official legitimacy for nursing care of victims of violence. The Canadian Nurses Association (CNA) has also issued its position on family violence in the document *Family Violence: Clinical Guidelines for Nurses*, which states that it is the responsibility of every nurse to be an advocate on behalf of any client suspected of being a victim of abuse (CNA, 1992, p. 4). The American Medical Association (AMA) made violence against women a priority issue in 1992. The American College of Obstetricians and Gynecologists (1989), the Surgeon General (USDHHS, 1986), have forwarded recommendations that all women be routinely screened for physical abuse and offered counseling, education, advocacy, and appropriate referrals. The Joint Commission on the Accreditation of Healthcare Organizations (JCAHO, 1990) has created new standards addressing violence. These standards require emergency departments to demonstrate that they assess for abuse of women and offer some interventions.

Nurses in every health care setting are seeing both victims and perpetrators of violence. Health care professionals encounter more than four times the number of cases of intentional injury than are reported to police (Ozmar, 1994, p. 515). This finding implies that the health care system may be the primary site for identifying victims of violence. Nurses need to know how to identify victims of interpersonal violence, appreciate potential risk factors for future violent injury, and understand some of the unique considerations related to the care of abuse victims (Ozmar, 1994, p. 515). Acts of violence often escalate in frequency and severity and may ultimately result in homicide.

Family violence includes spouse abuse, child abuse, and elder abuse ranging from verbal abuse, light slaps to severe beatings to homicide. It occurs in all strata of society; it crosses all racial, religious, ethnic, socioeconomic, and educational barriers, and it is not confined to any particular age group or occupation. It is a myth that domestic violence occurs only in poor minority families.

Although the focus of this chapter is domestic violence and physical abuse, emotional abuse is equally damaging (Fontaine, 1996, p. 565). Words can hit as hard as a fist, and the damage to self-esteem can last a lifetime. Emotional abuse involves one person shaming, embarrassing, ridiculing, or insulting a loved one. It may include the destruction of personal property or the killing of pets in an effort to frighten or control the victim. Emotional abuse may also include statements that are devastating to the victim's self-esteem, such as, "You can't do anything right," "You're ugly and stupid—no one else would want you," "I wish you had never been born" (Fontaine, 1996).

Abusive caretakers come from all walks of life but have certain traits or characteristics in common:

- Overpossessiveness: viewing family members in terms of ownership and property
- Excessive jealousy
- Desire to control and dominate
- Poor control of impulses
- Low tolerance for frustration
- Belief that physical measures are necessary to control children
- Dependence on an elder for financial support and accommodation
- Drug or alcohol use
- History of poor mental health or a personality disorder
- History of abuse as a child by own parents

Spouse Abuse

Most spouse abuse is perpetrated by men against women; however, abuse also is perpetrated by women against men and can occur between partners of the same sex. It is not confined to marriage relationships: couples who are dating or living together may also be involved in violence. Women are more vulnerable to violence because of their disadvantage in size and strength and their social and economic dependence on men.

In contrast to child abuse, which is unlawful and punishable, societal sanctions regarding violence against women have not historically been as stringent (Jezierski, 1994, p. 361). Traditionally, woman battering was considered a private a domestic matter, informally condoned by law. Before 1700, laws allowed a husband to chastise his wife with any reasonable instrument, such as a rod not thicker than the husband's thumb (the origin of the phrase "rule of thumb") (Henderson, 1992, p. 27). Spouse abuse has gained increased national attention only since the women's movement in the 1970s. Efforts were begun to establish resources for battered women. Since then there has been a continuing focus on providing shelters and counseling and on passing new laws to protect the abused spouse.

Abuse or woman battering is defined as the repeated subjection of a person to forceful physical, social, and psychologic behavior to coerce without regard to her rights (Herton, 1986). The intensity and frequency of attacks tend to escalate over time. Abuse can be categorized as physical abuse, sexual abuse, psychosocial abuse, and property violence. *Physical abuse* involves any physical harm or nonconsensual touching. It may involve pushing and shoving, dragging or pulling; kicking, hitting, or beating the woman with fists or objects; locking the woman out of the home or in a room or closet or abandoning the woman in a dangerous place; or biting, choking, physically restraining, or threatening the woman with a weapon. *Sexual abuse* involves any forced or nonconsensual sex. It includes sexually criticizing the person, hurting her during sex, and/or treating that person as property or a sex object. *Psychosocial abuse* can involve threats of harm to the woman and her children, abuse of pets, constant criticism and downgrading in front of others, insulting the woman's family or friends, keeping the woman from talking to or seeing friends and family, and threats to kidnap the children if she leaves. It may involve keeping the woman from working or going to school, censoring her mail, taking away her car keys or money, accusing her of having affairs, or forbidding her to use the telephone. *Property violence* is threatened or actual destruction of material possessions.

It is especially difficult for many victims to leave an abusive relationship. Women who do leave an abusive relationship attempt an average of three to five separations before finally ending the relationship. Some women are threatened with loss of children or with death if they do not return home. Social and cultural beliefs also play a role. Women have been socialized to be self-sacrificing for the good of others and feel responsible for keeping the

RESEARCH NOTE

How Does Physical and Emotional Abuse During Pregnancy Compare Among Adult and Teenage Women?

Health professionals have expressed increased concern about the frequency and severity of violence in pregnancy, the consequences of abuse on maternal and infant health, and the amount of violence that teens experience in intimate relationships. A study was conducted to compare the amount of physical and mental abuse experienced by a sample of 691 African-American, Hispanic, and white pregnant teenage and adult women. The subjects were interviewed in the prenatal setting. On their first visit, 182 women (26%) reported physical or sexual abuse within the past year. There were significant differences between the teens and adults, with a higher percentage of teens (31.6%) reporting abuse during the prior year than adults (23.6%). The rate of abuse during pregnancy was 21.7% for teens and 15.9% for adult women. Adult women scored significantly higher than teens on two measures of mental abuse. For all subjects,

mental abuse correlated significantly with physical abuse.

Implications: Pregnancy offers nurses an opportunity for assessing abuse because it is one of the few times that healthy women have frequent, scheduled contact with nurses. At this time, pregnant women may be motivated to use health-seeking behaviors as they concern themselves with the health and safety of the unborn child. The high incidence of abuse reported by teens in this study suggests that health care providers can intervene early in the cycle of violence and perhaps prevent a potential escalation of the abuse.

SOURCE: "Physical and Emotional Abuse in Pregnancy: A Comparison of Adult and Teenage Women" by B. Parker, J. McFarlane, K. Soeken, S. Torres, and D. Campbell, May/June 1993, *Nursing Research, 42*(3), 173–178.

family together at almost any cost, and cultural beliefs about loyalty and duty may reinforce the role of victim. In addition, many women are financially dependent on their abusive partners; if they have outside employment, they are unlikely to earn as much as their male counterparts. If there are children, the woman may desperately need child support, and many fathers do not honor this obligation and default on the payments. The burdens of child care have traditionally fallen entirely on the mother. Thus, lack of affordable and adequate child care facilities has become a major problem for the single mother seeking employment.

Many people believe that abused spouses can end the violence by divorcing their abuser or that the victim can learn to stop doing those things that provoke violence. These beliefs are myths and not supported by facts. According to the United States Department of Justice, about 75% of all spousal attacks occur between people who are separated or divorced. In many cases, the separation process brings on an increased level of harassment and violence. In a battering relationship, moreover, the abuser needs no provocation to become violent. Violence is the abuser's pattern of behavior, and the victim can't learn how to control it. Even so, many

victims blame themselves for the abuse, feeling guilty—even responsible—for doing or saying something that triggers the abuser's behavior. Friends, family, and service providers reinforce this attitude by laying the blame and the need to change on the shoulders of the victim. Many people who do try to disclose their situation are met with disbelief or denial; this discourages them from persevering.

Child Abuse

Children of any age, race, religion, or socioeconomic status can be victims of abuse and neglect. Surveys show that child abuse goes hand-in-hand with spouse abuse 50% of the time (Bowker, Arbitell & McFerron, 1988). Perpetrators of the abuse may be parents, siblings, or a live-in or babysitting boyfriend. Laws mandate the reporting of suspected child abuse. These laws protect health care professionals from any liability that might result from their reporting suspected cases of child abuse in good faith (Devlin & Reynolds, 1994, p. 31). Child abuse can take various forms, including physical abuse, physical neglect, sexual abuse, and emotional abuse and neglect (Srnec, 1991, pp. 475–477).

Physical abuse is nonaccidental injury of a child. This definition excludes spanking and slapping the hands and buttocks of a child over 1 year of age, a practice condoned by some parents as acceptable methods of discipline. Physical abuse is relatively easy to recognize and treat. The most common types of physical abuse are burns, bruises, fractures, abdominal injuries, and head or spinal cord injuries. The location and pattern of injury help determine the likelihood of abuse. For example, accidental scalds usually occur on the front of the body; scald burns on the back and feet are suspicious. Bruises over bony surfaces such as the shin, forehead, knees, forearms, and chin are common occurrences among active children; bruises on the cheek, abdomen, back, buttocks, and thighs raise suspicion of abuse.

Whiplash-shaking can lead to severe injury in infants. Cerebral damage, neurologic defects, blindness, and mental retardation can result. These findings are seen often without external evidence of head injury. Nurses should suspect **shaken baby syndrome (SBS)** in infants less than 1 year of age who present with apnea, seizures, lethargy or drowsiness, bradycardia, respiratory difficulty, coma, or death. Subdural and retinal hemorrhages accompanied by the absence of external signs of trauma are hallmarks of the syndrome.

Another common, often unrecognized, form of family violence occurs between siblings (Fontaine, 1996, p. 522). Many people assume that it is natural, and even appropriate, for children to use physical force with one another: "It's a good chance for him to learn how to defend himself," "She had a right to hit him; he was teasing her," or "Kids will be kids." These attitudes teach children that physical force is an appropriate method of resolving conflicts. Sibling violence is highest in the early years and decreases with age. In all age groups, girls are less violent toward their siblings than are boys.

Physical neglect is failure to meet the basic needs of children by those persons responsible for doing so. Basic needs include adequate nourishment, clothing, housing, supervision, and medical care. Nurses must exercise caution, however, "not to define as willful neglect a case in which an impoverished or uneducated family is providing ... the best care possible within their means" (Srnec, 1991, p. 476).

Sexual abuse is the occurrence of any sexual activity between an adult and child. In includes either *assaultive* abuse, which produces physical injury and severe emotional trauma, or *nonassaultive* abuse,

which produces minimal or no physical trauma. Nonassaultive abuse is often chronic and severely disruptive of the child's sexual development. Children who have been sexually abused may demonstrate the following clinical signs: perineal rashes, genital-rectal irritation or tissue trauma, frequent urinary tract infections, evidence of vaginal or anal penetration by a foreign body, presence of sexually transmitted disease, and an unusually mature knowledge of sexual terminology and slang. Some children may become involved in promiscuous sexual activities and juvenile prostitution or pornography. Because child sexual abuse most often involves the parent of the child, this form of abuse is the least reported.

Emotional abuse and neglect is failure to provide an environment in which the child can thrive, learn, and develop. Obviously, this type of abuse is more difficult to identify and manage than physical abuse.

Children who are abused manifest various characteristics (see the accompanying box). Childhood abuse may have far-reaching consequences for the victim's health; violent sexual abuse may lead to the strongest long-term consequence. Hall, Sachs, Rayens & Lutenbacher (1993, p. 317) report a high incidence of depressive symptoms in later life of adults who had been abused as children.

Behavioral Characteristics of Abused Children

The child may

- Be unusually aggressive, withdrawn, overly compliant, or attention seeking.

- Appear afraid of a parent or wary of physical contact with an adult.

- Be inappropriately clothed during winter.

- Manifest developmental delay and failure to thrive.

- Express violence toward pets.

- Run away from home.

- Demonstrate changes in school performance.

- Be habitually late for school or avoid spending time at home by arriving early and staying late.

- Verbalize fault for injuries: "I deserved it."

- Attempt suicide or abuse alcohol or drugs.

Elder Abuse and Mistreatment

The rate of elder abuse is unknown. As the proportion of older adults in the population increases, it is possible that elder abuse will become even a greater problem. Elder abuse may affect either sex; however, the victims most often are women who are over 75 years of age, physically or mentally impaired, and dependent for care on the abuser. The abuse may involve physical, psychologic, or emotional abuse; sexual abuse; financial abuse; violation of human or civil rights; and active or passive neglect.

When elder abuse involves physical neglect, victims may suffer from dehydration, malnutrition, and oversedation. The victim may be deprived of necessary articles, such as glasses, hearing aids, or walkers. Psychologically, the person may suffer verbal assaults, threats, humiliation, or harassment. Abuse may also include failure to provide appropriate medications or medical treatment, isolation, unreasonable confinement, lack of privacy, an unsafe environment, and involuntary servitude. Some are financially exploited by relatives who steal from them or misuse their property or funds. Others are beaten and even raped by family members. Most victims experience two or more forms of abuse.

Elder abuse or neglect may occur in private homes, senior citizen's homes, nursing homes, hospitals, and long-term care facilities. Many of the abusers are either sons or daughters; others include spouses, relatives (grandchildren, siblings, nieces, and nephews), and, in some instances, health care providers.

Older adults at home may fail to report abuse or neglect for many reasons. They may be ashamed to admit that their children have abused them or fear retaliation if they seek help. They may fear being sent to an institution. They frequently lack financial resources, or lack the mental capacity to be aware of abuse or neglect and to report the situation. Examples of crimes are assault and financial abuse of an older person who is physically or mentally incompetent and has no trustworthy friend or relative to help. In some instances, nurses can intervene by educating caregivers about the needs of older adults and resources available to provide increased home support. They should also report the situation to the appropriate person in the health care agency.

CONSIDER . . .

- the incidence of woman, child, and elder abuse in your community. What types of abuse are experienced by women, children, and older adults in your community? Are there societal or community practices that support or encourage abuse in your area?
- how a previous abusive relationship might affect the nurse's practice.
- what professional experiences you have had with abuse or victims of abuse.

ASSESSING ABUSE

Often the nurse is the first one outside the person's family to discover that the person is being abused. Some battered women may not disclose the abuse, or they may minimize its impact. However, it is the nurse's responsibility to assess for and be alert for signs of abuse and not deny the violence.

During the assessment interview, the nurse must ensure privacy. Assessment must always take place away from the male partner and children. It may be difficult for the client to admit to the reality of family violence until a trusting nurse-client relationship evolves. The nurse should assure the client of genuine desire to help the entire family system. The nurse should also approach this topic as if it were any other health risk, explaining that all women are assessed for abuse. In addition, the nurse can offer the option of answering questions about incidents of abuse with "sometimes" instead of "yes" or "no"; this may encourage the client to make a first step to acknowledge the abuse.

Battered women enter the health care system for a variety of conditions associated with abuse. For example, common physical complaints of abused women include chronic pelvic pain, headache, irritable bowel syndrome, arthritis, pelvic inflammatory disease, and neurologic damage. Psychiatric illness (e.g., alcoholism) may also be the result of a history of sexual or physical abuse.

Nursing History

Because domestic violence is so prevalent, many health care professionals now believe that questions concerning abuse should be part of any health history. To detect the presence of abuse, various assessment tools may be used. An abuse assessment screen has been developed by the Nursing Research Consortium on Violence and Abuse.

The Canadian Nurses Association (1992, p. 9) proposes that the nurse assess the frequency of family conflict and aggression by asking such questions as these:

> "Many times, families don't handle problems in the way that they would like to. How does your family handle problems?"

> "Has anyone ever used physical force? Who? When?"

The nurse must clarify vague or evasive answers and further explore any such areas by asking, for example, "What happens when you and your partner get angry?" or "Has anything happened to you that might have caused these symptoms?"

When assessing a child, the nurse may ask, "Moms and dads try to help their children learn how to behave well. What happens to you when you do something wrong?" or "Can you tell me more about this?"

If the response to initial questions indicate possible abuse, the nurse needs to conduct a detailed assessment. Most agencies supply nursing history tools for this purpose.

Physical Examination

Victims of physical abuse may suffer a variety of injuries. In general, small children may be retarded in their growth and development. During a head-to-toe assessment, the nurse observes for indications of abuse such as:

- *Head:* Bald patches on the scalp where hair has been pulled out; evidence of trauma from blows to the head, such as hematoma, facial bruises, facial fractures, bruised or swollen eyes, hemorrhages into the eyes; petechiae around the eyes from attempted strangulation.
- *Skin:* Swelling or tenderness, bruises, burns, or scars of past injuries on the skin, genitals, and rectal areas.
- *Musculoskeletal system:* Fractures or evidence of previous fractures, particularly of the face, arms/legs and ribs; dislocated joints, especially in the shoulder when the victim is grabbed or pulled by the arm.
- *Abdomen:* Bruises, wounds, or intra-abdominal injuries, especially if the woman is pregnant.
- *Neurologic system:* Hyperactive reflexes due to neurologic damage; paresthesias, numbness, or pain from old injuries.

If the nursing assessment reveals possible domestic violence, a team assessment needs to take place. The victim's medical condition and emotional state must be assessed. The severity and potential fatality of the situation must be considered, as well as the needs of dependent children and the legal ramifications.

Common *psychologic reactions* of abused women include fear of further abuse or death; low self-esteem; anxiety and depression; feelings of helplessness or hopelessness; repressed or expressed rage, guilt, or overwhelming apprehension or worry; suicidal thoughts, gestures, or attempts at suicide; impaired ability to make decisions; sleep disturbances; and panic attacks (Fontaine, 1996). Behavioral characteristics of abused children are shown on page 415.

CONSIDER . . .

- nursing and medical assessment instruments used in your practice setting. Are there areas or questions that specifically assess for abuse or violence? Do self-report instruments ask questions that would elicit a history of abuse?
- the possibility that abuse is underreported in practice settings whose staff are not attuned to the signs and symptoms of violence. How might the ignorance of health care providers exacerbate the problem of abuse?
- the responsibility of the nurse if evidence of abuse is detected during assessment.

DIAGNOSING ABUSE

Because abuse is complex and involves many aspects, a variety of nursing diagnoses may be appropriate. These include the following:

- **High risk for violence: Directed at others**
- **High risk for violence: Self-directed**
- **Health-seeking behaviors**
- **Rape-trauma syndrome**
- **Ineffective family coping: Disabling**
- **Ineffective individual coping**
- **Powerlessness**
- **Self-esteem disturbance**
- **Altered family processes**
- **Altered parenting**

Other nursing diagnoses may also apply, depending on the individual and family needs.

PLANNING/IMPLEMENTING INTERVENTIONS FOR THE ABUSED

The goals of treating abuse are (a) to empower the client to take control, (b) to support the client, and (c) to maximize the client's safety (CNA, 1992, p. 10).

Most people involved in intrafamily violence are disturbed by this behavior and would like it to end. Even though they want help to stop the abuse, they may not know how to seek the assistance they need. It is extremely important for nurses to be nonjudgmental in their interactions with all family members. The abusers may be distrustful of the motives of the nursing staff. Initially, the victims may be unwilling to trust the nursing staff because of family shame and fear of being blamed for remaining in the violent situation. The nurse should convey a nonjudgmental manner; in other words, the nurse should avoid blaming the victim or looking for pathologic elements in the victim's behavior. It is vital not to impose personal values on the family by offering quick and easy solutions to intrafamily violence (Fontaine, 1996).

Short-Term Interventions

Because the nurse may have the only contact with the client, it is essential that the nurse (a) determine the immediacy of danger, (b) convey that the person is not to blame and has the right to be safe, (c) explore options for help and, (d) provide information regarding available services.

It is important that the nurse avoid a judgmental attitude and support the person's choice about whether to leave the unsafe situation or return to the abusive relationship. See the discussion earlier about the difficulties women encounter in leaving an abusive relationship.

Because severely battered women are at risk for homicide, the nurse needs to inform the client about associated risk factors and determine the immediacy of danger. See the Danger Assessment Screen in Figure 21–1.

FIGURE 21–1 *Danger assessment screen*

SOURCE: Reproduced from "Nursing Assessment for Risk of Homicide in Battered Women" by J. Campbell, *Advances in Nursing Science, 8,* pp. 36–51. Used with permission.

Danger Assessment

Several risk factors have been associated with homicides (murder) of both batterers and battered women in research conducted after the killings have taken place. We cannot predict what will happen in your case, but we would like you to be aware of the danger of homicide in situations of severe battering and for you to see how many of the risk factors apply to your situation. (The "he" in the questions refers to your husband, partner, ex-husband, ex-partner, or whoever is currently physically hurting you.)

Please check YES or NO for each question below.

YES   NO

☐   ☐   1. Has the physical violence increased in frequency over the past year?

☐   ☐   2. Has the physical violence increased in severity over the past year and/or has a weapon or threat with weapon been used?

☐   ☐   3. Does he ever try to choke you?

☐   ☐   4. Is there a gun in the house?

☐   ☐   5. Has he ever forced you into sex when you did not wish to do so?

☐   ☐   6. Does he use drugs? By drugs, I mean "uppers" or amphetamines, speed, angel dust, cocaine, "crack," street drugs, heroin, or mixtures.

☐   ☐   7. Does he threaten to kill you and/or do you believe he is capable of killing you?

☐   ☐   8. Is he drunk every day or almost every day? (In terms of quantity of alcohol)

☐   ☐   9. Does he control most all of your daily activities? For instance, does he tell you who you can be friends with, how much money you can take with you shopping, or when you can take the car? (If he tries, but you do not let him, check here _____.)

☐   ☐   10. Have you ever been beaten by him while you were pregnant? (If never pregnant by him, check here _____.)

☐   ☐   11. Is he violently and constantly jealous of you? (For instance, does he say, "If I can't have you, no one can"?)

TOTAL YES ANSWERS _____

THANK YOU. PLEASE TALK TO YOUR NURSE, ADVOCATE, OR COUNSELOR ABOUT WHAT THE DANGER ASSESSMENT MEANS IN TERMS OF YOUR SITUATION.

The Holtz and Furniss Mnemonic Tool to Guide Immediate Treatment of Abused Women

A. Reassure the woman that she is not *alone* and that assistance and support are available from caregivers who can help.

B. Express *belief* that violence is not acceptable, no matter what she has been told by the batterer. Tell her that she should never be physically hurt.

C. Ensure *confidentiality*. Let the person know that her disclosure is private but will be documented on her medical record in case it is needed for legal purposes at a future date.

D. *Document* clear descriptions of all physical and psychologic symptoms; a history of at least the first, worst, and most recent incidence of abuse; what was said, done, and observed; date, time, and direct quotes of the client. Notes may be needed for legal purposes.

E. *Educate* the woman about (a) the cycle of violence and likely escalation of abuse and (b) assistance available for shelter or housing, jobs, legal issues, social services, medical care, crisis counseling, support groups (for victims and abusers), and other local agencies.

F. Ensure the woman's *safety*. Provide telephone numbers for a local shelter, the police, and telephone help lines. Discuss a safety plan for quick escape. Hide or place a suitcase containing personal belongings with a neighbor or friends. The suitcase should contain a change of clothes for the client and each child, a small amount of money, essential telephone numbers, a toy for each child, and copies of essential documents, such as marriage license, children's birth certificates, medical insurance number or plan, and, if possible, last income tax return. Explore all legal options, such as orders of protection or restraining orders.

SOURCE: Adapted from "Screening for Abuse in the Clinical Setting" by K. K. Furniss, 1993, *AWHONN's Clinical Issues*, *4*(3), p. 404.

Many agencies now provide protocols for health care professionals to follow. These offer specific guidelines for the identification, treatment, and referral of battered women seeking emergency care.

A simple mnemonic tool developed by Holtz and Furniss (Furniss, 1993) provides guidelines for essential interventions during this early contact of the client (see the accompanying box).

A collaborative team of nurse administrators and clinical nurses at Harris County Health Department in Houston, Texas, developed a screening and intervention triage tool for abuse. The triage structure facilitates appropriate intervention according to screening data. Each of the triage levels includes related interventions and essential documentation. See Table 21–1.

Abused children need to be encouraged to talk, but they must also be protected from having to provide multiple reports. Nurses need to tell an abused child that they believe the story, and they must reassure the child that he or she has done nothing wrong. The nurse should also avoid making negative comments about the abuser and to follow established protocols for mandatory reporting, documentation, and use of available support services (e.g., the police department, social service agencies, and child welfare agency).

Interventions for abused older adults include developing a positive relationship with both the victim and the abuser, exploring ways for the older person to maximize independence, and exploring the need for additional home care services or alternative living arrangements.

Nurses must familiarize themselves with agency protocols and resources available for victims of domestic violence. Most municipalities have crisis helplines and hotlines to provide assistance to victims of abuse. The nurse should also keep a record of telephone numbers for transition houses and rape crisis centers, alcoholic and drug abuse information, support groups, religious organizations, and legal services. There are also several national organizations that offer toll-free contacts, such as the National Organization for Victim Assistance, the National Coalition Against Domestic Violence (in the United States), and the National Clearinghouse on Family Violence (in Canada).

Long-Term Interventions

Goals for ongoing counseling and care may include (a) helping the client continue to choose to be safe from violence, (b) helping the client explore options for self-development, and (c) helping the client

TABLE 21–1 Screening and Intervention Triage for Abuse

| Steps | TRIAGE | | |
	Level I	Level II	Level III
SCREEN	No history or present threat of abuse.	Recent or present abuse.	Client presents with injuries.
INTERVENE	Group or individual education about domestic violence; give handouts and pamphlets of community resources to client.	Crisis intervention; individual counseling; assist client with escape plan; identify shelter and other emergency resources; assist client in contacting shelter.	Crisis intervention; notify police; refer client to hospital for treatment (call ambulance); notify shelter; transport patient to shelter.
DOCUMENT	Statement of no abuse or threat of abuse; give handouts/education materials to client.	Statement of present or recent abuse; counsel client; give numbers to shelter and police; plan escape route; note if client declines shelter assistance at this time, or if shelter should be contacted per client's request.	Give statement of medical care given; notify emergency services; note where client was transported and in what condition.

SOURCE: "Establishing a Screening Program for Abused Women" by M. V. Lazzaro, and J. McFarlane, October 1991, *Journal of Nursing Administration, 21,* p. 10. Reprinted with permission.

improve quality of life through increasing self-esteem (CNA, 1992, p. 14).

Usually, the best way to treat violent families is a multidisciplinary approach involving nurses, physicians, social workers, police, protective services personnel, and, often, lawyers. Most families are more open to accepting help during a time of crisis than at other times. They will most likely be willing to develop new behavior patterns for up to 4 to 6 weeks following a crisis. If they are not helped during that time, they will most likely return to previous behavior patterns, including violence.

Nurses should know the laws associated with reporting physical abuse. In the United States and Canada, nurses are required to report any suspected child abuse. The courts and child protective agencies make decisions in the child's interest. They may allow a child to remain in the home but under court supervision; they may remove the child from the home; and, in some instances, they may terminate parental rights if the abuse was severe.

State and provincial laws about reporting adult and elder abuse vary. Domestic violence is considered a violent crime; the victim has a right to be protected, and the perpetrator of the violence can often expect to be prosecuted.

When a nurse makes a report regarding family violence, it is important to inform the family that the report will be filed with the protective services. Nurses also need to keep families informed about what steps are being taken and offer counseling and support as required. The referral process is a vital component of nursing care because the family will need multidisciplinary interventions to halt the violence.

CONSIDER...

- resources available in your community for victims of violence. What shelters are available for abused women or children? What crisis programs are available to assist older victims of violence? What resources are available to offer respite for caregivers of older adults? What resources are available for abused older adults?
- that many agencies that provide services for victims of violence have small budgets and few paid staff. In your community, how many nurse volunteers provide care and support for victims of violence? Should such programs have a higher priority for funding?

PREVENTING ABUSE

Nurses in all areas of practice (e.g., maternal/child health; school; community and occupational health; mental health; primary and acute care; and academic settings) need to take a proactive role to prevent family violence. Early screening of vulnerable people and efforts to promote a change in attitudes and beliefs about family violence are essential.

If they are to assist victims effectively, nurses must be aware of their own feelings about family violence. Nurses who are unclear about their own feelings about family violence may deny its existence, blame the victim in crisis, or minimize the effects of the violence (CNA, 1992, p. 8).

Nurses can also be instrumental as advocates in developing policies and programs, and providing in-service training and education to health care professionals and the public.

Comprehensive violence prevention programs require a variety of different disciplines and organizations working together, such as state or provincial and local health care agencies, criminal justice agencies, and social service agencies (USDHHS, 1990, p. 240). The following strategies are recommended by the USDHHS in *Healthy People 2000* (1990, pp. 240–241):

- Public awareness programs that (a) dispel the myths about domestic violence, (b) publicize sources of shelter and support for battered women and their children, and (c) provide information about positive parenting, positive support, cues to suspect child abuse, and how to report child abuse to authorities.
- Coordination among domestic violence programs, child protection programs, substance abuse programs, mental health centers, the criminal justice system, and the medical community for referral, intervention, and case management. Provisions need to be made for linkages and continuity of care services, housing and other basic necessities, and job training.
- Expansion of (a) emergency shelter and support services for victims, such as respite care, child care, crisis facilities, help lines, self-help groups, and other natural helping networks; (b) transitional and low-income housing resources for victims to help them achieve safety and economic self-sufficiency; and (c) court-ordered treatment programs for abusers.

- Violence prevention and education programs, such as (a) school-based age-specific prevention programs for all school-age children; (b) projects for the prevention of alcohol and other drug-related abuse and neglect; and (c) multidisciplinary training programs for professionals in medical, legal, and social service fields who deal with potential victims and abusers or who are involved in the planning and implementation of prevention programs.
- Hospital-based or other health-facility-based information and referral services for victims and stressed family caregivers.

READINGS FOR ENRICHMENT

All, A. C. (1994, July). A literature review: Assessment and intervention in elder abuse. *Journal of Gerontologic Nursing, 20*, 25–32.

Current and projected demographic and societal changes warrant concern about elder abuse. This author discusses the extent of the problem of elder abuse, reviews current definitions, and reviews the research on assessment and intervention strategies for this segment of the population. Indicators for the detection of elder abuse, specific stressors identified as precipitants of elder abuse, characteristics of the victim and abusers, and interventions appropriate to the situation are included.

Chiocca, E. M. (1995, Jan./Feb.). Shaken baby syndrome: A nursing perspective. *Pediatric Nursing, 21*, 33–38.

This article was a winner of Pediatric Nursing's 1994 Writer's Award Contest. Shaken baby syndrome (SBS), previously called whiplash shaken infant syndrome, was first identified in the early 1970s. It is a leading cause of death and long-term disability in child abuse cases. This article includes the incidence, risk factors, mechanisms of injury, clinical signs, diagnosis, clinical management, nursing implications, prognosis, and prevention of SBS. The author also emphasizes that one of the nurse's most important responsibilities is to educate parents on the dangers of shaking infants.

Devlin, B. K., & Reynolds, E. (1994, March). Child abuse: How to recognize it, how to intervene. *American Journal of Nursing, 94*, 26–32.

This continuing education article includes key clinical and psychosocial factors to consider when examining a child who may have been physically or

➜

READINGS FOR ENRICHMENT

sexually abused. Information is provided about the types of injuries that suggest child abuse, indications of possible sexual abuse, and the nurse's legal obligations. Fourteen test questions are included.

Sheridan, D. J., & Taylor, W. K. (1993). Developing hospital-based domestic violence programs, protocols, policies, and procedures. *AWHONN's Clinical Issues, 4*(3), 471–482.

The authors share their experiences in developing two of the nation's eight hospital-based domestic violence programs. Implementing the suggestions contained in this article will enhance a hospital's successful compliance with the 1992 JCAHO guidelines for emergency and ambulatory services departments. The need for preprogram data collection, multidisciplinary support, client and staff safety, specific program services, and staff supervision is addressed. The article includes one of the most widely distributed examples of a battered woman's protocol developed at Chicago's Rush-Presbyterian-St. Luke's Medical Center. This protocol proposes a minimum standard of care for the identification, treatment, and referral of battered women seeking emergency care.

SUMMARY

The prevalence of violence and abusive behavior in North America is alarming. National health care organizations now view violence as a major health problem and are directing attention to its recognition, prevention, and treatment. Nurses need to know how to identify victims of violence, to appreciate potential risk factors for future injury, and to understand some of the unique considerations regarding care of victims of abuse. Acts of violence often escalate in frequency and severity and may ultimately result in homicide.

Family violence includes spouse abuse, child abuse and neglect, and elder abuse, neglect or mistreatment. It occurs in all strata of society. Abusive individuals have certain traits in common, such as overpossessiveness, desire to dominate, poor control of impulses, and a history of drug or alcohol use. Victims of spouse abuse most often are women, many of whom have difficulty leaving the abusive relationship largely because of fear, shame, guilt, and economic dependence. Child abuse goes hand-in-hand with spouse abuse about 50% of the time. Laws mandate the reporting of suspected child abuse. Elder abuse can involve not only physical, sexual, or emotional abuse but also active or passive neglect, violation of human or civil rights, and financial abuse. Those most vulnerable to elder abuse are females over 75 years of age, physically or mentally impaired, and dependent for care on the abuser.

Often the nurse is the first one outside the family to discover that a person is being abused. Appropriate assessment, intervention, and documentation are essential to prevent the abuse from continuing. The nurse needs to empower the client to take control, provide support, and maximize the client's safety. Treatment of violent families requires a multidisciplinary approach among nurses, social workers, physicians, family therapists, vocational trainers, police, protective services personnel, and lawyers.

If they are to assist victims effectively, nurses need to be aware of their own feelings about family violence. They also need to take a proactive role in preventing family violence. Nurses can advocate in developing programs and policies and provide in-service training and education to other health care professionals and the public.

SELECTED REFERENCES

AAN Expert Panel on Violence. (1993, March/April). Violence as a nursing priority. AAN Working Paper. *Nursing Outlook, 41*(2), 83–92.

All, A. C. (1994, July). A literature review: Assessment and intervention in elder abuse. *Journal of Gerontological Nursing, 20,* 25–32.

American College of Obstetricians and Gynecologists. (1989). *The battered woman.* Washington, DC: American College of Obstetricians and Gynecologists. ACOG technical bulletin no. 124.

American Nurses Association. (1991). *Position statement on physical violence against women.* Washington, DC: Author.

American Medical Association, Council on Scientific Affairs. (1992). Violence against women: Relevance for medical practitioners. *Journal of the American Medical Association, 267*(23), 3184–3189.

Bennett, L. (1993, Aug.). Growing up with violence. *Canadian Nurse, 89,* 33–36.

Bolton, F. G., & Bolton, S. R. (1987). *Working with violent families.* Newbury Park, CA: Sage.

Bowker, L. H., Arbitell, M., & McFerron, J. R. (1988). On the relationship between wife beating and child abuse. In K. Yllo & M. Bograd (Eds.), *Feminist perspective on wife abuse.* Newbury Park, CA: Sage.

Boychuk-Duchscher, J. E. (1994, June). Acting on violence against women. *Canadian Nurse, 91,* 20–25.

Brown, L. (1992a, Jan./Feb.) Family violence. Part I. Hidden secrets: Elder abuse. *Nursing BC, 24,* 18–20.

Brown, L. (1992b, March/April). Family violence. Part II. Hidden secrets: Child abuse and wife abuse. *Nursing BC, 24,* 10–15.

Bullock, L. (1993). Nursing interventions for abused women on obstetrical units. *Clinical Issues in Perinatal Women's Health Nursing, 4,* 371–377.

Campbell, J. C. (1992, Nov.). Ways of teaching, learning, and knowing about violence against women. *Nursing Health Care, 13,* 464–470.

Campbell, J. C. (1993). Woman abuse and public policy: Potential for nursing action. *AWHONN's Clinical Issues, 4*(3), 503–512.

Canadian Nurses' Association. (1992). *Family violence: Clinical guidelines for nurses.* Ottawa: Author.

Chez, N. (1994, July). Helping the victim of domestic violence. *American Journal of Nursing, 94,* 33–37.

Chiocca, E. M. (1995, Jan./Feb.) Shaken baby syndrome: A nursing perspective. *Pediatric Nursing, 21,* 33–38.

Committee on Trauma Research, Commission on Life Sciences, National Research Council and the National Academy of Sciences. (1985). *Injury in America: A continuing public health problem.* Washington, DC: National Academy Press.

Devlin, B. K., & Reynolds, E. (1994, March). Child abuse: How to recognize it, how to intervene. *American Journal of Nursing, 94,* 26–32.

Fontaine, K. L. (1996). Rape and intrafamily abuse and violence. Pages 555–584 in H. S. Wilson and C. R. Kneisl, *Psychiatric Nursing* (5th ed.) Menlo Park, CA: Addison-Wesley Nursing.

Frost, M. H., & Willette, K. (1994, Aug.). Risk for abuse/neglect: Documentation of assessment data and diagnoses. *Journal of Gerontological Nursing, 20,* 37–45.

Fulmer, T., & Ashley, J. (1989, Nov.). Clinical indicators of elder abuse. *Applied Nursing Research, 2,* 161–167.

Fulmer, T., McMahon, D. J., Baer-Hines, M., & Forget, B. (1992, Dec.). Abuse, neglect, abandonment, violence, and exploitation: An analysis of all elderly patients seen in one emergency department during a six-month period. *Journal of Emergency Nursing, 18*(6), 505–510.

Furniss, K. K. (1993). Screening for abuse in the clinical setting. *AWHONN's Clinical Issues, 4*(3), 402–406.

Greene, B. (1991). *The war against women. Report of the Standing Committee on Health and Welfare, Social Affairs, Seniors and the Status of Women.* Issue No. 31. Ottawa: Canada Communications Group, Publishing, Supply and Services.

Grunfeld, A. F., Ritmiller, S., Mackay, K., Cowan, L., & Hotch, D. (1994, Aug.). Detecting domestic violence against women in the emergency department: A nursing triage model. *Journal of Emergency Nursing, 20*(4), 271–274.

Hall, L. A., Sachs, B., Rayens, M. K., & Lutenbacher, M. (1993, Winter). Childhood physical and sexual abuse: Their relationship with depressive symptoms in adulthood. *Image: Journal of Nursing Scholarship, 25*(4), 317–323.

Henderson, A. (1992, Feb.). Critical care nurses need to know about abused women. *Critical Care Nurses, 12*(2), 27–30.

Herton, A. (1986, June). *Protocol of care for the battered woman.* White Plains, NY: March of Dimes Birth Defects Foundation.

Hoag-Apel, C. (1994, Sept.). Protocol for domestic violence intervention. *Nursing Management, 25,* 81–83.

Horsham, P. (1992, Sept.). Child sexual abuse: What parents need to know. *Canadian Nurse, 88,* 32–35.

Jezierski, M. (1994, Oct.). Abuse of women by male partners: Basic knowledge for emergency nurses. *Journal of Emergency Nursing, 20*(5), 361–372.

Johnson, T. (1991). *Elder mistreatment: Deciding who is at risk.* Westport, CT: Greenwood Press.

Joint Commission on the Accreditation of Healthcare Organizations (JCAHO). (1990). *Accreditation manual for hospitals.* Vol. 1. Chicago: Author.

Kennedy, L. (1994, June). Women in crisis. *Canadian Nurse, 91,* 26–32.

Lazzaro, M. V., & McFarlane, J. (1991, Oct.). Establishing a screening program for abused women. *Journal of Nursing Administration, 21,* 24–29.

Limandri, B. J., & Tilden, V. P. (1993). Domestic violence: Ethical issues in the health care system. *AWHONN's Clinical Issues, 4*(3), 493–502.

Lichtenstein, R. V. (1981a, July/Sept.). The battered woman: Breaking the cycle of abuse. *Issues in Mental Health Nursing, 3,* 651–653.

Lichtenstein, R. V. (1981b, July/Sept.). The battered woman: Guidelines for effective nursing intervention. *Issues in Mental Health Nursing, 3,* 237–250.

McFarlane, J., & Parker, B. (1991, Dec.). Preventing abuse during pregnancy: An assessment and intervention protocol. *American Journal of Maternal/Child Nursing, 19,* 321–324.

McFarlane, J., Parker, B., Soeken, K., & Bullock, L. (1992, June 17). Assessing for abuse during pregnancy: Severity and frequency of injuries and associated entry into prenatal care. *Journal of the American Medical Association, 267,* 3176–3178.

Mondor, E. E., & Wray, M. R. (1994, April). What's the matter with Johnny? *Canadian Nurse, 90,* 35–38.

Moss, V. A., & Taylor, W. K. (1991, May). Domestic violence: Identification, assessment, intervention. *AORN Journal, 53,* 1158–1164.

Ozmar, B. (1994, Sept.). Encountering victims of interpersonal violence: Implications for critical care nursing. *Critical Care Clinics of North America, 6*(3), 515–523.

Parker, V. F. (1985, Jan.). Battered. *RN, 58,* 26–29.

Parker, B., McFarlane, J., Soeken, K., Torres, S., & Campbell, D. (1993, May/June). Physical and emotional abuse in pregnancy: A comparison of adult and teenage women. *Nursing Research, 42*(3), 173–178.

Patterson, R. J., Brown, G. W., Salassi-Scotter, M., & Middaugh, D. (1992, Aug.). Head injury in the unconscious child. *American Journal of Nursing, 92,* 22–30.

Rose, K., & Saunders, D. G. (1986). Nurses' and physicians' attitudes about women abuse. *Health Care for Women International, 7*(6), 427–438.

Ross, M. M., & Hoff, L. A. (1994, June). Teaching nurses about abuse. *Canadian Nurse, 90,* 33–36.

Saveman, B. I., Hallberg, I. R., & Norberg, A. (1993, Sept.). Identifying and defining abuse of elderly people, as seen by witnesses. *Journal of Advanced Nursing, 18,* 1393–1400.

Sheridan, D. J., & Taylor, W. K. (1993). Developing hospital-based domestic violence programs, protocols, policies, and procedures. *AWHONN's Clinical Issues, 4*(3), 471–482.

Simon, M. L. (1992). *An exploratory study of adult protective services programs' repeat elder abuse clients.* Washington, DC: American Association of Retired Persons.

Srnec, P. (1991, Sept.). Children, violence, and intentional injuries. *Critical Care Nursing Clinics of North America, 3,* 471–478.

Starr, R. H. (1988). Physical abuse of children. In V. B. Vanhasselt, et al. (Eds.), *Handbook of family violence.* (pp. 119–155). New York: Plenum Press.

United States Department of Health and Human Services. Public Health Service, Health Resources and Services Administration. (1986). *Surgeon General's workshop on violence and public health.* DHHS Pub. no. HRS-D-MC 86-1. Washington, DC: Government Printing Office.

United States Department of Health and Human Services. (1989). Education about adult domestic violence in U.S. and Canadian medical schools, 1987–88. *Morbidity and Mortality Weekly Report, 38*(2), 17–19.

United States Department of Health and Human Services. (1990, Sept.). *Healthy people 2000: National health promotion and disease prevention objectives.* DHHS Publ. No. (PHS) 91-50212. Washington, DC: US Government Printing Office.

United States Department of Justice, Federal Bureau of Investigation. (1986). U.S. Department of Justice Crime Reports: *Crime in the U.S. 1985.* Washington, DC: Author.

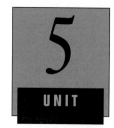

Visions for the Future of Nursing

22

Professional Empowerment and Politics

OBJECTIVES

- Discuss the role that power plays in nursing practice.

- Discuss the relevance of political action to nursing.

- Explain various strategies used to influence political decision making.

- Identify skills that are essential to political action.

- Identify ways in which nurses can participate in the political arena.

"Politics is the art of the possible; not the perfect. Often in the heat of battle we are unwilling to compromise, and therefore sacrifice all."
—B.J. Stevens, 1980

Nurses are actively participating in political processes to promote change within the profession and to influence policy making regarding nursing and health issues.

- The realities of the health care scene—increasingly scarce resources, more prevalent governmental regulation, an aging population, the emergence of health care as big business, technologic advancements, competition among providers for the health care dollar, and the developing political awareness of other health care professionals—demand that nurses become knowledgeable about and capable of influencing the development of health care policy and the delivery of client care.
- Nurses need to become more knowledgeable and skillful in the exercise of power to advocate more effectively for themselves, their clients, and their profession.
- Unless nurses develop their individual and collective political skills and use them to promote the profession and to advocate for clients, client care and the nursing profession will be jeopardized.
- Informed and concerned nurses can be effective in using the political process to promote change in the workplace, in professional organizations, in the legislative arena, and in the community.

POWER

Power is a concept that neither the public nor nurses themselves have traditionally associated with nursing. In fact, nurses often see themselves as powerless, particularly in regard to decisions involving clinical practice. It has been suggested that much of this powerlessness stems from the fact that nurses are predominantly women and that the majority of nurses work in hospitals, which have been male-dominated. However, in recent years more nurses have been appointed to senior administrative positions, and the picture is gradually changing. It is generally recognized, however, that nurses require more power commensurate with their knowledge and expertise as care providers.

Power has been defined in different ways. Ferguson describes power as "the ability to get things done on behalf of those whom nurses serve; at times, the goal may be to maintain, expand, give up, or share power" (1993, p. 120). Dennis describes power as "the ability to take action that regulates or manages other people; it is the ability to effect change or prevent it" (1992, p. 491). Both define power as an ability that can translate into an action. It should also be remembered that one *assumes* power; it is not *given*.

Often, the terms *power, influence*, and *authority* are used interchangeably, but they need to be differentiated. Power is the source of influence, whereas influence is the result of proper use of power. Authority is the official or legitimized right to use a given amount or type of power, that is, the right to act and the right to command (Claus & Bailey, 1977, p. 21). Authority may be either delegated or acquired.

Empowerment

Empowerment has been defined as the enabling of individuals and groups to participate in actions and decision making within a context that supports an equitable distribution of power (Mason, Backer & Georges, 1991, pp. 72–73). In this context, empowerment requires a commitment to a relationship between oneself and others, "...enabling individuals or groups to recognize their own strengths, resources and abilities to make changes in their personal and public lives. It is a process of confirming one's self and/or one's group" (Mason et al., 1991, p. 73). Obviously, empowerment requires the ability to recognize one's own strengths and to compensate for one's weaknesses—that is, to have a positive self-image.

Empowerment also means sharing power rather than grabbing it. Power grabbing connotes hoarding information and taking control and taking power away from others; power sharing, in contrast, connotes the values of equality and connectedness (Backer, Costello-Nickitas, Mason, McBride & Vance, 1993, p. 24). "Those people who wish to share power also wish to share influence, information, and control. They seek power *with* rather than *over*" (Mason, Talbott & Leavitt, 1993, p. 24).

To empower nurses for participating in policy making, Mason, Talbott, and Leavitt (1993, p. 24) suggest three processes:

1. Raising consciousness about the sociopolitical realities of a nurses' life and work within society
2. Developing a sense of self-efficacy or self-esteem regarding the nurses' ability to participate in policy making
3. Developing skills to influence policy making

Steps for Empowerment

1. *Nurses need to define themselves.* The dynamic environments in which many talented people work requires that nurses redefine and reformulate their work.

2. *Deliver the definable.* Doing work is not enough. Nurses need to determine whether society needs or requires that the work be done and whether they can ensure predictable outcomes.

3. *Determine that the work has been done well.* Continual evaluation is required. Excellence rather than mediocrity ensures that nurses remain strong in a highly competitive environment.

4. *Develop constituencies.* No one group or individual is powerful enough to control an agenda. Forming partnerships and taking united positions will help nurses be heard and heeded.

SOURCE: Adapted from "Perspectives on Power" by V. D. Ferguson, 1993, in *Policy and Politics for Nurses: Action and Change in the Workplace, Government, Organizations, and Community* (2nd ed.) by D. J. Mason, S. W. Talbott and J. K. Leavitt, Philadelphia: W. B. Saunders.

Ferguson (1993, p. 12) suggests that to attain maximum empowerment, nurses need to take four steps (see the accompanying box).

Sources of Power

Power theorists describe a variety of sources from which a person derives power. Understanding these sources of power is prerequisite to formulating a plan for developing one's own power and recognizing it in others.

French and Raven (1960, pp. 607–623) identified five sources of power: legitimate, reward, coercive, referent, and expert powers. Hershey, Blanchard, and Natemeyer added two more: connection (association) and information powers. Most leaders use all types of power at different times depending on the particular situation.

- *Legitimate* (or positional) *power* derives from one's formal position or title in an organization. It is associated with the authority that the position gives its holder to make and enforce decisions. The title "vice president for nursing"

RESEARCH NOTE

What Is Empowerment From a Client's Perspective?

The Mental Health Act Amendments of 1990 required that consumers be allowed to participate in decision making regarding their own care. As a result of this legislation, health care providers have had to reexamine the way services are delivered. Clients are being asked for their input, and many are taking the initiative in developing client-run programs. In one project, doctoral students obtained data from a focused group of chronically mentally ill clients who were involved in a client-run drop-in center in the Midwest. The students' goals were (a) to gain skill in conducting qualitative research and (b) to learn how the clients organize and manage services for themselves at the drop-in center. Data were obtained from 12 clients and 4 professional staff over a 5-week period through interviews, observation of participants, and review of documents. This qualitative analysis identified a major theme, empowerment, which had four process domains: participating, choosing, supporting, and negotiating. These domains represented four *levels* of empowerment for this group.

Clients at the first level of empowerment reported participating more than they previously had. At the second

level, clients were choosing and experiencing the consequences of their choices. At the next level, clients were supporting and helping each other, moving beyond their internal world. At the negotiating level, clients reported interacting on a more equal basis with staff and each other in order to meet their needs. Each level subsumes the previous levels; thus, someone at the supporting level also will be participating and choosing. A fifth domain, personal significance, described the effects of empowerment for each individual.

Implications: Although many authors have addressed the idea of empowerment, few have presented the client's perspective. If empowering clients is a desirable goal, then further study of the clients' perspective is needed. Nurses cannot hope to be advocates for clients unless they know what clients want and how they view empowerment.

SOURCE: "A Place to Be Yourself: Empowerment from the Client's Perspective" by L. M. Connelly, B. S. Keele, S. V. M. Kleinbeck, J. K. Schneider, and A. K. Cobb, Winter 1993, *Image: Journal of Nursing Scholarship, 25*, 297–303.

implies that the holder has power by virtue of the position, regardless of who holds that position or how effective that person is.

- *Reward power* is derived from the perception of one's abilities to bestow rewards or favors on others.
- *Coercive power,* by contrast, arises from the perception of one's ability to threaten, harm, or punish others.
- *Information power* is associated with persons who are perceived to control key information.

Reward, coercive, and information power all relate to the degree an individual can control the distribution of resources.

- *Referent* (charismatic, or personal) *power* is power derived from an individual's own vision, sense of self, and ability to communicate these so that others regard the person with admiration and are motivated to follow.
- *Connection (associative) power* derives from the perception that one has important contacts or relationships with others. These connections can be an aspect of both formal and informal networks.
- *Expert* (or knowledge) *power* is power derived from one's expertise, talents, and skills. One can include in this category Benner's (1984) vision of power in caring, that is, the positive power the nurse brings to the nurse-client relationship. This power enables the nurse to transform the client's life through advocacy and other means of caring.

Caring Types of Power

Benner (1984), in her classic work on clinical nursing excellence, describes six types of power that nurses can use when dealing with clients and significant others. These are powers that are associated with caring: transformative, integrative, advocacy, healing, participative/affirmative, and problem solving powers.

Transformative Power

Transformative power represents the ability of the nurse to assist clients to change their views of reality or their own self-images. Nurses display this type of power in caring for clients who have long-term illness. Providing compassionate care to clients who are unable to perform their normal hygienic care can help transform their self-image from one of worthlessness to one of value.

Integrative Power

Integrative power is the nurse's ability to assist a client to return to a normal life. In this process, the nurse helps clients integrate any disabilities into their lives and assists them back into the family and society.

Advocacy Power

Advocacy power enables the nurse to help a client and significant others deal with a health care bureaucracy. The nurse can explain to the client what services are available. In addition, the nurse can act as an "interpreter" between the client and physician. For example, a client may hesitate to express a concern to a busy physician. Recognizing that the physician may be able to ease the client's mind, the nurse may act as a liaison between the two.

Healing Power

Nurses can establish a healing relationship and a healing climate with a client. According to Benner, nurses can do this by mobilizing hope in themselves, the staff, and the client; finding an interpretation or understanding of a specific situation; and assisting the client to use social, emotional and/or spiritual support. Benner writes that an affirming and caring nurse-client relationship provides a basis for healing. A healing relationship empowers the client by bringing hope, confidence, and trust (1984, p. 213).

Participative/Affirmative Power

Participative/affirmative power is the nurse's ability to draw strength by investing it in others. Benner disputes the more traditional view that nurses have only so much emotional strength to draw on and suggests that involvement and caring permit the nurses to obtain strength (1984, p. 214).

Problem Solving

A committed person is more sensitive to cues than a less committed person, thus, a caring and involved nurse is able to solve problems at a higher level than a less involved nurse. Commitment and caring enhance the nurse's receptivity to cues and enables the nurse to recognize solutions that are not obvious. These abilities are due partly to intuition and feeling.

Traditional Types of Power

It is also important for nurses to be aware of the traditional types of power: physical, position, expert, and economic powers.

Physical power has been traditionally looked upon as the main source of power. Traditional male roles were based on men's superior physical strength: Men were responsible for providing food and shelter for the family because they were stronger. Now, as a result of technologic changes, many positions that formerly were available only to men because the job required physical strength are also available to women.

Position power is the power that results from an individual's title or position. For example, a nursing supervisor has specific responsibilities and power that other nurses do not have. Position power alone is not as strong as position power that is supported by expert or economic power.

Expert power is the result of demonstrated knowledge and competence. Nurses who have expert power and share it with others gain credibility and a sense of authority. Nurses who refuse to share their expertise lose power and are often considered selfish and unprofessional.

Economic power is the power people gain through providing or withholding resources. When nurses are involved in budget development, for example, they gain power through financial decision making. Traditionally, management controlled economic power in health care agencies; now, however, the advent of shared governance has distributed economic power more widely.

Laws of Power

Berle describes power as a "universal experience and human attribute of man with five discernable natural laws" (1969, p. 32).

Law 1 Power invariable fills any vacuum. People generally prefer peace and order and are usually willing to give power to someone who will restore order and thereby reduce their discomfort. When a problem arises, an individual will usually show the initiative to handle the problem and thus will exert power. Nurses should be aware that these are opportunities to assume power.

Law 2 Power is invariably personal. In many instances, people who effect change find common ground and come together committed to that change. To be successful, nurses must develop personal power, that is, the power one develops in oneself: self-esteem, self-respect, and self-confidence. Through their professional organizations, nurses can then exert personal power in the health care field.

Law 3 Power is based on a system of ideas and philosophy. When people demonstrate behaviors that indicate power, they reflect a personal belief or philosophy. It is this belief or philosophic system that gains followers and their respect. Nurses, however, have traditionally been comfortable "taking orders" and accommodating a hospital hierarchy rather than taking the initiative in such spheres as clients' rights and preventive care. Current problems in the health care system, such as increasing technology and cost (see Chapter 4), offer nurses an opportunity to fill a vacuum for change in the health care system and thereby offer solutions to these problems.

Law 4 Power is exercised through and depends on institutions. Individuals can feel powerless and unable to deal with many situations in a hospital, community agency, government agency, or other institution. By banding together with others through a state or provincial nursing organization, nurses can magnify their power and support changes in health care.

Law 5 Power is invariably confronted with, and acts in the presence of, a field of responsibility. Nurses in power positions act on behalf of other nurses or clients. Power is communicated to people observing the situation and is reinforced by positive responses. If group members believe that their beliefs or ideals are not represented, the vacuum will be filled by another person who can carry out the role and is supported by the organization.

CONSIDER . . .

- sources of power available to you as a clinical nurse. How can you enhance your expert power, your advocacy power, your healing power, your connection power, and your participative/affirmative power?
- how a nurse's self-image can affect that nurse's referent power.
- how expert power can enhance position power.

POLITICS

What is politics? For many people, the word *politics* evokes images of "crooked deals" hatched by men in "smoke-filled rooms," Watergate, the Iran-Contra dealings, bribes, and power brokers. More positive examples of political action are legislative initiatives to meet consumer needs and campaigns to elect nurse legislators. Although politics to some people connotes craftiness and lack of scruples, one can also view political astuteness as practical wisdom.

Politics can also be defined as "influencing—specifically, influencing the allocation of scarce resources" (Mason, et al., 1993, p. 6). Defined in this way, the word denotes more than action in the governmental arena; it is also applicable to every sphere of life where resources are limited and more than one person or group competes for them. "It is a process by which one influences the decisions of others and exerts control over situations and events. It is a means to an end" (Mason, et al., 1993, p. 6). *Resources* may refer not only to money but also to any number of cherished assets that are limited, such as personnel, programs, time, status, and power.

The allocation of scarce resources involves everyone in some way. Consider the following examples:

- A student applying for a college loan or competing with other students for his or her fair share of a teacher's time and attention.
- A client advocate competing for hospital education funds in order to provide more preoperative teaching.
- A citizen lobbying against the school board's proposal to divide one RN's time between two large schools.
- A member of a professional association seeking association action on a practice issue, such as care of clients with acquired immune deficiency syndrome (AIDS).

Nurses have always been involved in politics. For example, the founder of modern nursing, Florence Nightingale, used her contacts with powerful men in government to obtain needed personnel and supplies for wounded soldiers in the Crimea. Subsequent nursing leaders (discussed in Chapter 1) such as Lavinia Dock, Lillian Wald, Harriet Tubman, and Margaret Sanger—who were all skilled politicians and made significant contributions to the profession and society—may have been influenced by these wise words of Nightingale:

> When I entered service here, I determined that, happen what would, I *never* would intrigue among the Committee. Now I perceive that I do all my business by intrigue. I propose in private to A, B, or C the resolution I think A, B, or C most capable of carrying in Committee, and then leave it to them, and I always win. (Huxley, 1975, p. 53)

Political action refers to action by a group of individuals that is designed to attain a purpose through the use of political power or through the established political process.

Policy is shaped by politics. It refers to the values and principles that govern actions directed toward given ends; policy statements outline a plan, direction, or goal for action. Policies may be laws, guidelines, or regulations that govern behavior in government, workplaces, organizations, and committees.

Strategies to Influence Political Decisions

Many of the strategies used to influence political decisions will serve the nurse well in everyday professional activities.

Negotiating

Negotiation is a give-and-take process between individuals and groups to work out differences of opinion regarding the best solution to an issue. Guidelines to consider in negotiations are shown in the accompanying box. Two basic forms of negotiation are problem-solving negotiation and trade-off negotiation. In *problem-solving negotiation*, both parties confer to resolve a complex situation together. In *trade-off negotiation*, one party gives some concessions or "points" to the other party in exchange for other concessions or "points." Negotiating demands good communication skills of all participants. Before beginning negotiation, the

---

Guidelines for Negotiation

- Obtain all of the essential facts of the issue beforehand.
- Explore the other party's viewpoint. If the other party is a legislator, for example, obtain information about his or her views from news media and congressional records.
- Consider the consequences of the issue and how you can deflect those consequences in order to support your viewpoint.
- Verify the strength of your own viewpoint and ways to strengthen it further; then consider ways to counteract or weaken the other party's viewpoint.
- Determine any limitations surrounding your viewpoint, such as time constraints or other resources.
- Consider other groups that support your viewpoint or that of the other party.

nurse needs to know all the essential facts of the issue and conduct research to support a particular viewpoint. A familiar example of the negotiating process for nurses is the collective bargaining (contract negotiations) process between employees and employers.

Networking

Networking refers to a process in which people with similar interests and goals communicate, share ideas and information, and offer support and direction to each other. Network development builds linkages with people throughout the profession, both within and outside the work environment. Getting to know people helps build a trust relationship that can facilitate the achievement of professional goals: It is easier to access people one knows than it is to access strangers.

Nurses can develop networks by (a) attending local, regional, and national conferences; (b) taking classes for continuing education or toward an academic degree; (c) joining alumni associations and attending alumni meetings; (d) joining and participating in professional organizations; (e) keeping in touch with former teachers and co-workers; and (f) socializing with professional colleagues. Keeping an updated card file of colleagues and keeping in touch socially can keep the network fresh.

Political networks generally have three functions: (a) to provide information about legislative activities on particular issues, (b) to increase political action and awareness, and (c) to promote issues through the legislative process. These networks may be formal, with signed agreements and fee structures, or informal, requiring minimal monetary contributions.

Preparing Resolutions

Resolutions are formal statements expressing the opinion, will, or intent of an individual or group. Most nurses will be familiar with the specific format used to present resolutions at annual association meetings or conventions about nursing and health care concerns. Resolutions are an effective means of writing concise reasons and proposed recommendations for action, particularly for areas where services are inadequate. Nurses who present resolutions must, however, be well informed about the data presented, be prepared to offer additional data others might request, and be willing to consider amendments to the recommendations.

Establishing Political Action Committees

Political action committees (PACs) endorse candidates for public office, such as the Senate and the House of Representatives. Because tax laws limit nonprofit professional organizations from participating in various types of political activities, PACs provide an avenue for professional political action activities. Groups such as nursing organizations, women's groups, church groups, and civic groups may form PACs. Members of a PAC provide additional donations or pay dues to support the organization's activities because general membership fees in any nonprofit organization cannot be used to support such activity. Because they are used for political purposes, donations made to a PAC are not tax deductible.

The ANA Political Action Committee (ANA-PAC) is a political organization formed by the ANA. Many state nursing organizations also have political action organizations that serve similar functions on the state level as ANA-PAC does on the national level. PACs support legislative candidates based on their stands on key issues. For example, ANA-PAC would consider a candidate's stand on such specific health and nursing issues as national health insurance, third-party reimbursement for nurses, funding for biomedical and nursing research, elder abuse, and so on. Although nursing PACs have not created power equal to that of such groups as labor, education, and medicine, nurses are becoming more sophisticated in the political process and are gaining increased power.

Communicating with Legislators

Nurses can communicate with legislators through telephone calls, telegrams, face-to-face meetings, and written letters. For each method, the nurse needs to identify clearly the issue and the bill (by number if possible), explain reasons for interest in the issue, and provide constructive information and ideas. Telephone calls are usually received by a legislative assistant who keeps a record of all calls and the positions of the callers. In many regions, a toll-free number is available during the legislative session.

For visits to legislative officials, the nurse first needs to contact the local offices, which will provide assistance in arranging the visit and may additionally arrange other activities, such as tours of the legislature, attendance at committee hearings, and visits to a legislative session. Before the visit, the nurse should obtain information about the legislator's background, such as the legislator's occupation, previous professional and civic activities, political affiliation, voting record, and interests. Because only a few minutes may be allotted to the visit, the nurse should be prepared to be succinct in presenting personal ideas and facts, allow time for the legislator to answer questions, and leave a summary of facts and recommendations with the legislator to add to the perspective of the visit.

Letters are probably the most common mode of communicating with elected officials. Personal letters that reflect thoughtful and informed comments about an issue often receive more attention from legislators than form letters or postcards. When writing to legislators, the nurse should use a professional letterhead and address the public official appropriately. For example, in written communication, the President, Vice-President, senators, and state representatives are cited as The Honorable (full name) followed by their position (e.g., President of the United States) and the specific address. Salutations in letters are written as Dear Mr. (or Madame) President/Vice-President or Dear Senator (full name), or Dear Representative (last name). When communicating in person it is appropriate to say the following: Mr. or Madame President/Vice-President or President (last name); Senator (last name); and Representative or Mr./Ms. (last name). Elements to include in the letter follow:

- A statement of the request in the first sentence (e.g., "I request that you support Bill XY604") and a brief summary of the issue.
- A brief rationale for the request (e.g., "The bill is vital to improving..." or "the bill will adversely affect...").
- Factual data that support your viewpoint.
- A closing statement thanking the legislator for his or her concern and continuing support or attention.
- Appropriate closing. For a letter to the president of the United States, the appropriate closing is "Very respectfully yours"; for all other letters, "Sincerely yours."

Building Coalitions

Coalitions are alliances that distinct bodies, persons, or states form in order to achieve a common purpose.

Coalitions are like networks in function but differ in that the members of the coalition represent groups with numerous purposes and issues. The groups negotiate, compromise, and merge to achieve specific goals. Groups or organizations may be in coalition on one issue but adversaries on another. Building coalitions is a strategy to empower oneself; thus, nurses solicit organizations whose power is greater than their own. Groups with whom nurses may form coalitions are as diverse as the topics that are of concern to nurses; women's issues, child care, and the environment are only a few examples.

Lobbying

Lobbying is a process in which individuals or groups attempt to influence legislators to support or oppose particular legislation. Lobbyists monitor legislative activities and communicate the group's position to members of the legislature. Professional lobbyists may be employed by groups from various sources: public relations firms, management relation firms, legal firms, legislative consultants, and independent lobbyists, many of whom are former legislators. Which source is used depends on the issue. Law firms, for example, can provide legal advice as well as lobbying; public relations firms generally provide media resources for campaigns. Individuals and groups can lobby independently, but such efforts require considerable time, personnel, and funding. Lobbyists must follow various legal guidelines. Lobbying techniques include negotiating, media and letter-writing campaigns, testifying, endorsements, and donations.

Testifying

Decisions related to health care and nursing are often made by committees and commissions of various levels of government. These committees frequently conduct hearings to obtain information before making a decision. Hearings generally include people or groups with opposing views. **Testifying** refers to the presentation of information at a committee hearing, usually about controversial aspects of a proposed bill. Nurses may testify either as independent individuals or as official representatives of an organization. Opportunities to testify may be found in professional publications or newspapers. Guidelines for testifying are shown in the box on the following page. Most committees will accept written testimony if the individual cannot be present.

Guidelines for Testifying

- Confirm the time to register. In some instances, registration occurs at the meeting place on the day of testifying; in others, you must notify the committee of your visit to testify at a specified time before the hearing.

- Prepare your testimony concisely and clearly in advance. Avoid the use of professional terminology that may not be understood by the legislators, or explain any technical term used.

- Dress appropriately to convey your professional status, and introduce yourself. Make your position clear so that legislators know whether you are representing an organization.

- Maintain a courteous, professional composure throughout the hearing. Adhere to the rules of the proceedings.

- Verify any time limits for your presentation so that you can present essential facts and arguments first.

- Provide copies of your written testimony, including any graphs or other illustrations, to each committee member.

- Present your material without reading it to make the presentation more interesting for the listeners. Summarize the main ideas. Convey knowledge of the subject.

- Answer any questions completely. Be prepared to support any facts and figures you present with appropriate sources.

- Thank the committee for allowing your testimony.

CONSIDER . . .

- political strategies that you have used. Why were they effective or not effective? How would you alter them another time?

Developing Political Astuteness and Skill

By contributing to political activities in various ways, nurses can develop their political astuteness and skills. All nurses, as citizens and employees, can join and participate in organizations and participate in election processes. However, nurses who are employed by a governmental agency, such as the Veterans Administration or a public health department, must follow restrictions defined in the Hatch Act regarding their political activity. These restrictions do not apply to the general public and include serving as an officer or spokesperson of a particular political party. The major objective of the Hatch Act initiated in the 1930s was to prevent government workers from being forced to support political activities. Although these restrictions remain controversial, attempts to modify and repeal the Hatch Act have failed. Because each state has its own version of this act, nurses who are employed by state governmental agencies are advised to investigate specific limitations in their state of employment.

A discussion of when and where to engage in political action must be prefaced by a statement of three key assumptions:

1. *Individuals who are deeply concerned about a particular issue or cause are most likely to identify ways to take action.* Before becoming politically involved, an individual must make choices, including the conscious decision to set aside the necessary resources. For example, a student who wants her or his school to offer evening or weekend clinical practice hours may decide to seek election to the student council to work for this change from within.

2. *Political action in any sphere is best carried out by a group.* Individual activism is laudable, but group action is much more effective. It provides change agents with the collegiality and support necessary to sustain a vision for change and fosters creative thinking and planning.

3. *Successful political action requires the thoughtful application of change theory.* Before embarking on a project, the politically astute nurse will review the principles of change theory. Achieving goals for change requires thoughtful planning. Effective political activists plan strategy, much as nurses use the nursing process to evaluate clients' needs for care.

Nurses need certain knowledge and skills to increase their political astuteness and activity (Skaggs, 1994, p. 239; Ellis & Hartley, 1992, p. 359):

- *Keeping informed about health care issues.* Obtain information from sources such as the daily newspaper; television and radio news reports; professional journals (space about current legislative issues is routinely provided in both national and state and provincial nursing journals); open meetings of nursing organizations or other health-related organizations, which often sponsor speakers who are knowledgeable about the issue.

- *Ability to analyze an issue.* Identify all the relevant facts about the issue, look at the issue from all angles, and recognize how the issue fits into the larger picture.
- *Ability to speak out and voice an opinion.* Obtain knowledge of both the issue and the best person to whom to voice the opinion. After studying the dynamics of the organization, the nurse may choose a head nurse or supervisor who is a good listener and is concerned about the issue.
- *Ability to participate constructively.* Be a team player who encourages creative brainstorming and offers positive feasible alternative solutions to an issue, rather than offering only criticism.
- *Ability to use power bases.* Through discussion with colleagues and other professional experiences, identify people who influence decision making. It is important to remember that power does not always follow the hierarchical lines on the organizational chart and that the source of information is sometimes considered as powerful as the information itself. The nurse who uses many different channels of information gains power to choose among them.

Seeking Opportunities for Political Action

Nurses can exert political action in four spheres of influence: in the workplace, in nursing organizations, in the community, and in government.

Workplace

Nurses who successfully practice the politics of change in the workplace must analyze the structure and processes of this sphere to identify the available avenues for action (Talbott, 1985a). Nurses can influence both the outcome of client care and the nature of the workplace.

Nurses can exert expert, position, and economic power by negotiating the presence of nurse members on standing committees and the board of trustees and by becoming involved in the collective bargaining process.

In most hospitals, nursing homes, and public health agencies, a system of committees exists to deal with specific issues. For example, a nursing department has an equipment evaluation committee that selects and evaluates client care products used by the nursing staff. A pharmacy committee in the same hospital has representatives from nursing, medicine, and the pharmacy. In addition to formal standing committees, ad hoc committees or task forces can be appointed to deal with particular issues or problems. For example, a task force on a nursing unit might examine the best way to initiate a case management program and critical pathways.

Nurses who have an idea or problem they want addressed are advised to look for existing committees that might already be dealing with the concern or are likely to do so. For example, nurses concerned about staff safety in the parking lot may find that a hospital security committee is already looking into the problem.

Another way to generate interest in an issue is to write an article for the hospital or nursing department newsletter. Nurses who are present at nursing grand rounds also have the opportunity to inform their colleagues of an issue of mutual concern and enlist their aid in dealing with it. What can the nurse do if there are no newsletters or grand rounds? Form a task force of concerned nurses and, using a model for change, plan a strategy to establish ways of helping nurses communicate with one another through a newsletter, grand rounds, or possibly a support group.

The politics of client care impinges on the practice of every nurse. For example, the prospective payment system has drastically shortened hospital stays in efforts to reduce hospital costs. Preparing clients for earlier discharge has brought about the need for nurses to be "faster and smarter" in delivering client care and client education.

How can nurses ensure that cost-containment measures do not impair the quality of nursing care? One way is for nurses to collaborate with each other and other providers to delegate non-nursing tasks, such as answering the telephone, emptying the garbage, and transporting non-acute clients. Developing a demonstration project that compares cost and quality of care issues under different hospital unit structures can provide the necessary data and generate support from other providers and administrators for changing the role of staff nurses. This sort of "proactive" planning can empower nurses to take charge of nursing practice in ways that benefit clients and health professionals while conserving scarce resources such as money, time, and supplies.

Nursing Organizations

Powerful and influential professional associations, such as the ANA and CNA and their affiliated state/province and district associations, provide a collective voice for promoting nursing and quality health care. As such, these associations exert influence on the individual nurse as well as in the spheres of government, the workplace, the community, and the profession. Associations monitor and influence laws and regulations affecting nursing and health care. Their role in workplace matters ranges from studying practice issues to acting as the collective bargaining agent for nurses. Additionally, the professional nursing organization is often a visible presence in the community because it presents the nursing perspective on health care issues.

Professional organizations—including the ANA, CNA, NLN, and NSNA—publish articles on legislative matters and encourage nurses to take action on behalf of health care consumers and the nursing profession. Nursing lobbyists at the state and national level work to influence the development of health policy and legislation, but their success depends on the active support of nurses who back up these paid lobbyists by doing personal lobbying among their own elected officials.

The collective efforts of nurses influence the federal government through the political action committees such as the American Nurses Association Political Action Committee (ANA-PAC); see page 432. ANA-PAC also counts on nurses at the grass roots level to work for these candidates and to serve as congressional district coordinators (CDCs). CDCs are responsible for organizing nurses in their congressional districts for lobbying and campaigning. This effort has provided a mechanism for nurses to influence governmental politics collectively at the federal level.

Individual nurses can become politically active in local, state or provincial, and national organizations by participating in the activities of their professional associations, by serving as delegates at conventions, by becoming members of commissions, and by supporting national association efforts such as the ANA's Nursing Agenda for Health Care Reform. Student nurses can benefit from participation in the National Student Nurses Association (NSNA) by learning about the politics of professional associations.

Community

The community in which the nurse lives and works can include the local neighborhood, the corporate world, the nation, and the international community. The community encompasses the workplace, professional organizations, and government. Many nurses, including Lillian Wald, founder of the Henry Street Settlement and modern public health nurses, view the community as more than a practice setting. Nurses who live in the community where they work can understand and influence the complex interplay among individuals and groups that compete for scarce resources.

Many communities depend on expert nurses to help with a wide variety of health and social policy decisions, such as environmental pollution and health care for the homeless. For example, a nurse who serves as an elected member of the community school board can influence decisions that affect the health and health care of students, such as the hiring of nurses for the school system. Nurses' opinions on matters of the public health are frequently sought, and the enterprising nurse looks for opportunities to promote a positive image of nursing while serving the community.

Political involvement in the community often arises out of one's own interest in living and working in a community that is supportive of the health and well-being of its citizens. For instance, a nurse may become involved with an ad hoc committee to stop unlawful dumping of hazardous wastes in the neighborhood. As a member of such a group, the nurse wears two hats: She or he is both a concerned citizen and an expert on health issues. At the same time, the nurse's position in the group enables the nurse to extend networks and expand a support base for nursing.

As the self-help movement continues to expand, nurses are realizing how influential consumer groups can be. In many instances, such groups are founded by nurses who realize that customers, often their own clients, have a need for a self-help group. Sometimes nurses who have been clients themselves start postmastectomy support groups or similar groups. Nurses contribute their leadership skills to many organizations, including the National Alliance for the Mentally Ill (NAMI). The personally devastating experience of having a child with schizophrenia can be a powerful motivating force toward working in behalf of others through a group such as NAMI. The political power of groups with particular health concerns—including the Gray Panthers, the American Association of Retired Persons, and the Juvenile Diabetes Association—can generate extraordinary political influence on elected and appointed officials. Such groups offer nurses a variety of ways to learn about grass roots political activism. These groups can also be a community support base for nursing.

A variety of other opportunities for community involvement exist for nurses. Since many nurses are also parents, they can work on health issues through their school board. Those who ultimately run for government office have frequently begun their careers by running for the school board. Other nurses volunteer for community action groups, such as a community planning board or a fund raising committee for the city's art museum. Or, a nurse may get involved in the tenant's organization in her or his apartment building. Regardless of the issue, the same opportunity to organize and plan for change exists in the community as it does in the workplace, government, or professional association.

The Government

Numerous ways to influence governments personally are open to nurses. Of course, the most basic step is registering to vote. Voter registration drives are sponsored by a variety of organizations, including NSNA, which has developed a kit for nursing students to hold such drives. By voting, responsible citizens convey their opinions to elected and appointed officials on matters of concern.

The laws and regulations of local, state, and federal governments greatly influence nursing practice and health care. For example, federal laws and regulations establish funding of health care for the elderly, poor, and disabled (Medicare and Medicaid), authorize care services for special groups (including Native Americans, migrant workers, and veterans), set policies and formulas for reimbursement of health care services (as with prospective payment), and appropriate funding for special health care and social services (such as community health centers, the food stamp program, and the school lunch program).

State and provincial laws are responsible for defining and regulating nursing practice. Nurse practice acts in some states prohibit nurses from providing a broad range of services and can effectively limit nurses' ability to compete with other health care professionals in providing primary care services.

Nurses can become involved with political parties and local political clubs, work with elected officials, and accept political appointments as a means to influence health policy as well as nursing practice. Involvement in political parties and local political clubs enables the nurse to have some influence over affairs in the community and to develop a non-nursing support base for nursing and health care issues.

Nurses can also actively participate in campaigns of politicians who support nursing and health care, can become candidates for legislative offices, and act as information sources for legislative representatives.

CONSIDER . . .

- ways in which you have participated in political activities in the past—in the work setting, in professional organizations, in the community, and in government.
- how you would like to increase your participation in political activities.
- whether you believe nurses have an obligation to be politically active. Why or why not?
- selected political issues affecting nursing:
  a. Reimbursement of nursing services
  b. Equal pay for work of comparable value
  c. National health insurance
  d. Health care reform
  What sources would you use to obtain information about these issues? What political actions would you like taken in regard to these issues?

READINGS FOR ENRICHMENT

Bennett, S. L., Dodd, C. J., & Marshall, J. (1993). Analyzing your workplace. In D. J. Mason, S. W. Talbott, & J. K. Leavitt. *Policy and politics for nurses: Action and change in the workplace, government, organizations, and community* (2nd ed.) (pp. 241–253). Philadelphia: W. B. Saunders.

In every workplace there is a political climate, structure, and process that motivate, drive, and control the organization's effectiveness in producing its product. These authors discuss politics in the workplace, aspects of the organizational structure, the policy-making process, the role of outsiders, using the committee structure, assessing the role of quality in the organization, and analyzing financial resources. Such a political analysis of the workplace is essential to transforming its political climate to one that is supportive of creative change.

READINGS FOR ENRICHMENT

Foley, M. C. (1993). The politics of collective bargaining. In D. J. Mason, S. W. Talbott, & J. K. Leavitt. *Policy and politics for nurses: Action and change in the workplace, government, organizations, and community* (2nd ed.) (pp. 282–302). Philadelphia: W. B. Saunders.

The author introduces the nurse to the politics of collective action through collective bargaining in the private sector of the health care industry. It includes a brief review of nursing's history in collective bargaining, essential components of collective bargaining, negotiations, strikes and other labor disputes, and employer strategies.

Leavitt, J. K., & Barry, C. (1993). Learning the ropes. In D. J. Mason, S. W. Talbott, and J. K. Leavitt. *Policy and politics for nurses: Action and change in the workplace, government, organizations, and community* (2nd ed.) (pp. 47–67). Philadelphia: W. B. Saunders.

The authors discuss consciousness raising, getting started, the basic skills of politics, role modeling and monitoring, and learning through education. They state that "the most important factor in learning political skills is finding mentors who are politically involved and who will believe in us, support us, teach us, critique us, and then celebrate with us." The authors also recount political experiences of six nurse leaders to inspire and instruct the novice.

SUMMARY

Power is an invaluable instrument, the effects of which can be positive or negative depending on the way it is used and the ends to which it is applied. Power is assumed by a person; it is a skill that can be learned and effectively practiced. Sources or bases of power are described as reward, coercive, legitimate, referent, expert, connection, and information powers. An understanding of these sources helps nurses formulate a plan to develop their own power and to recognize it in others. Benner describes six types of power that nurses use when caring for clients: transformative power, integrative power, advocacy power, healing power, participative/affirmative power, and problem-solving power. Empowerment enables individuals and groups to participate in actions and decision making in a context that supports an equitable distribution of power.

Politics is the process of influencing the allocation of scarce resources in the spheres of government, workplace, organizations, and community. Political action in one sphere often affects other spheres. Strategies to influence political decisions include negotiating, networking, establishing political action committees, communicating with legislators, building coalitions, lobbying, and testifying.

As citizens, parents, and members of the nursing profession, all nurses can contribute to political activities in numerous ways—by voting, joining organizations, becoming members of committees, supporting deserving candidates, and so on. To make any effective contribution, nurses must keep themselves informed about health care and nursing issues, be able to analyze an issue, voice an opinion, participate constructively, use power bases, and communicate clearly. Nurses who value the nursing perspective on health issues recognize that a powerful voice for nurses is a powerful voice for health care consumers, the profession, and the nation.

SELECTED REFERENCES

Backer, B. A., Costello-Nickitas, D. M., Mason, D. J., McBride, A. B., & Vance, C. (1993). Feminist perspectives on policy and politics. In D. J. Mason, S. W. Talbott, & J. K. Leavitt, *Policy and politics for nurses: Action and change in the workplace, government, organizations, and community* (2nd ed.). Philadelphia: W. B. Saunders.

Benner, P. (1984). *From novice to expert: Excellence and power in clinical nursing practice.* Menlo Park, CA: Addison-Wesley Nursing.

Berle, A. A. (1969). *Power.* New York: Harcourt, Brace, and World.

Boykin, A. (Ed.). (1995). *Power, politics and public policy: A matter of caring.* New York: National League for Nursing. Pub. no. 14-2684.

Claus, K. E., & Bailey, J. T. (1977). *Power and influence in health care: A new approach to leadership.* St. Louis: Mosby.

Davidhizar, R, & Giger, J. N. (1994, Sept./Oct.). You have power, too! *NSNA/Imprint 41*(4), 64–66.

Dennis, K. E. (1991). Empowerment. In J. L. Creasia & B. Parker (Eds.), *Conceptual foundations of professional nursing practice.* St. Louis: Mosby-Year Book.

Ellis, J. R., & Hartley, C. L. (1992). *Nursing in today's world: Challenges, issues, and trends* (4th ed.). Philadelphia: Lippincott.

Ferguson, V. D. (1993). Perspectives on power. In D. J. Mason, S. W. Talbott, & J. K. Leavitt, *Policy and politics for nurses: Action and change in the workplace, government, organizations, and community* (2nd ed.). Philadelphia: W. B. Saunders.

French, J. R., & Raven, B. H. (1960). The bases of social power. In D. Cartwright & A. Zanders (Eds.), *Group dynamics: Research and theory* (2nd ed.). New York: Harper and Row.

Gilbert, T. (1995, May). Nursing: Empowerment and the problem of power. *Journal of Advanced Nursing, 21,* 865–871.

Hershey, P., Blanchard, K., & Natemeyer, W. (1979). Situational leadership: Perception and impact of power. *Group Organizational Studies, 4,* 418–428.

Huston, C. J., & Marquis, B. (1988, Summer). Ten attitudes and behaviors necessary to overcome powerlessness. *Nursing Connections, 1,* 39–47.

Huxley, E. (1975). *Florence Nightingale.* New York: Putnam.

Leddy, S., & Pepper, J. M. (1993). *Conceptual bases of professional nursing* (3rd ed.). Philadelphia: Lippincott.

Mason, D. J., Backer, B. A., & Georges, C. A. (1991, Summer). Toward a feminist model for the political empowerment of nurses. *Image: Journal of Nursing Scholarship, 23,* 72–77.

Mason, D. J., Talbott, S. W., & Leavitt, J. K. (1993). *Policy and politics for nurses: Action and change in the workplace, government, organizations, and community* (2nd ed.). Philadelphia: W. B. Saunders.

Skaggs, B. (1994). Political action in nursing. In J. Zerwekh & J. C. Claborn, *Nursing today: Transitions and trends.* (pp. 236–256). Philadelphia: W. B. Saunders.

Talbott, S. W. (1985a). Political analysis: Structure and processes. In D. J. Mason & S. W. Talbott (Eds.). *The political action handbook for nurses.* Menlo Park, CA: Addison-Wesley Nursing.

Talbott, S. W. (1985b). Political appointments: Getting appointed. In D. J. Mason & S. W. Talbott (Eds.), *The political action handbook for nurses.* Menlo Park, CA: Addison-Wesley Nursing.

Talbott, S. W. (1985c). Influencing your association. In D. J. Mason & S. W. Talbott (Eds.), *The political action handbook for nurses.* Menlo Park, CA: Addison-Wesley Nursing.

23

Advanced Nursing Education and Practice

by Jean Candela

OBJECTIVES

- Discuss education for advanced nursing roles.

- Differentiate among the various advanced nursing roles, including nurse educator, nurse administrator, clinical nurse specialist, and the advanced nurse practitioner.

- Describe the historical development of advanced practice nursing.

- Compare the various advanced practice nursing roles and their functions.

- Discuss certification and regulation of advanced nursing roles.

"New settings for practice, new kinds of patients, new roles and responsibilities all have generated a need for new ways of thinking, practicing and educating."

—Melanie Dreher, 1995

Graduate education provides specialized knowledge and skill to enable nurses to assume advanced roles in education, administration, research, and practice. It also prepares nurses for advanced practice in a variety of specialized roles in primary, secondary, and tertiary settings. Graduate programs prepare clinical nurse specialists, nurse practitioners, nurse midwives, and nurse anesthetists.

- Choosing a graduate nursing program involves identifying one's personal career goals and then selecting the best program to enable one to meet those goals.
- Nurses with graduate education can influence the health care system from within by assuming positions of leadership in administration, education, and practice. They can also influence the political system to effect needed change through the research process.
- The growth of advanced practice nursing occurs through education, professional role advancement, and legislation.
- Nurses prepared to assume advanced nursing roles bring new ideas, insights, and enlightenment to the total health care system. Their creativity, competence, commitment, and courage will influence the quality of care in a changing health system.

ADVANCED NURSING EDUCATION

Historically, basic education in nursing prepared the graduate to be a nurse generalist. Nurses obtained education for specialization after completing the basic program, usually through hospital-based postgraduate courses designed to provide knowledge and skill in a specialized area. This type of specialized preparation in the early part of the 20th century generally focused on obstetric nursing and private-duty nursing. As nurses acquired a greater body of knowledge in the sciences of anatomy, physiology, microbiology, chemistry, pathophysiology, and pharmacology, they became better able to make assessments about the nature of clients' problems. Nurses'

increasing skills enabled them to assume a more active role in the care of their clients. Knowledge and skill that had previously been the physician's domain gradually crossed over into nursing practice. For example, nurses acquired the skills to conduct in-depth physical assessments, venipuncture, suturing, ordering basic diagnostic studies, and administering life-saving medications under protocols.

As the nurse's role expanded, nurses became more specialized, and standards of practice required greater consistency in what nurses were permitted to do and could be expected to do. As the settings for practice became more specialized, post-basic specialty courses proliferated to include oncology nursing, critical care nursing, recovery room nursing, operating room nursing, rehabilitation nursing, and so on. These developments created a need for more formalized programs of study to ensure consistency of education and skill training.

Specialty education provided in universities and colleges at the master's degree level evolved during the 1940s and 1950s. The idea was greatly facilitated by the return of nurses from military service during World War II. These nurses often had GI benefits to return to school for advanced education. Passage of the National Mental Health Act in 1946 provided additional funds for education of nurses in the area of psychiatric/mental health nursing (Hamric & Spross, 1989, p. 4). During a 1952 conference sponsored by the National League for Nursing (NLN), it was agreed that the purpose of baccalaureate education was to prepare nurse generalists, whereas master's education was devoted to the preparation of nurse specialists. Master's level education was envisioned as the appropriate foundation for the preparation of nurses for specialty practice. Early graduate degrees in nursing focused on the functional roles of educator and administrator; for example, the degree offered at Columbia University's Teacher College focused on the preparation of nurse educators. The first clinical master's program was developed in 1954 by Hildegard Peplau at Rutger's University to prepare advanced practice nurses in psychiatric/mental health nursing (Sparacino, Cooper & Minarik, 1990; Hamric & Spross, 1989). At this time, nurses prepared with graduate degrees in clinical specialties were referred to as **nurse clinicians** or **clinical nurse specialists.** The primary purpose of the clinical nurse specialist (CNS) was to improve client care and nursing practice by functioning as an expert nurse in the practice setting. The clinical nurse specialist was considered to be an expert in a specialized area of nursing practice, usually in the acute care setting, and served as an expert care provider, a resource to novice nurses or general staff nurses for education and development, a consultant to the physician and other health professionals, and an active participant in research related to the specialized area of practice. Some believed that the clinical nurse specialist should not be used as a direct care provider, but rather as a clinical educator, consultant, or researcher. There was also concern that the role of the clinical nurse specialist was not clearly defined because nurses performed different roles and functions (educator, researcher, consultant, direct care provider, administrator) in different settings (Hamric & Spross, 1989, p. 7).

During the 1960s, the United States experienced a health care personnel shortage as a result of the Vietnam War. Also during this time, a maldistribution of primary care physicians exacerbated the problem. In response to this problem, Dr. Loretta Ford and Dr. Henry Silver (a physician) developed in 1965 the first nurse practitioner program at the University of Colorado focusing on the care of children. Within 9 years, there were 65 nurse practitioner programs in pediatrics; additional programs were developed that focused on women's health or family health. Nurses moved into other advanced practice roles of nurse midwives and nurse anesthetists (Wilson, 1994, p. 28).

Because of society's need to meet its health care needs and the lack of graduate-level clinical nursing programs, short-term certificate programs were created to prepare nurse practitioners to meet health care demands. There was no consistency in the educational prerequisites, the length of the program, and the goals and content of the program in these early nurse practitioner programs. Some programs required the nurse to have a baccalaureate degree for admission, while others simply required registered nurse licensure and varying numbers of years of nursing experience. Program lengths ranged from a few months to 2 years. Some programs were taught only by physicians; others were taught by both physicians and nurses. Today, most advanced practice education takes place at the graduate level, and American Nurses Association (ANA) certification at the advanced practice levels of clinical specialist and nurse practitioner require the master's degree.

There remains controversy related to the role of the clinical nurse specialist (CNS) and its differences

---

Clinical Nurse Specialist

Characteristics

Expertise in specific populations

Research projects—team member and evaluator

Case management

Staff development and teaching

Use of systems approach to problem solving

Strengths

Specialized knowledge and skills, in-depth knowledge, expertise

Systems skilled

Role flexibility—time and practice

Nurse Practitioner

Characteristics

Primary care, health promotion focus

Client-centered focus

Diagnosing and prescribing

Case management

Teacher

Strengths

Autonomy of practice

Cost-effective and reimbursable

Popular with consumers and legislators

Diagnostician

Holistic approach (prevention and wellness)

SOURCE: Adapted from American Association of Colleges of Nursing, 1994, *Role differentiation of the nurse practitioner and clinical nurse specialist: Reaching toward consensus.* Proceedings of the Master's Education Conference, December 1994, San Antonio, TX: Author, pp. 69–70.

---

from and similarities to the advanced nurse practitioner (ANP). The different titles and the various perceptions about these advanced practice roles cause confusion among health care consumers as well as health care professionals. In 1994, the American Association of Colleges of Nursing (AACN) held a conference on role differentiation of the nurse practitioner and the clinical nurse specialist. At consensus-building work groups, the participants identified the characteristics of the two advanced practice roles, their strengths, and the outcomes that might be expected if the two roles merged or remained separate (see accompanying box). The reasons cited for merging the CNS and ANP roles included (a) less confusion to the public; (b) clarification of competencies and titles, (c) greater professional and political power, (d) greater marketability of the advanced practice nurse designation, (e) guarantees that preparation of advanced practice nurses would occur at the graduate level, and, perhaps most important, (f) increased benefits to clients resulting from the more comprehensive preparation of their nurses. In a vote taken following the work groups, 68% of the participants voted to merge the ANP and CNS roles (AACN, 1994, p.71). Nursing schools are beginning to merge their existing clinical nurse specialist programs with nurse practitioner programs, providing all graduates with the knowledge and skills to achieve national certification and to be eligible for state licensure at the advanced practice level. (Regulation of advanced practice is discussed later in this chapter.)

CONSIDER...

- what knowledge and skills are shared by nurses and physicians. Which specific skills fall in the domain of basic nursing practice, which fall into advanced nursing practice, and which are specific to the practice of medicine?
- how the role of the primary care advanced practice nurse differs from the role of the primary care physician. How does the focus of care differ?
- the societal benefits of having advanced practice nurses provide primary care.

Master's Degree in Nursing Education

The earliest graduate programs in nursing focused on preparing nurse educators for schools of nursing. Today graduate programs in nursing education prepare nurses for teaching roles in schools of nursing, staff development, client education, and community health education. Because nursing educators are expected to have an area of clinical specialization, curricula in these graduate programs usually combine classroom education and clinical experience in a clinical practice area with course work in curriculum development, instructional strategies, and student evaluation.

Master's Degree in Nursing Administration

Graduate programs in nursing administration focus on preparing nurses for roles in health facility administration. Although most nursing departments are overseen by nurse administrators, some nurse administrators also assume responsibility for other institutional services, such as the dietary department, housekeeping, and physical plant. In many health care facilities, a nurse administrator is the chief executive officer (CEO) and has responsibility for all departments. Because of the need to provide instruction and experience in both advanced nursing management and sound business administration, some universities have created joint degree programs in nursing and business administration (MSN/MBA) or nursing and health services administration (MSN/MHSA). Nurses preparing for administrative roles in public health or community health settings may choose a joint degree program in nursing administration and public health (MSN/MPH). The importance of graduate preparation in nursing is the emphasis on preparing nurse administrators who are able to administer health care institutions by integrating sound business management principles with the standards of quality nursing care.

ADVANCED NURSING PRACTICE

The **advanced practice nurse** is described by Snyder and Yen (1995, p. 28) as "a nurse who has educational preparation beyond the basic preparation required to become a nurse and includes nurse practitioners, clinical nurse specialists, certified nurse-midwives and nurse anesthetists." The National Council of State Boards of Nursing describes the qualifications of advanced practice nurses related to education, knowledge and skill, and defines advanced practice as

the practice of nursing by nurse practitioners, nurse anesthetists, nurse midwives, and clinical nurse specialists, based on the following: knowledge and skills required in basic nursing education; licensure as a registered nurse; graduate degree and experience in the designated area of practice which includes advanced nursing theory; substantial knowledge of physical and psychosocial assessment; appropriate interventions and management of health care status.

The skills and abilities essential for the advanced practice role within an identified specialty area include: providing client and community education; promoting stress prevention and management; encouraging self help; subscribing to caring; advocacy; accountability, accessibility; and collaboration with other health and community professionals. (Mezey & McGivern, 1993, p. 5.)

In Canada, the Ontario Ministry of Health makes a special distinction that the "nurse practitioner should be seen to be a practitioner of advanced nursing and not a second-level doctor or physician's assistant." They describe a nurse practitioner as

a registered nurse with additional nursing education that prepares her/him to provide the public with services, within the role of nursing, in all five basic components of comprehensive health services (promotion, prevention, cure, rehabilitation and support) and at all levels in the health care system. The services she/he provides in the area of cure (diagnosis/assessment and treatment) are those that rest in the overlap between medicine and nursing and that can be safely and effectively given by either the physician or the nurse. (Mass & McKay, 1995, p. 7.)

Education for Advanced Practice

Education for advanced practice generally requires the baccalaureate degree in nursing and a specified amount of clinical nursing practice as prerequisites. Most advanced practice education takes place at the graduate level and includes at least 1 year of full-time study, which includes both didactic study and clinical practice. Graduate programs in the various advanced practice specialties are available throughout the United States. In Canada, the university schools of nursing in Ontario offer nurse practitioner educational programs (Mass & McKay, 1995, p. 9).

The **American Nurses Credentialing Center** (ANCC, 1995) states that approximately one-third of nurse practitioner education consists of theoretical study related to the field of practice, and two-thirds consists of clinical experience overseen by a preceptor. Clinical experiences include health assessment and management of clients with acute and chronic conditions, health teaching for disease prevention

and health promotion, research utilization, technical and decision-making skills, consultation and collaboration with other health professionals, and leadership skills. Many programs offer additional required or elective courses in entrepreneurship (to assist the graduate to set up an independent practice), small business management, cultural diversity, health care policy, and nursing informatics or health-related applied computer systems.

Regulation of Advanced Practice

The regulation of advanced nursing practice in the United States varies from state to state. Certification is a voluntary process "by which a nongovernmental agency or association certifies that an individual licensed to practice a profession has met certain predetermined standards specified by that profession for specialty practice" (Mirr, 1995, pp. 40–41). Many advanced practice nurses are certified by national professional organizations who have developed educational and experiential criteria for specialty certification. Many states require certification by a recognized national certification body before a nurse can function at the advanced practice level.

Legal authority for advanced nursing practice resides with the state boards of nursing, with the boards of medicine, or through a joint committee. Some states require a separate license for advanced practice nurses, while other states include such nurses under the RN license and describe the "scope of practice" to include what the nurse has the education and experience to do. Various legal titles are conferred by the states to designate the advanced practice nurse, including nurse practitioner (NP), advanced practice registered nurse (APRN), advanced practice nurse (APN), and advanced registered nurse practitioner (ARNP). In addition, certification titles such as certified nurse midwife (CNM), clinical nurse specialist (CNS), and certified registered nurse anesthetist (CRNA) only increase confusion in the public's mind about who advanced practice nurses are and what they do. This issue of advanced practice nurse titling is currently being studied by the state boards of nursing as well as the professional nursing organizations.

Advanced practice nurses, with the assistance of national professional organizations, have fought hard to obtain legal authority to practice, to be directly reimbursed for their service, and to prescribe medications. Whereas most states recognize the nurse anesthetist, the nurse midwife, and the nurse practitioner roles, many states do not recognize the clinical nurse specialist as an advanced practice role. Most states require the completion of a master's degree in nursing with an advanced practice specialty for licensure as an advanced practice nurse.

Advanced practice nurses have sought to receive direct reimbursement for their services from private insurers, Medicaid, Medicare, and other governmental funders of health care services. Whereas many states provide for some level of direct reimbursement from governmental sources, usually at a percentage of what a physician will receive for providing the same service, only 8 states provide full reimbursement for advanced practice nursing services. Some states authorize a percentage of reimbursement (usually around 80%) when the nurse bills directly, but will reimburse at 100% if the nurse bills indirectly through a physician/nurse collaboration.

The right to prescribe medications and other therapies is a third area requiring legal authority. Only 4 states deny prescriptive authority to advanced practice nurses. The majority of states allow advanced practice nurses to prescribe, but many require that such prescriptions follow physician protocols and be cosigned by a physician or include the physician's name and drug number on the prescription form. Some states require pharmacist approval. Many states limit the advanced practice nurse's prescriptive authority to certain classifications of drugs, often prohibiting the nurse from prescribing controlled drugs. Some states have developed a formulary of drugs from which nurses can prescribe. Some states grant prescriptive privileges only to nurses who are working in public health clinics, rural health facilities, or other underserved settings. In those states where advanced practice nurses have some level of prescriptive authority, they may be required to have a course in advanced pharmacology, some specified period of supervised clinical practice, or a master's degree in nursing. Some states mandate ongoing education in pharmacology to maintain prescriptive privileges.

In Canada, nurses performing advanced practice functions in British Columbia do so under the delegated authority of physicians through formal policies and protocols. Ontario is considering legislation that would authorize an extended class of registration for nurses who meet certain educational and experiential criteria to practice as nurse practitioners in expanded roles. Nurses holding this extended registration would be permitted to "communicate a diagnosis, prescribe and dispense drugs and apply and order the application of energy" (Mass & McKay, 1995, p. 8).

Types of Advanced Practice

There are four main types of advanced practitioners: the clinical nurse specialist, the nurse practitioner, the nurse midwife, and the nurse anesthetist.

Clinical Nurse Specialist

In 1980, the ANA (p. 23) described the **clinical nurse specialist (CNS)** as "a nurse who, through study and supervised practice at the graduate level (master's or doctorate), has become expert in a defined area of knowledge and practice in a selected clinical area of nursing." Sparacino and Cooper (1990, p. 11) describe the roles of the clinical nurse specialist as expert nurse clinician, consultant, educator, change agent, role model, and researcher. The clinical nurse specialist may also assume the role of administrator, although there is controversy about whether the CNS can maintain clinical practice expertise and effectively manage administrative responsibilities. The education and expertise of the clinical nurse specialist should be such that she or he is eligible for specialty certification on completion of the graduate course of study. The American Nurses Credentialing Center provides national certification of clinical specialists in the areas of medical-surgical nursing, gerontologic nursing, community health nursing, adult psychiatric and mental health nursing, and child and adolescent psychiatric and mental health nursing (ANCC, 1995). By 1995, the ANCC had certified 5653 clinical specialists in adult psychiatric and mental health nursing, 716 clinical specialists in child and adolescent psychiatric and mental health nursing, 1631 clinical specialists in medical surgical nursing, 601 clinical specialists in gerontologic nursing, and 294 clinical specialists in community health nursing (ANCC, 1995, p. 4).

The ANA describes the competencies of the clinical nurse specialist as

the ability to observe, conceptualize, diagnose, and analyze complex clinical or non-clinical problems related to health, ability to consider a wide range of theory relevant to understanding those problems, ability to select and justify application of theory deemed to be most useful in understanding the problems and in determining the range of possible treatment options, and ability to foresee and discuss short and long-range possible consequences. (1980, p. 23)

Nurse Practitioner

The American Association of Colleges of Nursing (AACN, 1993, p. 2) states that **nurse practitioners** (NPs) "conduct physical exams, diagnose and treat common acute illness and injuries, provide care to chronically ill adults and children, order and interpret lab results, and counsel patients on health promotion and health care options." In 1992, the American Academy of Nurse Practitioners described the qualifications of nurse practitioners as "registered nurses with advanced education and clinical competency necessary for the delivery of primary health and medical care" and published its standards of practice. The American Nurses Credentialing Center (1995) describes the nurse practitioner's practice as one which "includes independent and interdependent decision-making and direct accountability for clinical judgment." It further defines the nurse practitioner's role to include "participation in the use of research, development and implementation of health policy, leadership, education, case management, and consultation."

Certification of nurse practitioners is available from the American Nurses Credentialing Center (1995) in the areas of adult nurse practitioner, family nurse practitioner, school nurse practitioner, pediatric nurse practitioner, and gerontological nurse practitioner. By 1995, the ANCC had certified 326 school nurse practitioners, 1943 pediatric nurse practitioners, 5667 adult nurse practitioners, 7593 family nurse practitioners, and 1698 gerontological nurse practitioners (ANCC, 1995, p. 4).

Adult Nurse Practitioner The **adult nurse practitioner** is described by the ANCC (1995, p. 13) as a registered nurse "with a graduate degree in nursing who is prepared for advanced practice in adult health care across the health continuum." Adult nurse practitioners practice in both hospital and community settings. See the accompanying interview box for a description of one adult nurse practitioner's work.

Pediatric Nurse Practitioner The **pediatric nurse practitioner** is described as a registered nurse "prepared at the graduate level in nursing to assume a role as a principal provider of primary health care for children" (ANCC, 1995, p. 16). Primary health care includes "first contact care, comprehensive care,

INTERVIEW

Adult Nurse Practitioner
Bonnie Hammack, MSN, ARNP

What was your area of practice before you became an advanced practice nurse? "I practiced in medical-surgical nursing for about 4 years."

Why did you decide to become an advanced practice nurse? "I was working for some doctors and found I was performing some advanced practice skills. They encouraged me to become a nurse practitioner. I liked the independent practice, the ability to have more control over patient outcomes. I could give holistic care from a nursing perspective, not just medical treatment."

Where do you practice? "I work in the clinic and long-term care unit at the Veterans Administration (VA) Hospital. I also teach nursing in an associate degree program and an RN-BSN program. As a US Air Force Reserve nurse, I used my advanced practice skills when I was activated during Desert Storm to work in a military hospital emergency room.

What do you do in your area of practice? "I kind of fill in the blanks. When I'm working on the long-term care unit I provide follow-up care for patients with chronic health problems and deliver episodic care for acute problems. When I'm assigned to the outpatient clinic, I provide follow-up treatment and counseling. I practice autonomously and independently, but we're a team; the physician is available as a resource."

Describe your best experience as an advanced practice nurse. "I really like taking care of the elderly—it's like taking care of my grandparents. (I don't have any.) It's good to be able to answer their questions to put their mind at ease, to tell them that some things are a normal part of aging and some things can be treated. They don't always have to live with their discomforts; many of the discomforts can be treated.

What encouragement would you give to a nurse considering becoming an advanced practice nurse? "The sky's the limit! They can do as much or as little as they want; however, the advanced practice nurse must learn some business and consumer skills. They have to be the best and deliver quality care to clients, but they must also seek just compensation for their work."

coordinated or integrated care, and care that is longitudinal over time rather than episodic" (National Association of Pediatric Nurse Associates and Practitioners [NAPNAP], 1995, p. 97). Pediatric nurse practitioners use the nursing process in providing

INTERVIEW

Pediatric Nurse Practitioner

Sandra Levin, MSN, ARNP

What was your area of practice before you became a pediatric nurse practitioner? "I have been a nurse for 20 years, during which time I have worked as a pediatric staff nurse in the hospital setting and a classroom and clinical educator."

Why did you decide to become a pediatric nurse practitioner? "I always wanted to be a nurse practitioner, but there were very few programs available. I wanted a more autonomous role caring for children and educating their families about effective parenting."

Where do you practice? "I practice in an ambulatory pediatric setting in an urban community with a group of pediatricians. There is one other nurse practitioner and two physicians. We see children and families from across the socioeconomic continuum."

What do you do in your area of practice? "I perform many of the same things as a physician in relation to diagnosis and treatment of minor illnesses, but from a nursing view of health promotion, wellness, and holism. I prefer to work with well children assessing their achievement of developmental milestones. I then provide anticipatory guidance to parents about their child's development and related needs, such as safety, nutrition, immunizations, etc."

Describe your best experience as a pediatric nurse practitioner. "I like identifying subtle changes in a child that may indicate a larger health problem. I like working with parents helping them to recognize their child's potential and assisting them with their parenting skills. I especially like working with families who have a child with attention deficit/hyperactivity disorder. I like helping them plan behavioral interventions to help their child realize his/her full potential."

What encouragement would you give to a nurse considering becoming a pediatric nurse practitioner? "Go for it!" Especially in pediatrics there is a need for education of parents, helping them to have family harmony and have a child achieve his full potential."

direct and indirect nursing services to children from birth through adolescence and their families in the specific areas of health promotion, disease and disability prevention, health maintenance, and health restoration. The pediatric nurse practitioner's practice "builds on previous nursing knowledge and skill

and includes case management, client advocacy, and collaboration with other health professionals. Pediatric nurse practitioners promote the psychosocial, physical, and developmental well-being of the child and family and provide leadership in addressing health care trends and issues, professional issues and role development" (NAPNAP, 1995, p. 97).

The National Association of Pediatric Nurse Practitioners and Associates (NAPNAP) describes the many practice settings of the pediatric nurse practitioner to include private offices, schools, university health centers, community clinics, public health departments, nurse-managed clinics, health maintenance organizations, hospital-based acute care pediatric units, and pediatric intensive care units. National certification as a pediatric nurse practitioner can be obtained through the National Certification Board of Pediatric Nurse Practitioners and Nurses (NCBPNP/N), which was established in 1975, and through the American Nurses Credentialing Center (ANCC). The purpose of these certification examinations is to promote high-quality health care to children and their families by ensuring that pediatric nurse practitioners meet both knowledge and experiential standards. See the accompanying interview box for a description of a pediatric nurse practitioner's role and practice setting.

School Nurse Practitioner School nurse practitioners are described by ANCC (1995, p. 15) as prepared "to assume responsibilities in the health care of preschool, school-age children, and adolescents. Their practice builds on previous knowledge and skill in using the nursing process, and preparation in educational systems, school health, community health, health education, and planning for the needs of exceptional children in the educational system."

The school nurse practitioner incorporates many of the functions of the pediatric nurse practitioner but applies them in the school and community settings, often in collaboration with teachers, school officials, community agencies, and community leaders.

Family Nurse Practitioner The ANCC (1995, p. 14) describes the **family nurse practitioner** as "a registered nurse with a graduate degree in nursing who is prepared for advanced practice with individuals and families throughout the life span and across the health continuum." The functions of the family nurse practitioner include many of the same activities as the functions of the adult nurse practitioner and the pediatric nurse practitioner focusing on the integrated family unit. The family nurse practitioner provides care to clients across the many phases of the life span, including children, adolescents, pregnant women, adults, and older adults.

Gerontological Nurse Practitioner The **gerontological nurse practitioner** is described by the American Nurses Credentialing Center (ANCC, 1995, p. 16) as an "expert in providing primary health care for older adults and their families in a variety of settings." They "provide care and advocacy for the older adult to maximize functional abilities; promote, maintain, and restore health; prevent or minimize disabilities; and promote death with dignity." The gerontological nurse practitioner assumes many of the functions of adult nurse practitioner focusing on the elderly adult.

Psychiatric/Mental Health Nurse Practitioner The **psychiatric/mental health nurse practitioner** provides primary mental health care in inpatient and outpatient facilities, including ambulatory care centers, 24-hour crisis centers, alcohol and substance abuse clinics and residential treatment programs, schools, and social agencies. These specialists also provide care in collaboration with psychiatrists and psychologists in private practice. Many psychiatric/mental health nurse practitioners work with victims of domestic violence, including spouse abuse, child abuse, and elder abuse. Through hospice programs they provide counseling to clients who are terminally ill with AIDS or cancer. They assist clients in rehabilitation to overcome the psychologic effects of physical disability. They assist clients, family members, and other support persons who are dealing with the chronic problems of aging, especially clients with dementias, Alzheimer's disease, and other degenerative illnesses. A unique practice setting for the psychiatric/mental health nurse practitioner is "caring for the caregiver" in impaired nurse programs that provide substance abuse counseling and stress reduction and management education for professional

RESEARCH NOTE

What Type of Clinical Preventive Services Do Nurse Practitioners Provide?

The National Alliance of Nurse Practitioners (NANP) was one of five primary care provider groups that participated in a government-sponsored survey on clinical preventive services (CPSs). Two thousand randomly selected nurse practitioners were surveyed to obtain information regarding the percentage of their clients who "routinely" receive the specified assessment and intervention services based on 17 of the *Healthy People 2000* national health objectives for CPS.

Usable responses were returned by 892 (68%) of the sample. Analysis of the responses indicated that nurse practitioners already exceed the *Healthy People 2000* objective targets in some areas, including assessment of emotional and behavioral function, blood pressure, and cholesterol levels in adults; height and weight and hemoglobin and hematocrit in children; mobility and currency of medication lists in older adults; and family planning, preconception care, clinical breast examination, and Papanicolaou (Pap) smears in women of childbearing age. Areas where nurse practitioners are close to targets include assessment of exercise, cognitive function, sexual practices, and sexually transmitted diseases (STDs) in all age groups except infants and children; eye examinations and immunizations in children, mammograms in women of childbearing age, and mobility and falls prevention in older adults. Progress is needed in the areas of nutrition, seat belt/car seat use, smoking, alcohol and illicit drug use, occupational health risk and tetanus-diptheria boosters. Increased assessment and intervention is also needed in the areas of vision, hearing, speech, motor development, and parent/child relations in children; and hearing, vision, urinary incontinence, dementia, and influenza vaccines in older adults.

Implications: Nurse practitioners will continue to make a significant contribution toward achieving national health objectives as set forth by *Healthy People 2000*. With continued monitoring of achievement of objectives for clinical preventive services, nurse practitioners can improve their delivery of services, educators can improve curricula, and researchers can investigate the effective delivery of preventive care.

SOURCE: "Baseline Data on the Delivery of Clinical Preventive Services Provided by Nurse Practitioners" by K. B. Lemley, E. T. O'Grady, L. Rauckhorst, D. D. Russell, and N. Small, May 1994, *Nurse Practitioner, 19*(5), 57–63.

nurses to enable them to cope with practice in the changing health care environment. Psychiatric/mental health nurse practitioners are prepared to provide individual and family counseling, group counseling for families or support groups, and consultative services to other health care providers.

Certified Nurse Midwife (CNM)

A **certified nurse-midwife (CNM)** is a registered nurse who has advanced educational preparation in midwifery, which includes theory and extensive supervised clinical experiences in prenatal care, management of labor and delivery, postpartum care of the mother and infant, family planning, and gyne-

cologic care for well women. The focus of education is on normal obstetrics and newborn care. Most nurses who choose to become nurse midwives have extensive prior nursing experience in maternity and public health nursing. The majority of nurse midwifery programs in the United States offer the master's degree, and all are accredited by the American College of Nurse-Midwives (ACNM). The ACNM is also the credentialing organization that sets the standards by which nurse midwifery is practiced in the United States. Certified nurse midwives practice in all 50 states in the United States delivering babies in hospitals, in birthing centers, and in the home. Although most nurse midwives practice indepen-

---

INTERVIEW

Nurse Midwife

Terry DeFilippo, MSN, CNM

What was your area of practice before you became a nurse midwife? "I was a labor and delivery nurse and a childbirth educator for about 10 years. I was also a hospital inservice educator prior to becoming a nurse midwife. I started once to become a midwife, but the program didn't start as planned, so I went back to labor and delivery nursing and then returned to graduate school when the midwife program became available."

Why did you decide to become a nurse midwife? "After my experience working in labor and delivery, I wanted to extend my role and provide more total patient care. Midwifery was an extension of what I was doing. I didn't become a midwife to get out of what I was doing as a nurse but rather to go forward and provide more care to patients during the childbirth experience."

Where do you practice? "I work for a group practice which contracts to a large public hospital. We provide prenatal and postpartum care and family planning education in the clinic. We provide intrapartum and immediate postpartum care in the labor and delivery suite. We also provide care in a school setting for pregnant teenagers and for teenage mothers while they are finishing high school.

"My practice is somewhat different from the typical midwife. I previously worked in a private practice where we provided care for healthy women throughout life. My patients were primarily women who wanted a female practitioner or physician. Many were women who wanted a female practitioner for their daughters for their first pelvic exam."

What do you do in your area of practice? "I provide antepartum, intrapartum, and postpartum care for healthy

women and their newborns. I also provide some gynecologic care for healthy women, mostly family planning. I care for high-risk patients or patients with obstetric complications under detailed protocols with obstetrician/gynecologists. Most of my care is independent; some of my patients are co-managed with the physician who provides various levels of assistance depending on the patient's need. Sometimes the physician is simply reviewing the case and providing feedback.

"Studies have shown that nurse midwives are especially effective in prevention of preterm labor in teenagers because of personal support they provide and because they take time and show an interest in the patient. I think these patients identify more with the nurse midwife."

Describe your best experience as a nurse midwife. "I'm privileged to be present at a birth. I feel like I'm participating in a miracle every time I'm there."

What encouragement would you give to a nurse considering becoming a nurse midwife? "A nurse midwife has to be realistic about the personal commitment she is making. You have to be willing to put in the time/hours. You're not on a fixed schedule—you have to take call and be there when you're expected. This is especially so if you are in private practice; there may be no one else to cover you.

"You also have a great deal of autonomy and have a tremendous opportunity to have an impact on your patient, but with it comes a great deal of responsibility. The nurse midwife has the ability to empower women, which is very important. We need to give each other the respect we deserve. I assist patients in achieving what they want; they have choices, and they can make decisions about their care."

dently providing care for women and children, all maintain an affiliation with a physician specialist in obstetrics and gynecology for consultation and referral of clients with complications.

Nurse midwives also practice in Great Britain, Canada, Australia, Europe, Africa, and many of the island nations in the Caribbean. The education, regulation, and extent of practice of nurse midwives vary around the world. See the interview box on the previous page for a description of a nurse midwife's role and practice setting.

Certified Registered Nurse Anesthetist (CRNA)

The nurse anesthetist was one of the earliest advanced practice roles in the United States: Nurses started administering anesthesia as early as 1889. A **certified registered nurse anesthetist (CRNA)** is a registered nurse who has advanced educational preparation, including classroom and laboratory instruction and supervised clinical practice, in the delivery of anesthesia to clients in a variety of practice settings, including hospitals, ambulatory surgical centers, birthing centers, and clinics. The American Association of Nurse Anesthetists, founded in 1931, established a certification program for nurse anesthetists in 1945 and an accreditation program for educational programs for nurse anesthesia in 1952. A baccalaureate degree has been required for certification as a CRNA since 1987, and a master's degree will be required beginning in 1998. Nurse anesthetist working with physician anesthesiologists administer more than half of the anesthesia given to clients in the United States. In some settings, such as birthing centers and ambulatory surgical centers, nurse anesthetists may deliver anesthesia independently to clients with uncomplicated vaginal deliveries or minor surgeries. Nurse anesthetists maintain an affiliation with a physician anesthesiologist for consultation prior to or during the delivery of anesthesia to a client. See the accompanying interview box for a description of a nurse anesthetist's role and practice setting.

CONSIDER . . .

- the various roles and specialty practice areas of advanced nurse practitioners, especially the differences between the clinical nurse specialist and the nurse practitioner. What are the differences? What are the similarities?
- the practice of various advanced practice nurses

INTERVIEW

Certified Registered Nurse Anesthetist
William Maybury, MS, CRNA

What was your area of practice before you became a nurse anesthetist? "I worked in an intensive care unit for two years."

Why did you decide to become a nurse anesthetist? "I wanted to advance my skills beyond that of a floor nurse. Also, as a male nurse and knowing that someday I would be the main financial supporter of a family, I needed a job in nursing where I could earn enough to support a family possibly without having my wife work and be away from our children when they were young and in need of her."

Where do you practice? "I have been a CRNA for the past 25 years. I work for a group of anesthesiologists who contract to provide anesthesia services for a number of large and small public and private hospitals."

What do you do in your area of practice? "I administer anesthesia—general, regional, and local—and monitor anesthesia care. I do preoperative evaluations on patients to determine their most appropriate anesthesia needs during surgery. I give anesthesia to pediatric, neuro, obstetric, trauma, as well as other types of general surgery patients."

Describe your best experience as a nurse anesthetist. "My best experience is working one on one with patients as I give anesthesia. This means you use knowledge of all the specialties in medicine. You must know internal medicine, cardiology, respiratory, as well as other medical fields in order to administer anesthesia. As for myself, I enjoy pediatrics the most."

What encouragement would you give to a nurse considering becoming a nurse anesthetist? "As in any job or profession, you should advance in your knowledge and skills as far as you can. As you become an advanced practice nurse, you will have more knowledge and skills in that specific area. The job market for the future will be more open to an advanced practice nurse than a routine nurse, and the financial benefits are greater than those of a regular nurse."

whom you know. How does their practice conform to the roles and functions described in this chapter? What are their relationships with physician specialists in their practice area?
- client satisfaction with the advanced practice nurse. What client needs does the advanced practice nurse meet that the physician may not meet? What client needs does the physician

meet that the advanced practice nurse may not meet?

The Future of Advanced Practice Nursing

Advanced practice nurses fill a need for quality primary care services at an affordable cost to clients in both rural and urban settings. But as the functions of advanced practice nurses begin to overlap with those of primary care physicians, the need to delineate the nursing and medical roles becomes important to collegial and collaborative practice. More important, these roles must be delineated in order to decrease consumer confusion. There is a need for advanced practice nurses, physicians, private insurers, and public reimbursement agencies to keep a focus on the client: Which provider is best suited to provide which aspects of care?

Registered nurses, advanced practice nurses, and professional nursing organizations will need to educate not only the public but also the politicians and legislators in the proper role of the advanced practice nurse. The advanced practice nurse has a major role in preventing illness and promoting health for individuals, families, and communities.

Professional nursing organizations will need to ensure a high standard for those who aspire to advanced practice certification. Educational institutions will need to collaborate and cooperate with professional nursing organizations and employers of advanced practice nurses to ensure that the classroom and clinical instructional experiences prepare graduates to assume the advanced practice nurse role effectively. Recently there has been much discussion about merging the role of the advanced nurse practitioner with the clinical specialist to decrease professional and public confusion. Many educational institutions are already changing their curricula to integrate the two roles in graduate education. Some believe that by the year 2000 all advanced practice professional certification programs will probably require the master's degree.

CONSIDER...

- the future of advanced practice in your community, state (province, territory), and nation. How do you see advanced practice nurses solving some of the problems in today's health care system?
- whether advanced practice is a professional

career choice for you. Do you have the assertiveness required to perform in an independent role?
- the role differences between the registered nurse and the advanced practice nurse. Consider which nurses may not be appropriate for advanced practice roles. What will be the relationship between registered nurses and advanced practice nurses?

SELECTING A GRADUATE PROGRAM

Choosing a graduate program is an important decision for a nurse who is committed to lifelong work in nursing. Several factors must be considered, including professional career goals, personal and family factors, and characteristics of the proposed program (see the accompanying box).

Professional Career Goals

The nurse must first identify personal career goals. Graduate education is preparation for specialized practice. Not all graduate programs will provide the course work to meet the requirements for all

---

Criteria for Considering a Graduate Program

- Professional career goals
- Personal and family factors
- Program characteristics
  1. Type of graduate programs offered
  2. School's philosophy of nursing and education
  3. Accreditation status
  4. National standing
  5. Admission requirements
  6. Faculty qualifications
  7. Institutional climate
  8. Resources
  9. Clinical facilities
  10. Assistantships and other financial support
  11. Program graduation requirements

SOURCE: Adapted from "Graduate Education: Making the Right Choice" by G. W. Poteet, L. C. Hodges, and S. Tate, 1994, in *Current Issues in Nursing* (4th ed.) by J. McCloskey and H. K. Grace (Eds.), St. Louis: Mosby, pp. 182–187.

advanced nursing roles and all clinical practice settings. Some graduate schools of nursing focus on nurse practitioner roles; other focus on the roles of nurse educator and administrator. Some schools are highly specialized and may provide only a single program, for example, in nurse anesthesia. Some schools of nursing have become innovative and offer highly specialized graduate programs of study, such as nursing informatics, aerospace nursing, or forensic nursing. Some graduate schools of nursing integrate advanced clinical practice roles with functional roles of education or administration but still require that the nurse choose an area of clinical specialization, such as adult health or child health, women's health, gerontology, physiologic health, or psychiatric/mental health. Graduate study may include shared core or common courses that all students take (e.g., nursing theory, nursing research); however, the student must be assured that the program provides the course work and clinical experiences that the student will need to achieve personal goals. For example, the nurse who wants to become a teacher in a school of nursing should take courses in teaching methods and clinical evaluation of students; the nurse who wants to become a child health nurse practitioner must have clinical experience in pediatrics with appropriate faculty and preceptors.

The nurse must also decide whether to pursue a graduate degree in nursing, or a graduate degree in another field. For example, some nurses who want to become administrators in health care organizations may choose a graduate degree in business or health care administration. Nurses in psychiatric/mental health nursing may choose a graduate degree in mental health counseling. Before selecting a non-nursing graduate degree, the nurse should investigate the requirements for nursing licensure and certification in the desired field and consider possible future requirements. Currently, some national certification programs require the graduate degree in nursing (e.g., American Nurses Credentialing Center [ANCC] clinical nurse specialist in medical-surgical nursing or gerontologic nursing), whereas others do not (e.g., Association of Operating Room Nurses [AORN] nurse anesthesia). Many professional nursing organizations are developing or planning changes in certification requirements that will mandate the graduate degree in nursing. Many state boards of nursing are also developing rules that will mandate the graduate degree in nursing to practice in an advanced nursing role. (See page 444.)

Clearly defining professional goals enables the nurse to identify those graduate programs that provide the education and experiences to meet those goals. The nurse then considers personal and family factors and program characteristics to determine which program is most appropriate.

Personal and Family Factors

Several personal and family factors may affect the nurse's choice of a graduate nursing program. Is the nurse able to travel to another city or state to pursue graduate education? If there is a long commute to school, should the nurse relocate to be closer to school and its resources, such as the library or computer laboratories? Must the nurse support self or family while going to school? If so, the availability of employment opportunities are important. If the nurse is working while going to graduate school, the nurse may desire flexible school or work schedules to facilitate balancing study and work time. It may be best for the nurse to select a program that allows part-time study if work and family demands are heavy.

The nurse who is married needs the support of spouse and other family members while going to school. Working and going to school may limit the nurse's ability to fulfill spousal and parenting responsibilities. At the same time, children who see their parent continuing professional education have a role model for lifelong learning. The nurse who is returning to school needs to strategize with family members about how to meet family responsibilities.

Program Characteristics

Poteet, Hodges, and Tate (1994, p. 184) identify the following essential elements for assessing a graduate program: accreditation status, national standing, admission requirements, faculty qualifications, institutional climate, resources, clinical facilities, assistantships and other financial support, and program requirements. In addition, they recommend that the nurse should obtain information about what specific programs of study are offered and the school's philosophy of nursing and education. This information may be obtained from the institution's catalog or brochure, a telephone or in-person interview, or through discussion with a current student or graduate.

1. *Programs of study offered.* Does the school offer the specific program of study to enable the nurse to achieve professional goals? Are programs

offered on campus only or through distance learning techniques such as video conferencing, community-based learning, or correspondence?

2. *School's philosophy of nursing and education.* Does the school subscribe to the philosophy of one nursing theorist, or do they have an eclectic model, that is, an integration of several theorists? Knowing the school's philosophy helps the prospective student understand the foundational beliefs of the school, its faculty, and the curriculum. Is the school's philosophy of nursing and education consistent with the nurse's philosophy? Inconsistency between the nurse's philosophy and the program's philosophy may interfere with success in the program.

3. *Accreditation status.* Accreditation may be conferred by a state government; by a regional accreditation association, such as the Southern Association of Colleges and Schools (SACS); or by a professional organization, such as the National League for Nursing (NLN). In 1995, there were 234 graduate nursing programs in the United States accredited by the National League for Nursing (1995). Specialty nursing organizations may also accredit specific programs; for example, the American College of Nurse Midwifery accredits graduate programs in midwifery. Graduation from an accredited program may be important for the graduate to meet national certification requirements and to obtain licensure for advanced practice.

4. *National standing.* Programs may have a national reputation for excellence in certain fields of study. This reputation is usually based on the quality of the faculty, the facilities for learning, and the achievements of its graduates. Attending a program with a national reputation for excellence may enhance the graduate's opportunities for employment.

5. *Admission requirements.* Admission requirements may include a minimum grade point average (GPA) for undergraduate work, a minimum score on a national entrance examination such as the Graduate Record Examination (GRE) or the Miller Analogy Test (MAT), and successful completion of specific prerequisite courses such as physical assessment, statistics, or computer science. Most graduate nursing programs require completion of a baccalaureate degree in nursing. Some graduate programs allow nurses with a baccalaureate degree in another field to enter the graduate nursing program but require that the student complete any undergraduate nursing courses that were not previously taken (McGriff, 1996, p. 9). Because admission to graduate nursing programs is competitive, students need to be aware of specific admission requirements so that they can take action to meet or exceed the requirements; if they fail to meet the requirements, they may be denied admission. The student who is denied admission should question whether there are any admission waivers under which they might still qualify, such as a minority waiver.

6. *Faculty qualifications.* All faculty who teach at the graduate level should have a doctoral degree and a history of scholarly productivity. Students should expect to be taught by faculty who are expert in their fields. Students should seek a program where there are faculty who have expertise in the area of their interest.

7. *Institutional climate.* Prospective students may want to question students currently in the program about the climate of the school of nursing and the university/college. Do the university and school of nursing provide an environment of diversity where students can experience the value and strength of human difference? Is there an open climate in the school of nursing and the university community that allows scholarly inquiry without fear of retribution? Are relationships among faculty, students, administration, and other staff open and conducive to learning? Do faculty members have a reputation of being "student friendly"; that is, are they readily available for student consultation, or are they difficult to contact outside scheduled class times? Do faculty members challenge students to achieve their fullest potential in an atmosphere of academic rigor? Do faculty members teach most of the courses, or do teaching assistants or adjunct faculty teach a high percentage of classes?

8. *Resources.* What resources are available to support and enhance student learning? Are library materials adequate, including books and journals to support the student's field of study, computer services, and statistical consultation to facilitate student research? Are study areas, lounges, and dining facilities adequate? Students should also inquire about hours of operation, especially

evening, weekend and holiday hours, to determine whether resources are available when the student needs them. Is there on-campus housing available for the student who must relocate for graduate study?

9. *Clinical facilities.* Are adequate clinical sites and preceptors available to support students, especially those who are in programs preparing the advanced nurse practitioner? Clinical facilities should include primary, secondary, and tertiary settings that provide diverse practice opportunities. Preceptors should be available who are experts in the desired specialty and who like working with students. Clinical practice settings should provide opportunities for graduate students to demonstrate critical thinking in the delivery of care to diverse clients with complex problems. Some graduate programs may provide clinical opportunities that are international in scope, for example, clinical experience study programs to provide primary care in underdeveloped nations.

10. *Assistantships and other financial support.* What is the availability of financial assistance? Many graduate programs provide teaching or research assistantships, in which the student receives tuition assistance in exchange for providing either teaching or research support to faculty. For the student whose professional goals involve teaching or research, assistantships provide an opportunity to gain experience in the role while completing formal graduate education. Many professional nursing organizations provide scholarship assistance for graduate nursing students. Other financial assistance may be available, especially for the student pursuing a graduate degree as an advanced nurse practitioner. Students should inquire about opportunities for financial assistance from their professional organizations, the school of nursing, and the university financial aid office.

11. *Program requirements.* What are the requirements for degree completion—specifically, how many credit hours, what type of course work, how many classroom and clinical hours are required? Is a thesis required? Students may also want to ask about the average length of time for degree completion for full-time and part-time students.

CONSIDER...

- your professional goals as they may relate to graduate study. What would you like to be doing in 5 years, 10 years? What type of graduate program could enable you to accomplish your goals?
- graduate programs that you may be interested in attending. Do they provide the program you need to accomplish your goals? Use the listed criteria to evaluate the programs under your consideration. What are the strengths of the various programs you are considering? What personal and family factors should you consider in making a decision about graduate study?

READINGS FOR ENRICHMENT

Mezey, M. D., & McGivern, D. O. (1993). *Nurses, nurse practitioners: Evolution to advanced practice.* New York: Springer.

This book discusses the philosophical, historical, educational, and research perspectives of advanced nursing practice. Advanced practice nurses contribute chapters describing their practice and role in a changing health care environment. The authors also discuss legal aspects of advanced practice nursing and include a chapter on the role that the advanced practice nurse plays in the politics and policy of primary care.

The Nurse Practitioner: The American Journal of Primary Health Care.

This journal publishes an annual update (January issue) summarizing each state's position on legislative issues affecting advanced nursing practice, including the legal authority for practice, laws regarding reimbursement of advanced practice nurses by third-party payors, and prescriptive authority.

Snyder, M., & Mirr, M. P. (1995). *Advanced practice nursing: A guide to professional development.* New York: Springer.

This book is a resource for nurses who are considering advanced practice. The authors provide information on nurse practitioners, clinical nurse specialists, nurse midwives, and nurse anesthetists. Among the topics addressed are clinical issues (e.g., clinical decision making, developing clinical protocols and guidelines for advanced practice), professional issues (collaboration, consultation, independent practice), and legal issues (licensure and certification, prescriptive privileges, reimbursement).

SUMMARY

Nurses planning to pursue graduate study must determine their professional goals before choosing a program. After identifying specific programs that will enable the nurse to meet desired goals, the nurse needs to evaluate the programs based on personal and family needs and program characteristics. Graduate programs in nursing may focus on nursing education, nursing administration, or advanced practice nursing.

Advanced practice nursing has evolved from the early 1900s to become a well-defined area of practice that provides services related to disease prevention, health promotion, health restoration, and rehabilitation. Advanced nursing practitioners include nurse practitioners, nurse midwives, nurse anesthetists, and clinical nurse specialists. Advanced practice nurses work in a variety of practice settings across the health care continuum but are most suited to the delivery of primary care to rural and urban populations, especially underserved populations, such as the poor and the elderly.

Certification and regulation of advanced practice has been developed by professional nursing organizations and state boards of nursing to ensure safe practice by qualified practitioners. Increasingly, nurses are required to obtain education for advanced practice in graduate programs to be eligible for certification and/or state licensure.

The future of advanced practice includes redesign of graduate nursing curricula to incorporate the clinical specialist role with the nurse practitioner role. Continued legislative activity by advanced practice nurses will be needed to ensure equitable compensation and prescriptive authority. The advanced practice nurse will be a major contributor to the delivery of quality health care at an affordable cost to clients in a changing health care environment.

SELECTED REFERENCES

American Academy of Nurse Practitioners. (1993). *Standards of Practice.* Austin, Texas: AANP.

American Association of Colleges of Nursing. (1993, March). In search of the advanced practice nurse. *Issues Bulletin.* AACN.

American Association of Colleges of Nursing. (1994). *Role differentiation of the nurse practitioner and clinical nurse specialist: Reaching toward consensus.* Proceedings of the Master's Educational Conference. December, 1994. San Antonio, TX: Author.

American Association of Nurse Anesthetists. (1990). *The report of the National Commission on Nurse Anesthesia Education.* Park Ridge, IL: Author.

American College of Nurse Midwives. (1991). *Basic questions and answers about certified nurse midwives.* Washington, DC: Author.

American Nurses Association. (1980). *Nursing: A social policy statement.* Washington, DC: Author.

American Nurses Association. (1995). *Nursing's social policy statement.* Washington, DC: American Nurses Publishing.

American Nurses Credentialing Center. (1995). *1995 certification catalog.* Washington, DC: Author.

Boodley, C. A. (1994). Nurse practitioner educational guidelines: Program standards, curriculum, and graduate outcomes. *Role differentiation of the nurse practitioner and clinical nurse specialist: Reaching toward consensus.* Proceedings of the Master's Education Conference. American Association of Colleges of Nursing. December 8–10, 1994, San Antonio, TX. Pp. 59–68.

Cronenwett, L. R. (1994). Molding the future for advanced practice nurses: Education, regulation, and practice. *Role differentiation of the nurse practitioner and clinical nurse specialist: Reaching toward consensus.* Proceedings of the Master's Education Conference. American Association of Colleges of Nursing. December 8–10, 1994, San Antonio, TX. Pp. 1–20.

Ford, L. C. (1979). A nurse for all settings: The nurse practitioner. *Nursing Outlook, 27*(8), 521.

Ford, L. C. (1992). Advanced nursing practices: Future of the nurse practitioner. In L. Aiken & C. Fagin, *Charting nursing's future: Agenda for the 1990s* (pp. 287–299). Philadelphia: Lippincott.

Hamric, A. B., & Spross, J. A. (1989). *The clinical nurse specialist in theory and practice* (2nd ed.). Philadelphia: W. B. Saunders.

Jackson, R. A. (1995, March). The heartbeat of reform. *Canadian Nurse, 91*(3), 23–27.

Lemley, K. B., O'Grady, E. T., Rauckhost, L., Russell, D. D., & Small, N. (1994, May). Baseline data on the delivery of clinical preventive services provided by nurse practitioners. *Nurse Practitioner, 19*(5), 57–63.

Mass, H., & McKay, R. (1995, Aug./Sept.). Nurse practitioners: Expanding the role of nursing. *Nursing B(ritish) C(olumbia),* pp. 7–9.

McGriff, E. P. (1996, Jan.). Graduate education in nursing. *NSNA/Imprint,* pp. 9–11.

Mezey, M. D., & McGivern, D. O. (1993). *Nurses, nurse practitioners: Evolution to advanced practice.* New York: Springer.

Mirr, M. P. (1995). Legal issues: Licensure and certification, prescriptive privileges, and reimbursement. In M. Snyder & M. P. Mirr (Eds.), *Advanced practice nursing: A guide to professional development.* New York: Springer.

National Association of Pediatric Nurse Associates and Practitioners (NAPNAP). (1995, March/April). Scope of practice for pediatric nurse practitioners. *Journal of Pediatric Health Care, (9),* 96–97.

National League for Nursing. (1995). Baccalaureate and master's degree programs in nursing, accredited by the National League for Nursing 1995–1996. *N&HC: Perspectives on Community, 16*(4), 239–246.

Poteet, G. W., Hodges, L. C., & Tate, S. (1994). Graduate education: Making the right choice. In J. McCloskey & H. K. Grace (Eds.), *Current Issues in Nursing* (4th ed.). St. Louis: Mosby.

Ray, G. L., & Hardin S. (1995, Sept.) Advanced practice nursing: Playing a vital role. *Advanced Practice Nurse Sourcebook.* Springhouse, PA: Springhouse Corp.

Snyder, M., & Mirr, M. P. (1995). *Advanced practice nursing: A guide to professional development.* New York: Springer.

Snyder, M., & Yen, M. (1995). Characteristics of the advanced practice nurse. In M. Snyder & M. P. Mirr (Eds.), *Advanced practice nursing: A guide to professional development* (pp. 3–12). New York: Springer.

Sparacino, P. S. A., Cooper, D. M., & Minarik, P. A. (1990). *The clinical nurse specialist: Implementation and impact.* Norwalk, CT: Appleton & Lange.

Trofino, J. (1995, March). The brave new world of health care. *Canadian Nurse, 91*(3), 28–32.

Wilson, D. (1994, Dec.) Nurse practitioners: The early years (1965–1974). *Nurse Practitioner, 19*(12), 26, 28, 31.

CHAPTER

Looking Into the Future

by Dr. Fay L. Bower

OBJECTIVES

- Identify past events that have affected nursing.

- Discuss future events that will affect nursing.

- Identify anticipated changes in health care and nursing in the future.

"There is no more powerful engine driving an organization toward excellence and long-term success than an attractive, worthwhile and achievable vision of the future, widely shared."

—Nanus, 1992

This chapter is about the future. Some of the content is like what you see when you look into a crystal ball. Much of the content of this chapter is conjecture based on real issues; a bit of it is based on the author's hopes and wishes that flow from trends that are already observable. This chapter is offered as an image of what might be, could be, and probably will be if the trends of today continue and if what is written and believed about tomorrow comes true.

- Much has occurred in health care in the last decade. Changing demographics, changing economics, new diseases, new technology, new treatments, new drugs, and renewed concern about the legal and ethical issues of health care have provoked cries for change in health care delivery. These same factors have influenced change in nursing.
- To properly address the rapidly changing present and future, nurses need to review some of the significant events and the resultant outcomes in nursing and health care. Viewing these events in their appropriate context is important because so much that initiates change in nursing is created by the very issues and events that change society at large.
- To effect orderly evolution, rather than be swept along by chaotic change, nursing and the health care system must learn from yesterday and work hard today to create the vision for tomorrow's health care.

PAST EVENTS THAT HAVE AFFECTED NURSING

Events That Promoted Nursing's Growth and Development

Many events of the past spurred the growth and development of nursing as a profession; many events and public policy changes that were never intended to help or harm nursing's development nevertheless changed nursing. Social movements and technologic advancements also have propelled nursing into both favorable and hazardous positions.

A discussion about nursing's growth must include the impact of World War II on the quantity and quality of nurses in many countries. World War II and the period following were times of major change, both for health care and for women. Major medical and surgical advances were discovered (some by intent, others by accident), and new techniques for care were developed. Women played a major role in the military and performed valiantly in front-line medical units; some served as volunteers in the American and International Red Cross, while others entered the workforce in areas they had never before encountered. With most men at war, women were drawn into a work life that was new to them.

Nursing both advanced during this period and suffered. In answering the call to patriotic duty, many women chose nontraditional roles, particularly because the salaries available to "war workers" were higher. The changing work opportunities for women had a negative effect on nursing: The challenge of doing "men's work" attracted many women who might have otherwise pursued nursing. This shift in work choice caused a shortage of nurses in America, even after the war was over. In response to the shortage and in line with the desire of professional nursing organizations in the United States to advance nursing's professional standing, a 2-year associate degree nursing program was developed for the junior/community colleges. In the next several years, this model of education spread quickly, so that by 1994 there were 848 associate degree nursing (ADN) programs in the United States (National League for Nursing [NLN], 1994).

Although before World War II nurses were educated primarily in hospitals, the first university baccalaureate degree program in nursing (BSN) in the United States had been in existence since 1909. However, the number of BSN programs has not increased at the same rate as ADN programs; in 1994, there were 501 BSN programs in the United States, compared with 848 ADN programs. These changes in the education of nurses have significant implications for the future of professional nursing, which is discussed later in this chapter.

Another event that has affected nursing's growth and development is the position paper issued by the American Nurses Association (ANA) in 1965, which suggested that all education for nurses take place in institutions of higher learning. Although both ADN and BSN programs existed throughout the United States at that time, most nurses were prepared in hospital-based diploma programs, and the position paper met with much resistance and even anger. By 1978, the ANA issued another recommendation, one that was even stronger. The ANA recommended there be two levels of nurses prepared in universities or colleges: ADN and BSN nurses. In 1985, ANA went even further, suggesting different titles for the two levels of nurses. By then, several nursing organizations, including the NLN, had joined the movement. However, it was not long before the NLN withdrew its support in an attempt to avoid an intraprofessional fight. In 1995, the ANA reaffirmed its position and encouraged ways to move on the recommendation while preserving the integrity of the profession. As professional nursing moved toward the goal of requiring the baccalaureate degree as the minimum credential for professional practice, RN/BSN transition programs were developed to enable the ADN nurse to move upward. Although these developments have advanced nursing, the continued inability to reach consensus on the "entry to practice" preparation has resulted in divisiveness among nurses with different educational preparation.

In Canada, 2-year programs and 4-year degree nursing programs developed to augment the hospital training schools. In Australia and Great Britain, baccalaureate nursing programs emerged as those nations moved toward the goal of educating nurses in institutions of higher learning. It is interesting to note that individual nurses in the United States, Great Britain, Australia, Canada and other British Commonwealth nations elected to advance their own professional development by obtaining baccalaureate and master's degrees in other disciplines, most notably education, social work, and health service administration.

Another historical event that has affected nursing, especially in the United States, is the development of the role of the advanced nurse practitioner. In 1965, Dean Loretta Ford, in collaboration with Dr. Steven Silver (a physician) initiated a new kind of nurse preparation as a solution for the physician shortage in Colorado. Registered nurses were given 6 weeks of continuing education in which they learned assessment skills and then functioned as physician extenders. Almost immediately that education was increased, and currently most advanced nurse practitioners hold master's degrees and are certified by the ANA Credentialing Center or other specialty nursing organizations to function as advanced nurse practitioners. (For example, the American Associa-

tion of Nurse Anesthetists confers the title of certified registered nurse anesthetist [CRNA], and the National Association of Pediatric Nurse Associates and Practitioners certifies the pediatric nurse practitioner [PNP]). The development of advanced practice is another example of nursing responding to a societal need; and a resulting change in the practice of some nurses. This historical event has been an advancement and a problem: Nursing now struggles for legislation that will enable advanced nurse practitioners to receive third-party reimbursement and prescriptive authority.

In the United States in the mid 1990s, President Clinton's attempts at national health care reform and increases in the number of for-profit health care corporations also affected nursing. In an effort to avoid national regulation and the perceived problems associated with 'socialized health care' in other countries, insurance companies, physicians, and hospitals moved toward a system of managed care. This resulted in redesign of hospital-based client care delivery and consequent downsizing of both professional and support staff. To reduce costs, hospitals have instituted shorter length of stays, integrated systems, case management, and the use of unlicensed assistive personnel (UAPs). Other countries have implemented similar changes in order to provide their citizens with affordable health care.

A shift from curing illness to promoting health and preventing illness has, however, provided new opportunities for nurses. This shift in health care from the hospital to the community has increased the need for primary practitioners; more opportunities exist for advanced nurse practitioners and other advanced practice nurses, such as nurse midwives, nurse anesthetists, and clinical nurse specialists. This trend to involve more nurses in the care of the public outside the hospital setting has major implications for nursing education and for the future utilization of nurses.

Events That Have Indirectly Affected Nursing

Medical advances (e.g., new surgical procedures, the proliferation of diagnostic and monitoring instrumentation, and new pharmacologic preparations) have changed not only the physician's practice but also nursing practice. In the past, the nurse's hands, eyes, and ears were the principal tools for assessing clients; today, the nurse augments these tools with data from monitoring equipment that can provide more subtle and accurate information. Some of these advances have made the nurse's job easier; others, such as the development of new and more powerful drugs, have broadened the nurse's responsibilities. Knowing the drug's expected action, adverse effects, and compatibility with other drugs is a complicated responsibility. Nurses have significantly more responsibility and accountability today than they had in the past.

Cost-containment measures instituted by hospitals in many countries have also changed nursing practice. Changes that began as downsizing, or a reduction in staff to save money, quickly became a redesign of the entire hospital delivery system. Cross-training, focusing on the client, streamlining processes using continuous quality improvement (CQI), and the increased use of unlicensed assistive personnel (UAPs) or minimally trained support staff are only a few of the outcomes of the redesign. (See Chapter 1.) In some cases, the result was a redesign of the nurse's role; in other instances, an elimination of RN positions. RN and LPN/LVN ratios were shifted, and more management and delegation skills were required of the RN. Some RN activities were delegated to other, "cross-trained," health care workers (paramedics, respiratory therapists, phlebotomists, EKG technicians), and the RN was educated to assume additional responsibilities. Some RNs, for example, have returned to school to become respiratory therapists so that they might be able to provide total care to clients who have respiratory disorders or are ventilator dependent.

Managed care in the United States has been another cost-containment method that has affected the nurse's role. Managed care refers to a system in which hospitals (with subsidiary clinics, home care, skilled nursing facilities, and so on) and physician groups provide comprehensive care for groups of people who purchase their insurance and agree to use the program for health services. It is expected that free-market competition will provide the system with the lowest cost for care. And because the price for that care is based on the total number of members, the cost of caring for those who need care will be balanced by those members who are well and don't require services. Keeping members well so that they do not need the system is how costs are contained.

Case managers are needed as "gate-keepers" of the system so that only care that is deemed essential is provided. Cost for the care is determined proactively, so the system must be careful not to spend more than it is paid by capitation (numbers of those insured). Thus, in the new managed care environment nurses must have case management, coordination, assessment, health promotion, illness prevention, and cost-containment skills. The goal of keeping people focused on staying well and out of the hospital constitutes an entirely new paradigm of care. The way the goal is met and funded impacts the role expectations and responsibilities of the nurse.

Public policy has changed everyone's lives. Informed consent laws have increased the public's knowledge about and participation in decisions about their health care. The Self-Determination Act of 1991 has allowed people to make decisions in advance about their future health care, before they are unable to make such decisions. People have more choice about how and when health care will be delivered. These laws have also affected the role of the nurse. Monitoring the procedures for gaining consent and implementing procedures to ensure that the client's living will or durable power of attorney for health care is understood and documented are now a part of the nurse's responsibility. Issues such as the "right to die," assisted suicide, and other ethical dilemmas are of daily concern to the nurse in all practice settings. These and other added duties change the nurse's role, both in scope and accountability.

Social Movements and Technologic Initiatives That Have Affected Nursing

The women's movement that began in the 1960s has made a major impact on nursing. Predominantly a women's profession (about 10% of nurses are men), nursing has benefited from the recognition of women as a force for social change. As a result of the gains made by the feminist movement, nurses have gained better salaries, better working conditions, access to higher education, and access to opportunities as middle managers and executives in many occupations as well as nursing. Nurses have recently seized the opportunity to become entrepreneurs. Many nurses would have been unlikely to rise to such challenges if the women's movement had not opened the door to opportunity.

No discussion of the changes in nursing would be complete without indicating the impact of the information age and the way that computers have changed daily life. Computer technology is impacting health care by improving storage of and access to health care information. Nurses will be able to access and input client information at bedside computers or in the client's home through portable laptop computers. Computers will improve the accuracy and efficiency of documentation. By touching the computer screen, nurses record client information and make it available to the physician, the pharmacy, and any other service who is "on-line."

Clients can carry a card that contains information about their insurance coverage, status, medical history, medications, and demographic information. Insertion of this card into a computer sends that information to all who need to know; as a result, traditional health and medical records and files may soon become unnecessary. Instead of spending hours on manual recording, the nurse can spend that time with the client. Because the computer is often in the hospital room, at the clinic, or even in the home, the client can also share and participate in the development of the record.

Computers have also affected nursing education. Computer technology has facilitated supervision of students at a distance. Hand-sized computers provide information to students visiting clients in the home and act as vehicles for distributing client data to the college or clinic. Computerized instruction allows faculty to focus on the student's ability to think critically rather than on the ability to accumulate facts. A major advantage of computer technology is that it enables students to interact with information, classmates, faculty, and other nurses "on-line" at home, in the computer laboratory or library, in the classroom, or in the clinical setting. Thus, computerized instruction expands the instructional environment so that learning is portable, accessible, and always available. There are no constraints of time, person, or place. These advances in computer technology and their application to nursing and health care require that nurses broaden their knowledge still further, so that they become computer literate.

Through technology and travel, the world has become a smaller place. Immigrants and refugees readily cross national borders to seek opportunity in new lands. Nurses are more able to move rapidly to assist with the delivery of care to victims of natural and manmade health disasters. The shrinking of the worldwide community requires that nurses become more knowledgeable about and accepting of cultural

difference. Nurses need to be aware of different beliefs about health and illness and different cultural healing practices. The nurses of tomorrow need to be more than culturally aware—they need to strive for cultural competence in providing nursing care.

This overview of changes that have affected nursing and nursing practice is not meant to be comprehensive; there are many more good examples of events that have directly or indirectly changed nursing. Rather, this overview was intended to show that any changes in nursing in the past were usually linked to professional or societal change. As one considers the future, it is important to keep this point in mind.

CONSIDER...

- additional social movements or national events that have affected nursing as a profession, such as the civil rights movement, global human rights movements, the breakup of the Soviet Union, the space program, and so on. In what ways have these movements affected your practice of nursing and your own professional development?
- additional professional factors that have affected your practice of nursing and your own professional development, such as specialty certification, Nursing's Agenda for Health Care Reform, international professional nursing organizations, and so on. How have you responded to these professional influences?

FUTURE EVENTS THAT WILL AFFECT NURSING

Many factors will undoubtedly affect nursing in the future. Continued changes in the health care system, new regulatory methods, continued advances in technology and forms of treatment, and increased reliance on computers for managing, storing, and transmitting information will continue to shape and challenge nursing in the future. Both nursing practice and nursing education will be part of these revolutionary changes in health care. What nurses do, how they are educated, and where they will practice will change. In some instances these changes will be welcomed; in others, resisted. But change will occur; it always does.

Nurses must embrace these changes and be a part of the discussions that will shape the future.

This means that nurses everywhere and at all levels must accept that change is inevitable and that the role nurses once played is history. As nurses face the new century, it is clear that the 2000s are going to be years of rapid and unending change.

Health Care System Changes

As the health care system struggles to provide care for all people at a reasonable cost, it will undergo many changes. Although managed health care is only the latest attempt to reverse the escalating costs of care, time and the outcomes will determine its impact. However, while managed care is available there will be fewer professional nurses in hospitals and more multiskilled workers supervised by professional nurses. The term *multiskilled worker* refers to a person who is prepared to provide basic care under supervision but who is not licensed. Basic care will also change as technology takes over the measuring of vital signs and other parameters of assessment. The client's history, which is already on their personal computer card, will only need revising as new events occur and information is added to the computer record.

Because the length of stay for a hospitalized person will become shorter, the care provided will address the very acute phase of the illness episode and will be directed toward pain management, respiratory facilitation, cardiac support, and neurologic monitoring. Preparing the client for recovery at home will be a major aspect of the nurse's role. In order to plan and implement effective care, nurses will need to maintain and increase their knowledge of physiologic and psychologic functioning, technologic monitoring systems, client care, and computer systems.

Seriously ill clients confined to a hospital bed will require intensive care administered by professionals who will administer medications using equipment that is computer driven. There will be less worry about turning clients because the hospital beds of tomorrow will be designed to rotate the occupant periodically so that skin integrity is preserved. The professional nurse will assign dressing changes and other treatments to the multiskilled workers, so the cost of care will be contained by the number and level of the workers assigned to the units. Self-directed work teams made up of cross-trained professionals and multiskilled workers will direct, provide, and evaluate the care.

One of the most exciting possibilities for what might occur in the United States is described by Jef-

frey Bauer (1994), who proposes that the health care system be changed by breaking the monopoly held by physicians over the delivery of health care to American citizens. Bauer proposes that health care costs will not decrease until citizens are allowed to select the provider they want. He proposes that health care be placed on the free market so that maximum choice and quality competition are available. He believes we must "take the shackles off America's many competent non-physician providers and allow the American consumer free access to their services" (p. 19).

If Bauer's plan were to come into being—and there are good reasons to believe that it will—then advanced nurse practitioners, certified nurse midwives, dentists, pharmacists, certified nurse anesthetists, physical therapists, occupational therapists, and respiratory therapists, to name only a few, would be able to respond directly to the public's needs. The consumer would be free to choose from an expanded menu of qualified providers, a development that would bring the cost of care down while providing quality care for all. An example taken from Bauer's book makes his point:

At 75, Charlie is active, involved and very much interested in everything around him. His only real physical problem is adult onset diabetes, which he controls through proper diet and pills. A medium-built man who is very proud of his independence, he would rather spend time on his hobbies of gardening, bird-watching, and fixing bicycles for children than on, as he says, "going to the doctor like so many of these other old geezers." Nevertheless, he knows he has to be careful about his diabetic condition and realizes that his own at-home blood tests aren't always as accurate as he wishes.

Monopoly Model: Charlie makes a monthly visit to see his physician. Charlie and his doctor spend about two minutes discussing Charlie's health and about ten minutes discussing their common outdoor interests, after which Charlie gets a blood test. While Charlie likes his doctor, he nevertheless feels a little guilty that Medicare (and the American taxpayer) picks up the tab for what he largely considers to be a "social call."

Competitive Model: Charlie makes a monthly visit to a diagnostic center attached to his health clinic. He orders a blood test according to the health care profile that he and his geriatric nurse practitioner have generated and review every six months or so. Charlie receives the results within a few hours. If there are any problems, Charlie's nurse practitioner is immediately notified. Depending upon the severity of the problem, Charlie's nurse practitioner or a triage nurse from the clinic calls Charlie right away to discuss a course of action. Medicare is charged only for the blood tests and necessary clinic visits. (p. 168)

The difference between the two models, in terms of cost alone, is astounding. And the fact that Charlie has an active part in his health care is also important. The role of the advanced nurse practitioner clearly attests to ways that nurses in expanded roles can manage the care of clients in a cost-effective and quality manner.

However, even if the physician monopoly is not broken, nurses will be needed in increasing numbers in ambulatory surgical centers, diagnostic centers, home care, nursing homes, and skilled nursing facilities as hospitals become smaller and health care moves to the community. Those nurses with baccalaureate and master's degrees will have first choice as nonphysician providers because they are the best prepared for the role required of the nurse in the community. The nurse's role will include direct and indirect care; nurses will care for and manage others who provide care. In rural areas, advanced nurse practitioners will act as primary care providers as they assess, treat, and follow up on common, ordinary health care problems. Problems that require surgery or specialty consultation will be referred to physicians and other nonphysician providers. Physicians, nurses, and other health care providers will work together as interdisciplinary teams providing the consumer with the expertise of many care providers. Collaborative efforts will be necessary as the world of health care becomes more complex and technology continues to improve and change. The anticipated changes in the health care delivery system of the future require that everyone, health professional and consumer alike, must change his or her expectations and behaviors. The changing health care system requires more personal health responsibility on the part of the consumer and greater responsiveness on the part of health care providers to input from the consumer.

Regulatory Changes

One of the areas that has impeded nurse mobility and the development of advanced nursing practice and that has received much criticism is the fragmented regulatory system that licenses health care professionals (PEW Health Professions Commission, 1995). Currently, regulation is controlled by each state, so that in the United States 50 nurse practice acts control the practice of nursing. By applying for endorsement and paying the required fee, the nurse can be licensed in any of the 50 states because all 50 accept the NCLEX licensing exam as the measure of the nurse as a safe provider of care for entry to practice. Many nurses voluntarily elect also to become certified by the ANA Credentialing Center or other professional nursing organization.

Ongoing competency of nurses is measured by continuing education, which is mandatory in some states but not in others. The regulation of advanced practice is equally fragmented because, again, each state has its own regulations and ways of determining competency.

In the future there will probably be some major changes in the regulation of physicians and nonphysician health care providers. The National Council of State Boards (which is composed of representatives from each state's board) has proposed that there be national standards for licensing entry-level nurses and measuring the competency of nurses over time. The PEW Health Professions Commission (1995) went even further, proposing that the regulation of all physician and nonphysician health care providers be carried out at the national level and that the approach be an interdisciplinary one.

What would this mean? It could mean that regulations would be competency based, broad enough to allow for change, and yet definitive enough to assure the public that the provider, regardless of title, is qualified to offer the service. It could mean that quality control would be the key ingredient in determining universal standards for all health care providers, no matter where they practice or what title they hold. The state could provide the entry exam, and the professions could be held legally and financially responsible for the conduct of their members under state and federal guidelines based on general norms set across all health care disciplines. Would this work? Several professional organizations believe so, and there is enough pressure from legislators to indicate that kind of modification could occur.

The value of this kind of approach to regulation is that competency standards, not titles, would drive decisions; as a result, nonphysician providers would be considered equal partners in health care delivery.

Having the state control entry to practice based on national standards and the professions control certification based on their own specific practice expectations for general and advanced practice results in more meaningful recertification of providers with the least amount of government intrusion. These radical changes are becoming necessary to the removal of traditional practice barriers between physicians, nurses, and other health care providers. Advanced nurse practitioners have demonstrated that they are excellent primary caregivers (Aiken, 1993); but most state regulations, which generally are influenced by physician lobbyists, have kept legislators from making the changes needed for the legitimate use of advanced nurse practitioners. The argument of cost could be used to make the case for national, standardized regulation, but the argument that advanced nurse practitioners are adequately prepared and have demonstrated their value as primary care providers is a better reason to enact the changes proposed here.

Continued Medical, Surgical, and Pharmacologic Advances

Recent changes in hospital care, surgical procedures, and pharmacology have been nothing short of extraordinary. The use of lasers, scope surgery, and computer-driven diagnostic and surgical procedures has made surgery highly technical and very accurate. One wonders whether physicians, nurses, and anesthesiologists might soon be replaced by other, more sophisticated machines, robots, and computers.

The list of advancements in medicine is a long one. For example, it is possible to clone people (although whether to do so is an ethical controversy); treat highly infectious diseases with potent chemicals; keep people alive with machines that breathe for them and keep the heart pumping; and remove, sterilize, and replace a person's bone marrow to cure disease. It is possible to perform surgery while the client's blood is cycled through an artificial heart and lungs, transplant organs from human and animal donors, and replace old worn-out joints with new artificial ones. It is possible to save the life of a 26-week premature infant through mechanical breathing, intravenous feedings, and highly potent drugs. It is possible to replace amputated limbs with artificial ones and to provide computer and mechanical support that can enable a paralyzed person to pursue a career and be self-supporting. Many life-threatening

infectious diseases, such as polio and smallpox, have been eradicated; others, such as measles, mumps, chickenpox, and pertussis, could also be eradicated through widespread public immunization.

Although great progress has been made to eradicate infectious disease, AIDS, the Ebola virus, and other new infectious diseases still pose great problems, and even though there have been many strides in the fight against cancer, there is still no absolute "cure."

The development of medications that produce desired physiologic effects and change psychologic moods has prolonged life, made it more comfortable, and enhanced people's ability to enjoy it. Drugs can be a vital part of healthy living for those with chronic physiologic or psychologic illnesses. Some drugs, however, have also caused dependence, making people less able to cope or function without them.

Medical treatment of chronic conditions and acute phases of infection and much after-trauma care often centers around pharmacologic therapy. Furthermore, the number of nonprescription medications has increased in number as the Food and Drug Administration (FDA) releases many prescription drugs for over-the-counter purchase. The consumer now has even more choices than before. A trip to the drugstore or local supermarket or discount store allows the consumer access to a vast variety of remedies for a stuffy nose, sore throat, respiratory congestion, bowel problems, joint aches, heartburn, urinary discomfort, worry, or whatever else is causing distress. It is very easy to acquire drugs, and the public uses many drugs; in fact, polypharmacy has become a major problem in America because many people combine prescription drugs and nonprescription drugs in a haphazard manner.

Pharmacologic advancements have also had a significant impact on nursing. Nurses have had to expand their knowledge base of pharmacology and their skills in caring for clients who have had surgery or who are undergoing medical treatment. Keeping informed about the newest drugs means the nurse must consult the *National Drug Formulary* or other drug references more often. Moreover, it is becoming even more urgent for nurses to face the inevitable ethical dilemmas. The need for more information and more discussion about ethical issues will continue and escalate as health care in hospitals becomes more acute, as arguments rage over the distribution of financial resources for expensive "experimental treatment" (e.g., complex organ transplants) versus less expensive preventive care (childhood immunizations), and as more non-physician providers deliver care in homes, malls, the office or place of work, the school, the church, clinics, ambulatory centers, and nursing homes.

In the past, nurses have responded to the events that confront them; no doubt they will again. As nursing approaches the 21st century, however, their response will need to be quicker and more flexible. This means nurses will need more education and a greater understanding of the community and aggregate care. Nurses will also have to see themselves as "knowledge workers" and facilitators of care rather than individual caregivers. This is a major paradigm shift. Given nursing's historical record of responding to societal need, there is no doubt that nurses will come forth and meet the challenge.

Teaching, preparing educational materials, and teaching others how to teach will consume more of the nurse's time. Interactive video, distance learning, and using computers and other audio-visual equipment for learning will expand the market for instructional materials and good teachers. Because people will learn in their homes and at work, instructional materials will need to be portable and self-contained. Group learning will become as common as individual learning, and the use of the "information highway" will be a key mode of delivery. With satellites available and cables throughout the United States, North America, and the world, disseminating information will not be difficult.

Surgical procedures, medical treatment, and pharmacologic therapies will continue to advance. In fact, there is every reason to believe the advancements will develop even more rapidly, so that only those who are continuous learners will be able to keep pace. Nurses will have to be continuous learners if they expect to have a place in the new health care paradigm.

Historically, nurses have cared for the sick. In the new paradigm, nurses will focus on wellness and prevention. The nurse will be the primary person who works to help individuals stay well and do things that promote health. Nurses will have to increase their knowledge base about nutrition, exercise, vitamin replacement, and the effects of cigarette smoking and the use of alcohol. As "models of good health," some nurses will have to adopt healthier behaviors and life-styles. They will also have to keep abreast of the most recent research in the prevention and treatment of cancer, AIDS, and other infections.

Nurses will also need to take an active role in preparing healthy citizens for the future by teaching children about exercise, nutrition, safety, and other habits for healthy living, at a time when lifelong habits are learned. Teaching children about sex, sexually transmitted diseases, alcohol, and drug abuse will also be a challenge. In 1995, for example, the fastest rate of growth in the use of alcohol and cigarette smoking occurred among children 9 to 13 years old. Pressures from parents and organized religion have made it difficult to offer sex education in public and private schools. Nurses must be advocates for children and actively work to see that sex education becomes part of the school curriculum. Too many children become pregnant and have babies when they don't have the knowledge, desire, or resources to raise and care for them.

Computer Technology and Its Effect on Health and Nursing Care in the Future

Computers play an increasingly important role in health care. Computers have revolutionized surgery and diagnostic procedures. They have created a major change in nursing schools both as information managers and instructional tools. Hospitals have also been introduced to the value of computers not only as storage for information but also as conduits for recording and transmitting physicians' orders, for documenting nursing assessments and care, for completing audits, and for managing materials. It is difficult to remember how things were done without computers, although they were introduced only a few years ago. The potential applications of computers to health care are endless.

With careful planning, the computer should be able to simplify operations, save time, reduce effort, improve cost-effectiveness, and provide a paperless and fileless enterprise. The paper file of yesterday will be a computer disk or chip.

Physician and nonphysician offices should soon be able to access the hospital system so that they do not need a paper trail or their own electronic system. With managed care, the system should expand to connect the hospital, the insurance company (or payor), and the physician and nonphysician care providers. Soon, with a tap of the finger, a client's record can be accessed from any of those entities.

It will not be long before nurses will carry pocket computers on their uniform belts to record data and make assessments at the site of the client (whether in hospital, home, school, or job). These data will simultaneously be entered in the client's personal record and be available to any department in the hospital as long as the client is there. This capacity for simultaneous entry and distribution is already possible in restaurants, where the server enters the order in the computer at table side, records it, and notifies the kitchen without ever going near the kitchen until the order is ready. That same entry creates a bill that is ready for customers when they leave.

Similar activities will soon be part of every health care facility to ensure smooth, quick care and accurate accounting. The capacity is there; all that is necessary is to find ways to fund the systems and to put them in place so they "talk" to one another.

The computer systems of tomorrow will require that all health care providers be knowledgeable and practiced in the use of computers. It will take more than being computer literate to function in the computer world of tomorrow. Knowledge of word processing using several software packages, the ability to create spreadsheets, and the ability to adapt to ever-changing computer systems will be necessary. For a while, health care facilities will need to train their personnel, but eventually all workers will be expected to have computer skills when hired. This means that schools of nursing and other departments of colleges and universities will need to ensure that all graduates of their programs are able to access computers and obtain the information.

Virtual reality (the ability to simulate real situations via computer/visual technology) will also have a great impact on the preparation of health care providers. It is already possible to teach students using virtual reality, although on a limited basis, and it may not be long before people learn all psychomotor skills using virtual reality methods. Instructional laboratories that simulate the hospital setting will give way to a set of computers that can simulate the real world: the home, the clinic, the office or workplace, and the hospital. Interpersonal skills, cooperative decision making, and psychomotor skills will all be learned in a virtual reality framework. Initially, virtual reality software may be expensive, but over time it will probably cost less than the equipment now in use: Imagine the cost savings of eliminating laboratories that require many mannequins, simulated body parts, hospital beds, and other equipment. Also, the space occupied by laboratories can be allocated to other purposes.

Virtual reality can offer similar savings of cost and space for staff development programs. It is probably safe to say that the virtual reality experience would be more like the real one than would other methods using rubber or plastic models, for example.

Virtual reality can also make treatment simulation scenarios safer, eliminating the need to subject students to intrusive treatment while they play the role of the client.

In addition, nurses can use virtual reality to teach family members how to provide care for the client. Nurses can take them through the procedures in a safe and lifelike experience until they feel comfortable to perform the procedure on the family member. The entire process can be accomplished in the client's home or workplace. Today's laboratories force learning to occur at the hospital or the educational facility; tomorrow's laboratories that use virtual reality, in contrast, will be portable to almost any place where the client or student is located.

CONSIDER . . .

- what changes will be in store for nurses who were practicing in the health care system of the 20th century. What new attitudes, knowledge, and skills will those nurses need to acquire to remain current in their practice?

PAST LESSONS THAT CAN HELP NURSES IN THE FUTURE

From what has happened in health care, nurses can learn many lessons that may help them deal with the future.

1. The health care delivery system in the United States is remarkably flexible. Since the 1800s, the U.S. health care system has responded quickly to changes in technology, scientific discoveries, and new health threats. Medical science has undergone several revolutionary redefinitions; many infectious diseases have been conquered, and new ones have taken their place; more of the population has been able to survive to old age; the hospital has been redefined from a place for the poor to die to a place for anyone to be restored to health. For those who do die, the causes of death have changed. One hundred

years ago, the leading killers were polio and infectious diseases. Today's leading killers are heart disease, tobacco, AIDS, and violence. Health insurance, which was instituted in the early part of the century to support personal payment, now has become the main source of payment for health care.

2. Changes in the health care system have always occurred rapidly and sometimes without warning. Most of the changes outlined above took place quickly, and many of the advancements in medicine were unexpected or the result of war. Government and society did not set out to initiate Medicare or to institute diagnosis-related groups (DRGs) or, for that matter, to turn to managed care. These developments happened quickly as a way to solve an immediate problem. Clearly, the system is not driven by tradition or "cast in stone."

3. No one entity is in control of the health care system. Only a brief scan of any newspaper will reveal that no one body—neither physicians, federal or state governments, insurers or payors—controls the system, as President Clinton discovered when he tried to reform the system in the mid 1990s. Consumers are becoming more interested in how the system works and how to change it because it is their tax dollars that support it.

4. Health care providers, especially nurses, have made major strides each time the system changed. These most recent changes have clearly presented great opportunities for nurses and other nonphysician caregivers. New roles, roles most appropriately played by providers with an interest and preparation in prevention, are waiting to be filled by nurses.

As soon as one understands these lessons, the possibilities for the future become apparent. For example, it is possible for anyone to influence the development of tomorrow's health care system. Modifications will undoubtedly occur quickly and repeatedly as nations seek ways to provide quality health care for all. Control of the system will shift from one source to another. Because control has thus far resided with government, professionals, and insurance companies, it seems likely that consumers may be the next group to want and assume control.

VISIONS OF TOMORROW SUMMARIZED

Throughout this chapter several themes have emerged that provide the framework for a vision of tomorrow.

Health care will be provided mostly in the community. Whereas acute and critical phases of illness will be attended to in hospitals, most health care will be delivered within the community. During the 1960s, the number of hospitals grew rapidly because funding was available and because it was believed that the best care could be provided there. It has since been learned that hospital care is very costly, disrupts the family, and focuses on cure, not prevention. In the 2000s, care will be delivered primarily outside the hospital. Schools, churches, the workplace, home clinics, skilled nursing facilities, and nursing homes will be the sites for care.

Care is already provided in clinics, in nursing homes, in the home, and at skilled nursing facilities. In the next few years, there will be an increase in home health care (mainly because people will continue to be discharged from the hospital earlier to keep costs down). More health care will be also provided in schools and in the workplace. The rise of alcohol and drug abuse in the young, the increasing incidence of HIV in adolescents and young adults, and the increasing number of teenage pregnancies will require more preventive care in the school setting. The same is true of the workplace: Occupational health care is growing because prevention is less costly than illness care. Reducing absenteeism and tardiness increases productivity. Also, employees will avail themselves of services that are easy to access; accessing care on the job is often preferable to taking time from work to visit a clinic.

Churches are a natural place for health care, especially if there is a holistic approach. Much of what ails people is tied into their sense of self and how they cope. For many people, religious and spiritual resources can be integral to their ability to cope with illness or the threat of a health condition. Parish nursing is a new but growing field of nursing and has been particularly helpful in rural regions.

Health mobiles will bring primary health care and dental services and screening to special locations, such as farm workers' camps, retirement communities, and inner-city neighborhoods. Education to prevent problems will be a major focus for the homebound and the poor.

As the population grows older, Americans will receive more long-term care at home. Electronic monitoring equipment will be attached to telephones to allow those who are homebound to relay medical information to clinics or home health agencies. More and more follow-up will be done by telephone as reimbursement systems switch from fee-for-service to managed care and capitation.

Independent nonphysician providers, particularly nurses, will deliver the significant proportion of the nation's primary care. Because advanced nurse practitioners have responded so well to the country's need for more primary care providers, they will deliver a significant portion of the nation's primary care. Advanced nurse practitioners educated as family, pediatric, and geriatric care practitioners will complement physician family practitioners as the backbone of the nation's health care system. This linking will occur both in nurse-only practices and in collaborative practice arrangements with physicians. Nurse midwives will take over many of the primary care functions of obstetricians/gynecologists, including the management of low-risk pregnancies. Physicians will continue to do what they have been doing, but there will be much more collaborative practice with nurses and other nonphysician providers.

In the world of tomorrow, nurses will work collaboratively with physicians and other nonphysician providers. These groups of providers will offer their services in retail locations as small businesses (a major reason why all nurses will need a business education). Health "stores" will vary in size from small basic care operations located in shopping malls to free-standing buildings with huge clinics offering everything from dentistry and family medical care to physical therapy and life-saving emergency services.

The new providers (nurses, physicians, and other nonphysicians) will be much more attuned to what the consumer wants. The hours of service will change so the consumer can access the services in the evenings and on weekends. The larger locations will offer comprehensive wellness programs promoting healthy life-styles, provide facilities for weight control and exercise, and offer programs about nutrition and exercise. Illness care will be available, but the major emphasis will be on health promotion.

Nurses will take the lead in the development of these "health centers" because the framework for nursing throughout its history has been holistic and comprehensive. Nurses have always promoted health and focused on the prevention of illness. Moreover, nurses can lead the way to better health and cut costs by helping the public assume responsibility for their lives as healthy individuals.

Physicians will assume roles as co-providers, specialty-care providers, and consultants. Although many physicians may express serious concern about what is happening and will happen in the future, nurses and consumers can expect that many physicians will quietly lead the way into the new system. Many physicians will remain as specialty care providers because there will still be a need for physicians who are prepared to care for specific health care problems, such as oncologists, orthopedists, neurologists, psychiatrists, cardiologists, and so on. Other physicians will join collaborative practices with advanced nurse practitioners to provide comprehensive basic care. Some physicians will seize the opportunity to enter entrepreneurial businesses. There will be plenty to do in the new system, but everyone will need to change their expectations and responsibilities.

Physician activity will affect nursing as nurses seize opportunities for collaborative practice. Advanced practice nurses will need physician consultation in their independent practices, especially for their clients with more complex problems. Over time, physicians and nurses will work together in more ways and in better ways as it becomes more clear how the new system will unfold.

Informed consumers will become more self-directed and assume more responsibility for their health. One of the most exciting advances in the future will be "one-stop" diagnostic centers. Like a full-service gas station, these diagnostic centers will provide informed consumers access to urinalysis, blood tests, throat cultures, and even some radiographic tests. These diagnostic centers will be electronically linked to large, fully equipped laboratories for confirmation of diagnoses and to health databases that store consumer records. Educational services will also be available through interactive computer programs and video libraries.

Computer terminals in pharmacies will help consumers find answers to questions regarding health and illness. Pharmacists will be able to diagnose such common ailments as throat infections and skin rashes with the help of computer protocols and over-the-counter diagnostic tools. Women already can diagnose pregnancy at home using a simple diagnostic package purchased at a supermarket, pharmacy, or discount store.

For easy access, diagnostic centers will be located in health care clinics, supermarkets, shopping malls, and department stores. Consumers will also be able to authorize a pharmacist to access their personal medical records in order to check for allergies to prescriptive drugs or other medications. It is easy to see that consumers will have much more control, involvement, and accountability in their health care. This is perhaps the most exciting aspect of the new system.

Access to health care/consultation will resemble the market for other services and products. Because health care/consultation will be easy to access, it will resemble other kinds of services the consumer uses. The clinics, pharmacies, and diagnostic centers will remain open nights and weekends; some may even remain open 24 hours a day. Clearly, tomorrow's health care agencies will be much more attuned to the needs of the customer. Larger agencies will offer comprehensive wellness programs that promote healthy life-styles, including good nutrition and proper exercise.

Education and prevention will be the major product lines of the retail health and medical stores of the future. The focus of the new clinics will be on keeping people healthy as well as diagnosing and treating people who are ill. The dream of comprehensive care will finally become a reality.

Education for nurses will reflect the changes in the health care delivery system. Nurses' education, consistent with these many changes, will also change. The focus of the programs (regardless of the level) will be on the community and on prevention. Nurses will continue to teach how to care for the sick, but the major emphasis will be how to keep people well. Teaching, consulting, and learning referral skills will be essential for the nurses of the future, so much more time will be spent on helping students learn these skills.

Group work and a focus on working with aggregates will supersede the time spent on individual care. Since nurses will be in the community and focusing on prevention, it will be imperative that they can work with groups. Being able to work with parents, abused women, persons with AIDS, people with cardiovascular problems, and any number of other groups will be necessary if the nurse is to use time efficiently and spend it with the individuals who need the care. This means that the educational program must devote more time to developing nurses' group process skills.

Nursing students and nurses will also need computer skills. They will need not only word processing and spreadsheet skills but also the ability to use virtual reality equipment. Computer competence will probably become a prerequisite for admission to a nursing program in the future.

An important new focus for nursing education at all levels will be on the "community." Although students live in a community and read about communities, until they understand that a community is more than a geographic boundary, they will not be prepared for the health care of tomorrow. Much more time will be spent on the study of community and its impact on the health of the citizens. Nurses will also need to become more aware of the global community and become more geographically knowledgeable and culturally competent.

As geographic barriers become more passable, immigrants and refugees will move from areas with limited resources to areas with more opportunity. These immigrants will bring beliefs and practices about health care that are culturally driven; they also will bring illnesses that may be unique to their race or geographic homeland. Nurses will need to become more aware of global health problems and their impact on nursing practice. Through advances in technology, nurses have greater ability to communicate or travel to other countries and continents and are better able to network with the global nursing community.

Through technology, students will probably learn more at home than at the college or university. Student access to technology at home and the use of virtual reality will also change faculty behavior. Faculty will need to know how to manage distance education and keep abreast of ever-changing computer and video technology and the broadening concepts of community, prevention, health promotion, and the globalization of America.

An important and imperative looming change is a decision on the basic preparation of nurses. The ANA, NLN, and other specialty nursing organizations will take the lead and determine the basic preparation of professional nurses. This action will not only help correct the confusion for potential students, but also lay the foundation for advanced practice. Legislators, other professional groups and the public will finally know the scope of basic professional nursing practice. Statutes will be more clear, and regulations governing practice will be consistent. Nothing the profession can do will be as important or as necessary as this action.

The world of tomorrow is exciting. Health promotion, rather than medical care, will finally be the focus. With these changes will come a challenge for nursing. Nursing will need to grasp the opportunity and become the leader in the movement toward providing care that creates a better life for each citizen. Clearly there will be a need for more nurses prepared at the baccalaureate and master's levels to meet the demands of a community-based consumer population. New technologies will be available for nurses' use. The system is now ready and able to respond to the need, and the public is ready for the new ways. Nursing education and practice must seize the opportunity to make the necessary changes. The following story exemplifies the situation nurses are now facing and how they must respond if the world of tomorrow is to include a major place for nursing.

> Lions have a very successful strategy for hunting. The young lions are sent away from the den into the country, while the old, frail ones stay at the den. The old lions at the den begin to roar furiously, sending a very loud and frightening sound into the area. Hearing the roar, many of the animals begin to flee from the area of the den, and as they do they become prey for the young lions and are sacrificed as food. (Source unknown)

The moral of the story is simple. When nurses hear the roar, they should run toward it and not away if they want to remain viable. The roar is change; and nurses should not try to escape it but rather approach and embrace it.

CONSIDER...

- your own vision for the future of health care and nursing in your community, your nation, and the world. Is it consistent with the author's vision? Do you see different or additional changes that have not been discussed here? If yes, what are they?
- your emotional attitude regarding the anticipated changes for nursing and health care delivery. Are you pessimistic? Optimistic? How can you develop a positive attitude for the anticipated changes?
- your own professional future in view of the author's and your own visions for the future. What new knowledge and skills will you need to prepare yourself for the future? How will you go about obtaining these skills and knowledge?
- how through collegial support and participation in professional nursing organizations, the nurse can not only react to but also be proactive in planning the future of health care.

SELECTED REFERENCES

Aiken, L. H., Lake, E. T., Semaan, S., Lehman, H. P., O'Hare, P. A., Cole, C. S., Dunbar, D., & Frank, I. (Fall 1993). Nurse practitioner managed care for persons with HIV infection. *Image Journal of Nursing Scholarship*, 25(3) 172–177.

Bauer, J. (1994). *Not what the doctor ordered.* Chicago: Probus.

Mundinger, M. O. (1995). Advanced practice nursing is the answer … what is the question? *N & H C Perspectives on Community*, 16(5), 254–259.

National League for Nursing. (1994). *Nursing data review.* New York: Author.

Pew Health Professions Commission. (1995). *Licensure and regulation of health care providers.* San Francisco: UCSF Center for the Health Professions.

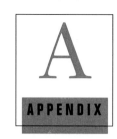

Selected Life-Style Assessment Tools

Name of Tool (Author)	Dimensions Measured	Comments
Lifestyle Assessment Questionnaire (National Wellness Institute, 1988)	Physical exercise, nutrition, self-care, vehicle safety, drug usage/awareness, social/environmental, emotional awareness/acceptance, emotional management, intellectual, occupational, and spiritual functioning.	Comprehensive tool with 11 dimensions and 110 items. Self-scoring.
Wellness Index (Travis & Ryan, 1988)	Nutrition, physical awareness, stress control, and self-responsibility.	Quick assessment tool with 4 dimensions and 16 items. Scoring focuses on the "balance" between the four dimensions.
Life Style and Health Habits Assessment (Pender, 1987, pp. 138–143)	Competence in self-care, nutritional practices, physical or recreational activity, sleep patterns, stress management, self-actualization, sense of purpose in life, relationships with others, environmental control to reduce risks, and use of the health care system.	Comprehensive tool with 10 dimensions and 100 items. Self-scoring.
Health Promoting Lifestyle Profile (HPLP) (Walker, Secrist, & Pender, 1987)	Nutrition, exercise, health responsibility, stress management, interpersonal support, and self-actualization.	Quick assessment tool with 6 dimensions and 48 items. Self-scoring.
Wellness Self-Assessment (Clark, 1986, pp. 36–42)	Nutrition, fitness, stress, relationships and beliefs, and the environment.	Quick assessment tool with 5 dimensions and 41 items. Self-scoring.
Self-Test for Health Style (U.S. Department of Health and Human Services, 1985)	Cigarette smoking, alcohol and drugs, eating habits, exercise/fitness, stress control, and safety.	Quick assessment tool with 6 dimensions and 24 items. Self-scoring.

Sources: Cited in Chapter 16, pp. 332–334.

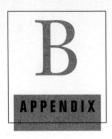

B

APPENDIX

Selected Family Assessment Tools Developed by Nurses

Name of Tool (Author)	Dimensions Measured	Comments
Calgary Family Assessment Model (Wright & Leahey, 1994, pp. 37–97)	Instrumental and expressive functioning: Internal and external structure: developmental stages, tasks, and attachment.	Based on a developmental-structural-functional framework. Paired with an intervention model.
Gordon Health Pattern Typology: Family as Client (Nettle, et al., 1993)	Patterns assessed: Roles/relationships, cognitive/perceptual, self-concept, physiological factors, values, health management, coping/stress tolerance.	Based on health pattern typology. Determines nursing diagnoses for a family.
Family Assessment Tool: Family Health Care Plan (Stanhope & Lancaster, 1992, pp. 780–789)	Family health care plan, family-community health nurse contract, health assessment guide, and family problem solving guide.	Developed for community health nurses. Assesses families for purpose of planning care.
Family Health Assessment (Friedman, 1992)	Identifying data: developmental stage and history, environmental data, family structure, functions, and coping.	Based on a developmental-structural-functional framework.
Family Health Assessment Intervention Instrument (Mischke-Berkey, Warner, & Hanson, 1989)	Family health impactors: Self-perceptions, caregiver perceptions of wellness activities, problem areas, and family stressors.	Based on a systems framework. Completed by each family member and the nurse.
Family Health Promotion-Protection Plan (Pender, 1987)	Family roles, community affiliations, communication/decision-making patterns, values, strengths, stressors, developmental transitions, self-care.	Assesses family health status, assists in the development of a plan to improve health.
Feetham Family Functioning Survey (Feetham & Humenick, 1982)	Functioning in household tasks, marital relationships, community involvement, family-children-friends interactions, sources of support.	Assesses factors that nurses could help change through care plans.
Family Assessment Tool (Holt & Robinson, 1979)	Home environment, family interaction styles, family and child health, and psychosocial history.	Developed for school nurses. Prioritizes family problems and strengths.

SOURCES: Cited in Chapter 16, pp. 332–334.

Index

cultural, 87, 362
ethical aspects of nursing and, 103
learning and differing, 166
respect for other's, 103
Variability, 210
Variables, 207–208
Variances, 131, 210
Veracity, 94
Verbal communication, 363–365
Violence, family, 411–424
"A Vision for Nursing Education" (NLN), 22
Visions for the future of nursing, 425–470
von Bertalanffy, L., 316t

Wald, Lillian, 13
Watson, Jean, 34t, 43–44, 318t
Weir, George M., 15
Weir Report (1932), 15

Well-being, 55
Wellness
defining, 54–55
dimensions of, 55i
Dunn's high-level grid for, 57–58
and health, 52–66
health care/promotion and, 147t
Wellness diagnosis, 263
Wellness Index, 320i, 471
Wellness models, 258
Wellness nursing diagnoses, 326–327
Wellness Self-Assessment, 471
Westerhoff, J., 316t
Western Interstate Commission for Higher Education (WICHEN), 213
Western Reserve University School of Nursing, 15
Wholly compensatory systems, 39
Willimon, W. H., 316t
Wills, 117–118

Withholding food/fluids, 101
Women
health concerns of adolescent, 329
Holtz and Furniss mnemonic tool for abused, 419
nursing and changing roles of, 9
spouse abuse against, 413–414
Women's movement, 460–461
Workplace politics, 192–193
Work-related social support groups, 303
World Health Organization (WHO)
health defined by, 53
health goals of, 71–72
on health promotion, 144
World War II, 10, 16, 458

Yale University School of Nursing, 15
Yoga, 386–387